American Medicine and the Public Interest

ROSEMARY STEVENS

American Medicine
and the Public Interest

NEW HAVEN AND LONDON, YALE UNIVERSITY PRESS

Originally published with assistance from the foundation
established in memory of Philip Hamilton McMillan
of the Class of 1894, Yale College.
Copyright © 1971 by Yale University.
Eighth printing, 1978.
All rights reserved. This book may not be
reproduced, in whole or in part, in any form (beyond
that copying permitted by Sections 107 and 108 of the
U.S. Copyright Law and except by reviewers for the public
press), without written permission from the publishers.
Library of Congress catalog card number: 77–151592.
International standard book number: 0–300–01419–8 (cloth)
0–300–01744–8 (paper)

Designed by Sally Sullivan
and set in Linotype Times Roman type.
Printed in the United States of America by
LithoCrafters, Inc., Chelsea, Michigan.

Published in Great Britain, Europe, Africa, and Asia
(except Japan) by Yale University Press, Ltd., London.
Distributed in Australia and New Zealand by Book & Film
Services, Artarmon, N.S.W., Australia; in Japan by
Harper & Row, Publishers, Tokyo Office.

This investigation was supported in whole by the United
States Public Health Service, through Research Grants
CH 00047 from the Division of Community Health Services
and HS 00374 from the National Center for Health
Services Research and Development.

CONTENTS

TABLES

PREFACE

This book is the second volume of a trilogy designed to explore the evolving patterns of medical practice in England and the United States. The first volume, *Medical Practice in Modern England: The Impact of Specialization and State Medicine,* was published by the Yale University Press in 1966. The third part of the study will concentrate on comparative aspects of health care organization in the two countries.

The study began with a single question, What is the effect of specialization in medicine on the organization and politics of health services, and how far is the effect one which is common to different countries at a similar stage of technological development? The question is simple; the potential answers are complex. Specialization in medicine is itself the by-product of a revolution in the science of medicine in this century which has not only transformed the structure of the medical profession but has had widespread implications for the costs, value, and organization of health services. Any study purporting to discuss the impact of specialization cannot reasonably ignore the scientific, social, and professional context in which medical care is provided. The original question thus led to explorations of the nature and underlying forces which shape health services in the two countries. The first book traced the evolution and existing structures and issues of the British National Health Service. This study analyzes the developing patterns of medical professionalism and health services which are intrinsic to the United States, and on which rests the success of future planning of health services in this country.

A study of the breadth of this book is dependent on the interest and goodwill of a large number of persons: to breathe life into the sometimes arid and often cryptic documentation of events, to allow access to unpublished documentation, to review and criticize the manuscript as it develops, and by no means least to sustain and encourage the researcher during the gradual unraveling of the work. I have been unusually fortunate in all these respects. Indeed, I cannot hope to do justice to all those who willingly offered their enthusiasm and advice. But I should like to thank all those who gave freely of their time and their opinions, while singling out those whose help was repeatedly and continuously available.

First and foremost I owe an immense debt of gratitude to I. S. Falk, professor emeritus of public health, Yale University School of Medicine. Not only was he the progenitor of the project; he has been a constant and invaluable critic throughout this study, managing to find time to read in great detail and with invariably helpful suggestions all the early drafts of this book. Since he participated in, and influenced so many of the events analyzed in this volume, his help was particularly significant.

The study has benefited greatly from the advice of other colleagues at Yale. Prof. E. Richard Weinerman, tragically killed in a plane crash in February 1970, was always generous with time for discussion of the potentials and attributes of the American health care system. I have also had the continuing and valued advice of John D. Thompson and of two other colleagues working in related areas of social administration in health services, David A. Pearson and Arthur J. Viseltear, all of the Department of Epidemiology and Public Health of the Yale University School of Medicine. Prof. Lloyd Stevenson, formerly of the Department of History of Science and Medicine, and George Rosen, professor of the history of medicine and public health, have offered valuable guidance in historical areas. (George Rosen's book, *The Specialization of Medicine, with Particular Reference to Ophthalmology,* stands alone as a detailed social analysis of the history of one specialty.) I am also indebted to Dr. Arthur Ebbert, associate dean of the School of Medicine, as well as to Profs. James Fesler of the Department of Political Science, Jerome K. Myers of the Department of Sociology, Robert B. Stevens of the Law School, and various other members of the Departments of Economics, History, Sociology, and Political Science, who contributed generously with their interest and time. Leonard Ross, editor of the *Yale Law·Journal* and now of the Harvard Law School, also made incisive comments on parts of the text.

During the academic year 1967–68 I was fortunate to be appointed as a guest scholar at the Brookings Institution in Washington, D.C. While there, Joseph Pechman, Rashi Fein, and Gerald Weber in economic studies, and Gilbert Steiner and Herbert Kaufman in governmental studies were all generous in their help. At this period, too, I was a visiting lecturer at Johns Hopkins University and benefited greatly from discussions with Dr. Kerr White and other members of the department of Health Care and Hospitals at the School of Hygiene and Public Health. Furthermore, Dr. George Silver (now professor of public health at Yale) and Dr. Richard Magraw, both of whom were then deputy assistant secretaries in the Department of Health, Education, and Welfare, nobly read and commented on a draft of the entire text. Many other persons in various divisions and bureaus of the federal government were unstintingly cooperative then and later. For all this help I am most grateful.

During the research, I was privileged to hear Dr. Willard C. Rappleye talk at length of his own role in developing the Advisory Board for Medical Specialties and other medical educational activities; he also commented on part of the draft and produced invaluable source materials. Dr. Robin Buerki reviewed his part in the development of the present structures of specialty boards as a past president of the American Hospital Association. Dr. John Parks, dean of the George Washington School of Medicine, and Dr. L. M. Randall of the Mayo Clinic, who is developing a history of the American Board of Obstetrics and Gynecology, kindly gave suggestions and advice. Generous assistance and documents were made available on numerous occasions by Dr. Victor Logan, who is preparing a history of the American Board of Internal Medicine.

These and other interviews and correspondence were of great importance in developing themes as well as substance in the working drafts of the book. Members and staffs of the twenty approved specialty certifying boards in medicine and other professional boards, committees, and societies were particularly helpful in providing initial reference points for documentary review, as well as information and advice. I should like to thank particularly for their continuing interest in the study over a protracted period Dr. Palmer Futcher of the American Board of Internal Medicine, Dr. John Nunemaker of the American Medical Association (now director of the American Board of Medical Specialties), Dr. Cheves Smythe of the Association of American Medical Colleges, and Dr. John Hubbard of the National Board of Medical Examiners. I must also thank the members of the faculties of many medical schools, from Alabama to Oregon, the officers of the many medical bodies mentioned in the text, and the innumerable practicing physicians, from Brattleboro, Vermont, to Austin, Texas, who have given their time to talk with me. I look forward to their continuing criticism and advice.

Besides interviews, an important source of information was access to unpublished materials. Through the kindness of Dr. Forrest Leffingwell, Dr. Robert D. Dripps, and Miss Charlotte Hickcox, the American Board of Anesthesiology allowed me to read the entire minutes of its meetings, from its founding to the present day, together with other related papers. Similar access was generously given by Dr. John Hubbard to the minutes of the National Board of Medical Examiners, and by Dr. Paul Sanazaro to extracts from the minutes of the Association of American Medical Colleges. Dr. Nunemaker provided materials from the records of the AMA's

Council on Medical Education, and President John Millis of Western Reserve University gave permission for me to see the background papers of the Millis commission on the graduate education of physicians. These sources are not always cited in the text, nor, for reasons of confidentiality, is the material fully used. Nevertheless, the insights and background they gave have been invaluable, and I greatly appreciate having been able to see them. The process of reading unpublished documents and records is after all one of the smugly satisfying incidentals of research such as this.

Another vast source of materials lay in contemporary publications. A systematic review was made of books and articles in the field of medical care and associated areas, of medical history, and of the development of the health professions. An analysis of relevant statistical data was also undertaken, most notably from reports published by the U.S. Public Health Service and from the American Medical Association. But quite the most fruitful source of published materials lay in the rich supply of figures, fragments, letters, and pieces of many kinds in the medical journals. The *Journal of the American Medical Association* was read from 1930 to 1970 and for other selected periods; and the *Journal of Medical Education* was read over the same period. In addition, other reports, journals, specialty publications, and association transactions of many kinds were reviewed for specific topics and for particularly relevant periods.

In this critical and time-consuming process, I was extremely fortunate in having as research assistants Mrs. Naomi Burns in the early phases of the research and Miss Joan Vermeulen in the later phases. They have both acted as outspoken and invaluable critics of the work as it has progressed and added to it their own perceptions as political scientists and experienced professionals in the health field. For the last two years of the project Joan Vermeulen devoted virtually her entire energies to the research necessary to develop what is intended to be a comprehensive volume. Without her the scope of the work would necessarily have been narrower. A number of students from the Yale Law School and School of Medicine have also contributed on a part-time basis to systematic journal reviews.

Special thanks should go to my secretary, Miss Kathryn Pettit, for deciphering and typing the many drafts of the text. She acted as my secretary for the whole of the five years (December 1965 to December 1970) while the book was being written. It was no mean feat and much appreciated.

All this advice and help are gratefully acknowledged. The errors that remain are of course my own. Some exclusions should however be mentioned. Osteopathic physicians have made a major contribution to American medicine, particularly in the provision of primary medical care. But the development of osteopathic medicine and its structure of specialties deserve a separate study and are thus not included. Specialization and public policy in dentistry and other health professions are, likewise, not covered in this book. The historical development of specific groups of physicians also deserve further study: in particular the place and contributions of Jewish physicians, black physicians, women physicians; and it is to be hoped that ultimately each specialty will generate its own professional history. Detailed descriptions and analyses of health care programs are not made available, for reasons of space and lest they distort the focus from the major themes of the book. In most cases, however, adequate materials are available elsewhere in the literature, and appropriate references made in the footnotes.

None of the book has been published elsewhere in its present form. Some years ago, part of the material of the first three parts of the book was incorporated in a dissertation for the Ph.D. requirements of Yale University. Portions of the last two parts were developed from public lectures delivered at the Health Sciences Center of the University of Minnesota and at the Johns Hopkins School of Hygiene and Public Health, as well as in a paper delivered at the 1970 meeting of the American Sociological Association. The latter paper, focusing on the manpower implications of specialized medicine, is published as "Trends in Medical Specialization in the United States" in *Inquiry,* March, 1971. Chapter 20, in expanded form, "Medicaid: Anatomy of a Dilemma," now appears in the symposium on medical care in the Spring 1970 issue of *Law and Contemporary Problems.*

My final thanks go to the National Center for Health Services Research and Development of the Department of Health, Education, and Welfare for the generous grant which made this study possible.

R.S.

Yale University School of Medicine
New Haven, Connecticut
December 1970

INTRODUCTION

The medical care system in the United States—using "system" in terms of the anatomy and physiology through which medical services are provided rather than implying a cohesive, centralized organization—is in the midst of upheaval. There are more persons working in health occupations than ever before, and increases in health personnel are, in relative terms, outstripping population gains. Each year more persons have insurance coverage for some part of their medical bills. Medicare, Medicaid, and other recent health programs have provided opportunities for the increased availability of medical services, for training additional personnel, and for affording the least advantaged more opportunities for adequate care. Yet the medical system is in a state of crisis, the numbers of physicians and other personnel are still too few; delivery of medical services is still—in many areas—grossly inadequate.

The sense of crisis has been brought about in part because of the rapidly rising costs of health services. The other, and equally important, side of the coin is a recognition of the expanding potential value of medicine. With the great advances in applied medical technology—in chemotherapy, in operating room hardware, in biochemistry, in therapeutics and surgery, and in many other fields—the ability to improve the quality of life, to delay death, to prevent sickness, has blossomed under the physician's hand. Indeed, it is a tribute to the rapidity of technological advance that some of the most important contemporary problems facing medicine are philosophical rather than physical: when life should be prolonged artificially, when organ transplants should be allowed (and when permission should be sought), how the physician can be taught to emerge from the shelter of charts and machines to converse naturally with the patient, and how the costs of medical care should be funded.

At the beginning of this century there was relatively little difference in the outcome of many conditions or diseases whether or not the patient was seen by a doctor. It is the technological revolution—part of the continuing industrial revolution in society as a whole—which has, in its potential to effect change, brought medicine firmly into the public domain. Rising consumer expectations and the growing value of medical services have created a situation in which deprivation of needed medical care, for economic reasons or because services are locally unavailable, has become morally and socially unacceptable. Health standards have been rising throughout the population, but medical services continue to be unevenly spread. Those in most need of medical care continue to receive the least attention. The poorer the family, the less money is spent on medical care, the less expenditure is covered by health insurance, and the fewer the medical and dental visits.

Such conditions are not new, but the changing social and medical environment has brought them into a new focus. The movement for equal opportunity and civil rights is now being matched by an awareness, both among consumers and in the health professions, of the gaps in basic health service, gaps which are particularly incongruous when contrasted with the sophisticated triumphs of the operating room. The current problems in medical care do not therefore represent a breakdown of preexisting situation, nor even less a sudden decline in health personnel and facilities. Rather, they derive from technological advance itself, and from the social demand for a more effective and equitable distribution of medicine's new capacity. Whether health is defined as a right or a privilege, or in some other way, it is becoming accepted by public and professionals alike that each member of the population should have accessible and effective medical care. The problems lie not in the lack of achievements but in the widening gap between what *can* be done for an individual under optimal conditions and what *is* being done for the individual under average and minimal conditions. The crisis is in the delivery, not in the potential, of care. In this sense medical care, whether provided through public or private agencies, is an essential social service.

A second essential ingredient of technological advance has been a rapid diversification of medical services and personnel. The full potential of medicine cannot be transmitted to an individual without a panoply of facilities bristling with equipment, and an army of specialized health personnel; and this is increasingly true of routine medical diagnosis as well as of esoteric treatment. Nor can health services be evaluated merely in terms of the distribution of doctors in relation to the population, the number of hospital beds, or the amount spent to purchase care. The person with curable cancer is unlikely to be reassured by the number of physicians and hospitals in his area if he has no timely access, either for financial or geographical reasons, to a qualified surgeon or radiologist or to a well-equipped radiotherapy department. The focus of medicine has thus expanded from the patient's bedside to a network of interlocking services; from the domain of one medical profession to an organizational system in which a multitude of specialists is equally involved; from an acceptance of medicine as an undifferentiated element in the market system to a situation where medical financing is one of the politically most prominent battlegrounds of the 1970s.

One vital feature of the health care crisis is the need for rational reintegration of services which have proliferated under the impact of specialism. Somehow the individual needs to be guided toward the appropriate service; equally, the service needs to be there, receptive to meeting his needs. This argues for two kinds of coordination: the first between health care specialists, and the second between each physician and the specialty diagnosis and treatment centers. Translated into organizational terms, this points to cohesive foci for medical practice (such as some form of group practice, or health centers inside or outside hospitals) and regional consultation and referral patterns. The transition is as yet only at the embryonic stage, but the group and the regional concepts are now widely accepted.

There are, however, implications other than increasing institutionalization in the rapid progress of medical specialism. Not the least of these is the impact of specialization on the medical profession. In 1931, 17 percent of all physicians in the United States were full-time specialists. Today the proportion is between 70 and 80 percent. The structure of medical education, training, and deployment has changed from one based on a general undergraduate training and general practice to a complex array of specialties and superspecialties, each with its own training and examination system. Medicine, as no other profession, is now functionally fractionated and internally stratified. This change is largely a product of the last thirty years.

Not only has the march of specialism lengthened the training of the medical student to the present eight or nine years; it also has created an unwieldly superstructure of specialty examining boards, a crisis in graduate medical education, a haphazard assignment of educational and training responsibility, and acute manpower problems. At the same time, the array of other health personnel has diversified, both along lines similar to those of medical specialism (laboratory and radiological technologists, for instance,) and in new or expanded specialist fields (occupational therapists, psychologists, microbiologists, medical social workers). Some 300,-000 physicians are joined by over 1.2 million other health professionals, and more than a million other health personnel.

This concurrent horizontal and vertical specialization—that is, specialism within one profession, and specialization which cuts vertically from one profession to another—has developed chronic stresses and strains within the older professions, most noticeably in medicine and nursing.

Each has to reconsider the kinds and length of education, the relationship between education and licensure, the delineation of specialists, the acceptance of differential ranks, and the evolution of new professional patterns. Broadly, each has to realign its professional structure around changing service ideals, which in themselves have been brought about through the changing content of the professional field.

In the United States as in England (and indeed most, if not all, industrialized countries), the shape of health services has been largely dictated by the particular modes of development of the medical profession. The role of the general practitioner, the relationship between generalist and specialist, the structure and nature of hospital staff appointments, the approach to cooperative and group practice—all these have been molded over many years in both countries by the evolving structure and ethos of the medical profession. In Britain the profession has divided itself into general practitioners and consultants; the United States lacks such division. Even before America's entry into World War I the major patterns of today's health services in this country were firmly established, and were distinct from those across the Atlantic. The richer members of the population used the services of generalist and specialist private practitioners, the poor congregated in clinics, and the remainder of the population fell somewhere in between. Physicians had a relatively open access to hospitals, compared with their European counterparts, with general practitioners frequently undertaking surgery; there was concern that the general practitioner was becoming obsolescent; the AMA's strong and unique role in American medicine was becoming set; specialist group practice (also an American phenomenon) was appearing; there was a flurry of activity over specialist qualifications and certification; and debates over compulsory health insurance included consideration of how far insurance would be effective if there were not also major improvements in the medical care system. These same issues appear today, although in a quite different technological and social context.

In both England and the United States the enormous scientific and technological changes in medicine, accelerating as they have in the last thirty years, have created common and acute organizational pressures. The role of the general practitioner early in this century may have been differently shaped in the United States and in Britain. Meanwhile, rapid specialization in medicine created similar problems on each side of the Atlantic for re-creating the concept of a generalist or primary physician, for grouping medical services to provide an appropriate base for the provision of well-coordinated specialist care, for reviewing the education and production of physicians in relation both to the development of other personnel and to some appropriate measurement of manpower need. This book follows the pattern of the British study in tracing the process of medical professionalism in its changing context from early professional identification, to the incorporation and shaping of the medical specialties, and on to current demands for health services which have sprung from the medical advances wrought by specialism but which call for changes in the older concepts of professionalism.

The book is divided into five parts. Part I describes the infancy of American medicine (with due reference to its European parentage), identifying the idiosyncratic strains of the American physician and his practice: the emergence of a standardized medical profession, the beginnings in the nineteenth century of the instrumental and laboratory innovations that were the basis of specialization, and the role of the American Medical Association as it became the one dominant medical organization.

Part II represents the childhood of specialism. Between 1900 and 1930, specialization became more firmly rooted; there was no professional hierarchy to contain it, nor organizational patterns of medical care to provide an answer. The quality of individuals holding themselves out as specialists became a matter of both professional and public concern; the graduate education of physicians was at issue; specialist licensing and professional and university certification were all raised as alternatives. In short, the problems of 1930 were similar to those of today. Their reanalysis clarifies many of the confusions of the 1970s.

In the next twenty years modern medical care developed its present outward forms. These are the subject of Part III. The public and professional institutions of an increasingly specialized medicine developed side by side. Such, however, was the political antipathy of organized medicine to discussion of the evolution of cooperative plans for medical care that specialist education and certification were divorced from interconnected manpower and organizational issues.

We are now in the stage of reexamination, reevaluation, and relinking of what developed independently as "political" and "professional" aspects of medicine. This process is the subject of Part IV. Generalism and specialism are terms applicable both to professional training and to the provision of medical service. The quality of care is of vital interest, though from different viewpoints, to those on both sides of the physician's desk. Regional distribution of facilities affect both the consumers and providers of medical care, as does any consideration of the future role of the hospital. Part V brings together the dominant themes and looks forward to alternative medical developments.

This study is only a beginning. If it stimulates others to undertake further research, it will have fulfilled one of its most important functions. However, it is to be hoped that the study approaches its primary goal: that of identifying and tying together in their evolving context the elements of today's health and professional crises.

PART I: THE PROFESSIONAL SETTING

CHAPTER 1

From Colonial Times to the Civil War

The First Two Hundred and Fifty Years

American medicine did not emerge as an entity until the turn of the twentieth century. Reliance on the scientific leadership of Britain, then France, and then (after the Civil War) Germany for a long time gave medical science in the United States an imitative rather than an original character. For most of this time, moreover, primary responsibility for giving medical care was in the hands of domestic or "irregular" practitioners. Experimental research did not begin to get under way until the 1890s. When it did, stimulated by an outstanding cadre of German-trained Americans, by drastic reforms in the medical schools, and by rich endowment from the fortunes of the nineteenth-century industrial barons, medicine was transformed; by 1920, the United States had replaced Germany at the hub of medical progress. American medical education, described by William Welch in the 1870s as "simply horrible," [1] had attained standards as high as any in the world. The medical profession was nationally organized in the American Medical Association, and the patterns of present-day medical institutions were already predetermined.

The late emergence of American research was in part the result, and in part the cause, of the slow and uncertain development of medicine as a profession in the seventeenth, eighteenth, and nineteenth centuries. There was both a scientific and a cultural, or attitudinal, lag between developments in Europe and their assimilation into American medicine; Harvard Medical School, for example, did not include the stethoscope as an object of instruction until thirty years after its discovery.[2] Hospitals, the product of a general humanitarian process, developed in Paris between 1750 and

1. James T. and Simon Flexner, *William Henry Welch and the Heroic Age of American Medicine* (New York, 1941), p. 113.
2. Abraham Flexner, *Medical Education in the United States and Canada.* A Report to the Carnegie Foundation for the Advancement of Teaching, Bulletin No. 4. (New York, 1960), p. 8 (hereafter cited as Flexner report).

1850, thus forming the nucleus for French medical sovereignty in the early nineteenth century. In Britain, general hospital expansion also began before 1850. But in the United States there was no widespread development before the 1880s. Nor were there before the late nineteenth century strong professional groups to initiate reform.

In Britain the structure of the medical profession derived from nationally focused and authoritarian guilds of physicians, surgeons, and apothecaries—themselves creating and maintaining three slowly converging branches of medicine, which were originally quite distinct. This unifying process was formally achieved in 1858, when a common medical register was established. Thereafter in Britain there was a common category of "doctor"; but some functional distinctions remained from the continuing guilds, the Royal Colleges of Physicians and Surgeons and the Societies of Apothecaries. And it was onto these preexisting distinctions that technological specialism was grafted. The nineteenth-century surgeon-apothecary became the twentieth-century general practitioner; the old physician and surgeon became today's specialist consultants; a system of consultation or "referral" between GP and specialist was built into the informal ethical system of the profession; and the GP had little or no direct access to the prestigious voluntary hospital.[3] These patterns were well developed in Britain by the early twentieth century; the American medical profession at that time was still seeking national unity and national focus. Organizational responses to the accelerating pressures of scientific medicine, of which the most obvious was the rapid development of medical specialties, were thus quite different in Britain and in the United States.

The American medical profession, like the British, sought unity. This was not, however, a question of integrating existing hierarchies but of bringing together diverse elements which were the product of independent local developments. Professional evolution in the United States, in medicine as in other fields, was a process of federation rather than of centralization. The American Medical Association, which had become by World War I the focus of a national profession, was built on state medical societies which depended on local associations. The Association of American Medical Colleges, spokesman for the teachers, became a federation of medical school deans; and the state licensing boards achieved their own loosely federated structure in the 1890s. These types of organization were totally different from the European guilds, which from their inception had been national in their authority and aristocratic in design.

The organizational structure of a profession both reflects and deter-

3. See Stevens, *Medical Practice in Modern England,* pp. 11–37.

mines the role of its practitioners. Whereas the medical professions of northern Europe developed in the context of an initially divided profession, with an inbuilt social ranking system, the American medical profession developed around, and out of, general practice. Attempts to create one "doctor" in America were focused not so much on one portal of entry to the profession (as in Britain, through the establishment of a medical register) as on achieving one standard of entry which would distinguish the "regular" from the "irregular" practitioner.

At the same time, however, there was periodic flirtation from the colonial years up to the twentieth century with proposals for establishing guildlike organizations in America to create a distinction between the better-trained and the less-trained medical practitioner. Posed by opponents in terms of elitism versus democracy, these attempts consistently failed. When attempts were finally successful early in the twentieth century to establish—on technological grounds—an American College of Surgeons and an American College of Physicians, these organizations were much more like voluntary specialist societies than the complex network of influence which characterized the British Colleges. During the nineteenth century, the medical profession did achieve a distinction between regular and irregular practitioners and laid claim to a professional monopoly of the practice of medicine. But within the regular profession the emphasis was placed more and more on leveling or averaging out distinctions, than on attempting to impose them at the level of training or of practice. There was thus no professional ranking structure whereby specialism in medicine might be contained. Questions raised by the emergence of a technocratic elite, including the wisdom of establishing organizations with educational and regulatory functions for medical specialties, had thus to be reexamined in a new context during the twentieth century.

THE PHYSICIAN IN THE COLONIES

From the start, medicine in the new colonies was structurally distinct from the stratified professional system that existed in Britain. The colonies began as separate entities, sometimes loosely interconnected, sometimes not at all; there were no major centers common to all of them, and even within the different colonies there was generally less emphasis on one or two centers than in England or the other countries from which the colonists came. The practitioners who emigrated were ship's surgeons, or apothecaries, together with men in other fields, such as the New England ministers, who acquired some degree of medical skill in Europe for the special purpose of their new life.[4] They filled the role of the English country surgeon-apothecary, rather than the city physician or the busy barber-surgeon. The divisions between the branches of medical practice in England were socially significant rather than functionally necessary, although specialization later offered a convenient rationalization for this arrangement. The new colonies could initially afford no such luxuries and, in most cases, were socially not disposed to encourage them.

In a colonial world dominated by unknown fevers, infections, malnutrition, and death, New England ministers and Southern planters alike acted as both lawyers and physicians. John Winthrop, the younger (1606–76) gave medical advice to settlers through correspondence, both before and after he became governor of Connecticut. Two presidents of Harvard College were in this same line of "domestic" rather than "professional" medicine, and in the scattered rural communities, schoolmasters and other educated men were also forced, from the lack of alternatives, to dispense medical advice. Indeed, the link between medicine and theology in New England lasted throughout the seventeenth century, and the terrible visitations of disease and death were fused into the religious life of the Puritan community.[5]

4. The first English practitioner to land on the American continent was Henry Kenton, a surgeon attached to the fleet of Capt. Bartholomew Gilbert, which was exploring the Virginia waters in 1603. A group of 120 settlers, other surgeons, and apothecaries arrived with the early Virginia colonists, but probably none of the practitioners working in Virginia prior to 1624 held a university degree. New England was served no better. Giles Heale, the ship's surgeon of the *Mayflower*, had served his apprenticeship and received his license as a barber-surgeon in London the year before the *Mayflower* sailed; but he returned to England with his ship in 1621, leaving the colony without a formally licensed practitioner. Deacon Samuel Fuller (1580–1633), who had probably studied medicine in Leyden, became the outstanding practitioner of the Plymouth colony. The first resident medical practitioner in New England was probably John Clark (1598–1664), who arrived in about 1638, claimed an English medical diploma for cutting for the stone, and set up practice in Boston. He became the founder of a long line of physicians handing down their skills from father to son, the last Clark dying in 1805. Wyndham B. Blanton, *Medicine in Virginia in the Seventeenth Century* (Richmond, 1930), pp. 3, 80–81; Henry R. Viets, *A Brief History of Medicine in Massachusetts* (Boston, 1930), pp. 14, 39–40. Materials on the early development of American medicine in general are drawn from Francis R. Packard, *History of Medicine in the United States* (New York, 1931); W. F. Norwood, *Medical Education in the United States Before The Civil War* (Philadelphia, 1944); and especially Richard H. Shryock, *Medicine and Society in America, 1660–1860* (Ithaca, New York, 1962).
5. During the first winter at Plymouth, about half the Pilgrims died, particularly in January and February 1621. The critical problems of infectious diseases continued in the next hundred years. In 1721 Boston experienced its sixth major smallpox epidemic: one in seven of the population died. By the end of the colonial period, however, vaccination was rapidly bringing smallpox under control. Viets, *Brief History*, pp. 14, 55–63; Daniel Boorstin, The Americans: *The Colonial Experience* (New York, 1958), pp. 226–27 and passim; Perry Miller, "The Scourge of Small-

Scientifically as well as socially, American medicine already had a distinctly non-European flavor. American attitudes to treatment, closely linked with botanical exploration in the New World, developed a strong emphasis on natural history, and on conservative common sense. For those cultured in physic there was neither the leisure for discussion nor were there universities at which to debate at length the dogmas of the causes of human disorders that engaged the "vitalists," "iatrochemists," and "iatrophysicists" in the European centers. Pride in the relative practicality of American medicine long outlasted the period of dependence on European theory; indeed it contributed to the often unproductive insularity of American medical science in the eighteenth and nineteenth centuries.

The different scientific emphasis, the absence of a metropolitan or university focus in the colonies, the prevalence of "domestic" medicine, and the parochial development of physician training through individual apprenticeship[6] discouraged the clear differences and disputes between physicians that distinguished European university-trained physicians and the non-university-trained surgeons and apothecaries. Nor was there in 1700 any Royal College, hospital, or medical school to reinforce or reinvent distinctions. There was some travel across the Atlantic during the seventeenth century, but the passage to England was dangerous and expensive. Consequently a self-perpetuating, decentralized system of medi-

---

pox," in *The New England Mind: From Colony to Province* (Cambridge, Mass., 1953).

6. The medical apprenticeship was formalized in a contract specifying the rights and duties of both parties. The apprentice paid a fee, lived with his preceptor, and provided services around the house and in the medical practice. Richard Townshend, after six years of faithful service to Dr. Pott in Jamestown, brought a petition to court in 1626 complaining that he was not being given instruction, an action he won. But the great majority of subsequent apprentices were apparently satisfied with their terms, even when they included "administering grease to the master's chaise, oats to his mare, or running errands for his wife." The standards of instruction varied widely—particularly where one erstwhile apprentice found himself training others. Preceptors often exploited the apprentices. In the days of the London Company (1607–24) the beginnings of hospitals had been made in Virginia; the first hospital (guest house) in America was constructed in 1612 in the new town of Henricopolis near the Falls on the James River. But with the dissolution of the company, these hospitals disappeared. Physicians and others who had acquired a reputation for nursing or who appreciated the business aspects would take seriously ill or emergency patients into their own homes for treatment. The apprentices were useful as pairs of hands and bedside nurses. Some practitioners had a veritable band of students. Dr. Thomas Hubbard of Pomfret, Conn., rode fast and furiously over the country followed by a pack of apprentices, known by his disapproving colleagues as "his hounds." Blanton, *Seventeenth Century*, pp. 24–25, 97, and passim; Walter Ralph Steiner, *Historical Address; The Evolution of Medicine in Connecticut, With the Foundation of the Yale Medical School as Its Notable Achievement* (New Haven, 1915) pp. 8–15; Norwood, p. 32 and passim.

cine began to develop. By the end of the seventeenth century there was still no medical school, nor were there licensing laws or medical societies in the colonies. A system of indenture for five to eight years to established physicians was common in Virginia; yet the only license required was a statement of professional skill. Massachusetts had enacted a law in 1649 requiring chirurgeons, midwives, and physicians to act only in accordance with the approved "Rules of Art," but it set up no educational or licensing provisions. Medical legislation in Virginia was aimed more at medical practitioners' "excessive rates and prices" than at their skill—an interesting comment on the patterns of the time.[7] There was no medical *profession,* no guild system as existed in England and other European countries, no effective medical elite, and virtually no public control over the standards of medical training or practice.

Not only were there no organizational pressures for a divided profession, but the apprenticeship system actively encouraged the development of one all-around bedside practitioner. The labels "chirurgeon" and "physician" in seventeenth-century Virginia connoted little difference in services performed. Surgeons were not also barbers, as were their English counterparts; there was little left to the seventeenth-century surgeon that physicians did not also do. The English custom of calling surgeons plain "mister" was lost, and the term "doctor" or "physician" was applied without regard to degree. Nor did the term "apothecary" have much use in a land where doctors dispensed their own drugs. As the settlements became more entrenched, and the simple local drugs gave way to imported products from England, practitioners began to open their own apothecary shops. By the 1770s there were numerous such shops in Williamsburg and other colonial towns, and there were few druggists who were not also physicians; indeed, for many doctors the drug business had become essential for financial survival. In a pattern that was to recur in the nineteenth century as a peculiarly American phenomenon, there had developed large numbers of physicians relative to the population—the outcome of an uncontrolled educational system. In the Revolutionary era the ratio of doctors to population was about 1 to 600. An estimate for New York in 1750 gives a ratio of about 1 to 350; and for Williamsburg in 1730 as many as 1 to 135.[8] There were thus in the eighteenth century relatively far more physicians than there are today.

The realities of this professional competition countered attempts by

7. Under an act of 1645 a physician might be arrested for unreasonable charges. Blanton, *Seventeenth Century,* pp. 250–51. For more information on the Massachusetts legislation see Viets, *Brief History,* pp. 45–46.
8. Shryock, *Medicine and Society,* p. 12; W. J. Bell, Jr., "Medical Practice in Colonial America," *Bull. Hist. Med., 31* (1957), 447.

colonial Americans trained in Britain during the eighteenth century to impose British professional and educational distinctions in the colonies. A 1736 Virginia law distinguished between "surgeons and apothecaries who have served an apprenticeship to those trades" and those who had studied physic in a university—the latter being able to charge twice as much.[9] Yet there is little evidence that the consultant in medicine ever developed, apart from a few isolated practitioners in the largest centers in the most sophisticated colonies. Instead, the pattern of combined practice seems to have developed concurrently and to have proved resilient all through the colonies. By the 1770s, even the distinguished and celebrated found it difficult to establish themselves as physicians without also dispensing drugs and undertaking surgery.[10]

Attempts to create an elite in the late eighteenth century had thus to be superimposed on a well-established pattern of general practice, and to run the danger of being attacked by the mass of doctors as well as by the public as the imposition of an uncalled-for monopoly. Moreover, since virtually all physicians had a similar type of practice (and there was little incentive for anyone to change), attempted distinctions between one doctor and another had to be molded out of educational backgrounds instead of functional differences—that is, between those trained wholly by domestic apprenticeship and the small but influential group of practitioners who by the outbreak of the Revolutionary War were receiving some kind of university education.[11] It might well have been an unequal

9. Packard, pp. 164–65.
10. A vignette of the situation can be given in the history of Dr. James McClurg, born in 1747. After studying at William and Mary College, McClurg went to Europe, decided on medicine as a career, and graduated from Edinburgh in 1770. Before returning to Virginia he studied in Paris and London, and in 1772 wrote a celebrated essay, "Experiments upon the Human Bile and Reflections on Biliary Secretion." McClurg settled in Williamsburg in 1773, establishing a considerable reputation. In 1779, during a stint in the Revolutionary army, he became the first professor of anatomy and medicine at William and Mary College (the second such chair established in the United States, the first being at Philadelphia). He was also prominent in public positions and was considered by Jefferson for a cabinet position. Even Dr. McClurg, however, found it impossible to make sufficient independent income without a surgical or apothecary practice. His solution was to practice solely as a physician and to live partly on his private income. But relatively few practitioners had this opportunity. Wyndham B. Blanton, *Medicine in Virginia in the Eighteenth Century* (Richmond, 1931), pp. 328–33.
11. The dominance of apprenticeship training continued until after the Revolution, except perhaps in the largest towns. Of the ten physicians in Boston in 1721, three had a liberal education (two at Harvard College), one was a surgeon from an English warship, one a Frenchman who had served in foreign wars. Only one, Dr. William Douglass (1691–1752), had received an M.D. At the outset of the Revolutionary War there were about 3,500 medical practitioners in the colonies, of whom not more than 400 had received any formal training, and of these only some 200 held

battle even if the British presence had remained. With independence and, more important, the changed social conditions of the beginning of the nineteenth century, the idea of an elite corps of consultants was doomed. What did develop, however, was an informal system of professional grading.

Until the establishment in 1765 of the first American medical school at the College of Philadelphia, university medical education meant a period of study in Europe. While this was rare in the seventeenth century, it had become common by the middle of the eighteenth. By the time of the Revolution, colonial medicine was thus strongly influenced by British thought and practice.[12] Edinburgh, which had established its medical faculty in 1726 and risen quickly to fame under the influence of the three Munros, became the focus of medical education for those who crossed the Atlantic; indeed the first Philadelphia faculty was composed entirely of Edinburgh graduates. There was also continued emigration of doctors from Europe to the colonies. While there was still little communication between the colonies, the ties with Europe were growing increasingly strong. During the century this trend was encouraged by the lack of a cultural and political center in the colonies, such as London provided in

---

degrees. The distinction of receiving the first medical diploma from an American university goes to Daniel Turner, who accepted an honorary Doctor of Medicine degree from Yale College in 1720—although there was no medical department at Yale until 1813. Turner's degree, given in return for his gifts to the college, was referred to by contemporary wits as "Multum Donavit." Packard, pp. 281–83; Viets, *Brief History*, pp. 56–57; Shryock, *Medicine and Society*, p. 9. Blanton estimates the proportion of Virginia doctors with degrees at the end of the eighteenth century to those without as about 1 to 9, of a total of about 500. Blanton, *Eighteenth Century*, pp. 207–08. The extra fees from apprenticeship continued to be welcome until apprenticeship finally disappeared in the late nineteenth century. Dr. David Hosack of New York expected an income from his pupils of $1,400 between 1826 and 1829. Henry B. Shafer, *The American Medical Profession, 1783–1850* (New York, 1936) pp. 33–34.

12. The British influence on colonial medicine began to be felt with the development of systematic teaching by those trained abroad. Dr. Cadwalader Colden in Philadelphia has credit for planning in 1717 the first known course of lectures. He planned to care for the poor of the city and to teach, while he hoped the city would pay him a salary. The aim, however, did not succeed. The first known lectures and anatomy demonstrations in Philadelphia were given by Dr. Thomas Cadwalader in 1750 to a small group of students. Cadwalader had been a pupil of Cheselden in London. Lectures were given by William Hunter (a relative of *the* William and John Hunter) at Newport, R.I., 1754–56. Lecture courses slowly became popular in major towns and remained even after the foundation of medical schools. Two other pupils of Cheselden, Silvester Gardiner and James Lloyd, together with William Douglass, exerted a marked British influence in Boston in the 1750s, and systematic teaching of his apprentices was attempted by Lloyd's pupil Joseph Warren before the Revolutionary War. Packard, pp. 286, 297; Norwood, p. 43; Viets, *Brief History*, p. 86.

England. The structure of the colonies encouraged parochial rather than centralized medical leadership and organization. Indeed, this important aspect of American medical development outlasted the colonial experience.

Those who returned to the colonies in the 1760s and after formed a cultural group whose interests lay in the encouragement of a well-regulated profession. Their Scottish experience bound them together; their training set them above the mass. The Edinburgh students petitioned the Virginia House of Burgesses, unsuccessfully, to restrict the practice of medicine to those who were licensed *and* held a doctor's degree.[13] John Morgan determined on returning to Philadelphia to practice medicine alone, "without turning apothecary or practising surgery." In his famous *Discourse* of 1765 he bitterly attacked "the levelling of all kind of practitioners." [14] But Morgan's crusade was bound to fail: an elite based solely on social distinction could not succeed in this country. The next best thing was an intellectual medical elite based on the universities. How far the American medical profession would be standardized to produce one acceptable product and how far and for which reasons a social, educational, or functional elite could be justified was to become a running theme in subsequent professional development. It continues today in the status struggles of specialists and generalists in modern medicine.

The foundation of the medical school in Philadelphia, stimulated by William Shippen, Jr., and realized through Morgan's vigorous canvassing in Europe, was a part of the movement by university-trained physicians to organize and rationalize medicine on a European model and to institute recognizable educational standards. John Morgan considered that even the best preceptors were unable to impart more than a "lame and insufficient" education to their apprentices and that the products of the system were not only poorly trained but dangerous—though how "danger" is defined is a matter of opinion in an era when preferred methods of treatment were sweating, blistering, purging, and bleeding, and when neither the theories nor the methods of medicine, even at Edinburgh, were of relevance to most of the diseases of the day.

The stimulating and intellectual discussions of theories of disease in which educated colonial Americans participated in Europe emphasized the cultural differences between men such as those on the staff of the

13. Blanton, *Eighteenth Century*, pp. 398, 401. The professional development of these different groups is analyzed in depth by Joseph Kett in *The Formation of the American Medical Profession. The Role of Institutions, 1780–1860* (New Haven, 1968).

14. John Morgan, *A Discourse upon the Institution of Medical Schools in America, 1765*, (Reprinted, Baltimore, 1937), p. vi.

Pennsylvania Hospital, who were almost all classical scholars and men of affairs, and the run-of-the-mill practitioner trained wholly by apprenticeship. The relative poverty of surgery, which was practiced by few men of standing in the American colonies and was an unpromising branch of medicine until after the Revolution, and the social inferiority of the apothecary in Britain were added reasons for those returning to the colonies to develop an educational milieu for a superior American physician.

Morgan's *Discourse* was based on a dissection of the state of medical education in the colonies and a detailed plan for the establishment of a medical school. His appointment as professor of medicine at Philadelphia in 1765 provided the opportunity to put the plan into effect. The Philadelphia school, to be developed on Edinburgh lines, divided medicine into five branches: anatomy, materia medica, botany, chemistry, and the theory and practice of medicine. Surgery, as such, did not appear. It was a *university* rather than a *hospital* medical school in the tradition of continental Europe, a tradition which Edinburgh then followed.[15] Thus the structure of the school—and of the leading schools which followed it— did not follow the English model, in which medical schools sprang from the hospital wards as a formal extension of, and background to, bedside teaching and had no university affiliation. Besides the debt to Edinburgh, however, leading physicians in the American colonies distinguished themselves from England by having available few general hospitals. While the Pennsylvania Hospital predated the Philadelphia medical school, King's College Medical School was established in New York at a time when only Bellevue (basically a poorhouse) existed as a resource for teaching patients; nor was there a general hospital in Boston when Harvard Medical School was founded in 1783. It was thus from necessity as well as choice that American medical education developed in the

15. Morgan could have founded his school on the Pennsylvania Hospital, already a flourishing center. The Pennsylvania Hospital in prosperous Philadelphia, the center of European influence in the colonies, was the first incorporated general hospital in America. Its foundation could be traced to Dr. Thomas Bond. Returning from surgical and midwifery studies in Europe in 1750, he interested other physicians and influential citizens in setting up a hospital for private patients. The hospital became a practical possibility when Benjamin Franklin lent his support, and it was chartered in 1751. It opened in 1755 as an institution for the physically and mentally sick, regardless of economic status, race, or creed. One of the purposes claimed for the Pennsylvania Hospital during the fund-raising campaign was the provision of training facilities for medical students. Physicians became accustomed to taking their apprentices round the wards, using them as dressers and assistants; and this system soon developed into requests from other students to walk the wards. Indeed, in 1763 it was decided to charge these students a fee for the privilege. Commission on Hospital Care, *Hospital Care in the United States* (New York, 1947), p. 438 and passim; Packard, pp. 322–25, 327.

eighteenth century from educational institutions, whereas at the same time English medical education was deriving increasingly from institutions concerned with patient care.[16] The patterns of professionalism in the two countries became increasingly distinct.

Morgan had intended that the Philadelphia school should accept only those with a college degree or evidence of other acceptable education. The medical school was thus, in modern terms, a graduate school. With the Revolutionary War, however, university medical education was disrupted and the postwar pattern was not the same. The charter of the College of Philadelphia was repealed in 1779 (although it was reinstated in 1783) and a rival (patriot) medical school was developed in Philadelphia. The two were finally joined as part of the University of Pennsylvania in 1791, but the dislocation caused by the war made it impossible to demand that all students have a premedical college degree. The earlier Philadelphia M.B. was discontinued in 1789 and the M.D. instituted, a degree which became customary for American medical students. A similar course was followed at the second medical school to be founded before the Revolutionary War: the Medical School of King's College, New York (Columbia), established in 1768.[17] Even without graduate selection, however, the Pennsylvania and the Columbia schools, followed before the end of the century by schools at Harvard and Dartmouth, provided a high-quality, competitive training. There was thus at last an effective alternative to going to Europe and an identifiable focus for further professionalism.

Infant medical societies were beginning to offer a second such focus. The first enduring societies were set up in the 1760s, and in 1766 the

16. The different development of voluntary hospitals in Britain and in the colonies emphasized the different approaches to physician education. Between 1700 and 1825, 154 new hospitals and dispensaries were established in Britain as charitable institutions for the sick poor. The Virginian, New Yorker, Bostonian, or Philadelphian returning home in 1750 had no such institution. There were some pesthouses for contagious diseases, some almshouses, and some houses of correction, but nothing approaching a voluntary general hospital. Neither the smallpox hospitals nor the houses of correction provided doctors with the kind of experience available in Britain or elsewhere—where the convenient collection of patients in rows of beds enabled the physician to classify and group his observations by signs and symptoms. Stevens, pp. 16–21; G. M. Trevelyan, *English Social History,* 3d ed. (London, 1948), p. 345.

17. King's College, founded largely through the impetus of Samuel Bard, also required an adequate premedical education or college degree, gave an M.B. degree, and probably had similarly high teaching standards. The M.B. was replaced as the basic degree by the M.D. in 1774. The Revolution interrupted the school's development. King's College was renamed Columbia, and the medical school was reopened in 1792; but it only limped along. A vigorous rival school was founded by the University of New York in 1807, and the two schools were merged in 1811. Packard, pp. 395–428. Harvard initially gave the Bachelor of Physic degree, but replaced it by the M.D. in 1811. Viets, *Brief History,* p. 113.

first state (provincial) society was established in New Jersey. Virginia had passed the first fee bill, setting maximum fees, in 1736. By the 1760s practitioners had revived the guild idea of regulating their own fees. The New Jersey society also pressed for licensing restrictions, which were passed by the provincial legislature in 1772. Both actions were followed when other state societies were set up in the years after the Revolutionary War. Developments in the late eighteenth century focused on continued professional grouping through the rapid growth of such societies and the development by these societies of journals and of restrictionist fee schedules setting out minimum fees.

By 1776, therefore, there were some distinctions, but not divisions, in the American medical profession. The average doctor practiced medicine, surgery, pharmacy, and midwifery. While there was no rigorous specialization, there was an informal grading of practitioners according to education and experience. Attempts to reimpose European distinctions had failed. Morgan's suggestion for a national college of physicians (on the model of the Royal College of Physicians in London), which would offer a license recognized throughout the colonies, was vetoed by Thomas Penn. The College of Physicians of Philadelphia was finally established in 1787, but it was not to play a role in licensing, as the English college did; it had no power to regulate the profession. If the leaders of the profession had failed to establish a formal stratification within the profession, they did have, in the new university medical schools, the foundation for an elite based on educational and professional attainments. Such a development offered a natural vehicle for the future growth of medical specialties. But the concept of an elite based even on educational superiority was unlikely to survive the social crisis of the post-Revolutionary years. What type of change might one expect from a profession so diffuse and in many ways so undistinguished when faced with the traumatic changes which were to follow in the period between Lexington and Fort Sumter?

THE POST-REVOLUTIONARY PERIOD

In the face of waves of immigrants, often with traditions and customs different from those of the original settlers, the growth of American professionalism was subject to new pressures. The combination of an overall population expansion of increasingly forbidding dimensions, with the excitement of westward migration, with increasing wealth, and the twin challenges of modern industrialization and Jacksonian Democracy, gave a more populist, less aristrocratic flavor to professional issues. The medical profession was to be concerned in the late eighteenth and early nineteenth centuries not so much with the restoration of distinctions within the profession, but rather with the more basic issue of who was a doctor and who was not.

Before the Revolution, the class of "regular" physicians had attracted those who wished to be called "urbane or English or fashionable," [18] rather than those who genuinely believed these physicians offered better treatment. In the years following the Revolution there remained a widespread unwillingness to use the services of orthodox doctors instead of cultists or quacks. In an era of continuing heroic treatments by orthodox physicians, the gentler methods of Thomsonianism and homeopathy flourished. But the unwillingness to seek out regular physicians was probably also due to the general fear of professional power, which was to grow rapidly after 1820, and to the specific fears concerning the activities of the medical profession. Public horror of dissection led to riots in Philadelphia, and in 1788 (after claims that an anatomist had waved the arm of a cadaver at a boy peering in through the window of the New York Hospital) to a "Doctors' Mob" in New York City, in which seven rioters were killed while trying to lynch the anatomist.

Nevertheless, despite this reluctance by the public to adopt modern medicine fully, a reluctance which was shared in other countries, the profession after the 1780s was slowly growing stronger. With the reestablishment of trade with Britain after the Revolutionary War and the shoring up of preexisting patterns of society, the old custom of educational travel for those rich enough to afford it was rapidly revived. John Collins Warren, James Jackson, Benjamin Waterhouse, Philip Syng Physick, Nathan Smith, and Nathaniel Chapman were among those who made the European tour in the late eighteenth and early nineteenth centuries.[19] Even

18. Daniel H. Calhoun, *Professional Lives in America; Structure and Aspiration, 1750–1850* (Cambridge, 1965), p. 3.
19. John Collins Warren (1778–1856), son of John Warren and instrumental in founding the Massachusetts General Hospital, graduated from Harvard, studied for a year with his father, and then went to London in about 1800, becoming a "dresser" to the famous surgeon Astley Cooper. Warren later spent one year in Edinburgh and another year in Holland, Belgium, and Paris, returning to Boston in 1802 with perhaps the most extensive medical education of any American physician of his time. James Jackson, Warren's friend, contemporary, and co-founder of the hospital, spent nearly three years in England, part of it with Warren at Guy's Hospital, partly studying the early cases of vaccination under Jenner's methods. Jackson returned to Boston in 1800 and shared with Benjamin Waterhouse the honor of being an authority on vaccination in America. Philip Syng Physick, born 1768, had four years of foreign study. Nathan Smith thought it so important to go abroad that he borrowed money to do so. Smith came of a relatively poor family, was trained by apprenticeship, and began practice in Cornish, N.H., in 1787. Realizing his own deficiencies he enrolled in the then recently established Harvard Medical School and received his degree in 1790 (the fifth man to graduate). He returned to

Ephraim McDowell, the pioneer backwoods surgeon who courageously and expertly performed the first ovariotomy in his own home in 1809, had studied for a year in Edinburgh.

The links with Britain took on a different, more tenuous form. Independence encouraged indigenous professional roots and education. In New England the old preacher-physician of the Cotton Mather type disappeared; systematic education finally began to replace European training, and medical societies began to grow stronger. At the outbreak of the Revolutionary War several states had recognized the need for surgeons and military hospitals.[20] Many such doctors had their knowledge tested by their commanders in the war—a factor that made examinations a familiar process and probably encouraged the development of licensing arrangements in the states after the war.[21] By 1780 an identifiable group of well-educated physicians existed in the major American cities: graduates of Edinburgh or Philadelphia, together with men such as John Warren of Boston who were not medical graduates but who had held military positions. As more medical schools were established, the size of this group continuously expanded and offered a nucleus of professionalism. At the same time, the Continental Congress and the establishment of the United States gave a feeling of unity throughout the colonies for the first time.

In this environment the idea of professional self-regulation, through developing medical societies or through the independent, degree-giving medical schools which rose rapidly in the early nineteenth century, superseded sporadic earlier efforts toward state licensing and control. New York had adopted governmental licensing of physicians as early as 1760;

his practice, but in 1796 approached the trustees of Dartmouth College with a plan to establish a medical school. While waiting for their reply, Smith went to Edinburgh and London, and returned not only with knowledge but also with books and equipment for the new college (established 1798). Smith was later instrumental in founding the schools at Yale, Bowdoin, and the University of Vermont. Nathaniel Chapman (1780–1853), the first president of the American Medical Association (1847), spent three years in Edinburgh and London just after 1800. After his return from Europe, Chapman became professor of materia medica—and later professor of medicine—at the University of Pennsylvania. Viets, *Brief History*, pp. 111, 128–29, 130–31; Samuel D. Gross, in Edward H. Clarke et al., *A Century of American Medicine, 1776–1876* (Philadelphia, 1876), pp. 128–31; Wyndham B. Blanton, *Medicine in Virginia in the Nineteenth Century* (Richmond, 1933), pp. 370–75.

20. Virginia, for example, passed an act as early as July 1775 that provided for raising two regiments with a surgeon and two surgeon's mates to each; the following year a further act was passed to provide hospitals and barracks and to appoint physicians and a director general of hospitals. Blanton, *Eighteenth Century*, p. 249.

21. Shryock, *Medicine and Society*, p. 11; and see Kett, *Formation of American Medical Profession*, pp. 10–20.

soon after its establishment in 1766 the New Jersey Medical Society had also successfully requested the provincial government to establish a licensing system. But licensing as a function of the legislature was largely overtaken in the early years of independence by professional controls. In 1800 six states had their own medical societies.[22] By 1830 there were medical societies in nearly all the states of the Union, each pressing to itself control of professional standards. The Massachusetts Medical Society was the first to be granted powers to license physicians by its own examination. By 1825 several other states had followed. Where there were no state societies, the states appointed district boards to examine and to license.[23]

An increasingly persuasive candidate for establishing the qualifications of a physician was the medical school. This possibility first seriously arose with the almost concurrent development of the Massachusetts Medical Society (1781) and the Harvard Medical School (1783). The Massachusetts Medical Society initially insisted that all Harvard graduates take its own licensing examination, but opposition was dropped after an impressive public examination; from 1803 *either* the Harvard degree *or* the society license qualified a man for practice.[24] Somewhat the same dilemma developed in Connecticut, where the Connecticut Medical Society was given power not only to examine and license physicians but also to confer degrees. When Yale University considered setting up its medical school, it had first therefore to win over the medical society. Agreement was finally reached in an act of 1810, the year the school was set up, in which the society and the university agreed to unite in forming the medical school. The medical school conferred degrees; the society gave the licenses.[25]

22. New Jersey (1766), Massachusetts (1781), Delaware (1789), South Carolina (1789), New Hampshire (1791), Connecticut (1792).
23. Ohio and Louisiana (1820), Alabama (1823), Florida (1824), Georgia (1825), Richard H. Shryock, *Medical Licensing in America, 1650–1965*. (Baltimore, 1967), pp. 17, 23–24; Donald E. Konold, *A History of American Medical Ethics, 1847–1912* (Madison, Wisconsin, 1962), pp. 2, 3.
24. Viets, *Brief History,* pp. 106–08; Shryock, *Medicine and Society,* p. 34; Shryock, *Medical Licensing,* pp. 25–26.
25. Apparently the movement to establish licensure had been prompted as early as 1763, "publicly to distinguish between the honest and ingenious physician and the quack or empirical pretender." An action group of 11 doctors had recommended that there should be examination and certification of physicians and that those not certified (except for those already in practice) would be legally restrained from collecting their fees. Even with a grandfather clause, this piece of restrictionism was defeated by the legislature. The creation of a state society was vigorously opposed by the public, as a potential private monopoly. The Connecticut Medical Society was finally formed in 1792, following societies in Litchfield (1764) and New Haven (1783). Thereafter public opposition gradually ceased; indeed, in 1800 the legislature voted to withhold the legal power of collecting debts from unrecognized practi-

Various patterns of professional regulation were thus emerging as distinct and rival possibilities. Given that some degree of regulation over physicians can ensure to the public a minimum standard of education or competence, and to physicians themselves an assurance of professional identity and solidarity, this may be obtained in different ways. Licensing by the state is one such way. Voluntary regulation by professional associations is another. Recognition of patterns of training through diplomas or degrees is a third. In more recent times other forms of regulation have emerged, in the form of approval of individual physicians by the increasing number and types of medical institutions which have become dominant features of twentieth-century practice—be they hospitals, health care systems, or payment schemes. In the early nineteenth century, however, medicine was still almost entirely a "loner" profession; the doctor practiced out of his own home, or in the homes of others. Coordination and regulation of practitioners—two essential features of emerging professionalism—had therefore to be approached either through the two places in which doctors did at some point come together, the medical school and the medical society, or through the external authority of the state.

THE RISE OF THE PROPRIETARY SCHOOL

Recognition of the medical degree as a gateway to practice created one set of circumstances when the degree was from the medical colleges at Pennsylvania, New York, Dartmouth, Harvard, or Yale; however, the opening of a rash of independent medical colleges in the early nineteenth century created a different problem. There could not be a standardized profession unless there was a standardized educational system; quality control thus became a real issue. In 1800 there were only 4 functioning medical colleges; in 1825 there were 18. Between 1810 and 1840, 26 new medical schools were founded; between 1840 and 1876, 47; and in the great wave of immigration at the end of the century (1873–90) 114 new schools were established. Altogether, it has been estimated, over 400 medical schools were founded between 1800 and 1900.[26] Many of these were short-lived; many failed during the Civil War. Each, however, had an impact on medical education and practice during the nineteenth century. Most of the early schools, founded while the social structure of the

tioners (repealed 1842). Meanwhile the medical society went to work to clean up quackery. Steiner, pp. 5, 8, and passim.

26. J. M. Toner, *Address on Medical Biography* (Philadelphia: Transaction of the International Medical Congress, 1876), p. 4; Henry E. Sigerist, *American Medicine* (New York, 1934), p. 133.

old colonies survived, were associated with liberal arts colleges. Many of the new schools springing up in the 1830s and 1840s were not. A precedent had been established in Maryland in 1812 when the state medical society sponsored a college of medicine, as part of the then nonexistent "University of Maryland." [27] This college and others which followed elsewhere were autonomous schools, granting their own degrees. The action of the South Carolina legislature in 1817 to accept as qualified to practice a graduate from any chartered medical school was followed elsewhere and became the general rule. The first privately owned and operated medical institution which pretended no allegiance to a college was set up at Castleton, Vermont, in 1818 by three local physicians.[28] It was followed rapidly by others. Legislatures apparently saw no difficulty in chartering such colleges since they similarly chartered the homeopathy and Thomsonian institutions which appeared in the 1830s.

No doubt these schools met an important social need, and without them the immigrants in the East and the pioneers trekking West would have received even worse medical attention than they in fact did. But such an educational base was barely what the leaders of the profession had been hoping for in the latter part of the eighteenth century. The patient, in the age of Jacksonian democracy, was to have the right to make his free choice between the trained and the untrained, and between the regular physician and the quack.

The university medical schools were rapidly outnumbered by the new proprietary schools. Nevertheless, though they found it difficult to maintain their standards in the face of this new competition, the university schools continued to remain in touch with the latest medical developments in Europe. The proprietary schools supplemented a local system of apprenticeship and provided a focus of training on a parochial basis for the country practitioner. Thus while the predominant pattern in England in the early nineteenth century was the hospital medical school and the earlier American pattern was the university medical school, the typical medical graduate in nineteenth-century America was the product either of apprenticeship alone or of a completely autonomous teaching institution. Standards of teaching thus ranged from inadequate to excellent. How to standardize the educational system and whether or not to divorce teaching from licensure were to become burning issues in the medical societies and schools of the middle and late nineteenth century.

27. Shryock, *Medical Licensing,* pp. 26, 28, and passim.
28. Its historian traces the use of the term "proprietary" to the use of the word "proprietor" in the founding document of Castleton. Frederick C. Waite, *The First Medical College in Vermont: Castleton, 1818–1862* (Montpelier, 1949), pp. 57–58.

The educational focus was changing—as the country was changing. The sudden growth of medical schools was but the top of the iceberg. The British pattern of medical practice, which had become a vague possibility between 1750 and 1810, was now totally out of the question in the political realities represented by the Age of Jackson. Westward migration and settlement, intensified after 1820, had begun in earnest. In 1800, there were about one million people living west of the Alleghenies; in 1810, there were 2.5 million; and by 1830 there were 3.5 million. The few medical schools on the East Coast could not produce enough doctors for the expanding territories.[29] The Eastern practitioner, who had grown up in urban Boston or Philadelphia, was probably loath, and unfitted, to migrate. The Midwesterner did not look to European traditions for his medical practice; and he almost certainly found himself less and less attracted to even the modified Eastern traditions. American medicine acquired a much more insular character.

In some cases the entirely American-trained doctor compared with the best in Europe. The remarkable William Beaumont (1785–1853) was trained entirely through apprenticeship. Daniel Drake (1785–1852) of Kentucky, another "Western American," began his medical career under a Dr. Goforth in Cincinnati, when that town had less than 1,000 people; after four years' apprenticeship he managed to go to Philadelphia, eventually attained his M.D., and in 1817 took the chair of materia medica at Transylvania, the first medical school west of the Alleghenies. The spirit of optimism, nationalism, and pride that distinguished early-nineteenth-century America affected medicine as other professions. An editorial in the first issue of the *Philadelphia Journal of Medical and Physician Sciences,* in 1820, admitted that American doctors might be less "erudite" than Europeans, but concluded that "in no country is medicine better understood or more successfully practiced than in the United States." [30]

JACKSONIAN DEMOCRACY AND THE MEDICAL PROFESSION

The issue of professional regulation, additionally confused as it was with the growth of proprietary medical schools, was even further complicated by the abandonment in the 1830s and 1840s of licensing regulations. After 1825, attacks on elitism at all levels of American society—and in all professional fields—led to demands for repeal of licensing laws and to the withdrawal of state recognition from medical societies. John Morgan had deplored any "levelling of the medical profession," but open

29. See Sigerist, *American Medicine,* p. 58 and passim.
30. Quoted by Shryock, *Medicine and Society,* p. 38.

competition was the essence of Jacksonian politics. In 1838 the Congress lifted restrictions on unlicensed medical practitioners in the District of Columbia. Massachusetts, Maine, and Connecticut made similar concessions. State after state repealed all medical legislation (Illinois, 1826; Ohio, 1833; Mississippi, 1834; Maryland, 1838; Texas, 1848; Michigan, 1851) or removed penalties for practicing without a license (South Carolina, 1838; New York, 1844) or exempted sectarians from existing laws (botanic practitioners in Alabama, Georgia, and Delaware; medicine vendors in Louisiana and Indiana). By 1845 there were at least eight states which gave their populations no guidance as to medical standards, and in many others, graduates of chartered medical colleges could ignore the remaining licensing provisions.[31] Just as England was preparing to entrench medical licensing by Act of Parliament, the United States seemed to accept the market as the sole criterion of professional skill.

There is evidence, however, that the physicians were not entirely unhappy with the demise of licensing. Many of the existing licensing laws were ineffective and confusing, and in some cases they were being used for those restrictive activities which were solely for the benefit of sections of the profession. The country was largely rural; the medical societies largely centered in the towns. In the latter, professionalism developed with enormous speed.[32] By the 1830s there was not only a mass of largely unenforceable licensing laws; there was also a network of medical societies concerned more with fighting quackery than with raising their own standards. Moreover, there was widespread public hostility to the medical

31. Konold, p. 7; Shryock, *Medical Licensing,* pp. 30–31. For analysis of the repeal movement in specific states, see Kett, *Formation of American Medical Profession.*
32. In Providence, R.I., for example, a medical School (Brown) was opened in 1811 and a charter for a medical society petitioned for by a group of 46 practitioners in 1812. The act thus passed gave the society licensing powers (exercised until 1895, when finally taken over by the state). In 1817, the first disciplinary action was taken—on ethical grounds—against a fellow of the society for advertising and selling a secret remedy. Dr. Usher Parsons, professor of anatomy at Brown University, was censured by the Rhode Island Medical Society in 1832; he had consulted with a physician who had been denied a license by the Northern District of the Rhode Island society because he was a member of the competing Central Medical Society. Such developments were going on all over the country, with greater or lesser enthusiasm, and with variation in the actual patterns of legislation, organization, and enforcement between one state and another. *Rhode Island Medical Society and Its Component Societies: 1812–1962* (Providence, 1962), pp. 15, 19. Virginia was an example of "lesser" enthusiasm. The Medical Society of Virginia was formed in Richmond in 1820, but although successfully incorporated it only survived four years, apparently because of professional apathy. The society was revived in 1841, but there was no real attempt at a statewide organization until 1846. This revived society was disrupted by the Civil War and had its second—and surviving—rebirth in 1870. The Virginian medical profession did not, therefore, attain licensing authority. Blanton, *Nineteenth Century,* pp. 75–81.

profession's overriding concern with fee schedules and other methods of controlling competition. There were charges that those who proposed restrictions did so "ostensibly for the protection of the sick, and the encouragement of medical science, but in truth, for the pecuniary benefit of a few aspiring physicians." [33]

The concurrent proliferation of proprietary schools may at least have encouraged students to go to a medical college and thus raised instead of lowered the average standards. But if restrictive legislation had survived, and been encouraged, the interest of both the profession and the public might have focused much earlier than it did on the standards of such schools. Georgia passed a law to restrict medical practice to graduates in 1821. But such legislation was unlikely to raise standards unless the schools were controlled, either by the profession or by the state, and they were not. As it was, the licensing laws were repealed before the pattern was set. Medical societies meanwhile were jealous of their *own* rights and authority over professional standards and restriction of entry.

With the repeal or weakening of medical legislation in the 1830s and 1840s professional interest in licensure declined. Instead there was a growth of new societies *without* licensing authority, which could separate regular from irregular practitioners without fear of being sued. Representative of this new type of society were the two important societies set up in 1847: the New York Academy of Medicine and the American Medical Association (AMA). But the time was not ripe for immediate reform. The American medical profession was in public disfavor and fraught with strife. College competed with college for students. Nathan Smith Davis, prime mover behind the AMA, complained of their "active rivalry, and a competition unrestrained by any mutual intercourse with each other, or social connection with the profession at large." [34] This lack of "social connection" proved a major stumbling block to those in the medical associations, as the schools continued to provide an alternative block of professional power.

But out of the seeming jungle of conflicting interests, some results, which were to have lasting effect, emerged. The AMA was one of the several attempts to bring together factious groups. A proposed meeting of all colleges, sponsored by the Medical College of Georgia in 1835, had been killed by the indifference of the older and more influential Eastern

33. This comment was inspired by the acquisition of a monopoly of teaching for the New York license by six physicians in New York and Fairfield. John F. Gray, *The Policy of Chartering Colleges of Medicine* (New York, 1833).
34. Nathan S. Davis, *History of the American Medical Association from Its Organization up to January, 1855* (Philadelphia, 1855), p. 19.

schools. Invitations in 1839 by the Medical Society of the State of New York to all colleges *and* societies to get together also received no response. Some physicians agreed that it might well be undesirable to link teaching with licensure, but they were even more concerned that if the state associations tried to force colleges to raise their standards, their students would go elsewhere. Nevertheless pressure was being exerted to set up a national convention. By 1846 there was a generally favorable response to the calling of a meeting of representatives of both societies and colleges throughout the Union. The AMA was formed in Philadelphia the following year. But the inbuilt differences in objectives remained. In the 1850s it was suggested that AMA membership might be used as a means of certifying practitioners, thereby replacing the devalued M.D. degree as a sign of competence. These suggestions came to nothing; and meanwhile the medical colleges began their own reform. The AMA did not acquire internal unity until medical college voting strength in the AMA was abolished in 1874 and did not attain real strength until direct hierarchical authority, from local through county and state to the national level, was established in 1902. Until then, this "national" organization of American medicine had no real power and was largely ineffective.

Indirectly, however, the AMA exerted influence on the foundation of other organizations. Following its organization, local medical societies began to appear or reappear in different parts of the country. The medical profession, even without the sanctions of licensure or the existence of guilds, was slowly being organized and was gaining a lead over its competitors: by 1860 there was only about one sectarian to every ten orthodox physicians.[35] Medical journals also flourished; by the mid-1840s journals had been started not only in the eastern cities but, following the rapid westward migration, also in Cincinnati and Columbus, Ohio; Lexington, Kentucky; Chicago; and New Orleans. As early as 1858, the *Pacific Medical and Surgical Journal* appeared, the first medical journal on the West Coast.[36] The existence of the societies and, perhaps to a greater extent, the development of the journals gave promise of greater

35. Kett, *Formation of American Medical Profession,* p. 185.
36. Medical journalism was the offspring of the numerous medical societies. According to Billings, the first medical journal in America was a translation from *Journal de Medicine Militaire,* published in New York about 1790. The first American journal was the *Medical Repository,* New York, 1797. Journals quickly followed in Philadelphia, Baltimore, and Boston. The first journal west of the Alleghenies, *Western Quarterly Reporter of the Medical Surgical and Natural Sciences,* came out in 1822. By 1876, 31 medical journals had been started in New York City, together with another 9 devoted to specialties and 6 reprints of foreign journals. J. S. Billings, in Clarke et al., pp. 329–37.

professional cohesion—not through medical guilds, as in Britain, but through political and scientific channels.

THE PROFESSION AT THE TIME OF THE CIVIL WAR

The doctor in 1860 could look back to very considerable changes in medicine. There was a decline in professional morale, as compared with the optimism of 1800, at least in the sense of medicine as an elitist calling. But the attitudes were perhaps more realistic as to the future needs for the provision of doctors and the future means of regulation. At least most practitioners now had some kind of formal education. There was a basic standard, low as it was, which most physicians met. There was a network of medical schools, poor as most of them were. There had been a resurgence of medical societies, although they remained weak. It was from this apparently poor but potentially fertile ground that the future structure of American medicine—and ultimately the future of specialization—was to emerge.

Nor had the substance of medicine stood still. The absence of hospital facilities for medical teaching outside one or two cities meant that teaching in all types of schools in the early nineteenth century was almost entirely didactic. Thus at the very time the Parisian school was teaching the importance of correlating clinical symptoms with pathological anatomy, the great majority of medical students in America had no systematic hospital teaching and little or no legal access to cadavers.[37] But Americans continued to visit the European schools. France rather than England had become the dominant foreign influence on American medicine; Bostonians such as James Jackson, Jr., and Oliver Wendell Holmes studied with the eminent physician Louis and others in Paris. America had discovered anesthesia for the world in 1846; it was used extensively during

37. Grave robbing was frequent and fashionable, and reprisals were sometimes severe. One of the most unusual tales of body snatching in this period concerns the Winchester Medical College in Virginia, extant from 1825 to 1829 and again from 1847 to 1861—a proprietary school of apparently high standards whose graduates consistently passed the examinations of the Army and the Navy medical corps. At the time of John Brown's raid, the entire student body from the college mounted the train to Harpers Ferry, prudently dismounting before the train reached the station. Here they stumbled on a body, which, with great presence of mind, they bundled in a box and shipped back to Winchester. The body was prepared and was soon joined by the two exhumed bodies of Shields and Copeland, executed after the battle. Unfortunately for them, the first body was of Owen Brown, John Brown's son. When the Federal army entered Winchester in 1862, Owen Brown's body was recovered and sent north, and the college buildings were burned to the ground. Many other proprietary schools perished during this period, but few so dramatically. Blanton, *Nineteenth Century,* pp. 16–19, 71.

the Civil War, with chloroform the choice of the Confederate army, ether of the Union. Urban practitioners had dropped their apothecary trade between 1790 and 1820 and were replaced by full-time druggists. The drugstore proliferated. Pharmacy was developing as an independent profession; schools were founded in Philadelphia and New York City in the 1820s, and in 1852 the American Pharmaceutical Association was established.

Hospitals were gradually being established for special diseases, especially in the large cities. Boston, for example, had the Massachusetts General Hospital in 1821, the Massachusetts Eye and Ear Infirmary in 1824, the Lying-In Hospital in 1832. Eye and ear hospitals were established between 1821 and 1830 in New York, Boston, and Philadelphia, and by the 1850s cities throughout the settled parts of the country had such hospitals.[38] In 1836 a hospital was established in New York for diseases of the skin, and a dispensary for skin diseases was set up in Boston in 1860. After 1800, moreover, influenced by the humanitarian treatment of Pinel in France, efforts were made to establish hospitals for the mentally ill. By 1844 there were twenty-two public and corporate and three private institutions for the mentally sick. This was also the year of the foundation in Philadelphia of the Association of Medical Superintendents of American Institutions for the Insane (now the American Psychiatric Association). Only the year before, Dorothea Lynde Dix had presented her famous memorial to the state of Massachusetts, in which she condemned the living conditions of the institutionalized mentally sick in almshouses, jails, and asylums throughout the state. Conditions were still poor in the 1860s, but public opinion was gradually moving toward a more enlightened view of mental health.[39]

As strides were made in medicine itself, specialist interests began to develop, although there were virtually no full-time medical specialists in 1860. The American physician was still a general practitioner—physician, surgeon, midwife. Under the impact of the French school, which replaced theoretical views of medicine with bedside experience, the physician now examined his patients instead of merely observing them. He might belong to a medical society and read one or two medical journals; he might live in the Midwest or Far West rather than the East; he might belong to the faculty of a proprietary college. But the typical practitioner in 1860, as in 1780, remained the rural private practitioner.

38. Viets, *Brief History,* p. 152; Shryock, *Medicine and Society,* p. 156.
39. See Samuel Hamilton in J. K. Hall, Henry A. Bunker, Gregory Zilboorg, eds., *One Hundred Years of American Psychiatry* (New York, 1944), pp. 73–76, Albert Deutsch, *The Mentally Ill in America: A History of Their Care and Treatment from Colonial Times* (New York, 1949).

Organizationally the patterns of professionalism were fluid. Voluntary regulation through a professional guild system, as advocated by Morgan, might have achieved a cohesive profession, but had failed. Compulsory regulation through licensing might have had a similar effect. As it was, the political pressures causing the breakdown of licensing laws after 1820 put licensing responsibility into the hands of the medical colleges; coordinating and accrediting the medical schools thus became another possible focus for creating a responsible unified profession.

In the event, neither the societies nor the schools were to have the regulatory function that both were able to retain and develop in Britain. Medical licensure in the United States was to become a function of the state legislature, under the Medical Practice Acts established from the 1870s. The idea of guildlike organizations was to reappear, but in the context of providing a regulatory mechanism for specialization, not as the basis for recognizing general physicians. The medical schools were to be standardized, but only after licensing laws were already in effect; indeed, it was to be largely through such laws that standardization was effected.

The basic issues as to which organizations were most appropriate in regulating standards of practice and as to how far professional or educational monopolies were justified in the interest of maintaining professional quality could not be objectively scrutinized in the uncertain turmoil of the 1860s. Professional development, as with other political processes, moves in a series of conflicts and compromises suited to the crises of particular times, rather than to any long-term and global rationalization. If, against the lowering menace of the Civil War, an American physician had been asked what were medicine's major dilemmas, he might have replied that there was a poor morale in the profession compared with earlier in the century (reflected in the journals and laments over medicine's "declining state"), that standards of education and practice were uneven, that there seemed to be a glut of doctors, and that "something would have to be done" to bridge the gap between the different types of medical colleges and the interests of the societies.

Taking a longer viewpoint, other peculiarly American patterns of practice were already evident. Specialization in medicine, already on the horizon, would be assimilated into a profession which was still struggling to establish standards for one medical practitioner. Outside a few major cities, hospitals were barely developed. When they were to be built in large numbers, from the latter part of the century, the context was again to be in relation to an undifferentiated and still largely decentralized profession, rather than—as in Europe—to one marked by hierarchical rankings and stratifications. As a result, the relation of generalism and specialism within the profession and the relationship between the physicians and the hospitals were to be radically different in the United States from those in Europe. While both professional specialization and the relative importance of hospitals came well after the Civil War, the basic influences of American medical practice by which their structure would be determined were already set; indeed, they were even then the product of a slow, 250-year gestation.

CHAPTER 2

Egalitarianism in Medicine and the Challenge of Specialism, 1860–1900

The years between the Civil War and the end of the nineteenth century were a period again of violent change, social and scientific. The evolution from a rural agricultural economy to a system of industrial capitalism was rapidly stimulated after the Civil War. Mass production techniques used in the war were applied to peacetime industries: railroads linked the East and West coasts; small towns became cities. In 1840, only 11 percent of the population lived in urban areas; in 1860 the proportion was 20 percent; and by 1900 it was up to 40 percent. The population itself rose from 31,443,000 to 75,992,000 in the same period, and immigration was approaching its peak. This rapid urbanization and immigration sparked the development of hospitals—a response as much to humanitarianism as to scientific pressures—and hospitals provided new foci for the institutionalization of medicine.

GROWTH OF PROFESSIONAL SELF-AWARENESS

The professions provided their own pioneers. In rural Kentucky in the 1880s, Dr. Robert Pusey, father of a celebrated dermatologist and AMA president, had the rather dangerous privilege of using a man-propelled tricycle on the railroad tracks.[1] When Dr. James A. Rankin arrived in the small town of Jamestown, North Dakota, in 1885, he found ten regular medical practitioners, serving a population of 3,500. As trails were made passable the doctor on horseback gave way to "a pair of leaping bronchos hitched to a buckboard," and then, in progression, to the typical horse-and-buggy doctor of the turn of the century.[2] The self-reliant general

1. William Allen Pusey, *A Doctor of the 1870s and 1880s* (Springfield, 1932), pp. 39–40.
2. For a good description of medical life in the Dakotas, see F. R. Smyth, "A

practitioner—often poorly trained in the chartered proprietary schools—bore a family resemblance throughout the states and territories. He provided the stereotype physician, and it was for his function that the medical schools continued to train.

But while the rural practitioner epitomized the virtues of independence, it was the practitioners in the growing cities who, in the second half of the nineteenth century, formed the core of an increasingly organized profession. The journals coming out of the cities created local, regional, and in some cases national foci. By 1898 at least 275 periodicals were being published, most of them monthly.[3] They brought the leaders of the profession into contact with the mass of the doctors and were an important vehicle for transmitting new discoveries and techniques.[4] Men such as William and Charles Mayo, who joined their father's practice in Rochester, Minnesota, in the early 1880s, relied, as did their contemporaries, on the medical journals for the latest techniques in operative surgery. The existence of journals, despite their varying quality, constantly reminded practitioners of their allegiance to a profession. Significantly, it was not until the American Medical Association organized its own *Journal,* first published in 1883, that the AMA began to exercise effective authority over the profusion of local and state societies.

The Civil War had impeded the development of a national medical association; Southern representation in the AMA ceased in 1861. In 1866 the AMA president voiced his regret that so few Southerners were present at the annual convention, but in the years that followed there was a gradual return of Southern membership, with the significant exception of black physicians. Virginia for a long while, however, showed no interest in the national association. As in many other parts of the country, there was as yet no effective state society.[5] Dr. Thomas M. Logan of California, who described himself as "under the incubus of seventeen years' isolation in the . . . comparatively sequestered city of Sacramento," had difficulty in finding a sponsor for his attendance at an AMA meeting of 1867 because, he claimed, there were no medical socie-

Great Half Century," *Lancet, 40* (1920), 304; James A. Rankin, "The Pioneers of Jamestown, ND." ibid., p. 315; V. H. Stickney, "The Pioneers of the Dakotas," ibid., p. 304.

3. James G. Burrow, *The American Medical Association: Voice of American Medicine* (Baltimore, 1963), p. 12.

4. "Away out on the borders of civilization, they watch the journals for some new thing, and whether it be carbolic acid or chloral, calabar bean or cundurango, their prescriptions for it are written long before the medicine can reach them through the channels of trade." H. Gibbons, "Annual Address to the California Medical Society," *Trans. med. Soc. Calif.* (1871–72), 16.

5. Blanton, *Nineteenth Century,* pp. 104–05.

ties at all in that state.[6] Indeed, many of the state and territorial societies were either not founded or did not become active organizations until after the Civil War.

Without regional bases on which to found a national profession, the AMA continued to be largely ineffective. Henry Bigelow noted in the 1870s the AMA's immature opinions, its "uncertain temper and impulsive action," its primarily social functions, and its lack of influence over either the local societies or the medical colleges.[7] John Shaw Billings, with more perspicacity, remarked on the usefulness of the national and state societies as vehicles for developing an esprit de corps among those engaged in general practice, through social gatherings and the dissemination of discussion on medical education and medical ethics.[8] These were lowly functions when viewed against the rapid strides in scientific medicine taking place in the German clinics and transmitted to the medical colleges on the Atlantic seaboard; but they were an important step toward professional identification. Indeed, to be a member of a medical society in the 1870s was for many a practitioner the only point of contact with his fellows, and it was the average physician's only hope for acquiring comparative distinction among his peers.

At the same time it was because of the primarily social functions of the (predominantly white) societies that black physicians were forced to develop their own organizations. There were some notable exceptions, such as the integrated National Medical Society of the District of Columbia (1870). By the 1890s, however, the separate development of associations and schools for black physicians was set. Its major symbol was the foundation of the National Medical Association in 1895.

Throughout the latter half of the nineteenth century physicians, particularly those from rural areas, found it necessary to develop a clearer notion of their professional identity. At a time when medicine was often primarily a matter of luck, and the cure as harsh as the illness, many sought a new approach to health problems as well as a more definite role for the general practitioner. One such attempt was made by Andrew Taylor Still, who, in searching for a more positive and unified approach to health, developed the theoretical foundations of osteopathy.[9] But,

6. Thomas M. Logan, "Annual Address to the California State Medical Society," *Trans. med. Soc. Calif.* (1870–71), p. 40.
7. He continued: "The American Medical Association is a body of medical gentlemen, practically volunteer delegates, having primarily in view the agreeable and commendable object of a journey to break the monotony of medical practice and give them an apology for leaving their homes and their patients at a pleasant season of the year." Henry J. Bigelow, *Medical Education in America*, p. 57.
8. John S. Billings, "Literature and Institutions," in Clarke et al., p. 347.
9. In spite of strong opposition from the medical profession, the first school of oste-

shunned by the existing medical schools, osteopathic medicine developed outside and not inside the regular professional institutions of medicine. The resulting osteopathic schools, associations, hospitals, and, eventually, licensing mechanisms and specialty boards grew as an independent, largely Midwestern phenomenon; the integration of osteopathic and non-osteopathic medicine is not finally complete even today. But osteopathy offered a different channel for individuals to enter medical practice. It did not give general practitioners trained in regular medical colleges any handle of distinctiveness over other practitioners.

A proposal was made at the 1871 meeting of the AMA in San Francisco for establishing a national academy of medicine: distinguished men would be elevated to the ranks of the academy, and a board of examiners would govern entrance to it. The following year, however, the subject was dropped.[10] This was a lonely echo of John Morgan's suggestion for a college of physicians. But it was also part of a continuing theme designed to provide an opportunity for professional eminence for the general practitioner—for grading above a standardized level—a desire which was to be transferred much later to demands for a general practitioner certifying board.

In the absence of a national academy, or an equivalent of the British Royal Colleges, the AMA had the functions both of educational upgrading and intraprofessional reform; it fell between two stools. The AMA was neither an autocratic elite based on educational leadership nor a representative of the majority of physicians. Henry Bowditch, AMA president in 1877, noted the complaint that it was "too democratic." [11] But it could be held equally that it was not yet democratic enough. The AMA had started with a convention of interested medical spokesmen joined by individual practitioners. In the conjunction of the schools and societies it sought to bring together two major interest groups, but in practice the AMA could represent the interests of neither. Attempts to stimulate educational reform were thwarted in the association by the influence of teachers in the proprietary colleges who had an obvious interest in maintaining the status quo. A report of 1872 regretted (in words which might be applied a century later) that "it seems much easier to show the defects in our present system than to advise a suitable and practical

---

opathy was started in Kirksville, Mo., in 1892, and by the turn of the century 12 such schools were in existence. See E. R. Booth, *History of Osteopathy and Twentieth-Century Medical Practice* (Cincinnati, Ohio, 1924); George W. Northup, *Osteopathic Medicine: An American Reformation* (Chicago, 1966).

10. Morris Fishbein, *A History of the American Medical Association, 1847 to 1947* (Philadelphia, 1947), pp. 81–83.

11. Ibid., pp. 93–94.

remedy," and after ten years of work the AMA's Committee on Medical Education, disillusioned, concluded that in the interests of harmony it would be better to discontinue the unequal struggle.[12]

The stresses and strains on the AMA in these early years pointed up the lack of effective organization in American medicine. In Britain the question of professional recognition had been accepted as a function of the State; the British practitioner was trained predominantly in the hospital schools. Thus neither licensure nor the details of training devolved wholly onto the shoulders of the medical profession. The American Medical Association had, in contrast, been born out of a professional sense of responsibility for training and licensure, whether through the medical schools—which were by now virtually an extension of the apprenticeship system—or through the medical societies. Educational and professional reform thus rested not only on a changed AMA organizational structure (although this, in itself, was an important factor) but also on the delineation of relative responsibilities among the professional societies, the schools, and the states.

In the societies and in the schools during the last quarter of the nineteenth century and the first years of the twentieth, the focus of reform was on upgrading standards of entry into the profession: to "level" the whole profession above a recognized base rather than to create an educational elite. In the twentieth century this process was to be known as standardization. It satisfied the urges of democracy while enabling the profession to simultaneously advance its standards and drastically reduce its ranks. At the same time, however, a new, and to some threatening, professional aspect was emerging out of the scientific advances of the middle and late nineteenth century. This was the creation of specialist interests and the parallel development of specialist societies. The growth of scientific medicine suggested for American medicine the emergence of a technocratic rather than a social or educational stratification. It became increasingly unlikely that an American national academy of medicine would draw distinctions among general practitioners; it was increasingly possible that interest in special aspects of practice would lead to specialist societies and journals, and eventually to regulatory groups.

SCIENTIFIC MEDICINE AND STANDARDIZATION

The development of scientific medicine, the growth of specialization, the reform of the medical schools, and the organizational pressures influ-

12. George H. Simmons, "What the American Medical Association Stands For," *J. Amer. med. Ass., 21* (1907), 1733.

encing the AMA were interwoven. As medical advances in Europe stimulated reform in the major Eastern medical schools, practitioners were
encouraged to develop special interests, and this, indirectly, led to the
establishment of specialist societies as rivals to the AMA. Observation,
examination, and diagnosis of patients—the heritage of the Paris school
—stimulated the invention and refinement of mechanical aids, around
which specialist interests began to grow. The stethoscope (1819), the
ophthalmoscope (1851), the laryngoscope (1855) charted the gradual
progress of medicine toward an exact science. The foundation was laid
also for the assimilation into medicine of bacteriological techniques after
1870; for the rise of abdominal and gynecological surgery in the 1880s;
and for the rapid and widespread use of radiological diagnosis at the turn
of the twentieth century.[13]

By the 1870s Germany had become the center of scientific development. Its large clinics, its laboratory orientation, the high preliminary
requirements for training, and the opportunity to move from one great
center to another lured American students by the hundreds, reaching a
peak in the 1870s and 1880s and only beginning to decline in the decade
before World War I. Between 1870 and 1914 about 15,000 American
practitioners undertook some serious study in German-speaking universities, first chiefly in Vienna, then in Berlin. It has been estimated that at
least a third and perhaps half of the best-known men and women in
American medicine in that period received some part of their training in
Germany, including virtually the entire faculties of the medical schools at
Harvard, Johns Hopkins, Yale, and Michigan.[14] The effect of this massive movement is still felt in the outlook and hierarchical structure of
American medical schools.

To have belonged to the American Medical Association of Vienna had
some of the same éclat as had membership in the Virginia Club of Edinburgh over a hundred years before. Men such as William H. Welch, John
Shaw Billings, Nicholas Senn, and John B. Murphy circulated with their
compatriots in the crowded specialist clinics, attended private courses,
undertook operations and autopsies, and pored over microscopes in the
laboratories. On their return to the United States they attempted to
introduce into their own centers the techniques and ideas learned in
Europe, Welch initially in New York, where in the late 1870s he and

13. See Rosen, *Specialization of Medicine,* pp. 14–30; Richard H. Shryock, "The
Interplay of Social and Internal Factors in the History of Modern Medicine," *Scientific Monthly* (Apr. 1935), pp. 221–30.
14. Thomas N. Bonner, *American Doctors and German Universities: A Chapter in
International Intellectual Relations, 1870–1914* (Lincoln, Nebraska, 1963), pp. 13–
14, 23, 32, 61, and passim.

T. Mitchell Prudden separately pioneered in the teaching of scientific pathology. Senn returned in 1880 to become professor of surgery at the College of Physicians and Surgeons in Chicago at the age of thirty-six. Four years later the twenty-five-year-old Murphy, filled with the implications of the new bacteriology on the practice of surgery, began his own teaching career in Chicago, at Rush Medical College. Chicago, like the other major American cities, particularly those on the eastern seaboard, was becoming well served with eminent medical teachers. The contrasts between men such as these and the average doctor emphasized a basic distinction between the domestic general practitioner and the new type of clinical scientist, who was increasingly also a specialist.

Teachers in the leading American schools were faced with the dilemma of defining what, in this context, was an appropriate course of medical education. In the 1870s (as now) the question was being raised as to whether it would be sensible to recognize different courses of education for different kinds of physicians. Prof. Henry Bigelow of Harvard was one who claimed that it was not necessary to give the future family doctor detailed laboratory training: "You cannot turn out medical men with the uniform perfection of Ames shovels or Springfield muskets." [15] Such teachers put practical and judgmental qualities above previous scholastic attainment or class attendance in evaluating the raw material of the physician and resisted the growing standardization movement.[16] One student who attended Harvard Medical School in 1869 noted that the professors judged students to be potentially safe country doctors by their characters as much as by their knowledge; and that promising students, the future teachers and research workers, were given special attention and experience.[17]

This early (and in modern terms, radical) track system was possible while the schools were responsible only to themselves, and while entrance and curriculum requirements were minimal. But it was swept away in the process of reform. Under the vigorous direction of President Charles

15. Bigelow, p. 13 and passim.
16. Most medical students of the 1870s had little more than a grade school education. This they followed by an apprenticeship supplemented by a short course at a medical school. Dr. Charles Warren wrote for the U.S. Commissioner of Education in 1870 that, while preliminary education should be improved, there was nothing in the content of medical training "that cannot be mastered in two years by any intelligent youth who has previously studied at a common school." *Report of the Commissioner of Education, 1870* (Washington, D.C. 1870), p. 393. See also Shryock, *Medical Licensing*, p. 47; Viets, *Brief History*, p. 171–73.
17. E. H. Bradford, "Medical Education Fifty Years Ago," *Boston med. surg. J.*, *189* (1923), 748–62.

Eliot, Harvard introduced a graded curriculum in 1871,[18] at the same time lengthening the course of instruction to three years and instituting regular written examinations; from 1877, all students seeking to enter the school had either to possess a college degree or to pass a qualifying examination in a foreign language (Latin, French, or German) and physics. The school that became the Northwestern University Medical School had introduced a graded curriculum in 1858, but the Civil War had interrupted further developments along these lines, and Harvard's reforms in the 1870s marked the beginning of a new movement toward a genuine university medical education—a movement which was to acquire a glittering symbol in the 1890s, in the form of the new Johns Hopkins school, and was to reach its apogee in the Flexner report of 1910. Under President Eliot's prodding, Harvard Medical College ceased to be indistinguishable from the mass of proprietary medical schools. Standards rose. The payment of student fees to individual teachers was abolished, and professors were paid part-time salaries instead.

These changes were followed by several other schools in the 1870s. But such programs were exceptional.[19] Yale did not move from the proprietary fee system until 1880, nor the University of Pennsylvania until 1896. As late as 1898 the University of Vermont's decision to assume full control over its proprietary College of Medicine—against the wishes of its dean—was termed "nothing short of revolutionary." [20] As elsewhere, however, continuous progress in clinical medicine was making it impossible for schools which valued their reputation to exist as purely didactic centers. The growth of specialization was making it impossible for general practitioners to be adequate teachers of the scientific subjects which had replaced the general apprenticeship as the first two years of medical education. Clinical medicine required patients; scientific pathol-

18. A graded curriculum meant specific courses assigned in logical order to each year of study. It was common elsewhere for the same courses to be mounted each year: first, second, and third year students sat side by side on the same bench. See Francis H. Brown, ed. *The Medical Register for New England, 1877* (Cambridge, 1877) pp. 109–18 and passim; Shryock, *Medical Licensing,* pp. 45–46; Viets, *Brief History,* pp. 133, 173.
19. Some schools followed more gingerly than others. Yale's bow to the graded curriculum in the late 1870s was a three-year course, the first year of which reportedly covered "the more elementary branches," the second "the more practical branches," and the third, a review of the courses and additional studies as might be required. Two full courses were required, running concurrently with a compulsory three-year apprenticeship to a private practitioner: this was the normal pattern of New England colleges at the time. F. H. Brown, *Medical Register,* pp. 142–43.
20. William A. R. Chapin, ed., *History, University of Vermont College of Medicine* (Hanover, N.H., 1951), p. 41.

ogy demanded laboratories. The best, and richest, medical schools began
to strengthen their links with hospitals in the 1870s and 1880s[21] and in
1893 the Johns Hopkins Medical School was established around the
specially designed Johns Hopkins Hospital. The influence of the German
clinics could be observed in the encouragement of such large patient
centers, previously almost unavailable in America.

The improvements made by a few of the medical schools in the 1870s
and 1880s widened the gap between the leading schools and the average
proprietary college. The variations were now between schools rather than
among the students in any one school. It was becoming accepted that
schools should admit students according to common educational criteria,
and that all students should pass through the same curriculum. The doctor as family adviser was overtaken by the doctor-scientist. As apprenticeship gradually declined toward the end of the century, mass production techniques began to take over: medical reform meant the production
of a standard, well-educated man.

RESPONSIBILITY FOR REFORM

The educational changes at Harvard and other leading colleges suggested
a *university* basis for education reform, and in 1876 twenty-two of the
better colleges set up their own organization—now the Association of
American Medical Colleges—to upgrade standards from within. The
association began to register colleges in 1879–80; but it lost many of its
members when it decided to require three, instead of the generally accepted two, full courses of lectures for graduation, and its effect was
negligible.[22] Some teachers may have resisted the pressures as being
reform for reform's sake; others may have feared losing students to competing schools. But whatever the reason, the universities did not rise as
the center of professional reform. The AAMC, strengthened in 1890,
gradually became the accepted spokesman of medical school deans; but
it did not rival the AMA in authority, even in the field of education, and
even today educational authority is shared between these and other
bodies.

While the leading medical schools were reforming admission standards
and curricula, the state medical societies were beginning to appreciate
the potential strength of licensing boards. If state examining boards were
established, a degree alone would no longer be regarded as a license, and

21. See e.g. George Blumer, *The Modern Medical School* (Albany, N.Y., 1916).
22. See Dean F. Smiley, "History of the Association of American Medical Colleges: 1876–1956," *J. med. Educ., 32* (1957), 512–25.

teaching would finally be separated from licensure. Graduates of poor schools would not pass the license examinations; thus the boards would provide leverage in reforming the schools. The argument for licensing boards was not—as in the pre-Jacksonian era—to separate regular from irregular practitioners (indeed, some of the new boards were for political reasons to include homeopaths, eclectics, and other sectarians, as well as regular physicians) but to iron out differences within the medical profession by measuring all physicians against an established norm. Under pressure from the expanding medical societies, state legislatures, beginning in the 1870s, established and in some cases reestablished examining boards. In the 1880s the Illinois Board of Health (the licensing agency) began to list American and Canadian medical colleges according to qualitative criteria. By 1893, eighteen states required an examination of applicants for license, and in seventeen others a school diploma conferred the right to practice only where the school had been declared "in good standing." [23]

Control of medical standards through the regulation of entry to the profession was to be the basis of the AMA reforms in the early twentieth century. But standardization went deeper than this. Above a defined minimum all physicians were to be equal; once within the sheltered confines professional democracy was to reign. The contrast with Britain was never more apparent. There the existence of different diplomas at the graduate level had perpetuated the older social distinctions. The profession had been reformed, in that entry was now through a common medical register; but it had not been standardized. Staff appointments to the major voluntary hospitals were retained by those who had gained the higher diplomas of the Royal Colleges. These men, after a common medical education, chose to become *either* physicians *or* surgeons, and as consultants were a different kind of physician from the general practitioner. The leading physicians and surgeons formed a social elite in control of the major hospitals and their related hospital schools. In the United States the response to the pressures of specialism was different from that in Britain, since the specialties in this country had to be assimilated into the prevailing egalitarianism of professional reform.

SPECIALISM AS COMPETITION

Before the Civil War medical specialism posed few professional problems. Nonmedical specialists were cultists or quacks—at least from the point of

---

23. Shryock, *Medical Licensing*, p. 48; *Report of the Commissioner of Education, 1892–93*, pp. 1617–20; William Carr, "The Appointment of State Boards of Medical and Dental Examiners," *J. Amer. med. Ass., 37* (1901), 5–7.

view of the regular practitioner. Some physicians in the cities were interested in special aspects of their practice or held specialist clinics in hospital outpatient departments or dispensaries, and some developed concurrent interests in what would now seem incongruous fields. But such interests were on the whole peripheral to general practice. Not until after 1870, under the stimulus of those returning from specialized clinics in Germany, did the specialties really begin to develop as scientific and social entities.

The social and pecuniary potential of specialization was evident quite early to the city practitioner. Even in the 1850s and 1860s local practitioners were resentful about specialist advertising. One offender was Julius Homberger, a New York ophthalmologist, who made extravagant but apparently credible claims for his treatments and skills. Homberger was censured by the state society in 1865, the society ruling that in his advertisements, cards, and other announcements he might put his name, the title M.D., his office location and residence, but not refer to any special skills. Dr. Homberger thereupon resigned from the AMA and continued to advertise. The AMA met in 1868 and expelled him.[24] But this alone did not solve the more general problem of whether, and how, special interests were to be allowed.

The problems of ethical regulation were thorny. While medical specialism was scientifically inevitable in the long run, and desirable, its appearance was an implicit slight upon the general practitioner. The ill-trained and self-styled medical specialist (the bonesetter, pile doctor, or clap doctor) was often little different from a quack; and the energies of the medical profession had long been devoted to stamping out such phenomena. The well-trained medical specialist, on the other hand, provided a more insidious form of competition because of his superior scientific skills. The rural general practitioner, even in the 1860s, could not hope to keep up with scientific improvements in medicine, however hard he tried; nor did he have the time to make his own scientific observations or to keep proper records. There was already a gap between the potential of medical science and the level of knowledge in the field. Specialism partially bridged this gap, whether it was through interest by general practitioners in such areas as the diseases of women, joints, blood vessels, or eyes, or through the more formal research interests of physicians in the major schools.

The AMA had recognized the division of medicine into certain legitimate areas of interest at its meeting at Louisville in 1859; this was the

24. Konold, pp. 35–36.

beginning of the association's scientific sections.[25] But the original sections were largely for research interests, rather than an endorsement of specialism in private practice. A report of the AMA Committee on Ethics of 1866 held that clinical specialism ran the danger of narrowness, a tendency to magnify unduly the diseases covered by the specialty and thereby to undervalue the treatment of special diseases by general practitioners. It also criticized specialism for a tendency to high fees and for leading to undue measures for gaining certain specialists a popular reputation—criticisms which were to be reiterated through the century and later. Nevertheless, specialization of one kind or another was becoming inevitable. The issue was not therefore to deny that medicine (and thus the patient) would benefit from subdivision, but to decide what reasonable subdivisions were, and what were their interrelationships. The AMA report concluded that most problems could be overcome if the specialist gravitated to specialism only after a period in general practice.

While there was awareness, even at this early stage, of the need to define relationships and boundaries in specialized medicine, there appears to have been no outstanding condemnation of specialism as a whole. After the Homberger case, however, a new AMA committee on specialties was appointed. The conclusions of the new committee, reported in 1869, revealed a consciousness of the competitive dangers of specialism to the ordinary physician, which became a continuous theme in the medical journals in the latter part of the century, and gave an added, restrictive dimension to the concept that all specialists should arise from general practice. One specific question was title, or rank. Was the specialist to be allowed, however legitimately, to enhance his status and income by flaunting his honors and degrees? As might have been expected from a body largely composed of generalists, the report said no; specialists would not be allowed ethically to adopt any title except M.D. On the one hand, this decision could be seen as an attempt to curb the development of freestanding and possibly irresponsible specialties, whose exponents might forget in their enthusiasm that while science could be subdivided, the patient could not. On the other, the recognition of the M.D. as the only sign of the physician protected both the general practitioner who eschewed special interests and the emerging unity of the profession. Specialism, it was alleged, was unfair in implying that general practitioners lacked competence to treat certain classes of disease.

25. Fishbein, p. 1092. The original seven sections were Anatomy and Physiology; Chemistry and Materia Medica; Practical Medicine and Obstetrics; Surgery; Meteorology; Medical Topography and Epidemic Diseases; Medical Jurisprudence and Hygiene.

But at the same time the role of general practice itself became increasingly problematical. If the M.D. degree showed evidence to the public of a willingness to practice in all branches of medicine, it followed, as an AMA judicial court pointed out in 1874, that specialism was simply a self-imposed limitation of the duties implied in the general title of doctor. The general practitioner saw himself as the kindly, responsible, bedside clinician, while the specialist was depicted as a mere technician who lacked basic psychological skills.[26] The generalists were battling in a highly competitive market against the emergence of a technological elite, but the problems had long-term implications. Could the general practitioner survive as the mainstay of practice with specialists providing limited skills?

These questions of personal, professional, and organizational relationships grew more acute as the century progressed. While the AMA was busy considering whether specialists should have the right to issue cards announcing their specialties, scientific specialism was beginning to blossom, and with it the establishment of specialist associations. The American Ophthalmological Society was formed in 1864, the American Otological Society in 1867, the American Neurological Association in 1875, both the American Gynecological Society and the American Dermatological Association in 1876, the American Laryngological Association in 1879, the American Surgical Association in 1880, the American Climatological Association in 1883, the American Pediatric Society in 1888, and others before the end of the century.

The societies were careful to follow the AMA's ethical suggestions. Both the Ophthalmological Society and the Otological Society carefully stated in the 1870s that members were not allowed to attach to their names any title, or to publish any indication that they gave attention to special practice.[27] These were scientific groups, usually limited in number, designed for the discussion of the latest research. Nevertheless the special societies, together with dispensaries and clinics, provided a focus for practitioners who were interested in new developments and techniques and in advancing their own practices; they were a nucleus for emerging specialist identities. Philadelphia, which apart from New York was prob-

26. See ibid., pp. 74–75; Konold, pp. 36–38. The term "family physician" was used in the nineteenth century in relation not to the physician, but to the content of books on medical first aid for the family; e.g. L. M. Day, *Improved American Family Physician, or Sick Man's Guide to Health* (New York, 1833); S. S. Fitch, *Family Physician* (Boston, 1866); *The Doctor at Home; Treating the Diseases of Man and the Horse* (Enosburgh Falls, Vt., 1844). The term, reflecting the wants of the family itself rather than the physician's own definition of his role, might usefully be so redefined today.
27. F. H. Brown, *Medical Register*, pp. 6–7.

ably the most outstanding center of specialist interests, included in addition to its general hospitals a maternity hospital (founded in 1836), a mental hospital (1841), a children's hospital (1855), and an orthopedic hospital (1867). Rapid immigration to that city as elsewhere was reflected in the establishment of the German Hospital (1860) and the Jewish Hospital (1865). There were also ten dispensaries, including specialized dispensaries and clinics for the eye and ear, chest diseases, gynecology, and dermatology. Philadelphia was also the home of four specialist societies: pathology (1857), obstetrics (1868), ophthalmology (1870), and odontography (1863).[28]

In the 1870s large hospitals began to give recognition to the specialties, usually first in the outpatient services and later within the hospital. The Massachusetts General Hospital, which had been divided as early as 1828 into divisions of "medicine" and "surgery," developed in quick succession departments of dermatology (1870), neurology (1872), laryngology (1872), ophthalmology (outpatient physician, 1873), and aural surgery (outpatient physician, 1886). Orthopedics followed in 1900, with urology and pediatrics in 1910. These changes were made reluctantly, in the teeth of opposition from the existing medical staff who were concerned that the special departments would monopolize special classes of patients. The first neurologist appointed to the outpatient department at the MGH was entitled the "electrician"; the first physician for diseases of the throat, the "laryngoscopist." Both titles indicated the status, if not the function, of a limited technician; both were changed in 1873.[29] By then it was clear that specialists could not be so casually treated. The creation of departments—and of the career route from physician to outpatients to full attending privileges—itself gave institutional impetus to specialist practice.[30]

THE SPECIALISTS

Although right up to the end of the century there were relatively few men exclusively in specialist practice, identification as a specialist was

28. Reuben Friedman, *A History of Dermatology in Philadelphia* (Fort Pierce Beach, Fla., 1955), pp. 199–223.
29. Frederic A. Washburn, *The Massachusetts General Hospital: Its Development, 1900–1935* (Boston, 1939), pp. 296–350. On the resistance by the profession to specialization, see George Rosen, "Changing Attitudes of the Medical Profession to Specialization," *Bull. Hist. Med., 12* (1942), 343–54.
30. Although progress was often slow, specialized hospital departments were common by the end of the first decade of the twentieth century. Mount Sinai Hospital in New York, for example, had no division into a medical and a surgical service until 1877 (surgery even there being hardly considered a separate practice, and the

becoming quite common. Louis Duhring, renowned for his work on cutaneous diseases, conducted a flourishing dermatological practice in Philadelphia from 1870 and reportedly became a millionaire. Abraham Jacobi (first special professor of pediatrics at New York Medical College, in 1860, and first president of the American Pediatric Society, in 1888) was recognizably a pediatrician, though he and his contemporary, J. Lewis Smith, both objected to suggestions that they were exclusively occupied with diseases of children.[31] Edward Jackson, founder of the *Journal of Ophthalmology* in 1884, was clearly an ophthalmologist, even though ophthalmology itself was considered a branch of the practice of ear, nose, and throat medicine to the end of the century. Francis Delafield, professor of pathology in the 1880s at the College of Physicians and Surgeons in New York, was a laboratory clinician, as was William H. Welch, who was appointed to the new chair of pathology at Johns Hopkins in 1884 and became the outstanding American influence in the development of his specialty. Indeed, such was the enlargement of pathology in the 1880s and 1890s through the development of bacteriology and the improvement in the microscope and laboratory techniques that by the end of the century pure pathology—laboratory specialism—was becoming a recognized complement to clinical specialism, rather than a young man's job before embarking on practice.

Specialism was not confined to the great Eastern cities. Dr. William H. Watkins of Portland, Oregon, announced his special attention to the diseases of the eye and ear in the 1860s.[32] A speaker addressing the University of Vermont alumni in 1876 spoke of specialism as "the fashionable spasm of the day," [33] and a Kansas journal exclaimed in 1880

attending physicians of all New York hospitals being primarily GPs). But the pressures for special services built up rapidly in the plans for a new hospital building in 1901, and it was envisaged that the following would be included: general medicine, four divisions; general surgery, two divisions; gynecological surgery, two divisions; one ophthalmic and aural department; one neurological department; one dermatological department; a children's department. Each of these services was to have its own chief and staff, and there would also be wards for accident cases, a service for tuberculosis and for convalescent patients, departments of pathology, anesthesiology, radiology, and hydrotherapeutics, as well as a dispensary. Joseph Hirsch and Beka Doherty, *The First Hundred Years of the Mount Sinai Hospital of New York, 1852–1952* (New York, 1952), p. 114.

31. Fielding H. Garrison, *History of Pediatrics* (Philadelphia, 1923), p. 105. See also R. Friedman, *History of Dermatology,* p. 121; G. E. Arrington, *A History of Ophthalmology* (New York, 1959), p. 195; Esmond R. Long, *A History of Pathology* (Baltimore, 1928), pp. 136–37; F. C. Shattuck, "Specialism, the Laboratory, and Practical Medicine," *Boston med. surg. J., 136* (1897), pp. 613–17.

32. O. Larsell, *The Doctor in Oregon: A Medical History* (Portland, 1947), pp. 156, 171.

33. M. H. Henry, *Specialists and Specialties in Medicine* (New York, 1876), pp. 1–11.

that "every cross-road village has its ophthalmologist, aurist or gynecologist, not mentioning the gentlemen who in a minor way make the rectum, urethra, throat, nose, pharynx, etc. their particular field of onslaught." [34] Complaints in the journals took on a modern ring. The patient, it was claimed, was no longer seen in his bed but in the specialist's anteroom; the specialist was often ill qualified, and the general practitioner was being bypassed. Despite considerable professional disapproval, specialist advertising continued. Virginia physicians in the 1870s advertised their prowess as "Specialty—Surgery," "Diseases of Females," "Diseases of the Urinary Organs," "Diseases of the Ear and Eye," and so on.[35] By the mid-1870s there was a recognized class of physicians in the cities whose prime concern was often to make money and advance themselves socially. Shrewd, practical, and often well educated, these men took up specialties because of the easier work and the more constant hours. Such specialism, entered into from self-interest as much as scientific reasons, posed a threat to general practice both in financial terms and in terms of relative social and professional standing.

PROFESSIONAL ROLES AND RELATIONSHIPS

The problems of professional relationships grew during the 1880s and 1890s, largely as a result of the concurrent rise of surgery, of nursing, and of hospitals. By 1900 medicine had become characterized by overlapping professional blocs: state and local medical societies, state licensing boards, medical schools, the AMA, the specialist societies, hospital staffs, hospital practice and private practice, and generalists and specialists. The relationships between these blocs bespoke shifting professional patterns and raised continual questions of definition. What was the function of the general practitioner in relation to the specialist, and how far might their relationships be formalized? How far might hospital outpatient practice expand before local practitioners would charge "hospital abuse"? And would a new guild system emerge?

Meanwhile, at the scientific level, surgical practice was being revolutionized by the acceptance of asepsis and antisepsis. The death rate from abdominal and pelvic surgery was 40 percent in the decade 1880–90; it fell to below 5 percent by 1900. Combined with the earlier acceptance of anesthesia, surgery became both more acceptable to patients and more challenging to practitioners. It became the first large medical specialty,

34. Quoted by Thomas N. Bonner, *The Kansas Doctor: A Century of Pioneering* (Lawrence, Kansas, 1959), p. 68.
35. Blanton, *Nineteenth Century,* p. 157.

and the first in which the delineation between a general practitioner and a specialist became a matter of acute concern. The American system, unlike that in England, had never identified surgeons as a separate caste; moreover, until the 1880s there was no living to be made from surgery alone. The opening of the abdomen changed this, first by providing much more surgery and second by providing a type of surgery which many general practitioners preferred not to attempt.

Drs. William and Charles Mayo began to develop their practice in Rochester, Minnesota, as a surgical practice in the 1890s. By the turn of the century, there were five partners—and the railroad was bringing patients from far and wide. The rapid development of the Mayo Clinic epitomized the expansion in medicine through surgery; by 1912 a total of 15,000 patients was being seen, and this figure more than doubled in the next two years.[36] Albert J. Ochsner of Chicago, Halsted at Johns Hopkins, and their illustrious contemporaries were first and foremost surgeons; and surgery itself was on the threshold of a new period of scientific subdivision, under men such as Harvey Cushing in neurosurgery and Hugh Young in urological surgery. Although surgery in general was still confined to the extremities and the abdominal cavity, its potential was everywhere evident. The journal *Surgery, Gynecology and Obstetrics,* launched by Franklin Martin in 1905, was an instant success.

Surgery was also a monetary temptation to the practitioner in an age when much of medicine as other professions, was distinguished by commercialism. From the early 1890s abdominal and pelvic surgery was practiced, in the words of the AMA *Journal,* by "as restless and ambitious a throng as ever fought for fame upon the battlefield." [37] It became common, particularly after 1900, for surgeons to "kick back" part of their fee to practitioners who referred patients to them. Fee splitting could be rationalized as a sign of the acceptance by the general practitioner of his professional limitations, and of an increasingly functional division of practice between those who did surgery and those who did not. But at the same time it put a fiscal, readily-abused transaction at the core of the generalist-specialist relationship. From California to New York, restrictive business practices proliferated.[38] In some part this trend was un-

36. Helen B. Clapesattle, *The Mayo Brothers* (Boston, 1962), pp. 387, 411, 464.
37. *J. Amer. med. Ass., 17* (1891), 947.
38. After 1880 medical societies began to warn members against criticizing other physicians. Doctors began to feel they had to cover up each other's mistakes in order to preserve the "general respectability of the profession." Medical men in a small Arkansas town in the early 1890s protected themselves financially by notifying each other of individuals who made unremunerative patients. Some physicians accepted secret commissions from druggists and drug firms for prescribing their

doubtedly due to the large number of doctors in relation to the population —the product of the large number of medical schools. The immediacy of competition as a problem for the average physician meant that questions of the number of medical students and schools were being given more attention by the turn of the century than the more fundamental issues of generalist-specialist relationships.

But while general practitioners were attempting to guard their interests in relation to specialists, both were affected by a third source of competition offered by the rapid growth of hospital clinics and outpatient departments. The dispensaries, designed to provide charity care for the poor, an expression of late nineteenth-century humanitarianism, were a rich source of teaching and research materials for interested physicians. There were thus both social and professional interests in their development. But as specialist clinics developed, the cries from other physicians became rancorous; the issue was similar to later professional hostility against private specialist group practice. Doctors who practiced outside the clinics objected to the competition. They were, it was claimed, being deprived of their legitimate fees by the use or "abuse," of the free facilities by middle-class patients.[39] In New Orleans, complaints of such "indiscriminate almsgiving" occupied the medical profession from the 1880s until 1926, when the Charity Hospital, then the fifth largest hospital in the country, finally submitted to the introduction of a means test.[40]

A similar battle over hospital abuse took place in Britain in the late nineteenth century, but the different terms of professional reference produced a different outcome. British hospitals had begun to develop rapidly before the emergence of specialization and were staffed by unpaid physicians and surgeons. These men retained their monopoly of the major hospitals when the inpatient and outpatient departments became specialized. The battle over patients in the outpatient clinics was thus in Britain an expression of the struggle between these hospital-attached specialists and the outside practitioners, who were largely general practitioners.

American hospitals had a much later development. Hospitals were few and far between until the late nineteenth century, when the conjunction of urbanization, a rapidly expanding population, the development of the nursing profession after 1870, and finally the emergence of surgery, had

---

products; others performed unnecessary services for the fees. Fee splitting followed a similar pattern. For example, see Konold, pp. 49, 65; "Medicine as a Profession," *Boston med. surg. J.*, *135* (1896), 637–41; *J. Amer. med. Ass.*, 17 (1891), 991–93.
39. See Michael M. Davis, *Clinics, Hospitals and Health Centers* (New York, 1927), pp. 60–61 and passim.
40. A. E. Fossier, *History of the Orleans Parish Medical Society 1878–1928* (Privately printed, 1930), pp. 105–29.

a phenomenal impact. There were estimated to be only 178 hospitals in
the United States in 1873. By 1909 there were 4,359 hospitals, with a bed
capacity of over 421,000.[41] Unlike British hospitals, which generally had
"closed" (i.e. limited) medical staffs, the many new American hospitals,
established in an age when there were still no formal distinctions between
one type of practitioner and another and often founded by practitioners
themselves, tended to open their facilities to all practitioners; moreover,
they provided the logical opportunity for general practitioners to undertake surgery.

As a result of these early differences, American and British hospital
staffing patterns remain different today. Out of the struggle over outpatients in Britain there emerged in the early twentieth century a recognized system of patient referral from general practitioner to specialist and
back. It became accepted that the specialist was to act as a consultant,
seeing patients only on the generalist's advice: he was not to accept
patients who came directly to his office. Over time, hospital outpatient
clinics became specialist consultation centers. The general practitioner
retained control of the patient, while the specialist had control of the major hospitals; and the two areas of monopoly acted as checks and balances. Fee splitting in such a system was unnecessary. Indeed, the small
cadre of physicians and surgeons on the staffs of British hospitals prevented the unlimited practice of surgery which rapidly characterized
general practice in the United States.

The "hospital abuse" question in this country did not have the same
overtones of professional delineation as in Britain. Hospital outpatient
departments in the United States continued to be general clinics as well
as to offer specialist services; they continued to be a potential reservoir
of competition to the private practitioner. Neither the general practitioner
nor the specialist monopolized either the hospital or the patient. In terms
of who was the patient's primary physician, what was the role of the
specialist, how he should be identified, and whether all physicians should
have hospital privileges, there was a general free-for-all.

A NEED FOR GUILDS?

The unrestricted practice of surgery and the failure of ethical sanctions to
prevent fee splitting or to encourage an open system of specialist consultation emphasized the absence of any regulating guilds in American medicine. The specialist societies remained scientific foci rather than regula-

41. On the development of hospitals, see E. H. L. Corwin, *The American Hospital*
(New York, 1946), p. 8 and passim.

tory agencies into the twentieth century; the organizational development of specialties was still at an early stage. In 1873 Samuel Gross and other AMA members, disappointed by the lack of AMA leadership and frustrated by the endless discussions on ethics, threatened to withdraw and establish a national scientific organization. However, this rebellion was put down when the association created the judicial council to streamline decisions on ethical questions. The AMA's own scientific sections were still developing only slowly, while professionally they were of secondary importance to the specialist associations. It was in this context that in 1879, Gross, then professor at Jefferson Medical College in Philadelphia, proposed a new association for surgeons. From this developed the American Surgical Association, a national society of distinguished practitioners, writers, and teachers. Fellows of the new society had to be graduates of a respectable medical college and have an established reputation; they were thus distinguished both by their special interest in surgery and by their relatively superior educational attainment.[42] The new association tried to provide the leadership which the AMA surgical section had not provided.

Its foundation and the precedent it offered for further segmented specialist groups disturbed the leaders of the American Medical Association, which was still struggling toward professional unity. Dr. N. S. Davis, an AMA founder, made a strong plea for such unity in 1883. Reviewing the development of the AMA as a representative body interested largely in improving standards of medical education, he urged that more physicians associate themselves with state and county organizations and asked that these organizations pay less attention to their purely social function and more to advancing medical science.[43] However, Davis failed to stimulate the AMA to change its focus, and there were controversies throughout the 1880s over the role and power of the AMA in relation to other groups. These included further disillusionment among eminent scientific leaders when the AMA did not assume scientific leadership in planning the International Medical Congress in 1885.

Meanwhile specialist societies continued to appear. The Association of American Physicians was established by a group of laboratory-minded physicians in 1886, with an exclusive membership and primarily scientific objectives. The focus of this association, like the American Surgical Association, was to advance medical knowledge and research rather than to promote the interests of the average member of the profession, and it provided a prestigious forum for debate. But inevitably this, like other

42. Fred B. Lund, "Fifty Years of the American Surgical Association," *Ann. Surg.,* 92 (Oct. 1930), 481–97.
43. Fishbein, pp. 110–11.

new associations, was also a reflection of the inability of the AMA to offer an appropriate umbrella for the development of specialism. The AMA was faced with the dilemma of unifying the general practice of medicine through common entry and educational standards at the very time that specialist interests were demanding a new fragmentation.

Efforts to bring the national specialist societies together into one large organization resulted in the American Congress of Physicians and Surgeons, which first met in 1888. The congress provided another platform for medical leadership outside the AMA and brought out yet more clearly the AMA's primary role as a political body, with only a secondary interest in scientific advance. The specialist societies detracted from the position of the AMA as the spokesman for medicine and weakened interest in its scientific sections. Although Dr. Claudius Martin, in addressing the 1891 meeting of the congress, stressed that there was no competition between it and the AMA, there clearly were clashes.[44] Membership in special societies accelerated, while interest in the AMA declined.

At the turn of the century, then, the AMA was forced to begin reconsidering its role as a scientific as well as medicopolitical organization. Could it encompass the dual role? Would it be possible to prevent the extension of specialist groups into self-regulating guilds? Would the AMA be able to serve the interests of both general practitioners and specialists? The forces of scientific subdivision were competing strongly with concurrent pressures for a homogeneous and standardized profession. The outcome was closely related to the future of the AMA itself as the central authority of the medical profession.

44. Pediatrics was a case in point. The newly constituted pediatric section of the AMA (1879) declined after a strong start under Jacobi and others: the AMA membership was not ready to accept pediatrics as a separate field. The momentum for organized pediatrics thus came from outside. The International Medical Congress, 1887, held a pediatric section which was attended by leaders of the specialty, and it was out of this that the American Pediatric Society was formed in 1888—taking the Association of American Physicians as a model. Jacobi became its first president. Urology was another example. In about 1891 the urologists in the American Congress of Physicians and Surgeons constituted themselves into a section on andrology, the male counterpart of gynecology. The AMA did not agree with this move, and the editor of the *Journal* predicted no future for the specialty as long as the general practitioners felt themselves competent to deal with such cases. H. K. Faber and R. McIntosh, *History of the American Pediatric Society, 1887–1965* (New York, 1966), pp. 7–8; "Andrology as a Specialty," *J. Amer. med. Ass., 17* (1891), 691.

CHAPTER 3

Reform Achieved

The AMA and
Medical Education, 1890–1914

American medicine between 1890 and 1914 moved toward professional maturity. The respective roles of the colleges, the universities, the state licensing agencies, and the professional associations crystallized into the forms we still know today. For the first time the societies, licensing associations, and a leading bloc of colleges had common aims: the upgrading of entrance standards to the profession, the specification of curricula in the medical schools, the suppression of the weakest proprietary institutions, and the reduction in the number of students graduating from medical schools. These aims interlocked. The reform movement was partly educational, partly restrictionist, having as its goal both more highly trained and fewer physicians.

The movement for reform coincided with social forces, such as expansion of the cities and more advanced communications in railroads and in the telegraph, which made a national effort possible. It also coincided with scientific pressures for change in the educational system and with the appearance of new financial resources. Medically speaking, the United States until the end of the nineteenth century was intellectually a European colony, influenced by Britain until about 1820, then by Paris, and after the Civil War by the university clinics in Germany. By the mid-1890s, however, the tide was beginning to turn. American private philanthropy, born of the great fortunes made during and after the Civil War, began to create the endowed foci of medical research without which American medical science could not have been self-sustaining.[1] Specialist

1. Rockefeller funds created the Rockefeller Institute for Medical Research (1902), the General Education Board (1903), and the Rockefeller Foundation (1913). The Carnegie fortune spawned the Carnegie Institution of Washington (1902), the Carnegie Foundation for the Advancement of Teaching (1905) and the Carnegie

societies stimulated the scientific interests of leading practitioners; the laboratory and the bedside began to replace the classroom as the focus of teaching. The era was distinguished by the establishment of the Johns Hopkins University Medical School, the outstanding model for American medical education; by the developing Mayo Clinic, which offered in its group of specialists a new practice form; by the successful restructuring of the American Medical Association as the dominant professional organization of medicine; and by the report of Abraham Flexner on medical schools in 1910, which was to be both the symbol and the basis for educational reform.

JOHNS HOPKINS—MODEL FOR REFORM

In the Johns Hopkins school, established in 1893, were crystallized the problems facing medical education in the last decade of the century: the need to concentrate medical education around patient and laboratory facilities; the growing expense of medical education, which could no longer be met wholly from student fees; the application of German clinical and departmental principles of organization, including the establishment of full-time professorships; and the upgrading of entrance standards—in this case by making medical education a graduate training course. Johns Hopkins achieved in the late nineteenth century the national leadership in university medical education which John Morgan had hoped for in the Philadelphia school before the American Revolution.

By the 1890s universities generally were beginning to introduce graduate studies.[2] Nevertheless the establishment of a graduate program of medical education was revolutionary. Curiously, it appears to have been incorporated almost by accident through a stipulation of Mary Garrett

Corporation of New York (1911). These foundations, though among the largest and most influential, were a few among many. In 1891, the medical schools possessed an estimated $500,000 in endowments. Between 1903 and 1934 nine foundations alone granted medical institutions about $150 million—half of what they gave for all purposes. Medicine became the chief recipient of foundation benevolence. Richard H. Shryock, *American Medical Research: Past and Present* (New York, 1947), pp. 88–101; Richard H. Shryock, *The Unique Influence of the Johns Hopkins University on American Medicine* (Copenhagen, 1953), p. 37.

2. University graduate education had begun at Yale in the 1850s. Harvard made a formal beginning in graduate studies in the 1870s, when Yale was reorganizing its graduate department. These schools were modeled on the philosophical faculty of the German universities. There was little real success in graduate education, however, until Johns Hopkins University began its program. Graduate education in the scientific fields was also developing at Rensselaer Polytechnic Institute, New York, 1824; Harvard, 1847; and the Sheffield Scientific School at Yale, 1859. See Charles F. Thwing, *A History of Higher Education in America* (New York, 1906), pp. 418–19.

and other major donors to the school that no student be accepted who had not achieved an A.B. degree or its equivalent, together with a knowledge of French and German and the fulfilment of certain premedical studies. Apparently, these standards had been in the minds of John Shaw Billings and William Welch as the long-term ideal; as immediate demands, they were received with consternation by the university trustees, and only reluctantly accepted. In fact William Osler is said to have remarked: "Welch, we are lucky to get in as professors, for I am sure that neither you nor I could ever get in as students." [3]

The combination of these high entrance requirements and a four-year curriculum put Johns Hopkins standards well above those of any other school in the United States, Britain, and probably in the world.[4] The school was also distinguished by being built around a major hospital. The Johns Hopkins Hospital, opened in 1889 and with a radically new type of nurse-training school,[5] was planned with specific educational functions in mind; hospital and medical school were part of an interlocking complex. The reputation of the medical staff and the organization of the school on the German departmental pattern completed the scientific lure of Johns Hopkins as a national medical focus. Each hospital unit was under the supervision of a permanent chief who held a corresponding chair in the medical school: medicine under William Osler; surgery under William S. Halsted; gynecology under Howard A. Kelly; pathology under William Welch. This formidable combination drew medical visitors from far and wide.[6]

3. Flexner and Flexner, p. 219 and passim.
4. Harvard and the University of Michigan were themselves moving to a four-year curriculum in 1893. But neither attempted at this point to limit entry to graduates. In 1884, 54 percent of Harvard medical graduates held previous degrees. This proportion actually declined through the 1880s and was only 23 percent in 1893, the year the medical school was established at Johns Hopkins. See Flexner and Flexner, pp. 221, 223; *Report of the Commissioner of Education, 1892–93*, p. 1625; A. Z. Reed, *Training for the Public Profession of the Law* (New York, 1921), pp. 329–30.
5. Nurses were trained in a graded two-year course (instead of the common pattern of one year of training followed by a year of nursing in private families), and graduate nurses, rather than students, were placed in charge of hospital departments. *Commission on Hospital Care*, pp. 474–77.
6. Dr. William Mayo made a special visit from Minnesota to Baltimore in 1894, introducing himself to Dr. Osler as "a young doctor from the West." A group of 200 surgeons from around the country were dazzled by the operating skill of Howard Kelly when the AMA met in Baltimore in 1895. One of the spectators described its impact on the noted Chicago surgeon Nicholas Senn: "Do you know what his expression reminded me of? The surprise that might have been seen on the face of an American Indian at the approach of civilization." Clapesattle, pp. 288–90; Franklin H. Martin, *Fifty Years of Medicine and Surgery: An Autobiographical Sketch* (Chicago, 1934), p. 234.

The organizational innovations adopted at Johns Hopkins reflected the research approach which had previously been applied to the creation of university graduate education in the arts. In Welch's words: "The medical school should be a place where medicine is not only taught but studied." [7] Experimental medicine thus stood at the center of educational reform. The role was established, too, of the university rather than, as in England, the hospital as the legitimate base for teaching a vocation. The idea of the use of the laboratory and the wards as an integral part of medical teaching was disseminated rapidly by the many students, residents, and visitors to Johns Hopkins in its early years. Medical schools one by one began to establish full-time clinical professorships and, more slowly, to replace the old system of part-time teaching by local practitioners.[8] The costs of such reforms were often prohibitive. The average proprietary school could not contemplate raising enough funds to lengthen its curriculum, let alone to provide adequate equipment or to pay its professors competitive salaries. There were therefore financial pressures for proprietary schools to close, merge, or seek university affiliation in the early twentieth century, quite apart from increasingly effective outside pressures to abolish or reform the weaker schools.

PROGRESS TOWARD NATIONAL STANDARDS

Pressures for such change took several forms. First, the power of the press was increasingly appreciated. The Illinois State Board of Health compiled a list of approved medical institutions in 1894 for the AMA *Journal;* in 1896 the *Journal* put out its first report on the medical colleges of the United States, with a statement on each, including fees, study hours, and officers; in 1901 it published its first educational number and presented a compilation of medical practice laws. The following year, reports were printed from the medical examining boards in thirty-two states, showing candidates, their school of practice (e.g. regular, homeopathic), their college, whether they had succeeded or failed the licensing examinations. In 1904 the first state board number of the *Journal* was printed. By this time the published information made possible comparisons of the various schools. It also disclosed which boards tended to pass candidates from schools in their own states at a higher rate than those from elsewhere. The AMA *Journal* had become an instrument of public exposure; and it was largely through such exposure that certain kinds of reform were to be achieved so rapidly.

7. Flexner and Flexner, p. 223.
8. The process was gradual. Many schools were still on the part-time system in 1916. See e.g. George Blumer, *The Modern Medical School* (Albany, 1916).

During the same period, the AMA succeeded in developing a close connection between itself and the state medical associations. A bylaw of 1882 enabled any affiliated society to join the AMA. In 1896 an amendment was introduced to make state societies branches of the AMA, but it was tabled. Finally, in 1901, following the report of a special committee, the present basic structure was established. Membership in the county society carried membership in the state association; the state associations in turn appointed delegates to the national association. George Simmons, who was then both secretary of the AMA and editor of its *Journal,* later defended this plan as being the only one on which the AMA could be organized if it were to represent the profession of the whole country.[9] Backed by the increasingly powerful *Journal,* the new organization had an immediate impact on the reorganization and federation of local medical societies. By 1905 all states except Virginia and Maine had fallen in line with the AMA plan; membership in medical societies rose from 35,-000 in 1901 to over 70,000 in 1908.[10] The medical profession was becoming centralized and unified, and the AMA, with its new organizational machinery and an effective *Journal,* was expanding to become for the first time an effective national force.

State licensing boards meanwhile were sufficiently developed to set up the National Confederation of State Medical Examining and Licensing Boards in 1891. Both the licensing boards and the Association of American Medical Colleges were prescribing higher standards of training for those presenting themselves for licensing. Representatives of sixty-six colleges attended a reorganization meeting of the AAMC in 1890. The following year the AAMC agreed, in conjunction with the Confederation of State Boards, to recommend a three-year medical course; and, following the success of Johns Hopkins, in 1894 the AAMC urged four years of study. Higher entrance standards were also vigorously endorsed. By 1896 the confederation was recommending high school graduation as a minimum requirement for medical education, and this was made AAMC policy in 1900.[11] If such guides had actually been followed, the attempt

9. George H. Simmons, "Some Fragments of the History of the AMA," pt. 2, "The Reorganization," *AMA Bull., 28* (1933), 124.
10. Burrow, pp. 30–31, 41–42. The strong opposition in Virginia centered on the fear that the movement was an AMA plot to control physicians and on the objections by members of local medical societies to paying fees to the state society. Southgate Leigh and Alexander Craig, campaigning for the AMA in 1915, urged the political advantages of combination, including the presentation of a united medical front: "No physician has a right to speak ill of a brother physician and his work." Raising standards of medical education and grouping into societies were thus also aspects of professional chauvinism. *Trans. Forty-ninth Annual Session Med. Soc. Virginia* (Richmond, 1916), pp. 110–16.
11. Dean F. Smiley, "History of the Association of American Medical Colleges,"

to set up a common national standard or at least a minimum standard of medical education, which was the crux of the standardization movement, could have been successful without AMA intervention. Through formal sanctions the licensing system could have provided the national unity sought by the leaders of the profession. But the state examining boards set up before 1900 had widely differing standards and procedures.[12] Some required an examination, some did not; some were thorough, others merely political pawns. The National Confederation of State Medical Examining and Licensing Boards began to force commercial colleges out of existence but did comparatively little to assimilate the standards of its own members: like the AAMC, it was not in its interest to antagonize its own membership; nor, indeed, was there unanimity within either organization about the desirability of requiring all schools to maintain the same level.

Instead, then, of change coming from within the colleges or licensing boards, the catalyst for reform ultimately became the reorganized American Medical Association. AMA spokesmen increasingly linked the raising of medical school standards with the reduction in the number of doctors, a philosophy which was attractive not only to the leading educators, whose search for foundation money for the schools was predicated on educational reform, but also to the struggling practitioner competing for his living in an already crowded profession.[13] For the last quarter of the

J. med. Educ., 32 (1957), 515–18. Lowell T. Coggeshall, *Planning for Medical Progress through Education* (Evanston, 1965) p. 49 (hereafter cited as Coggeshall report).

12. The motivation of the state societies in pressing for licensure, rather than for control of entry by the medical societies, was described by the Michigan State Medical Society in 1902: "The Society will avoid all political entanglements. . . . Far better retain the method of our past two periods and relegate to special boards all police duties in regulating the practice of medicine—said boards representing the several sects patronized by the people. We may do much to secure the best individuals on the boards and compel their obedience to the law. Such independent position will enable us to lead in all movements for the application of science to the common good, and have our leadership recognized." Leartus Connor, quoted in *Medical History of Michigan,* ed. Colonel Bell Burr et al. (Minneapolis, 1930), p. 403.
13. President Charles W. Eliot remarked in 1907 that since Harvard had demanded a degree for admission to the medical school, the university had received additional endowment of more than four million dollars: "Gentlemen, the way to get endowment for medicine is to improve medical education." *AMA Bull., 3* (1907), 263. In 1900, however, less than 10 percent of practicing physicians in the U.S.A. were graduates of genuine medical schools. About 20 percent had never attended medical school lectures. The majority were the products of apprenticeship or of the proprietary schools. Moreover it was feared that the proportion of ill-trained practitioners was increasing. The editor of the AMA *Journal* noted that while there were 90 medical schools in 1880, there were as many as 154 in 1904; and that these would produce twice the number of doctors required to maintain the already

nineteenth century there had been alarm at dwindling medical incomes and bogus medical degrees and diplomas. Educational reform was therefore politically feasible. The interests of Eastern professors and Midwestern general practitioners were, for a crucial period, the same.

One of the first actions of the reorganized AMA was the establishment of a committee to take up with the U.S. Congress the question of national medical licensing. Early in 1902 an editorial (attributed to Dr. William Rodman, the prime mover for national licensing standards and then a member of the AMA Board of Trustees) was published in the AMA *Journal,* pointing to the need to overcome "the present anomalous conditions regarding the regulation of the practice of medicine in the various states" and suggesting a national board to examine physicians for qualifications for any post in the federal government. It was suggested that this board should be appointed by the president, and that the standards should be made sufficiently high to encourage its recognition by the states.[14] But this idea was dropped as constitutionally difficult; licensing power was vested in the states, and the states were unlikely to press for the constitutional amendment necessary to set up a central or national examining agency. Also, the state medical societies, which had recently given up some independence in fusing with the AMA, were unlikely to countenance so soon the loss of their influence on the state examining boards. The National Confederation of State Medical Boards voted down the whole idea. Thus even the nucleus of a national licensing system was suppressed.

The state boards themselves were more interested in a system of reciprocity—that is, acceptance of one another's licenses without examination—which would maintain their independence while working toward common licensing practice. The American Confederation of Reciprocal Examining and Licensing Boards sprang from a meeting of four Midwestern states (Illinois, Indiana, Michigan, Wisconsin) in 1902, quickly

---

"absurdly crowded conditions." President Billings of the AMA in 1903 stressed the interlocking needs of elevating standards and reducing numbers: the obvious corrective action was through forcing the poorer proprietary schools to close. Meanwhile, numbers continued to rise. In 1910 there was one doctor for 568 persons; in large cities there was one for 400 or less, and many small towns of 200 or less had 2 or 3 doctors. *J. Amer. med. Ass., 45* (1904), 1205, quoted by Burrow, p. 33; Flexner report, p. 14. See also "An Overcrowded Profession: The Cause and the Remedy," *J. Amer. med. Ass., 37* (1901); and William Pepper, *Higher Medical Education: The True Interest of the Public and of the Profession* (Philadelphia, 1894), pp. 29–30.

14. Editorial, "National Board of Medical Examiners," *J. Amer. med. Ass., 38* (1902), 108–09. Dr. Rodman said later that the surgeons general of the army, the navy, and the Marine Hospital Service were willing to cooperate in such a board, and even to act as examiners. *AMA Bull., 9* (1914), 326.

broadened its interests to questions other than reciprocity, and became a small pressure group for licensing reform, adding its voice to the other professional reform groups. By 1904, twenty-seven states had some reciprocal licensing arrangements with other states, and this had increased to thirty-six in 1911.[15] Some success in state cooperation was thus achieved. It was strengthened in 1912 when the two confederations of state boards united to form the present Federation of State Medical Boards of the United States. But success was limited by the continued unwillingness of the state boards to achieve anything like a common standard (an unwillingness which continued until the 1960s). States with high standards resented reciprocating with states with poor standards. The state medical societies, which usually sponsored the legislation and frequently controlled the examining boards, resented threats of outside intrusion.[16] The further possibility of setting up uniform state legislation through a model medical practice act was discussed by the AMA from 1908 until 1917 when it too was dropped as unfeasible, although it was again raised abortively in the 1920s.

There was yet another alternative. During the earlier discussions of legal control or coordination of state licensing, a *voluntary* national examining board was suggested. Candidates would sit for an examination which, it was hoped, would be recognized by the states as qualifying for their license. This idea, vigorously sponsored by Dr. William Rodman and subsidized by the Carnegie Foundation for the Advancement of Teaching, resulted in the formation of the National Board for Medical Examiners in 1915.[17] The Federation of State Boards, which only the

15. N. P. Colwell, "Progress and Needs in Medical Education," *AMA Bull., 6* (1911), 78.

16. See e.g. James E. Egan, "Facts and Fallacies Concerning Interstate Reciprocity in Medical Licenses," paper read by invitation before the Illinois State Medical Society at Springfield, 17 May 1906; William C. Tait, "Medical Legislation in California," *Calif. Med., 1* (1903), 72–76. The potential of reciprocal arrangements between states as the basis for a national licensing system was meanwhile demonstrated in Canada, where there were similar constitutional difficulties over establishing federal jurisdiction: the provinces had licensing powers under the British North America Act of 1867, which serves as the Canadian Constitution. But in Canada, due almost entirely to the persistent efforts of Dr. T. G. Roddick of Montreal who, among his other activities, fought for and obtained a seat in Parliament in 1896 to advance his cause, a medical act was passed in 1912, creating a national medical council for Canada and a national medical register, with a formal reciprocal relationship with licensure in the Canadian provinces. This succeeded through the general agreement of the provinces, obtained after the many years of advocacy by Dr. Roddick and by the Canadian Medical Association, to amend the provincial constitutions so that those holding Medical Council registration would have automatic licensure within the provinces. See R. W. Powell, "Registration under the Canada Medical Act," *AMA Bull., 9* (1914), 321–25.

17. Dr. John M. Dodson, dean of Rush Medical College, argued persuasively in

year before had reopened the question of an examination under federal authority, endorsed the National Board, together with other leading medical organizations. While many of the state boards were suspicious of its purpose and some were antagonistic, continuous assurances that the new organization was only a qualifying body, would never have licensing power, and would not reduce the state boards' incomes (since they could still charge for reciprocity) broke down much of the resistance; careful selection of the board members also helped. Eight states accepted the National Board examinations in 1915. The number increased to twenty by 1921, and to forty-one by 1932.[18] During the 1930s, however, other restrictive measures—notably the inclusion by certain states of additional basic science examinations and the practice of charging large fees for licenses by reciprocity—were to be incorporated into the state licensing requirements. Total reciprocity with the National Board—Rodman's dream—was not to be achieved, and there is still no national licensing scheme.

THE COUNCIL ON MEDICAL EDUCATION

The earlier failure of the licensing agencies to provide an integrated national leadership strengthened the role of the AMA as a national agency working through the individual states. Its vehicle, derived from an educational committee appointed by the AMA in 1902, was a new, permanent, and largely self-sustaining council, the AMA Council on Medical Educa-

1906 for a voluntary national board which would be dependent for its success on proving its excellence. There was a further AMA editorial in 1914, but no real focus of reform until Dr. William Rodman's presidential address to the AMA in June 1915. Dr. Rodman announced a fait accompli: the National Board had been founded the previous month. The first board consisted of 15 members; of these, 6 were from federal government service (the surgeon general and a junior associate of the navy, the army, and the U.S. Public Health Service). The Federation of State Medical Boards had one representative, as did the AAMC and the American College of Surgeons. The board also included Dr. Louis B. Wilson of the Mayo Foundation, Drs. Rodman and Victor Vaughan from the AMA, and 3 members at large. Dr. Wilson later commended Dr. Rodman's careful selection, which included 2 deans of medical schools, 2 heads of university graduate medical schools, 2 internists who had been physiologists, and 2 surgeons. There was however some criticism that there was "too much government in it." Louis B. Wilson, "Work of the National Board during its First Quarter Century," *Proc. ann. Cong. med. Educ.* (1940), pp. 24–27; William L. Rodman, "Symposium: The National Board of Medical Examiners," *AMA Bull., 11* (1916), 137.
18. Everett S. Elwood (exec. secy. National Board), "State Board and National Board Relations," *Proc. ann. Con. med. Educ.* (1932), pp. 92–95; Womack, "The Evolution of the National Board," p. 820. For current requirements of the state boards see "State Board Number," *J. Amer. med. Ass., 200* (1967), 1055–72.

tion. The council was set up in 1904 with three functions: to make an annual report on medical education to the AMA House of Delegates; to make suggestions for improvement; and to act as the AMA's agent in its efforts to raise standards. In its design as a central regulating body for medical education, the council filled a function which under other conditions might have been regarded as the role of national government. In so doing, it immeasurably strengthened the AMA. While its effect was to restrict the supply of physicians (and thus to advance the interest of the average practitioner), the council's membership of five was impeccably educational. Under the chairmanship of Prof. Arthur Dean Bevan of Rush Medical College, the AMA's Council on Medical Education and not the AAMC became the main spokesman for the universities.[19]

With the resources of the AMA and its *Journal* behind it, and with a growing tide of public opinion in favor of medical reform, this formidable group could scarcely fail to have an impact. The council found itself with the power to present suggestions as if they were legally required. AMA presidents and trustees came and went, while the council continued to drive for reform.[20] Bevan remained chairman from 1904 to 1928; and the first secretary of the council, Nathan P. Colwell, remained in office until 1931. The AMA had created what was in effect a quasi-public agency—yet one which at the same time was ultimately dependent on the support of the AMA rank and file. While the aims of education and of the social and economic interests of the profession coincided, as they did before World War I, this structure had everything to commend it. But the council carried the long-term disadvantage of prescribing standards, an autocratic function which in other countries was the function of government or of professional guilds, while at the same time having to submit to democratic control.

The Council on Medical Education held its first conference in 1905. Bevan noted five "especially rotten spots": Illinois, Missouri, Maryland, Kentucky, and Tennessee.[21] Not more than six of the fifty-four medical

19. The four other eminent members were Prof. W. T. Councilman of Harvard University, Prof. Charles Frazier of the University of Pennsylvania, Dean Victor C. Vaughan of the University of Michigan, and Prof. J. A. Witherspoon of Vanderbilt University. Herman G. Weiskotten and Victor Johnson, *A History of the Council on Medical Education and Hospitals of the American Medical Association, 1904–1959* (Chicago, 1959), pp. 4–5.
20. Three of the first five members of the council themselves became AMA presidents: Witherspoon (1913–14), Vaughan (1914–15), Bevan (1918–19). Thus the educational and political structures were unified. On the authority of the council, see Arthur Dean Bevan, "Cooperation in Medical Education and Service," *J. Amer. med. Ass., 90* (1928), 1173–77.
21. "First Annual Conference on Medical Education," *J. Amer. med. Ass., 44* (1905), 1470.

schools in these states were considered acceptable. As a first move, the council that year adopted its own "ideal standard" for schools: preliminary education of university entrance level; a five-year medical course (one year of physics, chemistry, and biology, two years of laboratory sciences, two years in the clinical branches); and a sixth year as an intern. These standards were much higher than those required for membership in the Association of American Medical Colleges. At the same time the council realistically also set minimum standards: four years of high school for admission; a four-year medical course; and satisfactory performance in a state licensing examination (this being known through the lists of state board results by schools already being published in the *Journal*). Thus the existing movements of publicity and regulation were combined. Schools were divided into four classes on the basis of percentage failures in the home state licensing exams. The notion of ranking schools, which had already been initiated by the Illinois Board of Health, was continued on a national basis.

It was apparent that an extensive survey needed to be made of the schools. Inspections were begun by representatives of the Council on Medical Education in 1906, in most instances by both the secretary (Dr. Colwell) and a council member, and usually in company with representatives of the state medical examining boards. The visits alone in some instances had dramatic impact. In Louisville, Kentucky, Dr. Bevan and Dr. Colwell discussed the possibility of combining the seven medical colleges into one strong school, which might then use the Louisville Hospital. The seven schools, unwilling to be inspected at all, succumbed to Dr. Bevan's relentless drive; they followed just this course in the next few years. These and other schools had a pecuniary incentive to join forces, but the unfavorable publicity of the council ratings and a vulnerability to ridicule undoubtedly hastened the process.

Dr. Bevan observed that the council was "exceedingly lenient" in marking the poorer schools. Of the 160 schools inspected in 1906–07, 82 were placed in the council's class A (acceptable), 46 in class B (doubtful), 32 in class C (unacceptable).[22] The names of the schools were not published. Instead, each school was told of its rating, and the report was given to each state licensing agency. The state medical societies, now increasingly AMA constituents, were also encouraged to stimulate educa-

22. Council on Medical Education, *Third Annual Conference, April 29, 1907,* pp. 9–11. Weiskotten and Johnson, *History,* p. 9. In one instance, in an ingenious way of getting around the new AMA surveys, "a glib graduate of a cheap school has toured the country taking examinations with great success in many states and imparting to his alma mater a cosmopolitan character in the statistical summary." Henry B. Ward, "Address of President," *Proc. Ass. Amer. med. Coll.* (1908), p. 32.

tional reform: Dr. Bevan asked them to see that "the right sort of men" were appointed to the licensing boards. Thus the licensing boards became, in effect, if not formally, the council's agents. These activities stimulated the states to effect some reform, if only (as Dr. Colwell subtly suggested to them) to avoid being dumping grounds for poor-quality physicians.[23]

The process of educational reform strengthened the internal structure of the AMA and created the common national attitude which was necessary for professional unification. The identity of interest of the professional and educational movements was thereby emphasized. Compilation by the AMA of the first card index and medical directory of physicians in 1905 further strengthened professional cohesion. These activities also underlined the increasing *public* functions of the AMA, itself a *professional* association.

THE FLEXNER REPORT: TRIUMPH OF STANDARDIZATION

The reform movement was met, not unnaturally, with considerable resentment by the mass of medical colleges. Here, however, another trump card was produced in the increasing power of the large educational foundations. The Carnegie Foundation for the Advancement of Teaching, organized in 1906, in addition to undertaking the major task of setting up pension plans for professors in approved colleges, established a division for inquiring into the problems of higher education. This division was committed to investigating the profession of medicine, together with the professions of law and theology. From the records, it is not clear whether the foundation or the AMA Council on Medical Education took the first step in joining forces for medical reform; at a meeting of the council with Henry Pritchett and Abraham Flexner of Carnegie in December 1908 it was, however, agreed to pool their efforts. The foundation would, it was envisaged, be "guided very largely by the Council's investigation," [24] although in the subsequent report the council was not singled out for any more specific mention than were various other organizations. Dr. Colwell, the council's secretary, who had already made numerous investigations of medical colleges, revisited every school with Abraham

23. In 1900 only 6 boards had any kind of requirement for **preliminary** education— and of these, 5 required education below the high school level. In 1914, 42 states had some requirement, of which all but 2 required at least four years of high school. The big acceleration of standards was, however, to await the postwar period. Colwell, in *Report of Commissioner of Education, 1914,* pp. 203–04; ibid., *1916–1918,* p. 14.

24. Minutes of the Council on Medical Education, quoted by Weiskotten and Johnson, *History,* p. 10.

Flexner. The deans, contemplating the enormous monetary potential vested in Flexner as a foundation representative, opened up on their problems of staff, budgets, equipment, and curriculum. The result of the painstaking investigation was an extraordinarily frank document, laying bare the skeletons and drawing the issues as Flexner and the council saw them.

The Flexner report was published in 1910.[25] It provided for the first time a detailed exposure of the medical schools by name, and in so doing it brought to public notice the appalling conditions of many of the schools. Kentucky was delineated as "one of the largest producers of low-grade doctors in the entire Union"; Chicago "the plague spot of the country." The most devastating invective was reserved for the small proprietary schools: schools such as Bennett Medical College, a "stock company practically owned by the dean of the school"; and Jenner Medical College, an "out-and-out commercial enterprise." The National Medical University, also in Chicago, was distinguished by giving a free trip to Vienna to any student who paid fees regularly, in cash, for three years. Although the school occupied a badly lighted building, "containing nothing that can be dignified by the name of equipment," it claimed its top floor, where there were "two lonely patients," as a hospital. Terms such as "very weak," "wholly inadequate," "miserable," "dirty," and "utterly wretched" appear on almost every page of the Flexner report. Only Harvard, Johns Hopkins, and Western Reserve received clean bills of health. Some universities with mediocre medical schools were exhorted to do better. At Yale, where there were reasonable facilities, with the hospital "intelligently employed," instructors were overworked, postmortems were scarce, and the obstetrical-gynecological wards were not used for teaching. The report demanded that a more liberal policy be pursued, the laboratories be better manned, and the clinical facilities extended. To this end the need for large permanent endowment was stressed.[26]

The report capitalized on the groundwork of publicity carefully laid by the Council on Medical Education; and in turn it provided a stimulus to, and vindication of, the council's central role. Taking Johns Hopkins as the educational model for medical education, Flexner urged the provision of full-time staff, laboratory, and hospital facilities so that teaching and research could be combined in all schools. Medical education was strongly endorsed as a *university* function, thus denying any role for proprietary schools. The need for raised standards of admission and of teaching was

25. *Medical Education in the United States and Canada,* Carnegie Foundation for the Advancement of Teaching, Bulletin Number Four (New York, 1910).
26. Ibid., pp. 17, 199–200, 210–13, 216.

also emphasized. The Council on Medical Education could scarcely fault these conclusions. Even the deans cannot have thought the report would go so far, however, as to recommend no more than one (university-affiliated) medical school per city, the selection of schools for survival according to population criteria, and the drastic reduction in the number of schools from 155 to 31, each giving a four-year course and each with no more than seventy graduating students. In the immediate shock, Flexner's life was reportedly threatened, libel suits were mentioned, and in one case an action was brought claiming $150,000.[27]

The medicine was strong, but it was effective. Twenty colleges were said to have closed in order that their conditions would not be described in the Flexner report. Between 1904 and 1915, ninety-two schools merged or closed their doors in the face of higher state board requirements, financial difficulties, or the adverse publicity of the Flexner report.[28] By 1915, the number of schools had been reduced to ninety-five, and there were only eighty-five in 1920. In 1905 only five schools had required any college preparation for admission. Ten years later eighty-five schools prescribed a minimum of one or two years' college preparation; by 1932, every recognized medical school and most of the state licensing boards required at least two years' college work, many required three, and several a college degree. Medical education was becoming for the first time a truly graduate educational field. State licensing requirements rose with the higher entrance standards of the schools; by 1925, forty-nine boards required candidates for their examinations to be graduates of a medical college, and forty-six states refused to recognize low-grade medical schools as a preparation for the license.[29] Since the only national rating of colleges continued to be that of the AMA Council on Medical Education, the profession by then held effective monopoly control of educational regulation.

Much of the achievement of reform, however, was less the result of the stick of sanction than of the carrot of foundation subsidy implicit in the Flexner visits. Foundation money enabled the better schools to make the suggested improvements—and left the worse schools out in the cold.

27. Ibid., pp. 144, 151–54. For Abraham Flexner's own account of his experiences see his autobiography, I Remember (New York, 1940).
28. Fifty-two schools closed by merger; 40 became extinct. The former were largely the better schools, the latter the worse (i.e. those in the Council on Medical Education's "C" category). In 1904, 30 cities had between 2 and 15 medical schools; in 1915 there were 17 cities with 2 or more schools (including Chicago with 8, New York with 7, and Philadelphia with 6). And the process of merging was continuing. Report of Commissioner of Education, 1915, p. 197.
29. Commission on Medical Education, Final Report of the Commission on Medical Education (New York, 1932), table 88 (hereafter cited as Final Report).

Among other donations, Johns Hopkins Medical School between 1911 and 1936 received an estimated $10 million from the General Education Board (a Rockefeller foundation) and another $2 million from the Carnegie Corporation. The total foundation commitment to medical education up to 1938 has been estimated at $154 million; most of this went to the leading private schools.[30] Foundations were thus the most vital outside force in effecting changes in medical education after 1910, and for a long time they took the place of government support. The foundations injected money into the schools, fostered relationships between medical schools and hospitals, and stipulated the establishment of salaried professorships. Foundation support began to fall off during the Depression, but the modern pattern of large well-equipped medical centers was by then already set. There were closer relationships between medical schools and hospitals—partly through massive hospital construction—another result of foundation benevolence.[31] At the same time, medical education was put firmly, at least in name, under the wing of universities.

Even had there not been the concurrent sanctions and pressures of the state boards and the AMA, the proprietary schools could not have competed with foundation wealth and might well have withered away. But there were other stimuli for reform; medical schools were not the only professional schools coming under public scrutiny. The U.S. Bureau of Education joined the foundations in the early years of the century in a vigorous campaign to upgrade professional training standards and to correct the effect of a very rapid increase in the number of all types of professional schools from the 1870s. Between 1913 and 1914 alone there was a loss of three schools of theology, two law schools, and three pharmacy schools, as well as eight medical schools. Changes in medicine were, however, the most dramatic—not only because of fundamental scientific changes in medicine itself, demanding both social and professional readjustment and expensive institutions, but also because the educational background of medical students had been lower than that in theology or law.[32]

30. Hollis, Ernest V. *Philanthropic Foundations and Higher Education* (New York, 1938), pp. 211–17 and passim.
31. In 1906, 94 of the 162 medical schools had no access to hospitals. In 1926, 316 hospitals were affiliated with the 79 medical schools then existing. Of these hospitals, 50 were owned and controlled by the schools, 37 controlled but not owned by the schools, and 40 provided generous privileges. *Report of Commissioner of Education, 1914,* pp. 201–02; ibid., *1924–26,* p. 48.
32. In 1913–14, 37 percent of theology students had a university degree, as did 20 percent of law students. Medicine, despite rapid upgrading, could only claim 15 percent. *Report of Commissioner of Education, 1914,* vol. 1, pp. 6–7; vol. 2, pp. 315–16.

The success of the standardization movement in medical education was assured. Arguments against having one kind and level of doctor were swept away in the recognition of the need to establish a basic level of professional skill. Yet there were serious arguments against manipulating public institutions—the licensing boards, set up as agents of each state— for predominantly professional ends. Alexander Craig (who was to be secretary of the AMA from 1911 to 1922) was one who questioned whether this was a proper purpose of licensure: "It seems to me that the object should be to determine the minimum of qualifications necessary for the protection of the public." [33] Others saw a dangerously aristocratic trait in the use of the license not only to suppress the quack but also to remove variety within the profession. Such was the criticism that in 1914 the secretary of the Council on Medical Education felt moved to defend the licensing laws, which so clearly benefited the general practitioner:

> The medical profession approves the system which requires the same general professional education of all its members. The specialist upon the eye and the specialist upon the throat, the physician and the surgeon, must each undergo the same training and must pass the same State examination. One may select any specialty he chooses and may adopt any method of treatment which his educated judgment dictates. He may use large dose or small, massage or electricity. What the State requires for one body of practitioners it should not abate in favor of another.[34]

This egocentric view of democracy—egalitarianism within the profession, but an entry barrier against those outside—was to be transformed into a badge of belief. Those who complained that pressure for rigorous medical laws, set up according to the standards of the leaders of a profession, "would be the equivalent to establishing a state medicine, which is and ought to be as obnoxious to the body politic as the establishment of a state religion," [35] were quickly forgotten. The medical profession gained through the more important reforms; and so undoubtedly did the middle-class public.

Today's reader of the Flexner report might reach very different con-

---

33. Quoted in "Fourth Annual Conference of the Conference on Medical Education," *AMA Bull.*, 3 (1908), 294.
34. N. P. Colwell, "Medical Education 1913–14," *Report of Commissioner of Education, 1914*, p. 207.
35. Dr. J. W. Pettit of Illinois, quoted in *Second Annual Conference of the Council on Medical Education*, 12 May 1906, p. 67.

clusions from those grasped eagerly by the scientist deans of the university schools of the time. Flexner spoke of medicine as a public service, but the overriding message of the report proved to be the need to develop scientific excellence in the schools. The two goals were not incompatible, but they did not always coincide. One serious and long-term result of standardization was the closure of schools for black physicians. There were eight such schools at the beginning of the century, most founded after 1880. In the wake of the reform movement, four closed before 1914; a fifth (the large Leonard Medical School in Raleigh, North Carolina) shut its doors in 1915; a sixth (the Medical Department of the University of West Tennessee) finally capitulated in 1923. In their short life, these six schools graduated a thousand physicians, nearly half of whom passed their state board examinations. The demise of these schools, and the marked and continuing discrimination against black health professionals in white medical institutions, left Howard Medical School, Washington, D.C., and Meharry Medical College, Nashville, Tennessee, as virtually the sole source of black physicians; as late as 1947, there were only 93 black students in white medical colleges compared with 495 at Howard and Meharry, and even today the balance is not yet redressed. The number of black physicians tripled between 1890 and 1910, from 909 to 3,409; thereafter the flow was stemmed.[36] Howard and Meharry were saved from extinction largely through foundation support.

In other respects, too, the standardization movement had a stultefying social effect. The poor boy began to find it more difficult to enter medicine as costs rose, the curriculum lengthened, and the night schools disappeared.[37] There was concern that rigid entrance requirements would exclude potentially gifted students with unusual educational careers.[38] Another argument centered around the desirability of encouraging a system of medical education that would produce physicians for different purposes, including generalists and specialists and physicians for both

36. See Herbert M. Morais, *The History of the Negro in Medicine* (New York, 1967), pp. 60, 89–90, and passim.
37. Whether in fact poor boys did constitute a smaller proportion of the student body after Flexner was debated at the time. Claims of the decline came largely from the poorer schools, which had an interest in establishing sympathy. Henry Pritchett of the Carnegie Foundation dismissed claims by the Temple University night school of medicine that it benefited the poor boy by saying it was motivated purely by a desire to run a profit-making medical school. Henry S. Pritchett, "The Obligations of the University to Medical Education," *AMA Bull.*, 5 (1910), 219–92.
38. A. Lawrence Lowell, "The Danger to the Maintenance of High Standards from Excessive Formalism," *AMA Bull.*, 9 (1914), 288–93.

urban and rural areas.[39] But such arguments fell on deaf ears and are only now being revived. In the wake of the Flexner report medicine became a staunchly middle-class occupation, centered on the towns and cities.

If in the process the poor boy were denied access to medicine as a profession, if the standards were made so rigid that the gifted were sometimes excluded, if in the long run it might have been advantageous to the health care of the American people to continue to train a vast spectrum of doctors ranging from medical scientists to rural practitioners, these were small considerations at the time. Success was to be measured in the rising status of the doctor, in the excellence of the leading schools, and in the unification through the AMA of the professional institutions of medicine. [40] In these areas the standardization movement was a triumph indeed. The fundamental questions remained whether the public would always benefit from delegating to the profession vital decisions on profes-

39. E.g. Henry B. Ward of Lincoln, Nebr., AAMC president in 1908, considered that there ought to be different classes of schools, for if all men were trained at the level of the best eastern schools, "we should lack for those content to occupy the smaller fields in professional work." AAMC, *Proceedings of the Eighteenth Annual Meeting* (1908), p. 25.

40. Nevertheless, not all medical education was under the auspices of the medical schools. By the turn of the century there were 12 osteopathic schools in operation. With the formation of the American Osteopathic Association in 1897 an effort was made to close the most flagrantly unethical of these schools and to raise the educational standards of the more academically oriented institutions. These first attempts at self-regulation were initially unsuccessful, but in 1902 the AOA issued a memorandum to all osteopathic schools recommending that the minimum course of instruction be three years, with a fourth year, including surgery, to be made obligatory as soon as possible. Any college seeking recognition by the AOA was expected to meet this minimum. As a result, by 1910, 4 colleges had been forced to discontinue teaching operations. The remaining osteopathic colleges joined the mass of regular medical colleges in being roundly condemned in the Flexner report. The schools were found to "fairly reek with commercialism," making exaggerated claims as to both the healing and the earning power of osteopaths. There were no valid criteria for admission, overcrowded classes, insufficient numbers of rooms, poor facilities, no full-time faculty, and totally inadequate clinical opportunities. The report found that the osteopathic schools did not begin to approach even a moderately good medical school in quality and that the instruction furnished was "inexpensive and worthless." Flexner report, pp. 163–66. Like the AMA, the AOA made educational reform one of its primary objectives. After 1910 the schools of osteopathy, while decreasing in number, began to improve the quality of their educational program. Simultaneously there occurred a change in their professional philosophy—no longer were the schools satisfied with graduating practitioners of a separatist profession. Rather, they began an attempt to contribute to the general development of a valid concept of medicine. For a review of this process, see Arnold I. Kisch and Arthur J. Viseltear, *Doctors of Medicine and Doctors of Osteopathy in California: Two Medical Professions Face the Problem of Providing Medical Care*, U.S. Dept. of Health, Education, and Welfare, Public Health Service, Division of Medical Care Administration, 1967.

sional standards and what the primary purposes of such standards should be.

THE MEDICAL PROFESSION IN 1914: NEW PROBLEMS AND NEW ROLES

By World War I there was a standardized educational system geared to produce a highly trained medical journeyman and a standardized professional structure (the AMA) geared to exert influence over the colleges and licensing bodies as well as over the practice of medicine. The AMA's Council on Medical Education had developed its own standards which were regularly publicized (these included a student register to reveal the standards actually enforced by schools). It had the enormous prestige of the *Journal,* available by 1916 to some 75 percent of the medical profession; it had the backing of AMA membership, which increased from 8,400 in 1900 to 70,000 in 1910, and to over 83,000 in 1920;[41] it had regular meetings with the state licensing boards; and it cooperated closely with the Association of American Medical Colleges. Licensing boards had been brought together in some degree of reciprocity; from 1915 the voluntary National Board provided an obvious base for national standardization of licensing examinations. There was in short one unified medical profession, poised to become a politically active force. The whole process of unification, which had begun as soon as the first practitioners entered the American colonies, was complete.

On the other hand, there were new pressures and new problems. The educational movement had dominated the years between 1890 and 1914, but it had not obscured equally compelling issues. The increasing research orientation of the medical schools and hospitals accelerated the scientific forces which precipitated change. As a result, the movement toward greater medical specialization continued inexorably. Problems of guiding patients to the appropriate specialist, of which surgical fee splitting was the symbol, became acute. A new system of graduate medical education was developing even as the undergraduate schools were being reformed. The proper role of the general practitioner was in doubt, even as the Flexner report was creating a general education in the medical schools. The medical reform movement, curbing numerical competition, served to protect—perhaps fossilize—the independent general practitioner, even as technological changes were suggesting his obsolescence. As standardization at the basic level was achieved, fragmentation was becoming evident in the delivery of health service.

41. In 1920, there were about 145,000 physicians in the United States, so the AMA still had some way to go. Burrow, p. 49.

A new cycle of professional development was thus beginning. Out of it would flow new organizations, conditioned in turn by the practices and attitudes built up during the medical profession's long progress toward unity. Standardization of the profession was accomplished through the invocation of rigid state controls. It was not entirely strange, however, that the medical reform movement should be followed after World War I by AMA hostility to any other form of state or collective intervention. Individual members of the profession had suffered from the appearance in the late nineteenth century of free dispensaries set up by college faculties to provide teaching material, from the prodigious growth of community hospitals with their specialist outpatient clinics,[42] and from the growth of specialist medical societies. Not unnaturally such developments were seen more as a competitive threat to the private general practitioner than as an inevitable movement toward institutionalization, which was the natural outcome of increasing specialism.

42. In 1900 there were about 150 outpatient clinics in the United States; the number grew to over 5,000 in 1925. Michael M. Davis, *Clinics, Hospitals and Health Centers*, p. 5.

PART II: FORMAL RECOGNITION OF THE SPECIALTIES, 1900–1930

CHAPTER 4

Surgeons, Physicians, and General Practitioners

The Rebirth of the College System, 1900-1916

The specialist societies which were the outgrowth of scientific subdivision in the last part of the nineteenth century—the Association of American Physicians, the American Surgical Association, the American Pediatric Society, and many other national, regional, and local societies—represented one aspect of specialization. They were the embodiment of an increasing professional focus on a special field or interest. Providing a nucleus for intellectual stimulation rather than professional cohesion or the advancement of prestige, the societies represented the *specialty* rather than the *specialist*. From the practitioner's point of view, they signified a special interest, not a specialist avocation. By the early twentieth century, however, specialism had advanced in some fields to a second stage of professionalism: concern over the educational standards and competence of those claiming specialist skills.

Specialization of function was an inevitable and perhaps desirable outcome of a steadily widening, more effective body of medical knowledge. The problem was that there were no ready definitions of what was a "specialty," what a "specialist."

If "medicine" was to continue its development as one profession (and three centuries of evolution were not to be lightly ignored) at the very time that technological expansion demanded a variety of skills, professional tensions were only to be expected. There were no established routes to achieve a cadre of medical specialists. Some such defined routes were of increasing interest to those practicing a specialty, for reasons both of safeguarding their own interests and of safeguarding the general public from procedures which were often dangerous. One possibility was a new type of license, riding piggyback over the basic license but with the same exclusive intent. Only those with M.D.s would "practice medicine"; only those licensed as specialists would "practice surgery," "ophthalmology," or other defined specialist fields. But while this solution might appeal to those who would be licensed and to members of the public who were concerned with protection, it had little to offer those members of the profession who—because of the restrictionism built into licensure—would be restrained from entering or pursuing particular specialty lines. Even voluntary self-regulating associations threatened those practitioners likely to be excluded. The debate over regulating surgery in the first two decades of this century emphasized crucial (and continuing) aspects of professional specialism. Was formal regulation of specialists desirable? And, if so, could "general practice" continue to be the privilege of all practitioners, as guaranteed in the basic license?

THE RISE OF THE SURGEON

These questions achieved immediacy with the accelerated development of surgery in the last decade of the nineteenth century. Halsted's careful work at Johns Hopkins and the growing fame of the Mayo Clinic testified to the potential of surgery and precipitated the widespread establishment of hospitals in which surgery could be performed. Most of the hospitals now in existence were founded between 1880 and 1920, and the middle class for the first time entered hospitals on a large scale.[1] It became possible to be a "surgeon" rather than a general practitioner; for the first time in American medicine (although not in Europe) there was a split between those who practiced surgery and those who did not.

Under the dangerous assumption that surgery in the anti-microbe era was now relatively "safe," professional enthusiasm for performing operations escalated. Robert Morris led a public battle from 1908, when he spoke at the AMA Section of Surgery and Anatomy against the temptations of "the technique that inspires a feeling of security" and "surgical art for art's sake." Already, it was being claimed, the patient was being lost sight of, even by the experts, because of the natural tendency of the specialist to focus narrowly on the disorders of a certain part of the body.[2] But such warnings fell largely on deaf ears. While men such as

1. In Connecticut, for example, there were only 2 general hospitals in 1880. Eleven more were founded before 1900, and at the entry to World War I, Connecticut had 26 general hospitals. State of Connecticut, *Report of the Department of Public Welfare, 1923.*

2. Morris urged surgeons to look at their death and recovery rates and to compare them with those both of other surgeons and of spontaneous recovery with no surgery at all. Robert T. Morris, *Fifty Years a Surgeon* (New York, 1935), pp. 110–38 and passim. Also well worth reading, even today, is Harvey Cushing's analysis of specialization, reprinted in his *Consecratio Medici and Other Papers* (Boston, 1940), pp. 48–78.

Morris and Harvey Cushing pressed for a reunification of the art of medicine with the techniques of surgery, at least for a time the surgeon as engineer overshadowed the surgeon as physician.

By the early years of the twentieth century, surgery was expanding in all directions. The gynecologist of the early 1880s had been limited to the speculum, the sound, and the curette. With the introduction of anesthesia, the discovery of antisepsis, and the opening of the abdomen, gynecology rapidly became a surgical specialty. So rapid was the development that there were fears that gynecology would disappear as a separate field and be merged into general surgery; it was claimed in 1905 that "the specialty is so well advanced that there is not very much more progress to be made in it." [3] In the 1890s the focus of abdominal surgery had switched to appendicitis, and there were lengthy battles—especially in the Middle West—as to whether the appendix should be removed or conserved. Gastroenterostomy became possible. Dr. William Mayo performed sixty-five such operations in the second six months of 1905, with no deaths and no secondary operations. [4]

As surgical subspecialties developed, generalism in surgery began to disappear. The combined specialty of ear, nose, and throat thrived with the popularity of tonsillectomies. Urological surgery began to gain the technical skills and apparatus that would establish this field as a respectable focus for the physician, distinguished from the long ineptitude of the "clap doctor"; in Texas, where there were too few full-time surgeons—of any kind—to form an exclusively surgical society, Dr. B. Weems Turner of Houston was able, in 1913, to limit his practice to urology. [5] Harvey Cushing's interest in neurosurgery, itself underpinned by the rise of neuroanatomy and neuropathology, began at Johns Hopkins in the 1890s; his work led the development of this new specialty in the first two decades of the twentieth century. [6] These concurrent developments raised serious problems of coordination and interrelationships both between one surgical field and another and between the medical and surgical aspects of a given specialty.

3. Editorial, "The Future of Gynecology," *Surg. Gynec. Obstet., 1* (1905), 63.
4. Clapesattle, pp. 305, 328.
5. Robert S. Sparkman et al., *The Texas Surgical Society: The First Fifty Years* (Dallas, 1965), pp. 12, 18, 20. For the acceptance of urology as a legitimate field, see editorial, "Andrology as a Specialty," *J. Amer. med. Ass., 17* (1891); Hugh Cabot, "Is Urology Entitled to be Regarded as a Specialty?" *Trans. Amer. Urological Ass., 5* (1911), 1–10; and, for the longer view, Hugh Young, *A Surgeon's Autobiography* (New York, 1940).
6. See Francis Walshe, "The Evolution of Ideas in Neurology during the Past Century and the Future of Neurological Medicine," *J. roy Inst. publ. Hlth., 23* (1960). 37; W. Riese, *History of Neurology* (New York, 1959), p. 202.

When the Mayo Clinic, the organizational transformation of the Mayo group practice, was opened in 1914, Dr. William Mayo insisted that the subspecialties be grouped under general medicine or surgery. Even so, ophthalmology, otology, and orthopedic surgery were set up with their own organizations.[7] The Massachusetts General Hospital reorganized its surgical staff and surgical work in 1911 to bring together fragmented surgical departments under general direction, to increase proficiency in surgical specialization. Chiefs of service were appointed, and surgeons were assigned to have charge of cases falling within given surgical regions: brain surgery, stomach surgery, rectal surgery.[8] Generally, however, the surgical specialties were developing piecemeal, and a man with an interest in one field often had little knowledge of developments in another. General surgery was already declining. The good nose and throat man could not expect to be an equally expert rectal surgeon, and there was a growing feeling in the emerging specialties that the mere holding of an M.D. degree ought not to entitle any practitioner to enter these, or other, surgical fields.[9]

THE PLACE OF THE GENERAL PRACTITIONER

The questions of interspecialty relationships at major institutions such as the Mayo Clinic or the large university-affiliated hospitals were only a small and relatively minor aspect of the problems being generated by the explosion in surgery. Discussions of the relationship between general surgery and the surgical subspecialties were at a totally different level of sophistication from the widespread, and to the patient potentially much more dangerous, question of the relationship between surgery and general practice. The American general practitioner was accustomed to performing surgery. There had not been a traditional split in function—as in Britain, where the surgeon and physician came from different professional lines—between the practitioner who cut and the practitioner who prescribed. Before the opening of the abdomen and the rise of the surgical subspecialties there was relatively little surgery of a major nature which the general practitioner was called upon to undertake. With the development of procedures that made the ill-trained or incompetent surgeon potentially lethal, there arose crucial questions of the functional delineation

7. Clapesattle, pp. 500, 521, and passim.
8. Washburn, pp. 83–84, 89.
9. E.g. Thomas J. Hillis, "The Hospital Governor and His Staff," *Med. News* (*N.Y.*), 77 (1900), 7–8; editorial, "Specialism," *Calif. Med.*, 9 (1911), 492; James B. Herrick, "The Educational Function of Hospitals and the Hospital Year," *AMA Bull.*, 6 (1911), 107.

between one kind of practitioner and another. Implicit in such delineation was some kind of professional control.

There were various possible alternatives. The public might be educated to seek out the better trained. Informal control might be effective if general practitioners voluntarily sent surgical patients to a competent surgeon; or if only those who had received an adequate period of training held themselves out as surgically proficient. Formal control might be exerted by the hospital, as surgery began to move from the patient's kitchen table to the well-equipped operating room, through restriction of operating privileges to those deemed competent. Alternatively there might be a case for formal recognition of trained surgeons through the teaching system (a university degree or postgraduate diploma); through additional licensing for surgeons; or through professional endorsement via a specialty association or examining board. Regardless of the method, the intention would be to focus the practice of surgery on surgical specialists. The corollary would be to redefine, and thus restrict, general practice.

There was much discussion at the turn of the century of the role and the future of the general practitioner. The general practitioner, in becoming less and less omnicompetent, was allegedly becoming less useful to the profession, less equal to emergencies, and somewhat demoralized; and it was claimed that all doctors were, and should be, specialists of one kind or another, except in outlying rural areas.[10] General practitioners, lulled into a false sense of security in their own judgment by the environment of the gleaming operating rooms in newly opened hospitals, were criticized by surgeons for attempting to perform surgical operations which they were not competent or trained to do.[11] On the other hand, some were seeing an enhanced role for the general practitioner as a generalist and diagnostician in light of the narrowness of viewpoint of the specialist.[12] The general practitioner himself was developing his image as a family adviser and counselor, who would give advice on personal and family problems as well as on purely "medical" subjects and who would

10. See e.g. Washburn, p. 317; F. H. Davenport, "Specialism in Medical Practice," *Boston med. surg. J., 145* (1901), 81; and L. Duncan Bulkley, "How Far has Specialism Benefitted the Ordinary Practice of Medicine?" *Bull. Am. Acad. Med., 4* (1899), no. 2.

11. E.g. "It would appear to the uninitiated impossible in such a hygienic sanctuary, to commit a surgical sin, and yet one constantly sees in that operating room heinous crimes committed against the most fundamental surgical principles and technique which ought always to be kept inviolate." J. M. L. Finney, "The Duty of the Family Physician in the Management of Surgical Cases," *N.Y. St. J. Med., 12* (1912), 230.

12. See Carolus M. Cobb, "How Far Should the Specialist in Rhinology and Otology Presume to Treat the Systemic Condition of His Patients?" and discussion, *J. Amer. med. Ass., 41* (1903), 1517–20.

act as a foil to the scientific expert.[13] Indeed, problems facing the medical profession at the turn of the century were curiously similar to those of the 1970s.

But the question of restricting surgery and other aspects of specialism through a redefinition of *roles* could not be entirely successful unless there were incentives of one kind or another to encourage these roles to be created in an effective social framework; in other words there also needed to be a redefinition of *function*. The general practitioner might claim he was now a family adviser and would eschew surgery, but this would not help him if his patients decided to bypass his services and seek out the surgeon directly. Without effective consultation channels there could be no recognized demarcation of function or delineation of roles between the man who claimed to be a general practitioner and the one who claimed specialist skills. Consultation channels—a referral system such as that which was developing at the same time in Britain—could only be encouraged by the ethical sanctions or traditions of the profession, through organizational monopolies, or on the basis of financial incentives to the practitioners who referred and to the specialists who accepted such consultations.

The rapid growth of hospitals in the United States at the same time as the boom in surgery, and the predominantly egalitarian spirit of the American medical profession, made the development of hospitals as the monopoly of well-trained surgeons—at least at that time—an unrealistic solution to quality control, except in the large teaching centers. In Britain, general practitioners were gradually being excluded from the surgical staffs of the larger community hospitals; but they were retaining their own area of monopoly in the "gentleman's agreement" that patients should be referred to surgeons through general practitioners.[14] The outline of a similar system could be seen in the United States. General practitioner referrals to specialists, at least for the well-to-do, increased after 1900. Some large urban hospitals developed a closed-staff system similar to that in Britain, with a relatively small and carefully chosen attending staff. The municipal hospital authorities in Chicago went so far as to select

13. Konold notes that in the mid-nineteenth century the physician approached patients almost exclusively as a *medical* adviser. With the physician's involvement in public health, sanitation, nutrition, and personal hygiene, the practitioner began to feel qualified to give advice on personal and family problems. After 1890 the role of family adviser and counselor was idealized as the ultimate in the doctor-patient relationship; Konold, p. 46.

14. The British system was strengthened in the passage of health insurance legislation in 1911, which confirmed the general practitioner as the primary "doctor" of at least the working class. See Stevens, pp. 34–37.

their visiting surgeons through competitive examination.[15] But these patterns were by no means common. The great majority of the new hospitals were organized on an open-staff principle, often by the very practitioners who wished to use them; that is, such hospitals gave access to surgical facilities to all practitioners who felt themselves to be competent surgeons.

The arguments in favor of a limited staff were the achievement of high surgical standards and the advancement of scientific research. At the same time they were felt by those thus excluded to be "monopolistic and unfair" and not necessarily in the best interests of the patient.[16] The limited-staff pattern was not one likely to appeal to the American medical profession outside a few major cities. Thus control of surgical standards remained as a potential role for the hospital, but one which was only halfheartedly applied. How far the power of the hospital could and should be mobilized to prescribe standards was to become (and still is) a recurring and central topic in the debate over specialist regulation. Without a hospital monopoly, there was no institutional affiliation through which the relatively competent could be distinguished from the remainder.

Individual general practitioners developed their own consultation controls along pecuniary lines. The general practitioner would agree to send patients to a particular surgeon in return for part of the surgical fee. At a time when there was a demonstrable glut of physicians, the desire to split fees was apparent on both sides. Indeed, if the practice of dividing fees had been systematized and openly recognized, a consultation system might have been developed on this basis, with the AMA, for example, deciding what the respective proportions should be. Instead, fee splitting was the label of a surreptitious and commercial affair. Dr. William Mayo, in his presidential address to the AMA in 1906, roundly condemned fee splitting as a crying evil.[17] But the practice of fee splitting rapidly spread. Already, in 1902, the AMA had empowered county medical societies to expel those who split fees secretly, but few charges were made against such persons. Local medical societies were still trying to unify the profession locally rather than to split ranks. Indeed, an exposé of the fee-splitting racket in Chicago in 1904 by two members of the Chicago Medical

---

15. See Konold, p. 41; S. S. Goldwater, "The Hospital and the Surgeon," *Mod. Hosp.,* 7 (1916), 274, 377.
16. Goldwater, "The Hospital and the Surgeon," p. 376.
17. "The one secretly takes money from the patient without his consent, and the other, in order to complete the bargain, charges more than he should." William J. Mayo, "The Medical Profession and the Issues Which Confront It," *J. Amer. med. Ass., 16* (1906, 737–40. For an analysis of the approach to fee splitting as an ethical problem, see Konold, pp. 65–66.

Society brought down discipline upon their own heads and not upon the fee splitters.[18] The AMA Code of Ethics of 1912 clearly stated that it was both degrading and unprofessional to receive a commission or divide a fee "unless the patient or his next friend is fully informed as to the terms of the transaction." [19] While there were no immediate effects from this pronouncement, a few local efforts to control fee splitting were made. In 1913, the Los Angeles County Medical Association printed a list of members with an asterisk against the name of each member who stated he did not split fees, with the laconic comment: "Some of those who have so stated and whose names are so marked may lie, but at any rate they are known to be liars by at least one other person." [20] The Wisconsin legislature passed a law making fee splitting a misdemeanor punishable by the forfeiture of the diploma of any surgeon who gave a commission to anyone bringing him cases for operation.[21] But while this reportedly excited much comment, general professional acceptance of fee splitting continued. That fee splitting might be a symptom of the lack of other controls over the distribution of patients among generalists and specialists does not appear to have been considered.

In the absence of a controlling hospital monopoly, whereby only recognized surgeons would be allowed to operate, or an effective ethical pattern of consultation, whereby the general practitioner had an acceptable incentive to refer, the well-trained surgeon had few means of proving his worth. In turn, the general practitioner was virtually free to operate as he desired. The surviving egalitarian concepts of an earlier period might have it that the profession should continue as a standardized whole, with the public free to make its enlightened choice; but the public was scarcely in a position to keep up with the latest surgical developments and with their best and worst practitioners. William Mayo was probably right in his view that the people were more than two decades behind advanced medical thought.[22] Already the AMA was refuting the public's ability to recognize one product from another, in its concurrent battles against the uncontrolled production of patent medicines and in favor of food and drug legislation. While some questioned, "Are we living in America or

18. The society was particularly annoyed because Dr. John B. Murphy, a noted figure in many disputes, came out against fee splitting rather than in defense of a united profession. Loyal Davis, *J. B. Murphy, Stormy Petrel of Surgery* (New York, 1938), pp. 211–20.
19. "Principles of Medical Ethics, A Proposed Revision," *J. Amer. med. Ass., 58* (1912), 1792–93.
20. Editorial, *Calif. Med., 11* (1913), 254. And see ibid., *10* (1912), 222, 228–29.
21. *AMA Bull., 9* (1914), 165.
22. Mayo, "The Medical Profession and the Issues Which Confront It," p. 737.

Darkest Russia?" [23] it was clear that there were limits to be placed on free consumer choice, and that such limits would continue. Medical licensing already limited the public's choice of physician, in order, so the profession said, to protect that public. Did not surgery (and other specialties) logically demand that the public be protected by the further licensing of specialists? A remaining alternative in the case of surgery was the creation of a label to draw a line between one self-professed surgeon and another.

FOUNDATION OF THE AMERICAN COLLEGE OF SURGEONS

It was in this context that the American College of Surgeons was founded —the offspring of a dynamic man, Franklin Martin of Chicago, and a creature of its age. It came into being because of Martin; but it prospered because of the potential of a recognized group. If a well-trained group of surgeons were able to dominate surgery, they would offer a degree of skill which might eventually be demanded by the public as a right. They would also make enough money to practice without the dubious constraints and temptations of fee splitting. The College was to rise on both planks: the stipulation of a level of training and skill and an attempt to abolish fee splitting.

Franklin Martin's influence as a national surgical leader began with the establishment of the journal *Surgery, Gynecology and Obstetrics* in 1905. The stated objects of the new journal were to advance specialist knowledge, to give practitioners a review of the literature in their fields, and to bring together in an outstanding journal the divisions of surgery included in the title. The journal was an immediate success.[24] It gave Martin and other surgical leaders a vital line of communication with the ordinary practicing surgeon. Articles on the use of iodine in surgery, on bacteriological studies, on types and preferred methods of surgery, and on emerging surgical fields—such as Cushing's article on brain tumors in 1905—offered the practitioner a current operative text. But reading was not sufficient education; the practicing surgeon had to *see* operations for

23. Henry R. Strong, *The Machinations of the American Medical Association: An Exposure and a Warning* (St. Louis, Mo., 1909), p. 36. For an account of the AMA's role, see Burrow, pp. 67–92.
24. *Surgery, Gynecology and Obstetrics* had over 2,000 subscriptions in the first year. A British edition was published from 1908, and the *International Abstract of Surgery* from 1913. By the early 1930s, *SGO* had a monthly circulation of over 13,000. Franklin Martin's editorial, *Surg. Gynec. Obstet., 1* (1905), 62–63; Martin, *Fifty Years of Medicine and Surgery*, p. 291. Loyal Davis, *Fellowship of Surgeons; A History of the American College of Surgeons* (Springfield, Ill., 1960), pp. 26–30.

himself to learn how to do the new procedures and, at the lowest level, how to launch his own general surgical career. Thus Martin soon became involved in the development of what would now be called the surgical teach-in: the provision of some kind of machinery to provide practical demonstrations of surgical innovation.

Through the columns of his journal, followed up with 10,000 invitations to men listed in the AMA directory, Martin launched the first Clinical Congress of Surgeons in 1910, around the operative clinics of Chicago. Martin observed: "It was an innovation that the academic orators and medical politicians watched with amusement that they did not conceal, but it was immediately successful." [25] The 1,300 participants rushed to the well-known clinics of Albert J. Ochsner, John B. Murphy, Arthur Dean Bevan, and others—men who were not only prominent surgeons but also prominent in medical associations. Bevan was chairman of the AMA Council on Medical Education; Murphy, president-elect of the AMA. The AMA was thus in a peculiar relationship with the congress— and with the College, which grew out of it. Not only were some of its leaders involved, but it was providing the kind of postgraduate education which the rank and file demanded, and which the AMA had not offered.

The second Clinical Congress was held in Philadelphia in November 1911. This too was a great success and provided widespread publicity for surgeons. The congresses, indeed, were becoming so successful that some means had to be found to restrict membership to a manageable number. Martin had stressed the need to *democratize* surgical teaching and education; on his way to the third meeting in New York in 1912, he began to consider *un*democratic means of admission. Some of the better surgeons in New York were refusing to be scheduled on the programs with those they thought inferior—products of poor schools and limited experience. Selection of both the demonstrators and the observers thus raised questions of relativity. A crucial problem was emerging. Should the primary focus of surgical education be on upgrading the lowest common denominator to a standard of comparative safety; or should it be to create a relatively small, recognizable group of quality? In other words was there a case for surgical "standardization," as a parallel to the standardization of undergraduate medical education then taking place, or for a highly trained elite? Standardization might imply the introduction of a separate surgical license, mandatory for everyone who attempted surgery; the elite concept, on the other hand, might create a small intraprofessional group which, like the British Royal Colleges, exerted influence through its acknowledged high standards and through the acceptance of its fellow-

25. Quoted by L. Davis, *Fellowship of Surgeons*, p. 42.

ship as a qualification by hospital boards. The future American College of Surgeons was to be dogged by its indecision as to which line it would follow.

Martin pondered the problems of surgery on the train journey from Chicago to New York in 1912. It occurred to him that an organization might grow out of the Clinical Congress which would resemble the Royal Colleges of Surgeons in England, Ireland, and Scotland. The American College could specify professional, ethical, and moral requirements for *every* medical graduate who practiced general surgery or its specialties, would sponsor a supplementary degree for operating surgeons, and would allow special letters to indicate fellowship in the College.[26] The proposals were in essence a plea openly to recognize a distinction between those who were surgeons and those who were not, to provide in effect a form of surgical certification—which also implied a surgical monopoly. In his subsequent speech to the congress, Martin developed these ideas in terms of "standardizing" surgery. As one of his concrete suggestions, he spelled out the possibility of the congress's seeking "a means of legalizing under national, colonial, state, or provincial laws, a distinct degree supplementing the medical degree." [27] An important ingredient would be the establishment of a list, or of distinguishing marks in the directories of physicians.

These suggestions were eagerly welcomed by Murphy, Ochsner, Edward Martin, and other surgical leaders as a way out of the congress's difficulties. Murphy's enthusiastic supporting speech at the third Clinical Congress brought his 200 listeners to their feet, and a committee was appointed to set the plan into motion. The congress also agreed upon the need to establish standards for hospitals, with the intention of upgrading the many hospitals known to be inferior. The surgeon and his facilities would rise together. What is now the Joint Commission on Accreditation of Hospitals and what developed as the Fellowship of the American College of Surgeons (a model for the later specialty boards) had a common origin in concern over the standards and practice of surgery.

A third major area of interest brought up at the congress was the need for a publicity campaign on the early symptoms of cancer of the uterus. The three main prongs on which the College was to battle were now established, and the American College of Surgeons obtained its charter in November 1912. Franklin Martin's plan was to select founders from members of the faculties of all recognized undergraduate and postgradu-

26. Ibid., pp. 58, 61–62, and passim; Franklin H. Martin, *The Joy of Living: An Autobiography* (Garden City, New York, 1933), vol. 1, p. 410.
27. L. Davis, *Fellowship of Surgeons,* pp. 61–62.

ate schools in the United States and Canada, and from a list of other surgeons as the organization committee might designate. Immediately, therefore, the College became involved in an oligarchic process.

On a publicity tour for the new College early in 1913 Martin began to experience vehement opposition to such high-handed methods. Hecklers in Baltimore claimed that the universities and the AMA were attempting to provide higher standards and that there was no need for a College. Martin replied that the new organization, with the aim of attaining higher standards of surgery and the means whereby the public could discriminate in selecting a qualified surgeon, would strengthen their efforts. This elicited the question whether he had in mind "the establishment of a glorified surgical union, along labor lines," or an "exclusive Four Hundred in the profession." [28] In Philadelphia, also, it was claimed that the College would establish a class distinction in the United States in imitation of the undemocratic European systems. In New York only twelve or fifteen surgeons were present to listen to Martin's presentation, although others were rallied to support of the College over the telephone. In Boston, Martin gained the support of the deans of the Harvard Medical School (Edward H. Bradford) and the Graduate School of Medicine (Horace D. Arnold); Harvey Cushing and Frederic Cotton were already staunchly in favor. Los Angeles also seemed in favor. San Francisco was a disaster. The grand tour finished with successful meetings in Portland and Vancouver. There was in sum a very mixed reception, not only to Martin but to Martin's idea.

Objections to the foundation of a College included repeated charges of elitism: that it would usurp the position of the AMA; that the profession should not trust a small handful of men to select those to be regarded as qualified and that it was presumptuous to call the new organization the American College (thus claiming national importance); and that the distinguished regents of the College would be the puppets of Franklin Martin. There was alarm that Martin had divided his groups of surgeons who would be considered for fellowship into "classes" (A, B, and C)—a term with unpleasant elitist overtones. There was also the question of surgery versus general practice. If the College were to be limited to those who were full-time surgeons, or virtually so, the implication would be that the general practitioner had no right to continue to think of himself

28. Ibid., pp. 72–73; Martin, *Fifty Years of Medicine and Surgery,* pp. 302–03; *Joy of Living,* vol. 1, pp. 414–15 and passim. These sources provide a detailed account of the foundation of the American College of Surgeons and form the basis of the discussion of the College in this chapter.

as a first-class surgeon. And there were criticisms that the College was an ingroup "Chicago affair."

Nevertheless, in May 1913 the American College of Surgeons began its professional career: Dr. John M. T. Finney of Johns Hopkins was elected president. Although Martin expected opposition from the leaders of the specialist societies and the suspicion of the AMA, he was confident of success. The 450 surgeons who attended the first meeting were eager to have their ability formally recognized in the form of fellowship in the College. They were equally eager to exclude all fee splitters from their ranks. Fee splitting from the start became one of the central questions discussed by the College.

The AMA, which had itself previously passed a resolution against distinguishing marks for specialists, kept silent.[29] The Illinois delegation, reflecting the profession's schizophrenic reaction to the College, submitted two conflicting resolutions to the AMA in June 1914, one deploring the College "as violating the fundamental democratic principles on which the American Medical Association is based," the other heartily commending and endorsing it "as filling a long-felt want, which the American Medical Association has hitherto failed to meet." Both were disapproved by the house of delegates.[30]

The AMA itself was concurrently waging an autocratic war on the poorer medical schools. In principle the American College of Surgeons was not really doing anything different in its efforts to upgrade or eliminate the poor surgeon. The different emotions the two campaigns evoked were explicable primarily in what the general practitioner felt were his best interests. Medical school reform restricted entry to the profession. Its effects on existing practitioners were beneficial, through raising the caliber and image of the profession as a whole and, by no means least, by reducing the competition. Surgical reform was not so simple. It could not appeal to the practitioner who wished to do surgery, whose license entitled him to do so, and whose income and image would suffer should his surgery be taken away. The relative difficulty of regulating specialties through professional controls was even now apparent.

Martin and others saw the College as the logical next step in the movement begun by his journal and by the congresses. Others were not so sure. The *American Journal of Surgery*, while approving the basic purposes of

29. The AMA *Journal* reported the foundation of the College as a straight factual account, with no analysis, comment, or reaction. *J. Amer. med. Ass.*, 60 (1913), 1471, 1553.

30. *Proc. AMA House of Delegates* (June 1914), 44.

the College and even the use of the fellowship (FACS) on professional cards and in directories, noted that the next proposed step, encouraging legislation to define mandatory qualifications, would have the effect of "working hardships on capable practitioners and on the communities they serve." [31] The word monopoly was also being raised, and both general practitioners and aspiring specialists were rallying to defend their right to do surgery. Meanwhile, a bill was introduced to the Illinois legislature in April 1913 which would provide for mandatory licensure *as a surgeon* by the state board of health (the licensing body) before any but minor surgery in family practice or emergency surgery could legally be undertaken by an M.D.[32]

This bill, while unsuccessful, brought into the open the questions of limited or specialty licensing of physicians. The first question was whether such control was necessary; the second was whether it should be a public or professional responsibility. The College of Surgeons was establishing an American precedent—although not a European one—in allowing a type of professional qualification in medicine to be entirely organized by a voluntary group. Medical societies had in effect controlled licensure in the early nineteenth century, but the public held the ultimate power, as the abolition of licensing laws in the Age of Jackson had demonstrated. The question was now raised as to the basic level of competence at which the public ought to be protected. This in turn was contingent on the problematical but essential question of free choice.

Part of the difficulty, then as now, was what was meant by a "qualified" surgeon. Another difficult word was "standardization." Both terms were included as part of the policy of the College.[33] Dr. Finney acknowledged the difficulty of stating any definite standard for the surgeon; he was, however, in no doubt that if the profession did not accept the responsibility for standards, including the abolition of fee splitting, the public would.[34] An early College committee under Edward Martin considered

31. Editorial, "The College of Surgeons," *Amer. J. Surg., 17* (1913), 234–35.
32. Editorial, "A Bill to Restrict the Practice of Surgery," *Amer. J. Surg. 17* (1913), 235–36.
33. "The object of the College shall be to elevate the standard of surgery, to establish a standard of competence and of character for practitioners of surgery, to provide a method of granting fellowships in the organization, and to educate the public and the profession to understand that the practice of surgery calls for special training, and that the surgeon elected to fellowship in this College has had such training and is properly qualified to practice surgery." Report, "American College of Surgeons," *Surg. Gynec. Obstet., 18* (1914), 124. The same idea was expressed in William D. Haggard, "The Qualifications of the Surgeon," *Trans. Sect. Surg. Amer. med. Ass.* (1913), pp. 99–100.
34. J. M. T. Finney, "The Standardization of the Surgeon," *Trans. Sect. Surg. Amer. med. Ass.* (1914), pp. 211–223.

an examination for surgeons given by the Canadian and United States governments as the first step in centralized licensing; but this suggestion was too radical and was tabled. In the event, the College claimed to certify basic competence without having any restrictive powers: "An applicant who can meet all of the stipulated requirements," wrote Franklin Martin, "is fitted to do actual surgery." [35]

Meanwhile the battle against fee splitting became an integral, even dominant, part of the College's activities and assured its professional success. Those in the College were the most successful surgeons, most of whom had no reason for attracting referrals through splitting fees. At the first convocation of the College (November 1913) the fellowship was conferred on 1,059 surgeons. All had taken an oath which included a promise to shun "dishonest money-seeking and commercialism," "to refuse utterly all secret money trades with consultants and practitioners," and to teach the patient his "financial duty" to the physician. Finney's speech at this gathering stressed the aims of the College as being to elevate professional, moral, and intellectual standards; to foster research; and to educate the public to distinguish between "the honest, conscientious, well-trained surgeon, and the purely commercial operator, the charlatan and the quack." [36]

The College committee on the standardization of hospitals was also busy. A report of November 1913 approved the suggestion that the Carnegie Foundation investigate hospitals (and urged the foundation also to classify them) and recommended that the College encourage hospital trustees and medical staffs to follow up patients and to set up hospital efficiency committees. These proposals failed—as did attempts by the College in 1914 to put responsibility for hospital reporting onto the AMA, which declined on the basis of expense. In January 1916, however, the College did receive $30,000 from Carnegie for hospital standardization purposes (a move no doubt facilitated by the appointment of John G. Bowman, a close friend of Henry Pritchett and at one time Secretary of the Carnegie Foundation, as College director), and later that year it received the official cooperation of the American Hospital Association in that task. The first conference on hospital standardization was held in October 1917. Thus the American College of Surgeons became involved in its great task of upgrading the nation's hospitals—not merely from the standpoint of the surgeon, around whom standards had largely developed, but in terms of all the specialties.

The impressive convocation of 1913, with its rows of gowned surgeons

35. Martin, *Fifty Years of Medicine and Surgery*, p. 335.
36. L. Davis, *Fellowship of Surgeons*, pp. 121, 126–28, 481–82.

listening to an address by Sir Rickman Godlee, president of the Royal College of Surgeons of England, stirred up further dissension in the medical press. There were references to "the Royal Americans," the "latest product of medical snobbery in America." [37] It was claimed that the College was un-American and oligarchic, that it was a threat to the ordinary surgeon, and that the College would reduce the number of surgeons, in the same way that the AMA was reducing the number of all physicians. Had the College been entirely successful, it would of course have done just this. Such criticisms were, however, soon to disappear. By the end of 1914, 2,700 fellows had been admitted by selection; success in examination now became the portal of entry.[38] Prerequisites included a one-year internship, three years as an assistant, fifty case abstracts, visits to surgical clinics, and—for graduates of 1920 and after—two years of college before medical school. Not surprisingly, the Fellowship of the American College of Surgeons was interpreted by many as the granting of a supplementary degree. But the College, while specifying educational standards, did not teach; its examination was more nearly akin to the certification than to the educational process.

A new professional role had been established. A new and increasingly powerful organization had joined the AMA as a standardizing body. Specialist delineation had been achieved. The American College of Surgeons was much more than a specialist society; it had taken to itself the functions of labeling the surgeon and of grading the hospitals. While there was in the first years of the College much interlocking of leadership with the AMA [39]—indeed, the medical profession of the time was largely dominated by surgeons—there was potential conflict in their relations.

THE AMERICAN COLLEGE OF PHYSICIANS

With the founding of the American College of Surgeons, surgery could be claimed as a discrete and measurable segment of medicine. However,

---

37. Ibid., p. 130.
38. Ibid., p. 155. It should be noted, however, that other factors applied in one notable respect. Dr. Daniel H. Williams was the only black physician to be elected as a charter member. No other black physician was given the fellowship until 1934, and even then the southern membership of the College made further applications impossible. The situation changed only after a notorious incident in 1945, when the College informed a New York surgeon that fellowship was "not being conferred on members of the Negro race at the present time." By the end of the 1950s the College had more than a hundred black members (Morais, pp. 97, 135).
39. For example, Finney was chairman of the AMA Section of Surgery; William Rodman was prominent in the College while also president of the AMA. L. Davis, pp. 152, 158.

it was higher, in terms of education, training, and skill, than general practice. The Flexner report had outlined a basic undergraduate training for all physicians; the College provided an additional educational layer. In so doing it created a precedent for other specialties to follow and an unclear future for the generalist.

Internists were the next to distinguish themselves above the basic education for general practice. In a series of vituperative editorials against the American College of Surgeons in the *California State Journal of Medicine* in 1913, Philip Mills Jones had questioned: "And what in the world is the matter with the internists? Are they asleep at the switch? Are they going to let the surgeons, Murphy-Martin directed, put it all over them again? Are they not going to organize an American Royal College of Physicians? . . . Up and have at them!" [40] Jones was being deliberately sardonic. Heinrich Stern, however, after attending a meeting of the Royal College of Physicians of London in 1913, found the idea of a College for physicians appealing; he returned to New York fired with the idea of setting up a similar organization.

His own studies of metabolism having brought him national recognition, Stern, as did others like him, regarded himself not as a general practitioner but as a specialist in "internal medicine." The term was used, following the German model, for a practice consisting of nonsurgical disease, excluding dermatology. It also implied a focus on the physiological and chemical bases of disease rather than on the family, generalist, more folksy approach of general practice. Internal medicine in the United States was a relatively new concept, but its practitioners, with their scientific orientation, considered themselves specialists. The actual work done was probably similar to that of the English "consultant physician" who was usually a member of the Royal College of Physicians. Their view of the general practitioner bore some resemblance to the much earlier views of the "physician" which John Morgan and his colleagues held toward the average practitioners of his day.

Stern cherished the concept of an American college of physicians as eagerly as Franklin Martin identified with the College of Surgeons. But the internists had less reason than the surgeons to organize. They were already a fairly small and exclusive group; nor were they threatened with fee splitting, which seems to have been a surgical phenomenon. Stern received little support for his idea and only managed to set up the American College of Physicians in the early part of 1915. The purposes of the College included support for a federal law to provide a national medical

40. Editorial, "The American Royal Surgical Emporium," *Calif. Med., 11* (1913), 212.

license (although this plan faded into the background) and the specific encouragement of "biological medicine." [41] The College was to include the rank of fellowship, and above that, mastership (for distinguished service); administration was by a self-perpetuating council. It was decided, however, not to have admittance by examination—a crucial distinction between this college and the surgeons. Thus this college was much more of a specialist society than a quasi-licensing force.

Dr. Stern dominated the College until his death in 1918; by then there were 162 fellows, whose activities were chiefly confined to New York. The College had vaguely defined objectives and might well have died in 1919 had it not been for the enthusiasm of Dr. Frank Smithies, the new secretary-general. Dr. Smithies moved the headquarters to Chicago, which had become the capital of organized medicine, rallied support, and began to make the College a national organization. By the end of 1920 there were 518 fellows, and the College had established its own journal, the *Annals of Medicine*.[42]

But while these actions fortified the luster of the College as an organizational center for internal medicine, they did so in relatively narrow terms. The American College of Physicians was not to capture the primary allegiance of the nonsurgical specialists as a whole. American psychiatrists, pathologists, neurologists, and pediatricians had for some time had their own specialist societies, predating the establishment of the American College of Physicians. Their existence emphasized the College's role in *internal* rather than in *general* medicine. Whereas in England the nonsurgical specialties developed within or in reaction to the Royal College of Physicians—with pediatricians and other nonsurgical specialists expecting to take the general MRCP examination if they were to attain the heights of their profession—in America the College of Physicians was one among several competing forces.

THE COLLEGES AS GUILDS

While Franklin Martin's American College of Surgeons and Heinrich Stern's American College of Physicians consciously imitated the British

41. William Gerry Morgan, *The American College of Physicians: Its First Quarter Century* (Philadelphia, 1950), pp. 933–34 and passim. See also A. L. Bloomfield, editorial, "Origin of the Term Internal Medicine," *J. Amer. med. Ass., 169* (1959), 1628–29.
42. Only three issues were published. The *Annals of Clinical Medicine* took its place in 1922, and this in turn was replaced by the present *Annals of Internal Medicine* in 1927. W. G. Morgan, *American College of Physicians*, pp. 2–5, 135–36, 137, 151.

Royal Colleges, they came far too late to have a similar impact. The British Royal Colleges, dominating the development of specialist medicine in that country, continued to provide a superior cadre of physicians and surgeons through the Colleges' graduate entrance system: the examination for membership in the Royal College of Physicians and fellowship in the Royal College of Surgeons. Both examinations were of a higher standard than the basic medical course, were usually taken two or more years after graduation, were intensively competitive, and were reinforced through the operation of the medical practice system. They were in these respects well suited to become the basis of specialist identification—on the assumption that the specialist should be of high general attainment rather than of narrow technical skill, and that relatively few specialists would be required in relation to the body of the profession. In both the educational and the restrictive elements the Colleges appealed to those who sought the formal upgrading of specialism in the United States.

It is, however, one thing to appreciate the value of established institutions, and quite another to create these institutions anew. The time for guilds was past. The American College of Physicians was to be but a pale shadow of its British counterpart. That the American College of Surgeons became a powerful force in American medicine was due largely to Franklin Martin's passionate belief in its necessity. But its success also sprang from the obvious dangers of the new surgery in untrained and unpracticed hands and from the urge of leading surgeons to stamp out the practice whereby surgeons split fees with the general practitioners who sent them patients. Even with these incentives for public protection and private regulation, the American College of Surgeons was to compromise with the prevailing American attitude toward democratic rather than autocratic professionalism; and its role in the unfolding of surgical specialties was to be quite distinct from that of the Royal College of Surgeons.

Unlike that of the British surgical college, the American fellowship examination was designed not to admit only the cream of surgeons but to raise the minimum level of surgery. In its hospital standardization program, the College had potential access to developing a hospital monopoly by its fellows, and thus a distinctive organizational as well as an educational role. But the College was to stop short at creating a hospital-based surgical elite; in any event, the open-staff system of most hospitals would have inhibited such a development. Thus while the College concept was finally assimilated into American medical patterns, it was largely without the strong social and regulatory overtones of the British models.

Within the medical profession, the generalist-specialist relationship remained unsolved. It was clear that technological interests would continue to demand specialist skills, but no distinctions could yet be made about the strategy of specialist divisions within the profession. Each group of specialists developed around the technical exigencies of their interest and in so doing carved out a "specialty." By the time the American College of Physicians was founded, gynecology was both a medical and surgical specialty (although primarily surgical); urology, ophthalmology, and ear-nose-throat were also combined specialties. General surgery, on the other hand, was distinct from general medicine—a distinction recognized in the foundation of the College—and in neurology both medical and surgical specialists competed in the field. The American Colleges provided a basis for containment of further specialization, but had an indeterminate power.

The question remained as to how far a profession should guarantee the standard of competence of its members. Implicitly and explicitly, the College of Surgeons claimed through the establishment of qualifications for fellowship that licensure alone was an insufficient guide, for either the public or the general practitioner, to those claiming special skills or competence. The public, hospitals, and the general practitioner were still free to choose to use College fellows or to ignore their existence. In theory, then, the existence of a voluntary professional system encouraged rather than restrained enlightened choice. In practice, this argument would stand or fall by the effectiveness of the examining process, by the trust of the public in the profession's motives and methods, and in the use actually made of such diplomas.

The real issue was medicine's rapidly expanding technological efficiency: a two-edged sword of expertise and charlatanism which raised new questions of public protection, this time *within* the medical profession. Reform of the medical schools under the impact of the Flexner report was only a partial, nor necessarily relevant solution to the problems of translating scientific potential into service excellence. Indeed, secured by foundation support of research (as they were later to be lured by governmental benevolence), the schools became isolated from the conditions of practice—proprietary schools, whatever their deficiencies, had at least been firmly attuned to the average practitioner. The American College of Surgeons filled a major service need in that it offered the public a definition of a specialist.

Within the profession the gains were not so evident; for the existence of specialist qualifications in one field gave other practitioners an indeterminate status. The foundation of the College assumed that surgeons had to be more proficient than generalists. It was obviously not in the interest of the general practitioners (most of whom were trained in the pre-Flexner proprietary schools) to press for the introduction of a stratified caste system in which they would occupy the lowest rank. But in the long run there seemed to be little alternative. Thus even before World War I the generalist, clutching to himself the prerogative of part-time specialist interests, was beginning to feel confused and threatened. Nor were the surgeons and internists the only groups establishing elites. The ophthalmologists were also fighting a battle for recognition.

CHAPTER 5

Delineation of a Specialty

Ophthalmology, Optometry, and the First Specialty Board

Ophthalmologists were anxious, as the surgeons had been in the decade before World War I, to create standards of proficiency for a recognized specialist group. But the eye doctors' motivations and the questions raised by their efforts to do so were quite different from those of the surgeons. The well-trained surgeons battled against unethical specialists who indulged in fee splitting and against ill-trained and dangerous general practitioners performing surgery; the continued existence of both threatened their prestige and prevented them from being openly recognized as a special calling. The ophthalmologists' quest also rested on competition by "pretenders"; but in this case competition was also provided by those outside the medical profession.

Ophthalmology had developed by taking over a field already occupied by "quacks." Nonmedical opticians had not however died away. They were rising in authority at the end of the nineteenth century, and they offered the public an alternative to the medical eye specialist. In their battles to restrain the opticians, or optometrists, from entering their preserve, the physician ophthalmologists, concerned in developing their own field, claimed a monopoly of the supervision of eye conditions. In so doing, they raised not only the questions: What is a medical specialty? and How far should general practitioners be allowed to practice it? but also the fundamental questions What is the practice of medicine? and Should the medical profession have a monopoly of the healing art?

OPTOMETRY: THE PARAMEDICAL PROFESSION
AND THE MEDICAL MONOPOLY

While the center of clinical skill in the late nineteenth and early twentieth centuries was in Europe, certain practical and technical fields were developing independently and successfully in the United States. Optometry —the measurement for and fitting of eyeglasses—was one of these fields; anesthetics and dentistry were others. Dentistry was already outside medicine, yet dentists diagnosed, prescribed, and gave treatment. They were, in their field, engaged in medical practice; but they were focused on a limited area which was traditionally accepted as being outside medicine. Dentistry was not in the nineteenth century absorbed as a physician's specialty. The demarcation battles over surgery of the jaw were to be a mid-twentieth-century phenomenon. Both ophthalmology and anesthesiology, however, were recognized as part of the realm of the physician. Specialists in these fields came to believe in their exclusive rights over the specialty. The position of the medical ophthalmologist in relation to the optometrist bore similarities to later disputes between medical anesthesiologists and nurse anesthetists. The attitude of the ophthalmologist and anesthesiologist was hostile to his nonmedical colleagues, in marked contrast to specialties such as radiology and pathology where nonmedical personnel were welcomed, although presumably because they developed firmly under the physician's thumb. In the case of both ophthalmology and anesthesiology more was at stake than standards alone. The nonmedical practitioners in these fields provided active competition in lucrative fields of practice, and each attracted middle-class patients.

This last distinction may be observed by comparing the role of optometry with the rather similar, but far less disputed, position of nonmedical midwifery. European midwives were often more highly skilled in obstetrics than physicians, but midwifery had not developed along such lines in the United States, probably because in an overcrowded profession general practitioners had a greater incentive to retain obstetrical practice to themselves than did their European counterparts. Moreover, unlike optometry and dentistry, midwifery developed no new technological bases in the nineteenth century on which a new profession might rise. In the United States midwives were identified with the poor, the Southern Negro, and the Northern urban immigrant. To the average physician midwifery was thus largely an alien profession. It was also nationally unorganized. There was no effective pressure from the ranks of the midwives to offer a general alternative to medical obstetrics, and with the introduction of legislation to control the standards of nurse midwives before and after World War I their number rapidly declined. Indeed, midwifery appears only to have survived at all in the United States because of the higher costs of physician services, the scarcity of physicians in low-income rural areas, and habit and tradition in the populations served.[1] Generally, there

1. In New York City, 40 percent of all confinements were attended by midwives in

was little economic conflict between the midwives and the medical profession.

Optometry, on the other hand, was an expansive movement. Opticians were dispensing spectacles long before the medical profession became interested in the eye. Elisha North had opened the first American institution for the treatment of eye diseases in New London, Connecticut, as early as 1817. The New York Eye and Ear Infirmary had followed in 1820, and this was followed in turn by other eye hospitals and dispensaries. These provided centers for care and treatment and teaching in the urban areas, and foci for specialist interests by members of the medical profession. But it was not until 1860 that there were favorable social preconditions for the development of ophthalmology as a recognizable specialty. Two important scientific developments aided this process and brought physicians into competition with the optician. The first was the invention of the ophthalmoscope by Helmholtz (1851); this gave the physician visual access to the retina, proved useful in measuring refractions of the eye, and gave the "oculists" (as the medical eye specialists were termed) an instrumental focus for their specialty. The second was the work of the Dutch ophthalmologist Frans Cornelius Donder (1818–89) in the prescribing and fitting of spectacles, brought to the English-speaking world through his book *The Anomalies of Refraction and Accommodation* (1864).[2]

1909. The enforcement of educational requirements by the department of health and the restriction on immigration during and after World War I reduced this percentage; in 1928 midwives attended only 12 percent of the births. In New Jersey the percentage was reduced from 42 percent in 1918 to less than 19 percent in 1930. The number of midwives declined rapidly between 1920 and 1930 as states developed regulatory laws, both in the North and South: midwives in Birmingham, Ala., for example, reportedly delivered only 5 cases in 1928, as compared with 968 in 1917. A 1919 Illinois study showed that the highest use of physicians was by U.S. nationals (black and white) and by the Irish, German, and Jewish groups. Minnesota midwives, surveyed in 1923, were chiefly Scandinavians, Germans, Poles, and Finns. Immigrant midwives, however—some of whom were highly trained in European schools—grew old and died without being replaced. By 1930, 80 percent of the 47,000 midwives in the United States were in the rural South. Nurse midwifery—special training following the nursing diploma—has meanwhile developed, but, except for the notable Frontier Nursing Service in Kentucky, has not up till now substituted to any significant extent for the physician. Louis S. Reed, *Midwives, Chiropodists, and Optometrists: Their Place in Medical Care,* Publications of the Committee on the Costs of Medical Care, No. 15 (Chicago, 1932), pp. 5, 6, 17, and passim. States of Illinois, *Report of the Health Insuranace Commission of the State of Illinois* (Springfield, 1919), pp. 59–60.

2. Ophthalmology has received substantial attention from historians. Major sources of information for this chapter are. Alvin A. Hubbell, *The Development of Ophthalmology in America 1800–1870* (Chicago, 1908); James E. Lebensohn, "A Chronology of Ophthalmic Progress," *Amer. J. Ophthal., 59* (1965), 885–87;

The professionalization of ophthalmology was stimulated by the activities of Dr. Julius Homberger in New York in the early 1860s. (It was Dr. Homberger's inclinations toward advertising that caused the AMA to pronounce that physicians could not ethically publish their special titles or interests.) But Dr. Homberger had two other causes for fame. He founded the *American Journal of Ophthalmology* in 1862, the first special journal for the eye to be published in the United States, and he was also indirectly instrumental in the founding of the American Ophthalmological Society in 1864, out of a meeting of eight men held at the office of Dr. Henry D. Noyes. Noyes was a vigorous opponent of the practice of advertising by self-styled specialists, of which Homberger was the leading example. The new society took a firm ethical line throughout the century against any announcement by its members that they were in fact specialists in eye diseases, although whether this policy aided the patient who was trying to gain treatment for his eyes is a question of some doubt. As late as 1925 a candidate who later became a distinguished member of the society was excluded for allowing the use of the term "oculist" after his name in directories and on his stationery; and only in 1929 were the bylaws changed to allow members publicly to claim specialist interests.[3] Thus there developed the curious situation whereby surgeons wished publicly to proclaim their specialist status, including letters after their name so indicating their interests, whereas ophthalmologists spent long years dissociating themselves from the stigma of being an "eye specialist" because the name had originally been attached to those of an irregular medical persuasion.

The American Ophthalmological Society provided one professional basis for the specialty organization of physicians. In 1865 a request for a section of ophthalmic medicine and surgery was disapproved by the AMA. A combined section with otology and laryngology was, however, finally approved in 1877; in 1888 these sections divided, and ophthalmology was given a section of its own. This was the first section to publish its own *Transactions*. The Western Ophthalmic and Otolaryngological Society was founded in 1895—and became the American Academy

F. H. Verhoeff, "American Ophthalmology during the Past Century," *Arch. Ophthal., 39* (1948), 451; George Rosen, "New York City in the History of American Ophthalmology," *N.Y. St. J. Med., 43* (1943), 754; ibid., *Specialization of Medicine;* Arrington, *A History of Ophthalmology.*
3. Henry D. Noyes, "Account of the Origin and of the First Meeting of the American Ophthalmological Society," *Trans. Amer. Ophthal. Soc., 2 (1875)*, 11–16. See also Maynard C. Wheeler, *The American Ophthalmological Society: The First Hundred Years* (Toronto, 1964), pp. 110–12; Harry Friedenwald, "The American Ophthalmological Society: A Retrospect of Seventy-Five Years," *Arch. Ophthal., 23* (1940), 1–21.

of Ophthalmology and Otolaryngology in 1903. Specialty clinics and hospital departments continued to be established. There was pride in the precision of diagnosis and treatment possible in this field and in the American application of the best European techniques. Organizationally, ophthalmology had all the trappings of a specialty.

It was also gaining in numbers. By 1908, there were about 2,500 to 3,000 practitioners in the field of ophthalmology in America. There were thirty-five special hospitals, and many more departments in general hospitals.[4] The foundation in 1908 of the National Society for the Prevention of Blindness pointed also to a new concern with prophylaxis in the care of the eyes, and the detection and prevention of eye diseases in the newborn became an important function of public health authorities.[5]

As the span of ophthalmic practice was widening, however, medical ophthalmologists were faced with a number of critical questions. As with surgery, there was a group of well-trained specialists who had been to Europe, particularly to Germany and Austria, or who had emigrated from one of the European centers. Almost all the founders of the American Ophthalmological Society had spent considerable time studying abroad.[6] But there was no formal way of distinguishing such men from the poorly or partly trained practitioner—the so-called six-week specialist with a brief course in a proprietary school—or the general practitioner who dabbled in eye care. There were few residency training positions in the United States at the beginning of the twentieth century, and these few were in independent specialty hospitals rather than in university-affiliated institutions. Preceptorship provided an alternative, but was hard work; those trained as clinical assistants in private practice under this method often completed their training with three to six months in Europe, in order to become proficient in scientific subjects such as pathology. Since medical students were not taught to do refraction, there was an open field for such endeavor. It was a field on which the eminent student of Helmholtz or Von Grafe could scarcely look with equanimity, and it raised the old ethical question of what kinds of consultation should be permitted between the regular practitioner and outside specialists, whether they be optician, cultist, or quack.

4. Hubbell, pp. 193–94.
5. For example, Massachusetts in 1914 was presented with a bill giving the board of health authority, in addition to other methods of preventing blindness (including reporting), to advise the employment of an oculist for all neonatal cases, on the ground that treatment by a GP was often inadequate, and that cases were being brought to ophthalmic clinics only after the damage had been done. "Tenth Annual Conference on Medical Legislation," *AMA Bull., 9* (1914), 151. See also Lebensohn, "A Chronology," p. 889.
6. See Bonner, *American Doctors and German Universities,* pp. 89–90.

The European centers, concentrating on the pathology of eye diseases, were only peripherally interested in the lens aspect of the eye, which was the basis for refraction. As a result, many of the distinguished specialists had paid little attention to refractive errors. Yet the use of glasses, and of correcting eye defects by this means, was rapidly developing. The eminent eye specialist Edward Jackson observed in 1911 that more lenses were then being worn for correction of eye defects in a single city than were used sixty years before in the whole world. Jewelers and other shopkeepers rushed into a field in which substantial profits could be made: "Each party has pushed forward, proclaiming its superior right, by priority and fitness, to the field in question, like prospectors in a new mining camp." [7] The grinding of lenses and the making of glasses became a vast industry, largely cornered by the opticians. Leaders of the opticians, such as Charles F. Prentice of New York, considered eyeglasses as their vested right and looked on the growing interest of physicians in this field, from the 1870s onward, as "medical encroachment." [8] There were opticians who merely dispensed glasses on a physician's prescription (dispensing opticians); there were also those who prescribed for themselves (refracting opticians). The former posed no problem to the physicians: they were in a similar position in relation to medicine as were pharmacists. The latter, however, competed directly with the eye doctor. From the 1890s, battle was joined.

THE OPHTHALMOLOGISTS AND DEMARCATION DISPUTES

The disputes between the medical oculist and the nonmedical optician centered on New York City, the ophthalmological center of the country. Its chief protagonists were the noted ophthalmologists Henry Noyes and D. B. St. John Roosa (both founders of the American Ophthalmological Society) and the optician, or "opticist," as he preferred to call himself, Charles F. Prentice. Prentice was by no means the uneducated quack. The ensuing battle was thus of serious public and professional importance. An educated man, with a three-year training in mechanical engineering in Karlsruhe, Baden (1871–74), Prentice had entered his father's optical business in New York, devoting his evenings to the work of Helmholtz, Donders, and others and producing his own observations in optics. He also spent two winter semesters (1887–88) under the pre-

7. Edward Jackson, "The Optometry Question and the Larger Issues behind It," *J. Amer. med. Ass., 57* (1911), 265.
8. See Charles F. Prentice, *Legalized Optometry and the Memoirs of Its Founder* (Seattle, 1926), pp. 10–11 and passim.

ceptorship of the pathologist of the New York Eye and Ear Infirmary. According to his own account, Prentice became familiar with leading medical oculists. Dr. Noyes invited him to explain his suggested system of prism measurement before the Section of Ophthalmology and Otology of the New York Academy of Medicine in 1891. Hermann Knapp advised Prentice to study medicine, but he declined on the grounds that he had no desire to become an ophthalmic surgeon.[9]

The first skirmish was a friendly letter to Prentice from Noyes at the end of 1892. The question raised by Noyes was not of competence. Instead, Noyes objected to the charging by Prentice of a separate fee for examining the eyes, in addition to the charge for the glasses. Prentice apparently was free to prescribe, but he was not to take the credit for so doing. Noyes explained that it was a question both of economic competition and of an "injustice" to the public because it implied that Prentice had "the qualifications which entitle you to a fee for advice." [10] The issue was curiously similar to the much earlier disputes in Britain between physicians and apothecaries, over whether the latter could charge for giving advice as well as for drugs. It raised questions over what was and was not the "practice of medicine," and how far physicians should claim a functional and financial monopoly.

Noyes warned Prentice that he would antagonize physicians by assuming their functions. Prentice replied that his patrons were distinctly given to understand that he was not a physician and that he did not give medical advice. He claimed, no doubt truthfully, that he gave better services than the average optician and was appreciated quite as much as the "average rising oculist"; that to make an extortionate profit on the glasses alone would make him a charlatan; that he always referred patients to physicians when he discovered a disease condition; and that he did not care to ease the physicians' ethical problem by adopting the practice of some New York firms, of employing ill-equipped young medical graduates merely to write the optical prescriptions. Noyes passed this letter on to the more fiery St. John Roosa, and unwisely passed the Roosa comments back to Prentice. Roosa had no doubt that Prentice was deliberately cutting himself off from the oculists, that he was exceeding his proper functions merely to make more money, and that he was possibly violating the law by practicing medicine without a license. There was no

9. Prentice secured the copyright of the term "opticist" for well-qualified opticians, using it from 1886 until the optometry law was passed in New York in 1908. The term "optometrist" apparently originated in the New York legislature. Prentice disliked the term and thereafter called himself a physical eye specialist, as distinct from a medical eye specialist. Ibid., pp. 18, 233, 244–47.
10. Ibid., pp. 19–25.

thought now of assimilating men of Prentice's technical ability into the medical circle, of accepting them as well-trained technologists, or of leaving the public to make its choice. With the battle cry of protecting the public, the medical monopolists moved into action using, as they had previously used with such success against quackery, the machinery of medical ethics.

In 1895, after bitter remarks from Prentice to Noyes, it was reported to Prentice that Roosa had appealed to the New York County Medical Society to cease sending their patients to opticians to have glasses fitted on the grounds that it was an unethical practice. Reportedly Roosa also stated that "he would have the medical practice act so amended as to deprive men of Prentice's cult from meddling with ophthalmology." [11] Prentice's reaction was to mobilize opticians, so as to reach the legislature first, and to create a society which would, like the dental society, have powers to regulate opticians and to insure them against medical "molestation." On this basis the Optical Society of the State of New York organized in February 1896, although it had only eleven charter members, the dispensing opticians' withdrawing because of the opposition of the medical profession, on whom they depended for their livelihood. A bill was presented to the New York legislature the same year to incorporate the society. Cogent arguments were made by Prentice on the similarity between the optician and the dentist in relation to the physician. The same phrases appeared as were used of the American College of Surgeons. Prentice referred to the relationship between medical oculists and dispensing opticians as a collusion, a trust, and a concentrated and dangerous monopoly. The opposing opticians, on the other hand, objected to the bill as class legislation, granting peculiar privileges to the optical society.

The bill was defeated, but interest was aroused. Issues had been raised which applied to medical as well as optical standards. Prentice had emphasized that the medical degree alone carried with it no knowledge of optics, that many general practitioners did not know how to use an ophthalmoscope, and that opposition by the medical profession to educational improvement of opticians was not universal. He quoted Dr. Chalmer Prentiss of Chicago and Dr. Edward J. Brown of Minneapolis as being actually in favor of *qualified* opticians. Prentice also stated that his society would only approve those recommended by a regularly appointed

11. Ibid., p. 32. The following account of the dispute between the ophthalmologists and the opticians is drawn largely from Prentice's detailed quotation and description. See also Monroe J. Hirsch and Ralph E. Wick, *The Optometric Profession* (Philadelphia, 1968), pp. 124–47 and passim.

physician, at an eye infirmary of recognized standing. Training for a refracting optician was suggested as being two years of experience plus eight months at an eye infirmary, including use of the disputed ophthalmoscope (which was the badge of the medical oculist).[12] If this were done, the qualified refracting optician would be much better trained in refraction than the average general practitioner. Thus a new professional class would be born, with functions which cut across the traditional boundaries of medicine.

The battle was now raging, and it was no longer confined to New York. The medical law of Ohio (1896) was causing concern because of its broad scope in defining the "practice of medicine" to include any person prescribing for a fee any agency for any infirmity or disease. Whether the physicians should have a monopoly of all aids and prescriptions dealing with physical and mental health was a question barely debated by the physicians competing with each other in an overcrowded field. Prentice and others naturally took the opposite position: "Physics is not physic"; "A lens is not a pill"; "A lens treats light"; "A lens does not treat disease"; "Optometry is not medical science"; "Optometry is founded on optical science." [13] These slogans, invented by Prentice to illustrate what he called "tersely stated truths," appeared on buttons at optical meetings in the following years, in optical advertising, and in the numerous campaigns for optometry laws across the United States.

In the case of optics, where both medical and nonmedical specialists claimed expertise in a recognized technical field, there was a strong case for offering optical recognition outside preexisting professional boundaries, thus linking the two types of specialist through the specialty itself. This suggestion was made in 1897. A bill presented to the New York legislature in that year would have placed optometry under the Board of Regents of the State of New York, the controlling body for other types of licensure.[14] *Both physician and nonphysician eye specialists* would come under the proposed law. All unqualified persons would be subject to prosecution as in other forms of licensure.

This bill would have had three important effects: first, it would have created the first governmental specialist diploma for physicians; second, it would have linked medical and paramedical personnel within one structure; third, it would have restricted the basic medical license by

12. The society also wanted to control competition among its members, by ultimately fixing uniform prices for articles sold and by abolishing offers for free eye examinations.
13. The slogans are cited by Jackson in the "Optometry Question," p. 265.
14. For the text of the bill and a full account of its fate in the legislature, see Prentice, pp. 127–33.

excluding a specialist area—optics. Prentice saw the bill as the logical beginning of a unification of opticians with medical men, "to a point where in time their interests, both educational and otherwise, will have become so amalgamated as to have created the ideal eye-specialist." [15] The area of optics, like certain areas of medical physics and medical microbiology today, would thus have been recognized as a scientific field rather than a strictly professional preserve. General practitioners with an interest in the eye were, however, unlikely to take to such suggestions. The medical profession, set in its opposition, was not able to consider the bill coldly and objectively, even though it provided a basis whereby physicians might legally have dominated the opticians. The 1897 bill was defeated in the New York assembly by three votes; it died in the senate, after strong opposition not only from medical men but from some of the opticians whose interests also were threatened. After this date no state attempted to include physicians under their optometry laws. A golden opportunity was lost, and the two camps were fixed in mutual distrust.

Instead optometry developed as a separate profession, internally organized and supported by the public. The first state to pass an optometry bill was Minnesota in 1901; others followed rapidly. New York was the thirteenth state to do so, in 1908; twenty-six states had such laws in 1912; and the District of Columbia was last of all the jurisdictions to pass a law, in 1924. In some cases the medical profession withdrew its opposition to impending legislation. "We had the optometry bill up again," said a Connecticut delegate to an AMA conference in 1914; but since this bill was reportedly the least objectionable yet, the state medical society agreed to let it go, providing it include a caveat against the title "doctor" or its synonym being used by opticians, partly because Connecticut was becoming a dumping ground for those opticians who could not get licensed in other states.[16] The optometrists' cause was also upheld in the courts, the most notable decision being a U.S. Supreme Court case of 1904 (*Illinois Board of Health* v. *Lincoln Smith*) which ruled that optometrists were not engaged in the practice of medicine.

Columbia University established the first university-sponsored course in optometry in 1910. This was in the Department of Extension Education, not in the medical school and without its approval. Although such courses were naturally opposed by physicians, optometry was now a

15. Ibid., p. 143. In at least one place opticians were publicly accepted as eye specialists. The Board of Education of Syracuse, N.Y., used opticians in the 1890s to examine, prescribe, and furnish glasses to school children, which they had offered to do free of charge. Ibid., p. 138.
16. "Tenth Annual Conference on Medical Legislation," *AMA Bull., 9* (1914), 156–57.

legally recognized field. Four other universities followed. By 1930 Columbia was giving a four-year course in optometry (including two years exclusively devoted to the subject) for a B.Sc. degree; no university, however, gave optometrists a doctoral degree. Independent optometry schools on the other hand continued to flourish, to produce the most graduates, and to award doctor's degrees.[17] In demanding a doctoral title and in condoning inferior schools, the optometrists did little to advance their cause as a profession and much to fan the hostility of physicians.

Prentice, who had become president of the New York Examining Board for Optometry, had little support from either side in his continued efforts to establish better relationships with the ophthalmologists. The AMA had passed a resolution in 1899 that physicians should restrict their optical consultations to other physicians, "thus discountenancing the growing pretenses and assurances of the optician." In 1910 the AMA House of Delegates commended its Bureau of Medical Legislation for efforts to defeat "objectionable optometric legislation." [18] The same year the AMA Section on Ophthalmology voiced its disapproval of ophthalmologists serving on examining boards for opticians as being against the AMA ethical code. After a period of relative calm in the postwar years (coinciding with the reduction in numbers of physicians and thus a general attenuation of competition) resolutions concerning optometrists revived. In 1934 the AMA agreed to attempt to stop optometrists from prescribing glasses in hospitals; the following year it was declared unethical for any AMA member to teach or consult with anyone not associated with actual medical service. The AMA Section on Ophthalmology tried to reverse this position in 1941 (presumably because members were in favor of giving optometrists a good education and in collecting lecture fees), but the AMA House of Delegates tabled the request that year, and again in 1942. In the light of considered encroachment by optometrists, further efforts were made in the 1950s to cut off any contact between the two fields—except that ophthalmologists might accept (and retain) optometrist referrals. By 1966, however, M.D.'s were being encouraged to teach student optometrists "within the legitimate scope of optometric practice"; but there continues to be alarm from organized medicine lest

17. At the bottom of the scale in 1930 was the Philadelphia Optical College, which gave a doctor's degree after a three-month unsupervised course. L. S. Reed, *Midwives, Chiropodists, and Optometrists,* pp. 40, 42–43, 45. After 1935, however, most optometry schools had four-year courses, and since 1946 all have had five-year programs and some six. Frederick C. Cordes and C. Wilbur Rucker, "History of the American Board of Ophthalmology," *Amer. J. Ophthal., 53* (1962), 246.
18. This and the following AMA actions are reported in the AMA *Digest of Official Actions, 1858–1958,* pp. 538–40; and *Supplement to the Digest of Official Actions, 1959–1963,* pp. 215–17.

optometrists gain legislation authorizing them to diagnose or treat a disease or injury of the eye. The present relationship between the optometrist and ophthalmologist is better than it has been, but there remain two professional identities, instead of a unified concern with the care of the eye.

SPECIALIST INSIGNIA FOR OPHTHALMOLOGISTS

The optometry question stimulated ophthalmologists to put their own house in order. They were on weak ground so long as ill-trained general practitioners held themselves out as trained refractionists; and there was as yet no reputable mark of specialist skill such as the optometry laws provided for their rivals. At the same time, scientific developments were increasing the demand for highly skilled eye doctors. These included Crampton's development of the battery-handled ophthalmoscope in 1913, which made the ophthalmoscope a practicable instrument for internists, neurosurgeons, and others, but which required ophthalmologists to interpret the findings. Contacts were being made by leading ophthalmologists with a wide range of other specialties, and practice was no longer exclusively in or dependent on eye, ear, nose, and throat hospitals. The birth of neurosurgery and the developments in eye pathology increased the trend to separate development.

In his presidential address to the American Academy of Ophthalmology and Otolaryngology in 1908, Derrick T. Vail, Sr., raised the idea of a board similar to a state examining board to license ophthalmic practice for physicians after one or two years of graduate training. His proposal was designed to exclude the claims of the "six-week specialist," and other ill-prepared medical men.[19] Thus again the question of state licensure of medical specialists was raised, or some alternative form of qualification; but this time excluding the optometrists. This theme was taken up the following year (1908) by Alvin A. Hubbell of Buffalo in his chairman's address to the AMA Section in Ophthalmology. Hubbell recommended the establishment of required courses in ophthalmology for undergraduates, culminating in examination by both the medical faculty and a state examining board. Specialists ought, he considered, to have legally regulated graduate training, followed by a licensing examination conducted by expert ophthalmologists. These moves were designed both to protect the patient and to put a stop to the alleged injustice inflicted by the general practitioner "on the rights of his neighbor ophthalmologist, who has

19. Derrick T. Vail, "The Limitations of Ophthalmic Practice," *Trans. Amer. Acad. Ophthal. Otolaryng.* (1908), pp. 1–6. See also Cordes and Rucker, "History of the American Board of Ophthalmology," pp. 243–44.

qualified at much sacrifice of time, energy and money." [20] The idea of some sort of state examining board continued to be favored in 1911 and 1912, but no one was willing to take the enormous responsibility which its organization would require. Thus the question of specialist licensing in ophthalmology followed a course similar to that of the concurrent interest in setting up a specialist license for surgeons.

Edward Jackson of Denver, who became the leading influence for ophthalmic reform, stressed the need to build up "a definite class of practitioners especially trained to recognize and treat the defects and disorders of the eye";[21] in short to create a formally recognized specialty, although not necessarily through the licensing laws. As a move in this direction, Jackson recommended the establishment of a university degree such as the British Doctor of Ophthalmology at the University of Oxford, which had been set up in 1907 because of rather similar deficiencies in undergraduate medical education. Courses leading to a doctorate in ophthalmology were started about 1912 at the University of Colorado under Jackson himself, and also at the Universities of Pennsylvania and Minnesota.[22] The American Ophthalmological Society could not, however, make up its mind about university degrees. There was some doubt whether the doctoral degree in ophthalmology should be encouraged in all schools, because of the diversity of standards which would result. In 1913 the society formed a committee to consider raising membership requirements and to discuss the whole question of an ophthalmic diploma. This committee, whose members included Jackson, formulated a curriculum for a master's degree in ophthalmology; it had been decided that this would be preferable to a doctorate. The degree, it was suggested, would include both a thesis and an examination and would come under university (rather than medical school) auspices. There was also talk of combining forces with the AMA section and the American Academy of Ophthalmology and Otolaryngology to put maximum pressure on the medical schools to establish such courses.[23]

In 1912 Jackson also suggested differentiating the undergraduate medical course to include ophthalmology as an elective subject for medical students, so that some GPs would graduate as partially trained special-

20. A. A. Hubbell, "Ophthalmic Qualifications Which Should Be Demanded of the General Practitioner and of the Specialist, Respectively," chairman's address, *Trans. Sect. Ophthal. Amer. med. Ass.* (1909), pp. 9–20.
21. Jackson, "Optometry Question," p. 268.
22. S. Judd Beach, "American Ophthalmology Grows Up: Turbulent Years 1908–1915," *Amer. J. Ophthal., 22* (1939), 373–74.
23. See *Trans. Amer. Ophthal. Soc., 13* (1913), pt. 2, pp. 267, 275; Beach, "American Ophthalmology," p. 372; Cordes and Rucker, "History of the American Board of Ophthalmology," p. 248.

ists.[24] This idea—coming soon after the Flexner report and in the midst
of the national movement for standardizing the undergraduate curriculum
—indicated the speed of scientific change and of specialist acceptance.
The focus of the undergraduate reform movement was, however, more on
producing the generalist than the specialist, and Jackson's idea was unlikely to find general favor; indeed, only recently has the question of
specialist electives been seriously revived. Meanwhile the AMA urged the
establishment of one-year graduate courses in ophthalmology in the medical schools; and recorded the need for the establishment of standards of
fitness for practitioners in both ophthalmology and the related specialty
of otolaryngology (ear and throat).[25]

The movement to create a sign of specialist competence in eye diseases
gained momentum in 1913–14 in each of the three specialist organizations concerned: the AMA Section of Ophthalmology, the American
Ophthalmological Society, and the American Academy of Ophthalmology and Otolaryngology. Reform in ophthalmology thus came from
within existing organizations—unlike surgery, where reform came from
the creation of a completely new body. It seemed logical for the three
groups, which were already linked through Edward Jackson and were
concerned with the same problems, to cooperate. The academy resolved
in October 1913 to set up committees to confer with similarly appointed
committees from the other ophthalmological and otolaryngological societies, with a view to persuade the various postgraduate institutions of the
United States to adopt some manner of uniform curriculum and uniform
requirements for admission to ophthalmic and otolaryngologic practice.
Thus developed the concept of standardization in ophthalmology. One
wonders how far the optometry threat encouraged such remarkable unanimity; but it was a short step to the concept of a joint committee.

In this propitious atmosphere Edward Jackson presented the AMA
section's report on education in ophthalmology in June 1914. He suggested not only a joint committee but also a joint examining board.

THE FIRST MEDICAL SPECIALTY BOARD

Edward Jackson, like Franklin Martin, looked across the Atlantic for his
model of a new organization. He too lit upon the successful professional
monopolies long held by the English Royal College of Physicians and the
Royal College of Surgeons; but in this case the model was not the Col-

24. Edward Jackson, "The Proper Provision for Teaching Ophthalmology in the
Medical Schools," *Trans. Sect. Ophthal. Amer. med. Ass.* (1912), pp. 255–73.
25. AMA, *Digest,* pp. 536–37

leges themselves but the type of joint examining board set up by them to administer a common examination. The English Conjoint Board had been formed in 1884 to give combined examinations in medicine and surgery for the two Royal Colleges, as a basic medical diploma, legally recognized as a license. The functions of the Conjoint Board had been widened by the addition of postgraduate diplomas in public health in 1887 and tropical medicine in 1911 (other diplomas were to follow in 1920), but it was not in any sense a specialty board. Jackson's interest lay in its form as a professional examining organization, sponsored by more than one existing professional group, drawing its examiners from the medical schools, and giving a diploma—not a degree—which would be recognized by the profession and by public authorities as evidence of proper preparation for professional work. A conjoint board diploma in ophthalmology, sponsored by the leading specialist societies, would in Jackson's view "soon come to be sought by most of those desiring to enter on the practice of ophthalmology." [26]

Jackson thus turned away from two alternatives for professional recognition—licensure and the reliance on university degrees—as, indeed, had the American College of Surgeons. Discussants at the AMA meeting of 1914 raised the additional concern that there might be corruption where state legislatures were involved; there was also the unspoken danger of the state legislatures attempting to link up ophthalmologists with the new optometry laws. The chief difficulty with using university degrees as a standard of competence was that there was no way of standardizing or controlling the different degrees professionally. The AMA was only succeeding in upgrading basic medical degrees through its influence over the state licensing boards. Moreover, although there were by 1915 five universities with higher degree programs, these clearly would serve only a small minority of those who wished to be ophthalmologists. The surgeons were establishing a successful precedent for professional regulation of standards of competence through a voluntary mechanism, a nationally uniform standard, and a relatively high standard of entry. This concept was appealing, both in its practicability and in its ability to further the authority of the professional associations. As the surgeons would automatically turn their gaze to the standards of practical surgery in the hospitals, so a professional examining board in ophthalmology—under recognized leadership—would indirectly affect the experience in that specialty offered by hospitals and the training in the medical schools. It was

26. Edward Jackson, "Report of the Committee on Education in Ophthalmology," *Trans. Sect. Ophthal. Amer. med. Ass.* (1914), pp. 395–406.

recommended that the examination for recognition for fitness in ophthalmology should follow at least two years of graduate study and one year of supervised clinical experience. Thus the joint board would be both an examining body and a prescriber of training standards. Like the American College of Surgeons, formed only the year before, it would be a certifying agency but without any exclusive or legal powers.

In 1915 each of the three sponsoring societies was asked to adopt the report of the special conjoint committee which was set up following Jackson's earlier report.[27] The conjoint committee wanted all ophthalmologists to go through systematic courses, to be shown to be proficient, and to be given a certificate of proficiency. It was agreed that each society should appoint three members to the new conjoint examining board; that the board would appoint examiners, hold examinations, and determine requirements; that it would grant a certificate or diploma; and that the specialist societies should limit their membership to diplomates. The two specialist societies pledged not to admit members after 1920 unless they were board certified. The AMA section could not restrict entry, but agreed that from 1920 officeholders must be certified.[28] Thus the new certificate would have a direct relationship with society membership, as did the FACS with the American College of Surgeons.

The American Board for Ophthalmic Examinations, renamed the American Board of Ophthalmology in 1933, was formally created in 1916 and incorporated the following year. Edward Jackson was the first chairman. The first examinations were held in Memphis in December 1916, and two further examinations were held the following year; special stress was placed on refraction. At the three meetings, 120 certificates were awarded, of which only 28 were by examination. As with the American College of Surgeons, different methods of entry were used for different groups, including judgmental review alone of those with ten years' practice in ophthalmology; and as late as 1939 some eminent ophthalmologists were certified solely on their record.[29] The grandfather clause had become established. The board described its chief functions as being to establish *standards of fitness* to practice the specialty and to arrange, control, and conduct examinations to *test qualifications* and then confer

27. Quoted in full by Cordes and Rucker, "History of the American Board of Ophthalmology," pp. 250–51.
28. *Trans. Amer. Ophthal. Soc.*, 14 (1915), pt. 1, Minutes of Proceedings, pp. 30–33. *Trans. Sect. Ophthal. Amer. med. Ass.* (1915), pp. 230–232.
29. "Report for the American Board for Ophthalmic Examinations," *Trans. Amer. Acad. Ophthal. Otolaryng.* (1917), p. 213; Cordes and Rucker, "History of the American Board of Ophthalmology," pp. 251–53, 255, 260.

certificates on the qualified. It stated that it made no attempt to control practice by license or legal regulation: standards were to be maintained on a voluntary basis.[30]

The conjoint committee had not anticipated any wild stampede of candidates for the certificate. It did, however, hope to provide a widely accepted qualifying examination: a portal of entry to acknowledged specialist competence. Despite initial opposition and resentment against the idea of a self-constituted organization sitting in judgment over its peers,[31] the board was soon able to claim a sizable proportion of ophthalmic specialists—partly through judicious and continued use of the grandfather clause to attract leading practitioners into the group. The board had certified 501 physicians by the end of 1925. There were at that time about 900 ophthalmologists who restricted their practice to that specialty, and another 400 who gave it special attention; thus well over a third of those calling themselves specialists were board certified.[32]

The early diploma was intended to indicate a reasonable, even a minimal, standard of competence, not an advanced degree of skill. But the voluntary nature of the organization meant that those who chose not to enter the examination, or were not lured by the gift of a certificate, were outside the board's jurisdiction. The board was thus not able, at this time or later, to state categorically that those with the diploma were "safe" ophthalmologists and those without it were not. There continued to be a large group of inadequately trained ophthalmologists and a lack of legal or quasi-legal restrictions. This problem was inevitable in a system without sanctions, unless the medical schools, hospitals, and the public services were to restrict their appointments to those holding board certificates.

Thus began the first medical specialty board—a joint action of existing specialist associations, independent of the AMA, taking to itself responsibility for graduate education and qualifications in a self-delineated specialty. Meanwhile, graduate training was developing in the hospitals, and the AMA was being forced to consider its own role in regulating graduate as well as undergraduate medical education.

30. *American Board for Ophthalmic Examinations* (1925), p. 4; and reiterated in *American Board of Ophthalmology* (1950).
31. See e.g. the comments of Derrick T. Vail, in *Trans. Amer. Ophthal. Soc., 59* (1961), 329–41.
32. The figure of 501 comes from Cordes and Rucker, "History of the American Board of Ophthalmology," p. 263. Of the 501, about a third had passed the examinations; the others qualified on their record or through presentation of case reports. The number of specialists is estimated from Commission on Graduate Medical Education, *Graduate Medical Education,* p. 261, table 9.

CHAPTER 6

The American Medical Association and Specialization

The rapidity of organizational development in medicine before World War I epitomized the excitement and discovery of medicine itself. In quality, as well as in content, American medicine was transformed. One after another, physicians returned from the German clinics to practice, and to teach in American medical schools. Scientific experts jostled against the old-style practitioners. In the years between 1890 and 1914, American medical science was driven from mediocrity to eminence, paving the way for world leadership in medicine in the years following World War I. The change of emphasis from the largely commercialized practice of the turn of the century, fed from a multitude of second-rate schools to the specialized, university-dominated profession which characterized the years after World War I, was marked by overlapping, interweaving, and sometimes contradictory processes of organizational readjustment. In part, at least, this was because this rich period, by historical accident, marked the concurrent flowering of two potentially separate movements. On the one hand, reform of the medical schools, under the combined pressures of the AMA, the Flexner report, and state licensing regulations, was transforming the lackadaisical proprietary school into the modern medical center. On the other hand, the pressures to specialize were pushing physicians into new educational, regulatory, and practice forms. The proponents of both movements tended to be professors in the more progressive medical schools; but the aims were different, and there were some odd juxtapositions. Chicago, for example, was castigated in the Flexner report for the low state of its medical schools, yet at the same time it was developing as a center for surgery, as evinced by the popularity of the first Clinical Congress of American Surgeons. The prototype of the general practitioner might be thought of as the typical Midwestern physician, yet it was in Rochester, Minnesota, home of the Mayo Clinic, where much of the technical expertise of American specialization was to develop.

The professional organizations established in this crucial period reflected both the speed of scientific development and ambivalence as to where the practicing physician was headed. The AMA Council on Medical Education, the state licensing boards, and the voluntary National Board of Medical Examiners were engaged in realigning undergraduate medical education to produce a scientifically oriented all-around generalist. Yet of those graduating in 1915, only 23 percent would practice wholly as general practitioners; the remainder would either develop a specialist interest (36 percent) or limit themselves entirely to a specialty (41 percent).[1] As the medical colleges were reforming so as to produce a competent and modern general practitioner, the focus of medicine was turned to specialist skills. The premises of the Flexner report were thus rapidly becoming outmoded. The American College of Surgeons and the Board of Ophthalmic Examinations offered a prospect for further professionalism in the specialties. But while the future structure of specialist organization and specialty boards existed in embryo by the time of World War I, it was still far from clear who was to control specialist (graduate) medical education.

Signs of the inadequacy of undergraduate training alone as preparation for practice were evident in the rapid development of the hospital internship from the early years of the century, of the hospital residency for advanced students in specialties, of university programs, and of postgraduate courses and schools—the latter for general practitioners anxious to lessen their educational gaps and to acquire some specialist expertise. The examinations of the American College of Surgeons and of the Ophthalmic board were superimposed on this changing educational structure. As the basic licensing process was "solved," the scramble for specialization was on. The AMA had focused on the university as the center of medical training; it was doubtful whether it would be able to achieve the same domination of medical training at the graduate level which it had achieved so spectacularly in its undergraduate program. To do so would involve the extension of its influence over all aspects of medical practice, including the hospitals and the increasingly independent specialist groups.

THE AMA, THE INTERNSHIP, AND THE HOSPITAL

The first area of educational influence outside the university was the internship.[2] Following the example of Harvard in the 1870s, the medical

1. Commission on Medical Education, *Final Report,* p. 114, table 18.
2. The first use of the term "intern" in American hospital records is apparently in

schools had gradually abandoned their requirement of pre-medical-school apprenticeship. A postgraduate internship gradually filled this function by allowing the raw graduate to meet patients in a reasonably controlled institutional setting. Otherwise, since the didactic schools of the late nineteenth and early twentieth century had little access to clinical medicine, the young graduate learned bedside medicine (and surgery) on his first patients. For a number of reasons, including lack of work in the average hospital in the days before aseptic abdominal surgery and the appearance of a laboratory, and fear by the attending physicians of disputes between themselves and the house staff, there were few internships until the turn of the century. The Massachusetts General Hospital, for example, was without graduate house staff until 1911.[3] Those internships which did exist were competed for vigorously by the best students as the first rung on a ladder of distinction. The intern in a prestigious hospital might later be appointed to the outpatient, and then to the full attending staff, from which association he would draw professional recognition as an eminent specialist. House staffs tended to be divided between the medical and the surgical service, with training leaning primarily to one or the other. Such internships thus encouraged medical or surgical specialization. Medical internships were the more prestigious into the 1880s and went to the leading candidates. Howard Lilienthal, who in 1886 was the first intern at the Mount Sinai Hospital in New York ever to *choose* surgery over medicine, later remarked that his decision, even then, was received "as the equivalent of a social error." [4] The internship was thus part basic training, part an entry to specialization or consulting practice.

The boom in surgery at the end of the century had a radical impact on the role of the internship as well as in stimulating general hospital expansion. Aspiring surgeons sought hospital appointments for the necessary acquisition of operative techniques. In turn, the house officer became necessary to the hospital. He was needed to administer anesthetics, to act as "ambulance surgeon," to carry out simple laboratory tests, to serve in

---

the second annual report of the Board of Trustees of the Boston City Hospital in 1865—where the appointment of an ophthalmic intern is noted. Intern implied someone living in the hospital, extern someone living out. "Background and Development of Residency Review and Conference Committees," *J. Amer. med. Ass.,* 165 (1957), 60–64.

3. The Massachusetts General Hospital had been ahead of its time in appointing *graduate* house physicians and house surgeons as early as 1846. But three years later the older system was reintroduced, because the medical staff had become alarmed at the amount of authority the interns were assuming over patients. This shadow of professional competition continued at the MGH throughout the century. In 1877 it was declared that there was no work in the hospital for graduates to do; the hospital remained without a resident physician until 1911. Washburn, pp. 149–51, 156–68.

4. Hirsch and Doherty, pp. 77–78.

the increasing number of specialist departments and the clinics, and to help in the operations. By 1900 the house staff had become, at least in New York, the "real staff of every hospital in the city." [5] The competitive situation was reversed. Attending surgeons in New York City lured prospective surgical interns by promising them large numbers of operations. As even the lucrative major surgery was shared between them, a close relationship developed in New York between the younger attending surgeons and the surgical house staff. This had the effect of entrenching the house surgeon in the hospital system and of creating strong resistance to change.[6] The internship already had a twofold value; the provision of further education for the new graduate, who in turn would meet the staffing needs of the hospital.

By 1904, when the American Medical Association's Council on Medical Education first investigated the internship, it was thought that as many as 50 percent of new medical graduates went on to hospital training. Much of this "training" was, however, virtually unsupervised, and there were those who looked back with regret on the passing of the apprenticeship to a good practitioner.[7] The council recommended in 1905 that medical graduates take an internship in a hospital to complete their basic education. By 1914 it was estimated that 75 or 80 percent of graduates were taking an internship; indeed five colleges required an internship for the M.D. degree, and one state board (Pennsylvania) made it a requirement for licensing.[8] The four-year undergraduate curriculum suggested in the Flexner report included two years of clinical instruction and thus might be thought to obviate the need for an internship as part of a student's basic training. By 1925, however, twelve state boards had followed Pennsylvania's example; in 1932 the total was seventeen. In addition, fourteen medical schools required an internship before granting the M.D. degree, and over 95 percent of the graduates from schools which did not require internship—still the majority—were also said to be undertaking at least one year of hospital experience.[9] Since the internship was still regarded as the completion of the education of the general practitioner rather than the first rung on the ladder toward specialization, it was accepted as part of *undergraduate* rather than *graduate* education, and logically it should have been supervised by the medical schools. But only

5. Thomas J. Hillis, "The Hospital Governor and His Staff," *Med. News (N.Y.)*, 77 (1900), 4.
6. New York Committee on the Study of Internships and Residencies, *Internships and Residencies in New York City 1934–1937: Their Place in Medical Education* (New York, 1938), pp. 42–43.
7. Editorial, "The Education of the Interne," *J. Amer. med. Ass., 43* (1904), 469–70.
8. *Report of the Commissioner of Education, 1914*, p. 216.
9. Commission on Medical Education, *Final Report*, p. 141, tables 78, 80, 88.

rarely was this so. Instead, internships mushroomed at the whim of different hospitals, and there was clearly an argument for outside control.

The AMA Council on Medical Education made its first survey of internships in 1912. Although the council did not inspect all the hospitals, the survey was the first step to professional regulation. A list of approved training hospitals deriving from this survey was issued two years later, the first in a continuing series. The council's chairman, Arthur Dean Bevan, emphasized in 1913, when the purge of medical colleges was well under way, that the development of hospital teaching was "probably the most important active question before us in medical education." [10] As a result, the council began to shift its interest from the medical schools to the hospitals. The AMA had already developed a Section on Hospitals, which had as a major part of its responsibility a general listing of hospitals recognized by the association. It was, however, unable to exert the influence over hospitals which it had established over the undergraduate schools. A primary reason for this (over and above the increasing importance of hospitals themselves) was the interest in hospitals being expressed by other groups. During 1913 and 1914 both the AMA and the American College of Surgeons were considering hospital reform. The AMA hoped to receive a grant from the Carnegie Foundation to undertake intensive studies of hospitals in the thirty or forty largest population centers; but no grant was forthcoming. The AMA Board of Trustees turned down the suggestion by the American College of Surgeons that it take over responsibility for the expensive machinery of hospital regulation; Dr. Bevan himself raised no objection to the College's assuming the burden. Indeed, the relative poverty of the College in 1914 can have suggested to the AMA no great competition to its own activities in hospital standardization. But as a result, the AMA lost the initiative in the hospital standardization movement. The American College of Surgeons became the dominant force behind hospital reform, and Dr. Bevan was soon to regret his generosity.[11]

With the responsibility for hospital standardization—which meant, in effect, the specification of minimum standards of staff and equipment—established outside the AMA, the Council on Medical Education's role in hospital reform focused on the internship. In 1913 Dr. Bevan suggested that all internship programs be affiliated with medical schools, bringing the internship into the undergraduate educational orbit. In this way the internship would be in a similar relationship to the Council on Medical Education as was the undergraduate course; and in both, the council would act as a kind of guarantor of quality to the individual licensing

10. *AMA Bull.*, 8 (1913), 48–49.
11. Loyal Davis, *Fellowship of Surgeons*, pp. 157, 166–68, 175–76.

boards. He also suggested that internships might later be classified quali-
tatively as A, B, or C, along lines similar to the then existing classifications of medical schools.[12] However, these radical yet sensible suggestions
received little positive attention before World War I.

One of the difficulties which continued to beset the internship was that
it provided *experience* rather than education; it was also a necessary
corollary to medical school. By performing menial hospital jobs and
gradually working up to more responsible tasks, the raw graduate acquired a modicum of practical competence which otherwise he would
have had to gain on his own private patients. Even in the post-Flexner
schools the M.D. degree did not signify a "safe" general practitioner.
During World War I the surgeon general of the army required a year of
practical training in a hospital as a prerequisite to a commission in the
Medical Corps. Such safeguards were readily endorsed by the AMA. In
1919, the acting chairman of the Council on Medical Education noted
that the surgeon general's requirement had been a profound comfort to
parents with sons in the service: "One could not but shudder at the
thought of having his boy, seriously wounded perhaps, or desperately ill
with pneumonia, meningitis or some other serious disease, consigned to
the care of a young army surgeon, fresh from college, with no first-hand
experience at the bedside or in the operating room." [13]

With the internship established as a necessary part of medical education, the Flexner report's recommendation that medical education should
be a university function was in part frustrated. The products of the reformed medical schools were *not* on graduation complete physicians;
more and more, the final steps toward licensure were taken in hospitals,
most of which were independent of the universities. The aims of the M.D.
degree and the license thus diverged—and they have continued to do so.
Such divergence may however in the long run have strengthened the hand
of the medical schools, for as medical research centers they were no
longer solely concerned with undergraduate education and were gradually less interested in the general practitioner.

THE AMA, THE RESIDENCY, AND THE GRADUATE SCHOOLS

The concurrent growth of facilities for specialty training added yet another layer to the total system of medical education. For a chosen few
young physicians before World War I, there were residencies in the pres-

12. *AMA Bull., 8* (1913), 48–49.
13. Dr. John M. Dodson, "Fifteenth Annual Congress of the Council on Medical
Education," *AMA Bull., 13* (1919), 189.

tigious university hospitals, some of a standard to rival the more popular German training centers. The term "resident" was used at Johns Hopkins Hospital from the 1890s in the sense of a period of sustained specialty training following an internship, and the term gradually came into common use. Welch, Osler, and Halsted were influenced by the idea of the German university hospital "assistantship" for those likely to become specialists or professors. The structure was a pyramid; the weakest dropped out at each level. At Johns Hopkins a relatively large number of graduates were taken as interns, who competed for the residency. The resident could stay as long as he wanted; the others at his level usually resigned.[14] This system, which was adopted in other leading hospitals before World War I, was highly competitive, designed to produce researchers and teachers.

In the Middle West, the Mayo Clinic developed a similar system to that at Johns Hopkins, but based on private group practice rather than on the German type of university organization. In 1914, when the clinic itself was formally established, each senior clinician was made the head of a section in the division of medicine or surgery, while there was a centralized section of clinical pathology. The group already had a number of medical assistants. From 1912 on, these were called fellows; Dr. William Mayo had been unimpressed by the status of interns and residents in many Eastern hospitals: "They seemed to spend their days in subservient yessir-ing, in being flunkies for the permanent staff." [15] A three-year training plan was developed for the fellows, and from 1915 the Mayo Clinic was affiliated for graduate medical education with the University of Minnesota. The clinic was thus well prepared to meet the great expansion of specialism and graduate training in the years following World War I. It also established a strong precedent for *university*-based graduate education.

Outside the national centers, residencies were rare. Until 1920, they were usually found only in university-affiliated hospitals, and the main focus of specialist training remained in Europe. In the university hospitals, the resident could be part of a graduated team of chief, residents, interns, and students; the hospital thus had available to it a well-trained, full-time hierarchy of physicians. Even in university hospitals, however, the resident was generally regarded as a member of the hospital staff. He was not a university graduate student but more akin to an apprentice or a junior professional associate.

14. M. M. Davis, "The History of the Resident System," *Trans. Stud. Coll. Phycns. Philad.*, 27 (1959–60), 76–81.
15. Clapesattle, p. 521.

The existence of the hospital residency raised questions even before World War I as to the future locale of specialist training. The residency produced only a handful of specialists. By 1914 there were university graduate medical schools at Alabama, California, Tulane, Harvard, and Minnesota.[16] In addition, Abraham Flexner had counted thirteen independent postgraduate schools: they tended to give practical courses, chiefly in special areas, and to teach surgical and specialist techniques. These ranged from schools such as the New York Postgraduate School and Hospital (founded 1882) and the New York Polyclinic (also 1882) to their less reputable counterparts.[17] As the ophthalmologists' struggle had shown, there was considerable anxiety at the production of the "six-week specialist" from the latter, particularly where the organization offered a certificate or diploma which the graduate could display. Nor was this the sum of graduate training; postgraduate courses sponsored by various local medical societies offered a further channel.[18] It is impossible to distinguish how far such organizations and courses filled the need for what Flexner called "compensatory adjustment" and what is now called "continuing education," bringing the practitioner up to date, and how far they were in fact used as springboards to the specialties.

The generally uneven and confused patterns of specialist courses—from the medical society course to the three-year degree program in a medical specialty offered by the University of Minnesota—soon became a focus of attention for the AMA Council on Medical Education, thereby joining the AMA's interests in undergraduate medical education and in the internship. In December 1913, the Council on Medical Education appointed a committee, chaired by the dean of Harvard University Graduate Medical School, Dr. Horace D. Arnold, to investigate the status of

16. *Report of the Commissioner of Education, 1914,* p. 218.
17. The schools were in New York (4), Chicago (4), Philadelphia, Kansas City, New Orleans, and Washington, D.C. (2), the last for those accepted into the Army or Navy Medical Corps. Flexner report, pp. 174–77.
18. The AMA set up a postgraduate curriculum in 1907, planned to cover four years but so organized that it could be picked up at any point of the cycle. The course outline was printed in the *AMA Bulletin,* complete with references to journals and textbooks. The outline was designed for use by the county societies, as a formal program or a quiz class. It was thought that at least 200 local medical societies established postgraduate course in the first two years. These courses were intended to supplement the knowledge of the practicing physician. (They were also an encouragement to practitioners to join the medical societies.) These attempts were, however, sporadic and required constant local enthusiasm and supervision, often lacking. Continuing education went into a long period of apathy from which it is only just beginning to emerge. Editorial, "The Postgraduate Study Course," *AMA Bull., 8* (1912), 1–3; and see Burrow, p. 42 and passim.

graduate medical teaching. A preliminary report was made the following May. This committee, a mere four years after the Flexner report, conceded the inadequacy of a four-year medical course in giving the student any more than the elementary fundamentals of medicine. The burst of new knowledge had created a new educational crisis. Already elective courses were becoming common in the fourth year as a means of achieving a relative depth of study in one or two branches. The focus of vocational training was beginning to shift to graduate training; and here the need for standardization was as acute as it had been for undergraduates only a few years earlier. The question was how, and by whom, such standardization would be achieved. Dr. Arnold's committee, with its strong university orientation, recommended that the AMA regulate the graduate schools by approving them or not approving them—thus wiping out inferior graduate diplomas. The recommended philosophy was almost identical with the council's actions in relation to the undergraduate medical colleges. Commercialism in graduate medical education would be destroyed in the same way that it was being destroyed at the lower level; the graduate schools would be restrained from creating an undeserved elite. Graduate schools, it was suggested, would not be approved if they provided cram courses for licensing examinations, to make up deficiencies in undergraduate training of those from the poor medical schools. Thus the graduate schools would be brought into the AMA's network of rigorous educational upgrading and reform.[19]

In following these recommendations, the Council on Medical Education moved into the field of specialist education from a different point of view from that taken by the American College of Surgeons or the Board of Ophthalmic Examinations. Each of these organizations wanted to suppress the self-styled six-week specialist. But the council was extending its activities by proposing to eliminate the sources—the proprietary graduate schools—while the College set up an exemplary structure of fellowships which was designed to reduce the impact of the ill-trained man. The council's view would succeed only if the AMA could influence graduate education as a whole: not merely the proprietary schools, but the universities and the hospital training programs as well. To do this, however, standards for specialist training would first have to be set, and perhaps also a measurement and certification of accomplishment. Reporting in 1915, the council's Committee on Graduate Education recommended a systematic course of at least one year, for specialists, together with an-

19. "Preliminary Report of the Committee to Investigate Graduate Medical Instruction," *AMA Bull.,* 9 (1914), 313–18.

other year of supervised clinical experience, bringing the total educational period for specialists to seven years.[20] The AMA was emphatic that the basic responsibility for specialist education was, like undergraduate education, to be met by the universities, while the surgeons and ophthalmologists were seeking a predominantly professional solution.

PROBLEMS OF ORGANIZATIONAL OVERLAP

Both solutions implied the acceptance of a specialist label, be it certification by a specialist group or a higher university degree. There were, however, potential difficulties within the AMA if the Council on Medical Education went too far in the certification of specialists. The standardization movement had benefited the general practitioner by upgrading the status of physicians, thus promising to reduce his competition. AMA sponsorship of a caste system, however educationally justifiable and of however much public benefit, would run up against the GP's interests. There was a danger that a two-class system might develop. There was also an implicit problem in reconciling the aims of the general practitioner (the predominant AMA voter) with the aims of the professors on the Council on Medical Education. Was the much earlier split between teachers and practitioners to be revived within the AMA?

One aspect of the uncertain relationship between the general practitioner and the specialist in the years immediately before World War I was the role of the AMA specialist sections. The sections could be developed as associations of specialists (as they have since become); alternatively they could provide a forum through which specialist topics would be made available to all practitioners. In 1915 an AMA committee headed by Dr. Hugh Cabot reported that the latter function should be encouraged, to provide a scientific program for the general practitioner who otherwise had no scientific focus.[21] As a result, the Council on Scientific Assembly was established as an umbrella over all the sections. But the basic problems of the general practitioner remained, as did the AMA's organizational dichotomy and its commitment to a standardized profession.

There were also problems of relationship implicit in the AMA's attitude toward outside specialist groups. The American College of Surgeons had developed a close and overlapping membership with the association. But, in prescribing the standards for a surgeon, in assuming regulatory

20. See N. P. Colwell, "Medical Education, 1915," *Report of the Commissioner of Education, 1915,* Vol. 1, pp. 205–10.
21. Fishbein, pp. 287–88.

authority over his training, and in certifying competence, the College had annexed an educational area which the AMA had at the undergraduate level considered its own. The College had also accepted the responsibility for surveying and classifying hospitals. In many areas, then, the College had become a strong potential competitive force. In spite of this, open disputes between the College and the AMA did not arise until 1917, when Arthur Dean Bevan was AMA president-elect.

By 1917 the College was well established, with 3,800 fellows, a flourishing hospital standardization program, and the incomparable leadership of Franklin Martin. Martin, with his inimitable flair, stole the lead on the AMA by assuming medical leadership for wartime needs. He was one of seven members appointed by President Wilson (in October 1916) to his Advisory Commission of the Council on National Defense. He was the only physician on that committee, and thus an important spokesman for organized medicine. His appointment brought the American College of Surgeons into national prominence and gave it the ultimate seal of public respectability. Martin created the General Medical Board of the Council of National Defense, representative of the *entire* profession, and he set up the Volunteer Medical Service Corps without reference to AMA records. This was too much for certain groups within the AMA, including Dr. Bevan. The Chicago Medical Society (Bevan's home base) urged physicians not to join the Volunteer Corps, but this was hardly likely to provoke public enthuiasm. Nor was Bevan's unsuccessful appeal to President Wilson for Martin's removal.[22] The surgeons general of the army, navy, and U.S. Public Health Service were present at the sixth convocation of the College held in October 1917; the fellowship address was given by Sir Berkely Moynihan, colonel in the British Royal Army Medical Corps; the secretary of the U.S. Navy (Josephus Daniel) was a surprise speaker; President Wilson sent a telegram of greeting; and the final touch was the presence of John Philip Sousa and his band.[23] The AMA had been outmaneuvered in an area that could only bring national acclaim.

Dr. Bevan had good cause to be piqued by the success of the American College of Surgeons. The AMA, a democratic organization, could be weakened by the emergence of strong medical splinter groups. The undergraduate educational movement, which Bevan himself had led, was recognized as the purview primarily of the AMA Council on Medical Education; and graduate education was increasingly becoming the extension of

22. Loyal Davis, *Fellowship of Surgeons*, pp. 198, 214–15.
23. Michael L. Mason, "Significance of the American College of Surgeons to Progress of Surgery in America," *Amer. J. Surg., 51* (1941), 267–86. And see Loyal Davis, *Fellowship of Surgeons*, pp. 191–92; Fishbein, p. 300.

the undergraduate training period. Hospital services were not limited to surgery, as Bevan himself was quick to point out in 1917[24]; yet through its standardization program the American College of Surgeons was touching on all areas of medicine. In his inaugural address as president of the AMA in June 1918, Bevan asked pointedly, "Who represents the medical profession?" [25] If the AMA wished to reassert its leadership in the postwar period, it would have to offer a real challenge in the graduate field. The AMA had risen because of its educational reforms; its political force would be diminished if it lost its leadership in training.

Professional politics apart, there were strong reasons for some national group to organize the graduate field. There was a very real danger of fragmentation of professional qualifications if there were not one general educational leadership. The creation of the ophthalmic board emphasized this point. If the AMA Council on Medical Education could achieve its goal of university-centered specialist qualifications, a goal reiterated in 1917 despite the disappointing results of a survey of graduate education made by the AMA between 1913 and 1915, there would at least be common educational foci for all specialties.[26]

But the AMA was not alone in this concern. While the Council on Medical Education was approaching specialist training through the medical schools, the state licensing of surgeons and other specialists was being discussed. Licensing legislation itself was not passed, but the fragmentary movement in specialization presaged by the American College of Surgeons suggested to the National Board of Medical Examiners that it too might have a role here. Even before the National Board was founded in 1915, Dr. William Rodman had perceived the potential of a national structure which would conduct examinations not only at the standard of licensure but also in relation to specialist functions. Rodman spoke in 1914 of the possibility of a specialist who wished to move from one state to another being given not the whole licensing examination but a thorough examination in his own specialty[27]—an idea, incidentally, which reappeared as novel in 1968. This was only one aspect of the desire for specialist identification; but it was one of practical importance, and it linked the questions of licensure, training, and certification. As early as 1917, the National Board—a qualifying rather than a licensing agency—

24. "Conference on Hospital Standardization," *Bull. Amer. Coll. Surg., 3* (1917), 16–17.
25. Arthur Dean Bevan, "The Organization of the Medical Profession for War," *J. Amer. med. Ass., 70* (1918), 1806.
26. See Horace D. Arnold, "The Problem of Higher Degrees in Medicine," and discussion, *AMA Bull., 12* (1917), 207–12.
27. *AMA Bull., 9* (1914), 326.

began to consider offering specialist examinations.[28] It was in a strategic position to do so. It was already an examining agency; it was not troubled with the increasing medicopolitical problems of the AMA; and in its examinations of undergraduates it covered the whole field of medicine.

By 1917 the AMA, the American College of Surgeons, the Board of Ophthalmic Examinations, and the National Board of Medical Examiners were thus all actively concerned in one way or another with the graduate education of physicians. None could claim preeminence.

THE IMPLICATIONS OF WORLD WAR I

It was at this indeterminate stage that the United States entered World War I, and the problems of specialism were thrown sharply into focus. Indeed, specialism thrived in wartime conditions, and the general practitioner continued to lose ground. Organizational foci for specialism developed in the European base hospitals. Public awareness of the existence of well-trained specialists increased. At the same time, German preeminence in specialist training was brought to an abrupt halt, and large numbers of so-called specialists in the armed forces were revealed publicly as inadequately trained. The army acted as a filtering system for quality. No one reached the medical training camps unless they were initially felt to be desirable (thus eliminating the obviously incompetent, the sick, those of bad character, alcoholics, drug addicts, and so on), were from reputable medical colleges, were licensed to practice in the state in which they lived, were already in active practice, and had passed an examination before a local board. At the camps many more were rejected; physical unfitness rather than professional incompetence was used as the reason for rejection wherever possible, to avoid embarrassment.

Specialist qualifications received searching examination. The surgeon general's office card-indexed men whose reputation seemed to warrant their acceptance as specialists, but so many were found to be overrated that the specialists' divisions agreed to make specialist appointments conditional on examination. The results were appalling. Some of the "specialists" examined were found to be unfit to practice any branch of medicine in the service. A study of the examination results at Camp Greenleaf in 1918 revealed only one medical officer in three qualified to do independent surgery, and only about 6 percent were rated as high-class surgeons; there was a similarly small proportion of really high-grade men in internal medicine. Seventy percent of the otolaryngologists, 51 percent of the ophthalmologists, and 38 percent of those who said they were plastic

28. Minutes of the National Board of Medical Examiners, 7 June, 1917, p. 97.

and oral surgeons were rejected.[29] Thus the extent of educational deficiency was glaringly acknowledged—and at the same time directly linked with the potential danger to the public if such practices were to continue.

All these factors were to deepen concern over the preparation and role of the specialist in postwar prosperity, not only in relation to the kinds of intraprofessional questions which had stimulated the surgeons and ophthalmologists to develop separate organizations but also in relation to the provision of high-quality medical care to the public.

THE AMA TAKES STOCK

The Council on Medical Education determined after the war to expand its graduate educational role in relation to the internship, the hospital, and the universities. The council was at a pivotal position. The AMA had succeeded in its general organizational development and membership expansion in large part through the council's successes; the council therefore had more than an educational importance—it had become the focus for reform. Now, however, its work in undergraduate education had reached the routine stage; the crucial problems of education were clearly at the graduate level. At the end of the war it was obvious that the structure of the medical profession had changed, and changed toward specialism. It was also clear that medicine had increasingly to be regarded as a public concern. But the AMA had lost its momentum. In 1918 it was engaged in a power struggle over the position of president-elect; its general political functions were in need of revival; and some of the earlier enthusiasm for the association had waned.[30] Thus the desire to extend the council's work was part of a general reassessment of the AMA's role, and of its functions in public policy and in relation to other professional organizations.

In 1918 Arthur Dean Bevan announced that the Council on Medical Education would broaden its role to include hospital standardization—a direct challenge to the American College of Surgeons. Franklin Martin was furious. William Mayo attempted to bring peace to the profession through constructive meetings between the College and the AMA; the result was that in 1919 the two secretaries, Colwell (of the Council on Medical Education) and Bowman (of the American College of Surgeons) were directed to keep in touch with each other. But the College continued to bear the increasingly heavy responsibility for approving and upgrading

29. Col. Edward L. Munson, MC, U.S. Army, "The Needs of Medical Education as Revealed by the War," *AMA Bull., 13* (1919), 204–13.
30. Burrow, pp. 51, 65, and passim.

hospitals; and the AMA continued to complain. In 1919 the American
College of Surgeons produced its first list of approved hospitals and
adopted a code of minimum standards. But the list, which followed Bowman's visits in 1918 and 1919, was suppressed by the College because of
the horrifying conditions he had encountered; many of the larger, and
supposedly better, hospitals could not meet the standards Bowman regarded as minimal. In May 1920 the Carnegie Foundation, which had
already bestowed an initial grant of $30,000 on the College for its hos-
pital program, gave it a matching grant of $25,000 a year.[31] The Council
on Medical Education may well have been annoyed by the action of the
foundation which had previously supported its own activities. The AMA
organized a rival hospital conference, but the American College of Surgeons declined to participate on the reasonable grounds that it was unnecessary. But the AMA refused to be edged out of the hospital field, and
in June 1920 the council was renamed the Council on Medical Education
and Hospitals.[32]

Meanwhile the council was busy reassessing graduate education. In
1919, it brought out for the first time its own standards for internships,
"The Essentials of an Approved Internship," which were to be observed
by hospitals before their intern posts would be approved by the council.
The Essentials gave the council a legitimate role in general hospital approval—albeit one restricted to the needs of medical education rather
than of the patients being served. Simultaneously, the council launched a
reinspection of the graduate medical schools. This was done during 1919
by Dr. Bevan, accompanied by Dr. Louis B. Wilson of the Mayo Foundation and assisted in some cases by other members of the committee.[33]
The high-powered graduate committee, which included Finney of the
American College of Surgeons and Edward Jackson of the Ophthalmic
Board as well as other university educators, reported in February 1920.
It found that most of the graduate courses offered were short (from two
to twelve weeks) extension courses rather than complete specialist training. It was also found that the only real university graduate work in medicine was being done in association with the undergraduate, not the graduate, medical schools. In the class A undergraduate medical schools
2,014 graduates were found: 414 in the laboratory branches, 929 in surgery, 671 in fields of medicine. Even their position was not satisfactory.
There were too few positions, meager stipends, too much routine work,

31. Loyal Davis, *Fellowship of Surgeons,* p. 230.
32. The council was entitled the AMA Council on Medical Education and Hospitals from 1920 until 1964, when it reverted to the name Council on Medical Education.
33. *J. Amer. med. Ass., 73* (1919), 1955–57.

poor grounding in basic sciences, and a "self-satisfied provincialism." [34]
The graduates typically worked as apprentices to the great men on the
medical school faculty and were in little direct relationship with the university.

There was thus no ready system for the development of specialist education. If the universities were even to make up the deficiencies caused
by the decline of German specialist education, great expansion was necessary. During 1919, the Mayo Foundation (the graduate educational link
between the Mayo Clinic and the University of Minnesota) received over
1,000 inquiries for graduate work. In the country at large there were already some 4,000 long-term graduate students in medicine. It was also
estimated that another 6,000 graduates would seek short-term courses,
either to round out their undergraduate training or to learn a specialist
technique.[35] Could the universities cope with this expansion? On the evidence, it seemed unlikely—unless perhaps there was financial subsidy to
the schools for graduate education of similar magnitude to that received
from foundations for undergraduate education following the publication
of the Flexner report.

Dr. Wilson's committee, following his own success at the Mayo Foundation, suggested the establishment of strong university graduate medical
departments with a separate faculty and access to both general and special
hospitals, and staffed by full-time teachers. The Council on Medical Education concurred with the Association of American Medical Colleges,
which had also been studying graduate degrees, that university graduate
medical education should be restricted to the M.S. and the Ph.D., the
latter being for independent research. This was the pattern already in
operation throughout the Mayo Foundation except that the Ph.D. was
also granted for clinical work.[36] In essence, therefore, the views of the
Council on Medical Education were imitative. Undergraduate medical
education had been modeled on Johns Hopkins; graduate education was
to follow the Mayo Clinic.

But the pronouncement of ideals was not the same as their implementation. The basic issue in specialist training—as it was later to be in the
certification of competence—was the continued lack of professional or

34. Louis B. Wilson, "Report of Committee on Graduate Medical Education,"
AMA *Bull., 14* (1920), 58–67. Dr. Wilson, who was then chairman of the council's
special committee on graduate medical education, was to be a dominant figure in
the structural emergence of specialist education in the 1920s and 1930s. He played,
in relation to graduate education, the central role which Bevan had asserted in the
undergraduate reforms.
35. Ibid., pp. 65–66.
36. *Proc. Ass. Amer. med. Coll.* (1919), pp. 32–38.

university leverage. The amount of specialization depended on the exercise of the individual choice of each physician. It could not be entirely controlled, as could undergraduate training, through regulation of the medical schools. If only a small minority of physicians wished to specialize, as the leaders of the profession seemed to think, then expanded university graduate program might suffice; all specialists could be university trained. If not, many specialists would continue to train outside the direct auspices of a university. Without licensing, or quasi-mandatory certification (such as the limitation of hospital or public appointments to university-trained specialists) the AMA had no means of controlling the numerical balance between those content to be general practitioners and those striving toward specialization.

CHAPTER 7

The Public Interest and the Profession

The medical profession was not developing in a vacuum and its problems were not unique; they were part of a rapidly changing medical environment. The impact of the advanced technical skills, equipment, and knowledge in medicine developed before and during World War I made medicine more valuable to society, and also more expensive for the individual. The interests of the medical profession and the public were thus inextricably intertwined. Public concern over standards of health in the population was demonstrated in the establishment of programs and associations for tuberculosis, venereal disease, and public health nursing in the early years of the century.[1] That concern was aggravated by reports of the low health standards of school children and of the large number of men rejected by the draft.[2] The federal government entered the business of providing medical care for the armed services on a large scale during the war, and its programs for veterans set up after the war created a new dimension in the public provision of health services.[3] Expenditures in-

1. Among the earliest voluntary health agencies were the American Public Health Association (1872) and the National Tuberculosis Association (1904). By 1930 there were 20 or more such agencies of national scope. On public health nursing see "Report of the Committee for the Study of Nursing Education" and "Report of a Survey by Josephine Goldmark," *Nursing and Nursing Education in the United States* (New York: Macmillan, 1923), pp. 40–42 and passim.
2. About 25 percent of the draftees examined were rejected for military duty; however, over 46 percent were revealed to have some physical or mental defect. Quoted in Commission on Medical Education, *Preliminary Report,* p. 22.
3. Before World War I medical care of veterans was limited to domiciliary care of those disabled during or because of their service. In 1917, however, Congress gave disabled veterans the right to receive medical services irrespective of their domiciliary status. The new legislation initially included hospital care and orthopedic appliances for service-connected disabilities. Services were expanded in 1922 and 1924 to include hospital care for veterans of all wars for conditions which were not associated with their experience in the armed services. The construction of veterans hospitals, the establishment in 1922 of a new government agency, the United States Veterans Bureau, to supervise federal expenditures for veterans, and the extension of medical care entitlements brought the federal government into a potentially vast

creased. The provision of medical care to the population as a whole was beginning its long transition from a luxury to a necessity, from a privilege to a right.

Medicine was no longer the private profession it had been. Its organizational spokesmen were forced to consider not merely traditional professional functions—the ethical and educational regulation of the medical profession and the safeguarding of the profession's interests—but to involve themselves with the whole panoply of the organization, financing, and delivery of medical services. Medical education was central to this process. The training and certification of specialists was part and parcel of organizational considerations. Any system for delineating who was a medical specialist (and thus, by implication, who was not) had long-term ramifications in respect to overall manpower development, the means for coordination of specialist and generalist skills, and the optimal geographical and functional distribution of physicians. By no means least, there was the assumption that the profession would guarantee to the public that medical specialists were in fact well trained and of acceptable competence. The greater the public interest in medical care, the more important these issues would be.

THE PUBLIC'S INTEREST

Professionalism in medicine had developed around the private practice of medicine, whose model was a one-to-one relationship between practitioner and patient and whose financial transaction was an individually determined fee. Schematically, the health service "system" so represented could be drawn as a series of unconnected dots—each dot being one physician—scattered across the surface of a map, with concentrations of dots in the major cities. The boom in hospital building in the late years of the nineteenth and the early years of the twentieth century modified the pattern by offering many physicians a link in their common use of facilities; the hospital became a potential future coordinator of health services. But, with very few exceptions, independent solo private practice on a fee-for-service basis remained as the design of medical care through World War I—and was to linger for long after.

Such a system was well suited to medicine so long as it remained the province of the family doctor. Even before World War I, however, the family doctor was fast disappearing. There were, it is true, still large

---

field of general medical provision for one sector of the population. See Bernhard J. Stern, *Medical Services by Government:* Local, State and Federal (New York, 1946), pp. 175–79.

numbers of general practitioners, but except in isolated rural areas, these were no longer acting as the patient's only, or even primary, medical adviser. Both the mobility of the population and the desirability of medical specialization undermined what was later regarded as the traditional relationship between one doctor and one patient. Abraham Jacobi's description of the family doctor, "the chum of the old people, the intimate of confiding girlhood, the uncle and oracle of the kids," referred to a vanishing breed.[4] People who could afford to, increasingly chose specialists—internists, obstetricians, pediatricians, skin specialists, ophthalmologists, neurologists, orthopedic surgeons—in many cases calling on the specialists directly and not searching them out through the offices of a general practitioner. At the other end of the social spectrum, burgeoning hospital dispensaries and clinics offered specialist services to the poor, who in turn provided teaching and research opportunities for specialists to advance their skills and practices. The mass of wage earners, excluded from the dispensaries by the operation of their means tests and often unable to afford private specialist fees, fell into some kind of no-man's-land. It was this group who, virtually by default, made the most use of general practitioners.

There were thus already, before World War I, pressures on the traditional organization of medical care. The success of scientific medicine was pushing physicians and others toward specialization, yet specialist care was largely uncoordinated; hospitals and dispensaries were beginning to offer institutional foci for medical services, yet were being used by only part of the population. The future roles of the hospital, the family doctor, and the specialist were in doubt.

The expansion of new health professions added to the confusion. Besides optometrists there were X-ray technicians and laboratory workers, in private and in hospital practice. Social workers were appearing in hospitals; there were over 100 social services departments in hospitals and dispensaries by 1912.[5] Orthopedic surgeons, particularly in Boston, New York, and Philadelphia, were training young women graduates of schools of physical education to care for patients in their offices or in hospitals; these were followed by formal courses in physical therapy at the outbreak of World War I.[6] Following the example of the Mayo Clinic,

4. Quoted by M. M. Davis, "The Organization of Medical Service," *Amer. Labor Legisl. Review, 6* (1916), 16–20. And see this article for an excellent review of the status of medical practice at the time.
5. Ida M. Cannon, *Social Work in Hospitals: A Contribution to Progressive Medicine* (New York, 1913), p. 3.
6. These women treated thousands of "paralyzed" patients in the East Coast poli-

nurse anesthetists were being trained in the larger teaching centers, initially in the Midwest, but spreading rapidly throughout the country; of four formal programs established before World War I, one was in Portland, Oregon, and one in New York City.[7] These and other aides provided a type of vertical specialization which, while expanding the individual doctor's reach, contributed to increasing organizational complexity. Solo private practice by general practitioners was already becoming out of date; today's organizational issues in medicine were, on a small scale, already evident.

Organizational complexity was one result of the enormous strides in pure and applied medical science which in turn demanded specialization. Before about 1915, it has been suggested, the average person had little more than a fifty-fifty chance of benefiting from an encounter with the average doctor.[8] Under the impact of new knowledge, the rapid improvement of the medical schools, and the proliferation of hospitals and clinics which in turn generated new information, medicine was becoming vastly more efficient. Its efficiency was, however, frustrated by organizational and social constraints. The orthopedic surgeon might prescribe a brace; then the social worker would discover that the patient was starving himself to pay for it. The clerk or production worker might choose not to buy expensive drugs and avoid a needed specialist because of additional medical bills. The net health gain was thus lower than technological improvements alone would indicate. In the long term, the replacement of an uncoordinated system of general practitioners by an uncoordinated system of specialists would demand radical organizational realignments. In the short term, the *cost* of medical care was the most vital issue. To the individual, this was a question of how he could pay his medical bills. To society in general, denial of medical services meant increased welfare payments and lack of production due to time lost from work through sick-

---

omyelitis epidemic of 1916. But the aides were neither formally trained nor organized until World War I. A course in physical therapy was given to nonmedical personnel at Walter Reed Army Hospital soon after war was declared; this was followed by 14 other wartime courses, all producing "Reconstruction Aides." Some 800 physical therapists were produced, but many returned to other kinds of work after the war. In 1921 the American Women's Therapeutic Association was founded, becoming the American Physiotherapy Association in 1922, and in 1948 the present American Physical Therapy Association. American Physical Therapy Association, historical pamphlets and personal communication.

7. American Association of Nurse Anesthetists, *Notes on the History and Organization of the American Association of Nurse Anesthetists* (Chicago, 1966), pp. 6–7.

8. Lawrence J. Henderson quoted by Alan Gregg, *Challenges to Contemporary Medicine* (New York, 1956), p. 13.

ness; and the misery of unalleviated sickness which, while not translatable into dollar terms, was inevitably a loss of happiness.[9]

Public responsibility for the protection of health had been expressed in the second half of the nineteenth century in the provision of public health departments and services in the booming cities: in sewage systems, the reporting and prevention of communicable disease, and clean water supplies. In the early years of the twentieth century—as the political climate of the country changed from the laissez-faire individualism of the nineteenth century to a mood which at least tolerated collective action in the public interest, personified especially by the Progressive movement in the second decade of this century—these environmental programs were joined by more direct forms of health protection, under the stimulus of increasingly powerful consumer groups. Federal legislation regulating the food and drug industry was passed in 1906, after seven years of exposures of food and chemical processes in the popular press, and with support from a number of voluntary organizations, including the AMA; the same year a meat inspection act was passed. It was largely due to the efforts of women's groups that the Childrens Bureau was established within the Department of Labor in 1912.

Meanwhile numbers of organizations were studying the development of European social security schemes which were beginning to cover the working population for accident insurance, old-age pensions, sickness insurance, and health benefits. With the encouragement of President Theodore Roosevelt, the first federal workmen's compensation act was passed in 1908, for civil employees of the government. Between 1910 and 1915, workmen's compensation laws were enacted in thirty states.[10] The American Association for Labor Legislation, organized in 1906, established its own Committee on Social Insurance in 1912. Health insurance was considered the next logical step after workmen's compensation in the provision of a comprehensive social insurance program, and from 1913 became the focus of the committee's efforts.[11]

The health insurance movement, which flourished between 1913 and 1918, was thus the product of two converging developments, the tech-

9. For a contemporary analysis see Haven Emerson, "The Social Cost of Sickness," *Amer. Labor Legisl. Review, 6* (1916), 11–15.
10. Herman M. Somers and Anne R. Somers, *Workmen's Compensation* (New York, 1954), p. 34.
11. Excellent reviews of the development of the early health insurance movement are Odin W. Anderson's "Health Insurance in the United States 1910–1920," *J. Hist. Med. Allied Sci., 5* (1950), 363–96; and Arthur J. Viseltear's "Compulsory Health Insurance in California 1915–1918," ibid., *24* (1969), 151–82. For the social insurance movement as a whole see Roy Lubove, *Struggle for Social Security 1900–1935* (Cambridge, Mass., 1968).

nological and the social. Changes in the content, organization, value, and costs of medical care pointed toward some kind of insurance or group payment for medical bills, irrespective of prevailing political attitudes. The individual could predict neither his future needs for medical care nor the costs he would incur. Spreading the financial risks over a large number of people was thus logical; the arguments for health insurance were similar to those for life or fire insurance. From 1911, insurance companies began to offer "group coverage" for large industrial populations under a blanket policy, usually associated with life insurance, which included specified protection against accidents and sickness, and typically including nursing service. A few industrial and railroad companies had set up their own medical plans covering specified medical benefits, as had a number of unions, fraternal orders, and other organizations. Prepaid practice was also operating on a small scale at Johns Hopkins and the Massachusetts General Hospital.[12] The total amount of voluntary health insurance and contract practice was, however, minute before World War I, and it was into this vacuum that compulsory health insurance fell— part of a broader Social Security movement, which was itself a reflection of collective public activity in the Progressive era to safeguard individuals against loss of earnings. On the one hand, therefore, specialization in medicine was indicating the development of a more organized system of medical services. On the other, proponents of compulsory social insurance were arguing for organized group *payment* for medical care, irrespective of whether the services themselves were reorganized.

Under the leadership of the American Association for Labor Legislation, and with the support of the AMA, official investigation of health insurance was organized in eight states between 1915 and 1918, and a standard health insurance bill was introduced in fifteen states in 1917. Lengthy reports from the AMA's own Committee on Social Insurance, organized in 1916 with Isaac Rubinow as its secretary, provided detailed information on insurance schemes in other countries and were favorable in tone. The committee noted in 1916 that Lloyd George's Health Insurance Act in England (1911) had "unquestionably improved the condition of the working classes which have come under the law." [13] Interest in health insurance had, however, passed its peak by 1918. No health insurance act reached the statute books.

In the meantime opposition to compulsory health insurance had rallied,

12. Pierce Williams, *The Purchase of Medical Care through Fixed Periodic Payments,* Committee on the Costs of Medical Care Abstract no. C2 (Washington, D.C., 1932), pp. 14–15.
13. "Report of Committee on Social Insurance," *AMA Bull., 11* (1916), 354 and passim.

not only within the medical profession but also from commercial insurance companies, employers' associations, organized labor, and other groups. Both workers and employers were chary of the contributions which they would be required to pay under health insurance. But the objections were not merely financial. The Progressive tide was ebbing. Belief in direct governmental intervention to guarantee the individual's economic position was challenged by those who regarded an enlarged governmental role as undesirable paternalism. Compulsory health insurance was attacked from different quarters as being class legislation, socialistic, tyrannical, and, in the surge of nationalism as the United States entered the war, as "un-American" and "German."

The attitude of the medical profession toward health insurance reflected the confusion which existed both in medical practice itself and in the larger political debates. Before 1920, the American Medical Association was by no means against government intervention in health. The association had fought vigorously on behalf of food and drug legislation. From 1905 its Council on Pharmacy and Chemistry worked closely with the Department of Agriculture's Bureau of Chemistry to obtain legislation to put down medical quackery. The AMA campaigned for a national health department and favored the establishment of the Children's Bureau.[14] Until 1920, moreover, the AMA appeared to be in favor of legislation for compulsory social insurance. Overall, however, the AMA's position on public issues was not clearly defined. The impetus for social reform, even in areas touching medicine, was largely from outside the medical profession. With much of its energies absorbed by its own program of internal consolidation and professional education, the association acted more as a reactor to pieces of legislation than as an initiator of social change.

At the same time, there was growing realization that compulsory health insurance programs were a threat to private practice—and thus struck at the very basis of medical professionalism. Health insurance would require participating physicians to accept fee schedules, regulations, possible work reviews. It would set up an organization outside the doctor-patient relationship, over which the individual physician would have no control. It might limit the patient's choice of physician. One physician described the proposed California legislation in 1916 as "an assault upon the rights of every man practicing medicine in the State of California." [15]

14. For a review of AMA activities vis-à-vis federal legislation, see Burrow, pp. 54–131, 139.
15. D. M. Gedge, "The Proposed Social Health Insurance Act," *Calif. Med.*, 14 (1916), 445–47; quoted by Viseltear, "Compulsory Health Insurance," p. 164.

Thus the interests of professionalism diverged from the pressures for social action.

It was only, however, after World War I that AMA opposition to compulsory insurance was fully articulated. From 1918 an increasing number of articles antagonistic to health insurance appeared in the AMA *Journal*. The Committee on Social Insurance was reorganized in 1919, giving it a more conservative outlook; Rubinow was removed. While arguments both for and against health insurance were presented at the AMA meeting in Atlantic City in 1919, the following year the seal was set. The publication of articles by Malcolm Harris (a member of the Social Insurance Committee strongly opposed to legislation) in 1920, the failure of a health insurance bill in the state of New York (leaving no state with compulsory insurance as a live issue), and an AMA resolution at its annual meeting in New Orleans opposing compulsory health insurance solidified the profession against such government intervention.[16] Health insurance was seen not only to threaten the individual practitioner but also to divide the hard-won unity of the profession. Opposition to it during the 1920s and after provided the AMA with a new rallying cry for its organizational dominance of medicine.

SPECIALIZATION AND GROUP PRACTICE

Compulsory health insurance failed in the United States at a time when it was becoming commonplace in western Europe. The organizational implications, however, remained. In England, the health insurance scheme shored up the position of the general practitioner as the patient's doctor of first call, providing one element in the continuance of a relatively large number of general practitioners in England to this day. This mechanism was not available in the United States. Instead of the European medical care system, in which one physician would (at least in theory) provide the patient's primary point of reference and be the conduit between the patient and the specialists, there had developed in the United States a system in which generalists and specialists competed for the same patients.

Questions of the future coordination of these largely disconnected physician services were intensified during World War I. There were approximately 148,000 physicians in the United States in 1918. During the war, nearly 35,000 of these—a fourth—served in the army or navy; over 18,000 were sent abroad.[17] They included eminent specialists as

16. See Burrow, pp. 141–51.
17. Lewis Stephen Pilcher, "The Influence of War Surgery upon Civil Practice," *Ann. Surg., 69* (1919), 565.

well as young graduates: Hugh Young organizing urological services in
Europe, Harvey Cushing establishing a base hospital in France, George
Crile working in Rouen, W. H. Welch advising Surgeon General
Gorgas.[18]

Techniques and specialties were improved, particularly in psychiatry,
orthopedics, and plastic surgery, and the phrase "physical medicine and
reconstruction" came into general use for the first time—heralding the
mixed blessing of machine therapy in the 1920s.[19] But of greater long-
term significance than the technological advances was the social change
imposed upon physicians in wartime: upon the surgeons rather than upon
surgery. Physicians from all parts of the country were brought together,
evaluated, sent through medical camps, and commissioned in a large,
highly organized medical system based on hospitals. The younger generation of physicians, affected by the specialization, teamwork, and organizational efficiency of wartime medicine, might be expected to return to
peacetime conditions with a different view of medicine from that of their
older, pre-Flexner colleagues.

The increasing specialization of physicians made some form of practice coordination logical. By 1923, over 15,000 physicians listed themselves in the AMA directory as being full-time specialists; six years
later the figure was over 22,000. If those who regarded themselves as
part-time specialists are added in, some 30 percent of all active physicians
were at least partial specialists.[20] By far the largest specialty group
throughout the 1920s was general surgery. But specialty interests ranged
wide. There were now anesthesiologists, pediatricians, orthopedic surgeons, proctologists, radiologists, dermatologists, neurologists, ophthalmologists, and pathologists. There were specialists who confined themselves to obstetrics, others who were gynecologists, and a third group who
practiced in both areas. The specialties of eye, ear, nose, and throat appeared in various combinations. The fragmentary motion of modern
medicine was already evident. In all, twenty-three specialist fields could
be counted by 1923. While there was every argument for an individual
physician to work up special interests so that he could advance his own
competence and skills and thus offer potentially better care to his patients,
there was little coordination and cross-reference of such skills.

18. See Hugh Young, pp. 272–312; John F. Fulton, *Harvey Cushing,* pp. 419–21;
Flexner and Flexner, pp. 370–96; Grace Crile, ed., *George Crile: An Autobiography*
(Philadelphia, 1947), vol. 1, pp. 247–306; vol. 2, pp. 307–68.
19. See Harry E. Mock, "The Council on Physical Therapy of the American Medical Association," *Proc. Ann. Cong. med. Educ.* (1933), pp. 22–27.
20. Commission on Graduate Medical Education, *Graduate Medical Education,*
table 9, p. 261.

The typical solo practice of before World War I had relied on informal consultation and referral (sometimes formalized between general practitioner and surgeon by fee splitting). The patient presented himself to a physician, after making a choice of specialist on his own judgment, or he was referred from one physician to another. In the course of a year, a person might call upon four or five different specialists—even before World War I—and there might be little coordination of treatment among these specialists.

Group practice by specialists existed before World War I, the Mayo Clinic being the outstanding example, but groups were few and far between. A team of physicians in several fields working together out of one facility, with the convenience of interspecialty consultation and the use of common services, could offer to the patient both the wide array of interests available under the whole rubric "medicine" and the technical efficiency of specialists. Specialization could thus be continued in an organizational form which would substitute for the old general practitioner. Such patterns of cooperative practice were experienced by many physicians during World War I. Dr. John Dodson, acting chairman of the Council on Medical Education in 1919, was one who thought the wartime patterns marked a new mode of delivery and that returning practitioners, having experienced the accurate scientific work possible in the wartime group practices of specialists, would disdain solo practice in the postwar world.[21] Arthur Dean Bevan, who was then president of the AMA, also seemed to favor hospital-based group practice, but he was careful to include the general practitioner in the design; he thought the proportion of generalists to specialists should be about nine to one.[22]

After 1918, then, the idea of group practice began to flower. By 1930 there were about 150 such groups in the United States, involving 1,500 to 2,000 physicians, with concentrations in the West and Middle West. In Minnesota, it was claimed, there were few towns of 10,000 or more inhabitants without one or more private group clinics.[23] The typical group practice had up to 10 full-time physicians, included internal medicine, surgery, eye, ear, nose, and throat, and other fields, was organized as a partnership (some were organized as a corporation), depended on

21. John M. Dodson, "Remarks on Medical Education," *AMA Bull., 13* (1919), 185–91. Dodson was acting chairman while Arthur Dean Bevan was president of the AMA.
22. Discussion, ibid., p. 247.
23. C. Rufus Rorem, *Private Group Clinics: The Administrative and Economic Aspects of Group Medical Practice, as Represented in the Policies and Procedures of 55 Private Associations of Medical Practitioners,* Committee on the Costs of Medical Care Publication no. 8 (Washington, D.C., 1931), pp. 11–18, 33, and passim.

close affiliation with a hospital, and employed lay and other professional personnel. Few included general practitioners.

As a movement, however, specialist group practice was unsuccessful, and its development met with widespread professional resistance. Despite —or because of—its logic, specialist group practice represented potent competition to other physicians. The supposedly greater efficiency of a group presented competition to specialists who remained in solo practice; the concept of a multispecialist group presented a threat to the continuation of general practice. Initial enthusiasm within organized medicine was replaced by a spirit of caution, followed by hostility. Group practice, noted a speaker at an AMA conference in 1921, might be desirable, but it had its own dangers. These were categorized as "machine-like routine," the possibility of commercialization, and, most telling of all, the exclusion of the general practitioner.[24] The AMA attitude toward group practice began to crystallize into wary watchfulness. An editorial in the AMA *Journal* in 1921 raised the specter: "Does it mean that the family physician is being replaced by a corporation?"[25] While the Council on Medical Education and Hospitals concluded in 1922 that group practice was not a movement which would foster closed associations or denial of patient choice, and that it had a positive value in preventing physicians from doing work for which they were unfitted, the AMA House of Delegates could not agree. The interests of the educators and of the practitioners in the AMA had been similar in its great period of educational reform; now they were beginning to diverge. AMA leadership was passing from medical school faculty to the practitioner, and from progressivism to conservatism. The same year, the AMA's Principles of Medical Ethics were amended to denounce advertising by an individual or a group. Under the watchful eye of the AMA Judicial Council, multispecialist group practice has remained to this day in the background rather than in the vanguard of health services, a possibility rather than the model for organizational reform.

MEDICAL POLITICS AND "STATE MEDICINE"

Both compulsory health insurance and the informal voluntary development of group practice were expressions of a cumulative process of medical change from solo fee-for-service practice to cooperative payment and practice schemes. Challenging the position of the independent practi-

24. James B. Herrick, "Relation between the Specialist and the Practitioner," *AMA Bull., 15* (1921), 90–97.
25. Editorial, *J. Amer. med. Ass., 76* (1921), 452–53.

tioner, such schemes were actively resisted by the average physicians whose interests the AMA represented. Opposing the development of contract prepayment practice by corporations, urging physicians to avoid contact with hospitals which adopted any system of collecting medical fees, struggling against group hospital insurance schemes, and resisting any signs of governmental encroachment in medical care, the AMA sought to sustain a pattern of practice that looked not to the future but to the past. Suggestions for organizational reform of medicine continued to come more from outside than inside the medical profession, and they were looked upon as political threats rather than as adjustments to new forms of professionalism.

Having declared its opposition to compulsory health insurance by the states, the AMA was almost immediately faced with a new federal governmental role in the Sheppard-Towner Act of 1921; this provided the battleground for a major confrontation between organized medicine and government throughout the 1920s. The act authorized federal appropriations to states for the maintenance and improvement of the health of mothers and children and was administered by the Children's Bureau.[26] The AMA opposed Sheppard-Towner in 1921, as well as its proposed renewal in 1926. The association produced accusations of hasty hearings, threats to states' rights, and dangers to the fabric of the American home. Maternal and infant mortality rates in the United States, it was claimed, were no higher than in other countries, and even if they were, they could not necessarily be lowered through legislative, and particularly federal, action.[27] The Sheppard-Towner program was extended from 1927 until 1929, but, under the impact of the increasingly effective opposition mobilized by the AMA, further efforts failed. Attempts at revival in 1931 and 1932 were equally unsuccessful; not until the Social Security Act of 1935 were federal-state programs for maternal and child health reborn.

In its brief life (1922–29) the Sheppard-Towner program set a pattern for important aspects of federal financial aid to the states which was to be followed by other welfare programs: a closed-end appropriation dependent on state matching funds, the specification of standards on

26. For the background and development of the Sheppard-Towner Act, see Harry S. Mustard, *Government in Public Health* (New York, 1945), pp. 71–74; Nathan Sinai and Odin W. Anderson, *Emergency Maternity and Infant Care* (Ann Arbor, 1948), pp. 7–12.

27. But there was also opposition from those who were concerned that the administrative separation of services for children from other aspects of medical provision would inhibit the eventual establishment of a coordinated federal health program for all age groups. There was thus opposition from both conservative and liberal elements. See William C. Woodward, "The Sheppard-Towner Act: Its Proposed Extension and Proposed Repeal," *AMA Bull., 21* (1926), 136; Fishbein, p. 331.

which grants would be made, the acceptance of a grant system for categorical programs. But of even more importance, the Sheppard-Towner
Act also emphasized the growing social implications of modern medicine.
The Children's Bureau had developed not from scientific pediatrics but
from the social work movement at the beginning of the century; its establishment was supported primarily by social service and labor organizations. The emphasis of Sheppard-Towner had similar social aims: to
reduce infant mortality as well as to treat and prevent childhood diseases.
Those physicians who regarded themselves as pediatricians and obstetricians could not ignore the social issues of their specialties, and both
developed during the 1920s at the center of the child welfare movement.
But the trend toward publicly subsidized clinics and care was alien to the
interests and attitudes of those entrenched in other types of practice. A
new type of medical organization demanded a psychological and financial
reorientation on the part of individual practitioners which was difficult if
not impossible for the majority to accept.[28] Thus, while members of the
AMA Section on Diseases of Children favored Sheppard-Towner, they
were told that the section could not take a position opposed to that of the
house of delegates[29]—a clear case of the political insignificance of the
AMA specialist sections in relation to organized medicine as a whole,
and of the prevailing influence of the private practitioner over those willing to experiment with other organizational forms.

At its sessions in 1922 the AMA House of Delegates put on record its
opposition to all forms of "state medicine." This term was defined as any
form of medical treatment given, controlled, or subsidized by any form
of public agency; exceptions were however made for health services
organized by the army, navy, and U.S. Public Health Service, for control
of communicable disease, for treatment of the "indigent sick," and for
any other service which was approved by county or state medical societies.[30] Only the year before, Dr. Bevan had reminded the profession that
the best deterrent to governmental encroachment was vigorous action
by local medical societies to encourage the development of well-equipped
community hospitals as medical centers.[31] But by now, any institutional
form of medicine was becoming suspect. A philosophy was developing
that institutional medicine and private practice were mutually irrecon-

28. For a good contemporary review of the issues involved in professional change
in the 1920s see Bernhard J. Stern, *Social Factors in Medical Progress* (New York,
1927), p. 33 and passim.
29. Marshall C. Pease, *The American Academy of Pediatrics: 1930–1951* (New
York, 1951), p. 275.
30. *Proc. AMA House of Delegates* (May 1922), p. 44.
31. "Remarks by Arthur Dean Bevan," *J. Amer. med. Ass.,* 76 (1921), 1765.

cilable and that the profession's very integrity was threatened by anything savoring of government interference—a term which was rather widely defined, and whose interpretation was to be left to organized medicine.

THE HOSPITAL AND MEDICAL INSTITUTIONALISM

Nevertheless medicine was becoming inexorably institutional. Less and less did the doctor see the patient at home. Physicians' and dentists' offices sprang up in downtown streets away from urban residential areas. In the late 1920s nearly half of the physicians of Dallas, Texas, were located in one building.[32] Private office practice in hospitals was also developing, supplementing the increasing use of hospital outpatient clinics. A survey of private practitioners in Philadelphia in 1929 reported that the average full-time specialist spent only 6 hours on house calls out of a working week of over 50 hours, compared with 21 hours in his office, 16 hours in hospital practice, and 9 hours in clinics.[33] In New York and Chicago, the average doctor, generalist or specialist, spent up to 30 percent of his time in hospitals and clinics.[34] The medical institution was becoming necessary for a successful practice, particularly for the full-time specialist. By 1929, seven of ten physicians had some kind of hospital attachment.[35] Medicine was becoming an institutionalized, collective occupation.

Hospitals steadily increased in size during the 1920s, forming nuclei around which the medical profession clustered.[36] Concurrently, individual hospitals were expanding their departments, services, and auxiliary staff, such as nurses, physiotherapists, X-ray technicians, laboratory technicians, dietitians, and medical and psychiatric social workers. Taking

32. I. S. Falk, C. Rufus Rorem, and Martha D. Ring, *The Costs of Medical Care: A Summary,* Committee on the Costs of Medical Care, Publication no. 27 (Chicago, 1933), pp. 388–89.
33. Nathan Sinai and Alden B. Mills, *A Survey of the Medical Facilities of the City of Philadelphia,* Committee on the Costs of Medical Care, Publication no. 9 (Chicago, 1931), p. 37.
34. Michael M. Davis, *Clinics, Hospitals and Health Centers,* p. 5.
35. In 1929 there were 152,500 physicians, but of these about 9,000 were retired. An estimated 98,491 physicians were attached in some way to hospitals—after making allowance for duplicate appointments: attending and courtesy staff, 84,579; salaried hospital residents, 3,244; residents in specialist training, 1,921; physician superintendents, 2,442; interns in approved appointments, 5,310; other interns, 995. "Hospital Service in the United States," *J. Amer. med. Ass., 94* (1930), 929.
36. In 1909 there were 4,359 hospitals listed by the AMA with a total of 421,065 beds. By 1923 there were 6,830 hospitals, with 755,722 beds. Thereafter, the number of hospitals began to decline, but their size increased; by 1932, U.S. hospitals provided over a million beds. "Hospital Service in the United States," reprinted from *J. Amer. med. Ass., 155* (1954), table A.

health personnel as a whole, physicians were by the late 1920s vastly outnumbered by a great army of paramedical workers, many of whom were based on hospitals or clinics and whose functions were becoming vital to efficient diagnosis and patient care.[37]

The hospital provided an institutional focus of some magnitude; but it was in some respects an organizational threat. The threat was not so much of federal control versus professional control—only 220 of 6,830 hospitals were federally owned in 1923[38]—it was of hospital versus private practice. Questions of so-called hospital abuse by those considered potential private patients were by no means dead. Indeed, social and economic conditions caused many persons to seek institutional care; and the proliferation in the 1920s of clinics and outpatient departments offering free or subsidized medical services created a major alternative to private practice for as much as a fourth of the urban population.[39] An estimated 3 million persons passed through general outpatient departments in 1921; the estimate was up to 6.6 million in 1929.[40] Thus even in the prosperous twenties there was evidence of diverging trends between professional practice expectations and the actions of the public. It was not surprising that the mood of the AMA changed after 1920, and that conservatism replaced its budding progressive policies of the prewar decade.

Seen from the point of view of the general practitioner who had been trained in a proprietary or university school at the end of the nineteenth

37. A review of the scattered and imprecise data on health personnel by Peebles, who used figures referring as nearly as possible to 1929, gave a grand total of about 1,500,000 people engaged in health work in the U.S., of whom only 143,000 were physicians. Allon Peebles, *A Survey of Statistical Data on Medical Facilities in the United States: A Compilation of Existing Material,* Committee on the Costs of Medical Care, Publication no. 3 (Washington, D.C., 1929), p. 16. Of the 6,665 hospitals approved by the AMA in 1929, 4,026 reported laboratories; 4,394 X-ray departments; 1,799 outpatient departments; 2,160 schools of nursing; and 2,016 dental departments. "Hospital Service in the United States," *J. Amer. med. Ass., 94* (1930), 929. Over 2,000 also had departments of physical therapy. Ibid., *J. Amer. med. Ass., 96* (1933), 1017. About 1,000 had social service departments. Ibid., *J. Amer. med. Ass., 98* (1932), 2072.

38. The total number of government hospitals (federal, state, and local) was 1,736 in 1923 and 1,795 in 1929. These were chiefly state mental and tuberculosis institutions, which did not pose a direct threat to private practice. The federal government itself operated 220 hospitals in 1923 and 292 in 1929; the average number of patients was, respectively, 34,937 and 46,033. "Hospital Service in the United States," *J. Amer. med. Ass., 94* (1930), 926.

39. In the large cities, it was estimated in the mid-1920s, probably 20–25 percent of the population received their ambulatory care in part or whole in organized clinics and outpatient services. Commission on Medical Education, *Preliminary Report,* p. 21; and see Michael M. Davis, *Clinics, Hospitals and Health Centers,* pp. 5–9.

40. In 1921 an estimated one person in 35 was a hospital outpatient; the proportion dropped to one in 18 in 1929, and one in 13 in 1933. "Hospital Service in the United States," *J. Amer. med. Ass., 102* (1934), 1010; ibid., *96* (1931), 1021.

century and who had begun practice at a time when there was little question of the profession's monopoly of the whole health field, the physician was indeed threatened. He was threatened by increased specialization. He was threatened by the hospital as a potential center for a medical elite. He was threatened by the public's growing interest in the standards of medical care. And all these threats were heightened whenever the government, particularly the federal government, hinted that it might lend them aid.

The war had emphasized the vast gap between the average general practitioner trained many years earlier and the young scientific specialists from the reformed medical schools. As a result, by the early 1920s relations between general practitioners and specialists were strained. Almost three of every four graduates in 1920 claimed they would eventually limit their work to specialist practice.[41] Potential specialists were also less inclined to follow their elders in choosing a preliminary period in general practice.[42] The absence of an accepted referral or consultation system between the generalist and the specialist gave the general practitioner no well-defined social function. Nor was he incorporated into group practice. By the late 1920s, even in rural areas, the general practitioner no longer attempted major surgery and had often given up the practice of obstetrics, nose and throat diseases, and venereal diseases.[43] He was no longer even a "general" practitioner. Could general practice survive? General practitioners themselves—still by far the majority of the medical profession and the backbone of the AMA—were committed to the view that it could. It was this commitment which dominated the actions of organized medicine from the 1920s.

In retrospect, the general practitioner would have been well advised to favor both compulsory insurance schemes and group practice in the

41. Of graduates of 1915, 41 percent said they restricted their practice to a specialty. Of those of 1920 (who had only been graduated six years) 35 percent were already full-time specialists. Of the 1915 graduates 66 percent, and nearly 74 percent of those of 1920, said they intended eventually to limit their work to a specialty. The response rate to the questionnaire sent to all graduates of 57 class A medical colleges was 76.7 percent; even if all who did not reply were generalists, the results would be indicative of rapidly growing specialist interest. H. G. Weiskotten, "Present Tendencies in Medical Practice," *Proc. Ann. Cong. med. Educ.* (1928), pp. 74–79.
42. On behalf of the Council on Medical Education, Dr. Horace Arnold questioned 230 specialists who were regarded as representatives in their fields; only 14 percent reported experience in general practice, and only 6 percent advised such experience. *AMA Bull., 14* (1920), 64–65.
43. See, for example, Allon Peebles, *A Survey of the Medical Facilities of Shelby, Indiana, 1929,* Committee on the Costs of Medical Care, Publication no. 6 (Chicago: 1930), p. 26 and passim.

1920s, and thereby to have established his central coordinating role in medical care and made it financially advantageous not to specialize. But such a suggestion did not meet the realities of contemporary medical politics. The AMA, in its attempts to remold the profession to keep up with a fast-changing scientific world, chose to concentrate on professional education instead of organizational reform. As a result, the relationships between generalist and specialist were to be discussed as questions of professional ethics and of curriculum, and in terms of traditional professional responsibilities rather than of what their respective roles should be. The often restrictionist policies of the AMA from the early 1920s toward group payment and group service plans were not merely reactions to potential governmental intervention but also to the accelerating development of public and quasi-public medical organizations which challenged the concept of private solo practice.

CHAPTER 8

The Specialists and Professional Regulation

In the absence of adequate organizational or functional responses to specialization in medicine in the years following World War I, the emerging structure of the medical profession was dictated largely by professional controls over the physician's education. These centered on differentiating the specialist as someone of identifiably superior skills, a process which demanded a more formal stratification of the profession into specialty groups. Differentiations might have been achieved through specified training, through professional certification of competence, or through specialist licensure. All were live issues in the 1920s. Through one or the other of these means it was intended to standardize specialist training, as basic general training had been standardized in the prewar era.

Underlying these debates were unresolved questions of what kind of profession was appropriate to postwar medicine. We are accustomed today to rapid changes in the content of medicine, but the changes in medicine and medical institutions between 1890 and 1920 represented virtually a revolution. There were few guides. The indecision, confusion, and lost opportunities of the 1920s were symptoms of a new movement toward professional self-definition in specialized medicine. How should medicine be stratified? And what should the purposes of regulation be?

GRADUATE MEDICAL EDUCATION

By the early 1920s it was clear that the question of specialist training had to be linked with the medical educational spectrum as a whole, from new medical student to recognized specialist. The AMA had reformed medical schools and was suggesting university-affiliated internships and a university base for specialist studies. If the AMA were able to ensure the production of well-trained specialists through the existing educational system

—by using the same kinds of pressure that had proved so successful in the reform of medical colleges—there would then be only a secondary role to be played by professional certification agencies. The AMA might not have all the control it would like if the universities became the foci of graduate education, but such an arrangement would at least undermine the rationale for the widespread development of independent specialty organizations, or at least those which claimed anything more than scientific or fraternity concerns. The AMA at least subconsciously accepted the maxim that if there is a good and standardized system of training, there is less need for outside measures of competence.

There was not, however, a formal specialist educational system. Specialist training was spread over a large number of institutions. The internship was the responsibility of many independent hospitals; the residency was also beginning to develop under hospital auspices; and formal training courses were given by a variety of postgraduate hospitals, schools, and universities. It was comparatively simple to suggest the elimination of proprietary postgraduate colleges, but this would not result in the automatic concentration of àll graduate training in university-affiliated programs. It was possible that the AMA might achieve a university focus by encouraging a rapid expansion of university graduate courses. To be effective, however, the AMA would have had to extend its influence over hospitals on the one hand, and over universities on the other. There was no coercive measure, such as licensing, whereby the AMA could achieve these aims, although specialist licensing had been suggested. Nor was there the outside competitive pressure for reducing numbers which had distinguished undergraduate reform.

The American College of Surgeons and the Board of Ophthalmic Examinations had developed one set of answers. Neither specified university graduate education. Each, however, required candidates to have an approved background of training and experience, in one kind of institution or another; and each tested the level of competence and issued a certificate which had moral rather than legal force. The system was a compromise between a specified training program for all specialists, which was not yet possible, and a formal, quasi-licensing examination. If standardized, high-quality training programs were introduced for specialists through the universities (or through some other means), or if a system of specialist licensing had been established, there would be no place for voluntary professional regulation along the lines of the surgeons and ophthalmologists. The specialist would be recognized by his additional university degree, or by his additional license. If a graduate degree from a recognized university became the accepted route for specialist training, there would be little case for either licensing or professional certification. If the developing health service system had contained its own inbuilt incentives or controls through the operation of group practices, an effective system of referral to specialists, or assumption of responsibility for the quality of care by hospitals, there would have been little reason to consider other types of regulation at all.

These, then, were the conditions and problems of future specialist regulation. By 1920 neither the AMA nor the American College of Surgeons, or the National Board of Medical Examiners or any other group, had a central, unifying role. The Council on Medical Education was dedicated to reforming the structure of graduate education—the internship (now being taken by more than 90 percent of all graduates), the graduate school, and later the residency. In taking this line, the AMA was able to assert its responsibility in the area of training without compromising its organizational philosophy of democracy and standardization. The council kept aloof from the organizational danger of establishing formal specialist groups; but, if such groups were to be established, it was ensured an influential voice.

As part of its commitment to standardizing specialism through the educational process, in 1920 the AMA Council on Medical Education and Hospitals organized fifteen separate specialist committees, each with nine members and each including eminent university teachers and practicing specialists from major organizations and from all parts of the country. The committees were to develop suggested curricula in their clinical and preclinical specialties from undergraduate courses to programs designed to mark specialist skills.[1] In retrospect, the structure of separate committees could not but emphasize the fragmentation which had already taken place within the medical profession and the extent to which specialism had become important to the whole educational process. The committees reported in March 1921.[2] The clinical specialty groups agreed that there should be a four-year undergraduate course; all except the committees on internal medicine and on pediatrics also recommended at least one year of general internship. Specialty training was thus to follow five general educational years. Most of the committees specified one or more minor fields supporting the major specialty (psychology supporting

1. The specialties were internal medicine, pediatrics, neuropsychiatry, dermatology and syphilology, surgery, ophthalmology, otolaryngology, orthopedic surgery, urology, obstetrics and gynecology, public health and hygiene, anatomy, pharmacology and therapeutics, physiology, and pathology and bacteriology.
2. "Graduate Education in the Specialties," *AMA Bull.*, 15 (1921), 17–82.

neuropsychiatry, physical therapy supporting orthopedics), to be pursued half time for a year, or full time for six months. Opinions varied as to how long the training for the major specialty should take. Orthopedic surgeons and otolaryngologists recommended one and a half years, public health physicians and ophthalmologists two years; internists, pediatricians, and surgeons as much as three years. Under this scheme the pediatrician would spend a total of eight years in training. Would all of this be feasible within the university? If not, how would it be regulated and controlled?

Discussion of standardizing or certifying specialists at the end of their training revealed no clear acceptance of one method or another. Dr. Louis B. Wilson restated the advantages of his own University of Minnesota–Mayo Clinic method: certification by the chief of service and success in a thorough examination for a Master of Science degree.[3] This was, however, possible as a general method only if all specialists could be included in universities. The committee on internal medicine favored recognition of specialists through a degree (including the granting of honorary degrees, where their qualifications justified it to those already in practice) or certification by a body similar to that of the American College of Surgeons—perhaps through the AMA's Council on Medical Education and Hospitals. Some members of the pediatrics committee were against the granting of a certificate under any circumstances, while others favored the kind of board set up by the ophthalmologists, with cooperation between the American Pediatric Society and the AMA section. Neuropsychiatrists considered that qualification to practice as a specialist should be left to the state and national boards of examiners, possibly advised by the national specialist societies. The surgery committee, realistically noting that Yale was the only university with a graduate course leading to an M.S. or Ph.D. degree in the specialty, favored a Ph.D. degree under the auspices of a multiuniversity examining board for the favored few working in university hospitals, but was undecided as to what to do about those working outside university hospitals. The ophthalmologists recommended their own board system. The otolaryngologists, who were then considering setting up their own examining board, also favored a certificate, which could be displayed in the doctor's office. The obstetricians shared this view on the grounds that specialists should not be certified by a university, because the subject matter was not that of a university degree; they recommended as the ideal solution certifi-

3. Louis B. Wilson, "Summary of Reports on Graduate Training in Specialties," ibid., pp. 88–90.

cation by the American College of Surgeons or, pending this arrangement, by a joint committee of the Council on Medical Education and Hospitals and the gynecological societies. Dermatologists, on the other hand, thought certificates "a cheap form of distinction, easily imitated and open to many abuses";[4] and the orthopedic surgeons agreed. Pathologists urged a national committee to develop graduate training to certify competence and also to advance the practical and financial interests of pathologists.

In summary, the alternatives, although not yet expressed in such concrete terms, were regulation through university degrees, state licensure, the National Board of Medical Examiners, the Council on Medical Education and Hospitals, specialty boards similar to that of the ophthalmologists, or some new national structure. Despite the different approaches, there was clearly a desire to differentiate the well-trained specialists in some way. Since the committee membership represented the leading practitioners in each specialty, any other conclusion would have been surprising.

The 1921 committees provided a watershed in the development of the Council on Medical Education's interest in graduate medicine. The purely educational solution to specialist recognition, as advocated by Dr. Louis B. Wilson and Dr. Arthur Dean Bevan (chairman of the council) was joined by a growing demand for nonuniversity forms of certification. The delineation by the committees of training requirements in the various specialties also openly admitted the existence of educationally, and thus professionally, distinct graduate channels. In effect, therefore, the committees gave official recognition to the separate existence of specialist groups. In the clinical specialties these included internal medicine, pediatrics, neuropsychiatry, dermatology, surgery, ophthalmology, otolaryngology, orthopedic surgery, obstetrics-gynecology, and pathology. Of these, only surgery and ophthalmology had established a system of formal recognition through training and examination; their committees and the curricula set out gave other specialist groups an anchor and an impetus for separate development. The committees were therefore in a sense the forerunners of the specialty boards which were to proliferate in the 1930s; they looked to organizational fragmentation rather than to ultimate professional unity.

Meanwhile, Dr. Wilson, and his colleagues on the Council on Medical Education and Hospitals, endeavored to stimulate the idea of university education for the specialist. Dr. Bevan suggested that the AMA should ask twenty or more of the strongest university medical departments to

4. Ibid., p. 31.

establish graduate courses, and that the AMA also later contact the state licensing boards with plans whereby the practice of specialties might be restricted to recognized men.[5] If these policies had been followed, specialist education would have had the same structure and controls as the basic general training. Moreover, not only would the medical profession have had a monopoly, but each specialty would have had its own monopoly. The issue was whether the egalitarianism of American medicine would tolerate such a change.

GENERALISM AND SPECIALISM IN MEDICAL EDUCATION

The recommendations of the specialist committees came at a time when the role of the general practitioner was being assailed from all sides; they raised questions of the relative balance of generalism and specialism in medical education. One line of thought, held by the educators, was that general practice was a baseline from which specialisms diverged. In this case, general practitioners would continue to have both numerical domination over specialists and a legitimate claim to represent medical breadth, as contrasted with the narrowness of specialism. This was the view of Dr. Bevan and the Council on Medical Education during the early 1920s. It was thought that a mere 10 or 15 percent of all practitioners would later take up full-time specialist practice,[6] and that general practitioners would be able to handle 90 percent of all medical complaints without resorting to specialists.[7] Without any profesional sanctions to limit manpower distribution, this view was only realistic if no account were taken of the career intentions of younger men, or of the proliferation of part-time specialty interests. But the concept of 10 percent assumed enduring qualities in the balance between generalism and specialism. Perhaps no one really believed in the magic concept of 10 percent, which appeared with regularity throughout the 1920s and 1930s (and still appears from time to time) either as an ideal proportion of consulting specialists or as the proportion of work to be done by specialists. But it had a comforting ring of assigning relative weights.

The idea that every specialist should be a general practitioner of medicine before he could begin his specialist practice was one answer to organizational fragmentation. Dr. Bevan, for example, delineated two "safe plans for a specialty": either the specialist going straight into specialist

5. Ibid., p. 13.
6. "Remarks by Arthur Dean Bevan," *J. Amer. med. Ass., 76* (1921), 1764–65.
7. Commission on Medical Education, *Preliminary Report,* pp. 32, 51, and passim. The commission set up its own study of general practitioners of the classes of 1915–22 in communities of 50,000 or less; the 90 percent represented their opinion.

practice would act as a member of a group practice, taking patients referred to him by, and under the supervision of, a general physician who acts as "captain of the group" or the specialist would have a broad base of general medicine.[8] The prevailing mood made the second alternative the more acceptable one to general practitioners, and the easier one from the point of view of exerting professional influence. Resolutions in favor of a compulsory period in general practice before specializing appear regularly over the years in the *Proceedings* of the AMA; they were one way in which general practitioners could ensure both that general practice would continue and that specialists would remain numerically relatively small. (But in the long run this was a less workable argument than the alternative, organizational solution—that the generalist be the coordinator of care or captain of the team.)

At the same time this position weakened the generalist's position vis-à-vis the specialist; for if the specialist had first to be a generalist, then general practice was the lower of two ranks. And there were already general practitioners who resented being regarded as having a junior level of skill. At the AMA meeting in Atlantic City, June 1919, a resolution was introduced by a member from California asking the house of delegates to "encourage the designation of the practice of general medicine or 'family physician' as a distinct and dignified specialty" in its own right.[9] The action, which failed, was the first public step on the long road toward the recognition of general practice as an equal among the specialties.

The lack of definition of "general practice" dogged the discussion of specialist education throughout the 1920s. Was it a phrase for general medical education before specializing, a description of a past mode of practice, or a needed and new coordinating role (and thus a specialty) in modern specialized medicine? The educators seemed to regard general practice as the physician's basic education. In May 1922, the AMA House of Delegates agreed to a request by the Council on Medical Education to urge medical schools to revise their undergraduate curricula to provide a thorough training in general practice, delaying specialist courses until graduate school.[10] The same year Dr. Louis B. Wilson began the third council inspection of graduate medical schools. This led to the adoption in 1923 of principles for grading graduate schools, the decision to publish a list of approved schools, and efforts to eliminate

8. Arthur Dean Bevan, "The Organization of the Profession for the Practice of Modern Scientific Medicine," *AMA Bull.*, 15 (1921), 12.
9. *Proc. AMA House of Delegates* (June 1919), pp. 54, 58.
10. *Proc. AMA House of Delegates* (May 1922), pp. 27–29, 40.

the six-week specialist diplomas and certificates.[11] The chief concern was the supervision and facilities provided in the schools; however, stress was also laid on the nature of specialist training through an assistantship whereby, under the supervision of an expert, the graduate would gradually assume responsibility for diagnosing and caring for the sick. All the council was trying to do, it insisted, was to arrange graduate courses in a graded series, in an improved teaching environment, and also to control the intake to graduate schools, since this intake was much more uneven than the intake at the undergraduate level.[12] But, in the face of general practitioner interest in maintaining their access to some specialist training, the council had to make it clear that it was neither intending to limit postgraduate opportunities for general practitioners nor trying to assume authority over any individual or graduate school.

From 1924 the Council on Medical Education also began to investigate those hospitals claiming to offer residencies or "higher internships," designed to give increased knowledge and skill in the specialties. This move was separate from the efforts to grade courses in medical schools and was linked with the previously existing listing of approved hospitals for internships. No general hospital was approved unless it also had approval for internships. The first list of residencies was published by the council in 1927. A total of 1,699 residency places was approved in 270 hospitals.[13] In 1930 the council included 349 hospitals on its approved list, providing 2,069 residency positions. The council was by then firmly of the view that it was no longer necessary for a hospital to have a medical school affiliation, and that there was a sufficiency of good teachers outside the university centers.[14] Thus two types of specialist training were crystallized: first, the thorough work being done at university graduate medical schools, such as the Universities of Pennsylvania, Minnesota, Columbia (which was merged into a graduate center with the New York Postgraduate Medical School), and others, with programs of from three to five years; and second, an increasing number of residencies in non-university hospitals, usually of only twelve months' duration. For special-

11. Ibid., June 1923, 27–29, 30, 40; June 1924, pp. 26–28.
12. Any institution offering specialist work was, under the council's principles, to provide review courses in the relevant basic sciences, teaching clinics in hospital wards and outpatient departments, technical courses, and carefully selected assistantships. Courses would be graded so that the student could either go through a continuous two or three years' training or take the same work in segments over a longer period of time. Editorial, *J. Amer. med. Ass., 81* (1923), 1810–11.
13. *J. Amer. med. Ass., 88* (1927), 828–32.
14. "Hospital Service in the United States," *J. Amer. med. Ass., 96* (1931), 1019–20.

ist training, the ascendancy of the hospital over the university graduate school was already apparent.

THE ROLE OF THE COUNCIL ON MEDICAL EDUCATION

By the late 1920s, then, the council's listing of approved internships and of its standards for internships was matched by similar programs for residencies. In 1928, the AMA House of Delegates approved the council's codification of standards for residencies under the title "Essentials of Approved Residencies and Fellowships." It was only a step from approval of residencies to consideration of the content of training in those residencies, and to endorsement of specialty status.

Already the council had expanded from being purely a training agency to an accrediting agency of laboratory and radiology departments. Another branch of the AMA was also busy supervising physical therapy equipment. These specialties were therefore already under the AMA umbrella. Here again, it was only a step from supervising departments and equipment to advising on specialist standards. While the step had not been taken, nor was it generally recognized that it should be, the potential was there, and the AMA, willing or unwilling, had a foot in the door of the specialist certification process.

The AMA created its Council on Physical Therapy in 1925 not to recognize medical men but to combat the dangers of "machine therapy." Locked in combat with a vast industry, the Council on Physical Therapy sought to educate general practitioners in choosing rationally between one enticing apparatus and the next. Physical therapy had been recognized as having definite scientific value during World War I. After the war physical therapy equipment rapidly became a fad exploited by manufacturers and their salesmen:

Mysterious, high priced electrical applicances in mahogany cabinets became, in fact, the tail that wagged the dog, so that the term "physical therapy" was apt to call to mind, not heat, water, massage and exercises, the fundamentals of physical therapy, but the paraphernalia of the charlatan.[15]

15. F. J. Gaenslen, "Who Should Teach Physical Therapy?" *Proc. Ann. Cong. Med. Educ.* (1933), p. 20. Included among the council reports during the 1920s and 1930s were reviews of ultraviolet radiation, sunlamps, shortwave diathermy, artificial respiration, and hearing aids. The council publicized its views (stressing the virtues of massage and manual therapy) in the AMA *Journal* and in its *Handbook of Physical Medicine,* organized speakers, exhibits, and consultants, and advised on

Both nonmedical physical therapy aides and physical therapy machinery antedated full-time specialty interest in physical medicine by physicians: indeed, physical medicine as a rounded diagnostic and treatment specialty did not become established until the 1930s, and only began to flourish after World War II. The council's function was thus to act as the guardian of a specialty. Indeed, if physical medicine had been recognized earlier as a medical specialty, the council would undoubtedly have been responsible for the standards of its specialists.

Somewhat along the same lines, the Council on Medical Education expanded its work in 1926 to include the compilation of a list of approved clinical laboratories, and two years later it included the inspection, appraisal, and listing of X-ray departments.[16] It soon became obvious, however, that the character or training of the pathologist and radiologist was the vital issue in determining departmental standing—and the focus of inspection began to shift from equipment to specialist recognition. In the early 1930s the council was to prepare and publish lists of physicians specializing in radiology and pathology. Thus the council was becoming involved, admittedly by a circuitous route, in the direct determination of who was and who was not a qualified specialist in certain specialties, while at the same time expanding its involvement in programs of education and training in all specialties.

REGULATION OF SPECIALISTS THROUGH PROFESSIONAL ENDORSEMENT

Meanwhile, the certification of specialists by other professional groups remained a live issue, although the formation in 1924 of an examining board by the otolaryngologists—the only specialty board to be formed in the 1920s—was the extension of prewar thinking rather than any new movement. Otolaryngology had developed side by side with ophthalmology and shared its problems. Some 4,700 physicians limited their practice to the specialties of eye, ear, nose, and throat in 1925 (the great majority, 3,100, combined all four areas).[17] The establishment of the Board for Ophthalmic Examinations had distorted the training process for those in combined fields; it also posed problems of entry into the

---

education and research in the specialty. See Harry E. Mock, "The Council on Physical Therapy of the American Medical Association," *Proc. Ann. Cong. med. Educ.* (1933), pp. 22–27; Fishbein, pp. 923–35.

16. The first "Essentials of an Approved Department of Radiology or Roentgenology" were approved by the AMA House of Delegates in 1929. AMA *Digest,* pp. 442, 601.

17. Commission on Medical Education, *Preliminary Report,* p. 81.

American Academy of Ophthalmology and Otolaryngology which, after 1920, restricted membership of ophthalmic specialists to those who were certified by the board.

The popularity of tonsillectomies and submucous resections (and the profit to be made from them) made otolaryngology a tempting field for the general practitioner who wished to specialize. The 70 percent rejection rate of otolaryngologists during World War I, the high incidence of ear defects in drafted men, and the increasing involvement of otolaryngologists in the public health aspects of deafness emphasized the need to upgrade standards in otolaryngology.[18] The overemphasis by many practitioners on the surgical rather than the medical approach also caused alarm. G. E. Shambaugh described the type of specialist training in surgery in the early 1920s as producing "carpenters in oto-laryngology" instead of broad-minded specialists.[19]

After World War I each of the five national specialist societies in otolaryngology set up committees to consider "higher standardization": a two-year curriculum, leading to a university degree, was suggested by the academy in 1919.[20] Between 1920 and 1923, however, the five national societies of the specialty were all moving toward the same goal of a joint examining board. The National Board of Examiners in Otolaryngology was finally established in 1924, with two members from each of the societies. It was proposed that the board's examination would be accepted by the constituent societies as an entrance requirement; it would thus function on similar lines to the ophthalmic board.[21] The examination would be a gateway to a professional group as well as a badge of competence. As with the ophthalmologists there was a grandfather clause; of 1,368 physicians certified by the end of 1928, 354 were certified by

18. Diseases of the ear accounted for 4.5 percent of rejections for the draft. The chief public concern, however, was over children. A study of children in Missouri up to 1920 showed 38 percent with enlarged tonsils, 11 percent with adenoidal defects, and 4 percent with defective hearing; 24 percent were said to be mouth breathing. An estimate of the physical and mental condition in U.S. school children in 1918 produced a figure of 1 million children in the U.S. with defective hearing and 3–5 million with diseased tonsils or adenoids or other glandular defects. Similar high figures of defects in the population were given in the 1919 report of the Illinois Health Commission. Commission on Medical Education, *Preliminary Report*, pp. 75–77.
19. *AMA Bull., 15* (1921), 41.
20. *Trans. Amer. Acad. Ophthal. Otolaryng.* (1919), p. 405. The five national societies were (1) the American Otological Society, (2) the American Laryngological Association, (3) the American Laryngological, Rhinological, and Otological Society, (4) the AMA Section on Laryngology, Rhinology, and Otology, (5) the American Academy of Ophthalmology and Otolaryngology.
21. *Trans. Amer. Acad. Ophthal. Otolaryng.* (1924), p. 465.

invitation.[22] There were by then three specialist examining bodies, including the American College of Surgeons, each determining membership in national specialist associations. And the obstetricians and gynecologists were beginning to move toward the same solution. The first concrete suggestion for a board in that combined specialty apparently came from Walter Dannreuther in 1927 before the American Association of Obstetricians and Gynecologists; in the following year the American Gynecological Society agreed to cooperate.[23]

What was the function of such boards? Dr. W. P. Wherry, the first secretary of the Board of Otolaryngologists, said that board was primarily conceived "as a means of protection to the various national societies." [24] The examinations were welcomed as a means of limiting society membership, and thence the numbers (and quality) of those practicing in the specialties. Dr. Wherry urged certified otolaryngologists to canvass hospitals, colleges, and societies to accept as applicants only those holding the certificate. It was hoped that, as a result of these actions, the status of the specialty would be propelled upward, to a "major rather than a minor rating in the domain of medicine." [25] On the educational side, it was hoped to produce a safe and sane man to practice in the specialty.[26] As with the educational reform movement of the AMA, limitation of numbers would be accompanied by upgrading standards; both the professional interests of the physician and the quality of his education could be protected and justified at the same time. The otolaryngologists, like the ophthalmologists and surgeons, emphasized that they had no legal power, no licensing function, and were not attempting to confer a degree. However, by attempting to influence hospital trustees only to appoint diplomates to hospital appointments, and by cutting off access to the major societies to those without the certificate, the specialist groups involved were on the way to creating the type of professionally controlled

22. W. P. Wherry, "The American Board of Otolaryngology: History—Plan of Operation—Purposes," *Ann. Otol. (St. Louis), 37* (1928), 1067.
23. Clyde L. Randall, "Responsibility for Excellence," *Trans. Amer. Ass. Obstet. Gynec., 75* (1964), 5–14.
24. Wherry, "Otolaryngology," p. 1072. For other, similar comments, see e.g. *Trans. Amer. Acad. Ophthal. Otolaryng.* (1919), p. 401; (1922), p. 501; (1925) p. 420; Thomas J. Harris, "Graduate Education in Medicine in Relation to Training in Oto-Laryngology," *J. Laryng., 44* (1929), 301–08.
25. Wherry, "Otolaryngology," pp. 1072–73.
26. See Ross Hall Skillern, "American Board of Otolaryngology: Experiences and Conclusions in the Field of Preparation for the Specialty," *Ann. Otol. (St. Louis), 37* (1928), 1072–77. Dr. Skillern noted that the early candidates for the examination were often impatient, defensive, and surly; but by 1928 "covert enmity" had been transformed into a "spirit of fellowship and cooperation."

specialist monopoly which already existed in England and other parts of Europe.

The actions of the ophthalmologists and otolaryngologists were important because of the extent of specialization in these well-defined and often lucrative fields. Together, ophthalmologists and otolaryngologists outnumbered all other specialties; of the 15,400 physicians who claimed they were in full-time specialist practice in 1923, more than 30 percent limited their practice to these areas. In second place was surgery (22 percent), and in third, internal medicine (13 percent) (see table 1). If the surgeons and internists had joined the eye-ear-nose-throat men in pressing for numerical limitation and high-quality standards, a small specialist elite might well have been established. The boards might then have been used as instruments to attain the 10 or 15 percent of experts in the specialties that Bevan and other leaders seemed to think a desirable ratio and to ensure that general practice, at least numerically, really did remain the cornerstone of the profession.

Herein lay a major dilemma for the American College of Surgeons. The College, though it too used its examination as an admission process to a professional organization, had much wider interests than the two specialty boards. In the early 1920s it was involved in its ambitious program of hospital standardization; it established a committee on industrial surgery, and it set up a bone sarcoma registry and committees on fractures and on the radiological treatment of malignant tumors. In 1925, the College engaged a pathologist to direct its clinical research program. The College began its formal interest in surgical training in 1919, but training was felt by its critics to be among the least of its functions.[27] Over the long term, however, the purpose of the College was in some doubt. It had been Franklin Martin's intention not to create a surgical elite but to provide in the fellowship a sign of basic competence in surgery: to set minimum standards for surgery, rather than to specify the kinds of graduate training in the specialties that were involved in the Council on Medical Education's specialist committees of 1921. There were 6,181 fellows of the College in 1924, many more than the number of physicians said to be restricting their practice exclusively to surgery and a comfortable majority of all those said to be practicing as surgeons.[28] The assumption in standardization was that large numbers of practitioners might wish to practice surgery, and that the lure of College fellowship would be the incentive to take a training which they might not otherwise bother to acquire. The

27. See Loyal Davis, *Fellowship of Surgeons,* p. 273 and passim.
28. Ibid., p. 265.

Table 1. *Number of Full-Time Medical Specialists by Field of Specialty, Selected Years, 1923–1966*

Specialty	Number of full specialists							
	1923	1929	1934	1940	1949	1955	1962	1966
Total	15,408	22,166	26,756	36,880	62,688	84,444	129,828	151,930
Anesthesiology	107	132	159	285	1,231	2,453	5,555	7,476
Dermatology; syphilology	361	544	705	974	1,609	2,020	2,660	2,964
Hosp. admn./admn. medicine					273	366	979	2,620
Internal medicine	1,958	3,377	4,452	6,449	12,490	17,608	27,379	30,948
Obstetrics; gynecology	696	1,180	1,691	2,551	5,074	7,198	11,680	13,861
Ophthalmology; otorhinolaryngology	4,703	5,925	6,297	7,608	9,224	9,664	10,871	11,560
Orthopedic surgery	326	504	722	1,078	2,035	3,083	4,881	5,921
Pathology; bacteriology	317	408	652	987	1,730	2,514	4,501	5,941
Pediatrics	689	1,333	1,734	2,416	4,315	6,567	10,507	12,558
Physical medicine					234	374	632	682
Psychiatry; neurology	945	1,280	1,601	2,400	4,720	7,048	12,378	15,224
Pulmonary diseases	305	412	526	620	1,053	1,055	1,164	874
Public health; aviation medicine	315	676	836	1,555	1,567	1,680	2,664	1,971
Radiology; roentgenology	588	897	1,169	1,589	2,866	4,249	6,410	7,659
Surgery, occupational medicine	3,336	4,305	4,787	6,645	12,074	15,816	23,930	25,605
Urology	762	1,193	1,425	1,723	2,193	2,746	3,647	4,085

Includes specialists in active private practice, hospital practice (other than interns and residents), and other forms of practice.

Source: *Building America's Health*, III, table 209 (1952); 1955 and 1962 figures from *Health Manpower Source Book*, sec. 14, Medical Specialists, table 6, which also duplicates the above 1949 figures, thus establishing a base of comparability of data; 1966 data from American Medical Association *Distribution of Physicians, Hospitals and Hospital Beds 1966*, vol. 1, table A; 1966 figures refer to primary interest rather than to full-time devotion the specialty. The 1949 and earlier figures include occupational medicine under "surgery." To provide comparability, occupational medicine has also been added to surgery for the later data.

College movement was thus aimed at the average man, not the resident in the university hospital. It was inclusive rather than exclusive, whereas the two specialty boards had deliberately restrictive aims.

From the early 1920s, however, this position was severely challenged. Dr. Dean Lewis, a colleague of Arthur Dean Bevan, petitioned the College in 1924 to reduce the number of fellows and to take their geographical distribution into account; he also asked for more rigid examinations and for stringent qualifying criteria. A similar petition was sent from the Éclat Society, an association of young surgeons which had been formed in wartime France.[29] The figures might bear out Martin's aim, now reiterated by its board of regents, that the College was a democratic organization, concerned more with basic standards than with the certification of competence. But it could not satisfy the university-trained surgeons who were themselves seeking specialty recognition. It was for this reason as much as because of other criticism then being made of the College—of its publicity seeking, its focus on fee splitting rather than science, and the continuing dominance of Franklin Martin[30]—that surgical specialty associations in the United States were later to seek certification outside rather than within the American College of Surgeons.

The question remained as to what the impact of specialty certification would be if it were developed as an all-engulfing system, perhaps including the general practitioners who had unsuccessfully sought their own specialty recognition in 1919. The American medical profession had been traditionally opposed to the establishment of elites (at least within the profession), under whatever guise they appeared. By the mid-1920s hospitals which had followed a closed-staff policy for years were being forced by local practitioners to consider the implications of closed-staff structures in setting up a privileged class of practitioners and arousing in those excluded a natural resentment. This resentment was in part an outcome of the increasing usefulness of hospital facilities as part of private practice. Without a hospital connection, a physician of ordinary talents could not, it was observed, "mentally thrive." [31]

But if board certification were not to be used for accepting and denying entry to hospital staffs, what was it for? One answer was for delineating function *within* the hospital: that is, in assigning particular types of hospital privileges or activities. Another might be to enable the public

29. Loyal Davis, *Fellowship of Surgeons,* pp. 256–57, 492–93.
30. Ibid., pp. 246–47.
31. S. S. Goldwater, "The Extension of Hospital Privileges to All Practitioners of Medicine," *J. Amer. med. Ass., 84* (1925), 933–35. See also S. S. Goldwater, "The Specialist: What Shall We Do with Him?" *J. Amer. med. Ass., 88* (1927), 1691–93.

to select a specialist known to be well trained. These functions were purely qualitative: they assumed the boards to be guides of competence rather than symbols of professionalism. If the boards were, however, to develop as agents of the public rather than of professional groups, was the conjoint structure of specialist associations, or the College concept, an appropriate vehicle? These questions became acute in the late 1920s as new specialties began to coalesce, as other professional solutions were presented, and as specialist licensure became for the first time a real possibility.

REGULATION OF SPECIALISTS THROUGH LICENSURE

The question whether licensure should be used to signify specialist competence continued through the various discussions of the 1920s. State licensing had been used effectively as a vehicle for abolishing low-grade colleges between 1904 and 1920, and also in attempts to control non-medical practitioners. The examining boards had not hesitated to extend their function to regulating medical school curricula; during the 1920s they saw no reason why they should not make basic science examinations an additional requirement to ensure uniform training of all practitioners.[32] The basic science laws implied that there was a common pool of knowledge applicable as a minimum to all who were legally enabled to diagnose patients. Specialist licensure would also imply basic levels of knowledge and skill which should be recognized before a physician could treat in certain areas. Ought the public to have this kind of protection? In the face of apparent professional inability to deal with fee splitting, illegal and unnecessary surgery, and exorbitant surgical fees,[33] it appeared that the public should.

Discussion of licensure for specialists was no longer entirely academic. Alberta introduced specialist licenses under an act of 1926: no person was to hold himself out as a specialist, or as being specially qualified,

32. Basic science laws were enacted in Connecticut and Wisconsin (1925); Minnesota, Nebraska, Washington (1927); Washington, D.C. (1928); Arkansas (1929). By 1937, nine states and the District of Columbia had basic science boards, whose primary effect was to make it more difficult, if not impossible, for osteopaths, chiropractors, and other "irregulars" to be licensed. A good review of this development is *The Basic Sciences, Their Relationship to the Control and Regulation of the Healing Arts,* Kansas Legislative Council, Research Dept., Publication no. 58 (Feb. 1937).
33. There were "rumors of fee-splitting in nearly every city or town in any state of the union." The "ugly stories" among the laity about professional conduct in this and other respects had the sympathetic ear of many professional leaders. Editorial, "Unprofessional Conduct," *J. med. Soc. N.J., 26* (1929), 326–27.

without a certificate from the General Faculty Council of the University of Alberta to show he had completed one year of general internship and two and a half years of hospital specialist training.[34] In 1929, a bill was introduced into the New Jersey legislature to "regulate the practice of surgery," and the various arguments for and against specialist licensing had to be marshalled in political terms.[35] The New Jersey bill would have controlled the practice of general surgery, its subspecialties, and related fields—including, inter alia, obstetrics-gynecology, ophthalmology and otolaryngology, radiology, pathology, and anesthesia—that is, the great majority of specialists in the state. A state board of surgical examiners would have been set up by the governor, and this board would have approved training, conducted written examinations in the surgical sciences and in each of the specialties, and conferred licenses. The license would itself have carried a title appropriate to each field: for example, M.S. for a surgeon. While it would have had training connotations similar to those of the existing university degree programs, its big difference would have been in its mandatory and exclusive powers. Persons found guilty of practicing surgery without a license would have been fined $100 or jailed for up to 300 days, or both.

The bill passed the assembly (the lower house of the legislature) in April 1929 and proved a source of acute embarrassment to the medical profession, which found itself in opposition to a measure supposedly designed to raise medical standards. In a political climate marked by allegations of malpractice and complaints against physicians, the editor of the *Journal of the Medical Society of New Jersey* wrote that "the public will not be asking anything unreasonable if it demands that surgeons, general and special, shall present evidence of fitness before being allowed to practice in their respective fields.[36] At the same time there were serious questions about licensure, in the distinction to be made between the practitioners of clinical medicine and the surgeons and other specialists specified in the bill, in the fact that the "family doctor" would be prohibited from performing any major operation and many so-called minor ones, in the rigidity of licensing compared with the fluidity of scientific development, and—by no means least—in the as-

34. D. Sclater Lewis, *The Royal College of Physicians and Surgeons of Canada, 1920–1960* (Montreal, 1962), pp. 144–45.
35. State of New Jersey, Assembly no. 290, An act to regulate the practice of surgery, to license surgeons, and to punish persons violating the provisions thereof, introduced 26 Feb., 1929. For a review, see "Annual Report of the Society," *J. med. Soc. N.J. Suppl., 26* (1929), 8.
36. Editorial, "Regulating the Practice of Surgery," *J. med. Soc. N.J., 26* (1929), 772.

sumed relationship between licensing and quality. There was also undoubtedly concern that such a licensing system would be completely outside the medical society's control. The state medical society lobbied successfully in the New Jersey senate and prevented the bill from appearing on the senate floor. Effective lobbying resulted in the defeat of the bill by one vote when it reappeared in the state assembly in 1930; in 1931 the bill did not reach the floor, reportedly being "side-tracked by a clever trick." [37] Specialist licensure then disappeared from the legislative process in that state. But the problem of specialty recognition remained.

The solution of the New Jersey profession was to develop an alternative scheme of medical society endorsement of specialist qualifications, and this was presented to the Tri-State Medical Conference of the New Jersey, New York, and Pennsylvania medical societies in 1931.[38] The plan was to set up a state credentials committee to accredit specialists on the basis of experience, training, specialist society membership, board certification, or appointment at a recognized special department in a hospital. This plan offered certain advantages to the profession. Its standards were more flexible, indeed lower, than those suggested in the legislation. General practitioners with proper qualifications could be endorsed as specialists; and the society intended no absolute restrictive purpose. Thus, while no member of the medical society would be allowed to call himself a specialist unless so endorsed, any general practitioner could still attempt major surgical procedures. The reasoning might be tortuous, but the plan was politically appealing and was in fact put into effect for a short time. Meanwhile a number of other state medical societies were considering plans for certification of specialists in the states.

While state licensing, however, had obvious flaws, so did control by state medical societies. Should specialist recognition be vested in the states at all? There were 22,000 full-time specialists in the United States in 1929. When these were divided into specialties and states the components were very small. Only 132 self-styled anesthesiologists were listed for the whole country; only 504 orthopedic surgeons, and 408 pathologists.[39] If each state developed its own set of specialist standards, some might license only three or four men in certain specialties and prevent all other physicians from practicing in these fields. This would

37. Dr. Henry O. Reik of New Jersey, discussion of E. G. Waters' "Certification of Specialists by the State Society," *AMA Bull., 28* (1933), 10.
38. Edward G. Waters, "Specialists and Specialism: A Plan for Proper Control by State Societies," *Penn. med. J., 35* (1932), 491–93.
39. See table 1.

create not only a narrow monopoly but also real problems of what good-quality medical care should be. What was to happen to the patient who happened to need major surgery several hundred miles from the nearest licensed surgeon? or—more tellingly—to the patient who could not afford the specialist's fees?

In the last analysis the professional and public aspects of specialist qualifications could not be disentangled. Educating the public and the profession to make an enlightened choice of doctor instead of putting a stamp on all physicians would undoubtedly have had a larger political impact on standards than the more restricted methods of the specialty boards. The American College of Surgeons had, however, failed to provide the basic public education which would have allowed informed choice of specialists and reduced the allegations of dangerous surgery. The limitations of the free choice of doctor were put succinctly by one of the founders of the Board of Otolaryngology: "If I were taken ill in some distant city, I would have difficulty in selecting a specialist despite the fact that my opportunity to acquire knowledge of specialists in all lines, all over this continent, have been of an exceptional character." [40] In part, therefore, regulation was more a question of providing both doctors and patients with the means to recognize those who were well trained, than necessarily a legal exclusion of the inadequate.

NATIONAL SPECIALIST QUALIFICATIONS

The National Board of Medical Examiners was yet another body which had begun to develop an interest in specialist regulation, and which stood between licensing and certification. The board's examinations were already accepted as full or partial qualifications for basic licensure by many of the states; it was a national organization, and it was independent of the existing specialist groups and boards. If it were to take responsibility for specialist qualifications, specialist licensing might still be achieved by means of reciprocity between the states. Specialist training would then be nationally standardized.

The National Board reportedly received many requests in the early 1920s to extend its functions in this direction.[41] In September 1922, the year after the specialist committees of the Council on Medical Education had reported, the board set up its own committee inquiring into specialty qualifications. Its members were Dr. Louis B. Wilson, Dr. Walter

40. Discussion of Dr. Water's proposal, *Penn. med. J., 35* (1932), 496.
41. Louis B. Wilson, "Work of the National Board of Medical Examiners," *Proc. Ann. Cong. med. Educ.* (1940), p. 26.

Bierring, and Dr. J. Stewart Rodman. But the various specialty organizations indicated a general disapproval of attempts by the National Board to set up its own specialty examinations, apparently because graduate medical education was still so generally disorganized. Dr. Wilson recommended no further action until something had been done by the AMA about the graduate schools. National Board spokesmen conferred with the otolaryngologists in 1924 on the possibility of combined action in that specialty; but nothing was done.[42] The board's executive committee invited special society representatives to a meeting in May 1924 to discuss the whole issue of specialty qualifications. But interest again languished, until with Dr. Louis B. Wilson back on its qualification committee in 1926 the National Board decided it was opportune to raise the question once again with the special societies. But still no action was taken. Dr. Wilson himself stated in 1927 that the proper time had not yet come for the National Board to assume a function which might well be beyond its financial resources.[43] During the 1930s the National Board remained interested in offering specialty examinations—perhaps examining in the fundamental sciences, with the specialty organizations examining clinical knowledge. But any impetus would have had to come from the specialist groups themselves. The moment for leadership had been lost. In hindsight, so had the movement for specialist licensure.

REGULATION UNRESOLVED

The logical order in developing a system for training medical specialists would have been to build graduate education as a second stage, linked with the undergraduate program. However, although the medical schools had been upgraded, the issues of undergraduate education were by no means resolved. The AMA standardization program had created problems of curriculum rigidity in the medical schools. In their zeal, the state boards had developed detailed curriculum requirements, some even prescribing the number of hours to be devoted to specific subjects. Such requirements may have forced out the worst type of proprietary school, but they also imprisoned all schools in a rigid conformist system in which experimental teaching methods were virtually impossible.[44] If this were true for undergraduates, it might also be true if specified training

42. Minutes of the National Board of Medical Examiners, vol. I, 4 Mar. 1923, p. 191; 1 Dec. 1924, p. 240.
43. Ibid., 8 Mar. 1925, p. 254; 4 May 1925, p. 275; 27 May 1925, p. 278; 24 Oct. 1926, vol. II, p. 30; 15 May 1927, pp. 55, 63.
44. See Walter L. Bierring, "Consistency versus Chaos in Medical Education and Licensure," *Proc. Ann. Cong. med. Educ.* (1936), pp. 8–11.

criteria were demanded for graduate education—which needed even more experimentation. Abraham Flexner, still an *éminence grise* of medical education, had made this point in the discussion which followed the presentations by the fifteen committees on graduate instruction in 1921, advising caution and deliberation before the medical profession committed itself to any rigorous graduate system.[45] In part, therefore, the development of specialist training had to be delayed until medical schools had been reevaluated, and until the overlapping roles of the various agencies concerned—the AMA, the Association of American Medical Colleges, and the Federation of State Medical Boards—were disentangled.

One product of the medical colleges' growing concern over their role in the educational system was the organization of the Commission on Medical Education by the Association of American Medical Colleges in 1925, to examine the various organizational relationships in undergraduate medical education. At its first meeting a truce was called between the Federation of State Boards and the AAMC for a limited number of years, during which the federation would not impede experiments in medical education. This agreement marked the end of the federation's detailed educational functions, and in a sense, therefore, the end of rigorous methods of producing educational reforms which had been the hallmark of the AMA's success. The original standards of the Council on Medical Education for undergraduate education, taken up as the responsibility of the Federation of State Boards, were now assumed by the universities themselves.[46] The wheel had come full circle.

Meanwhile, as problems of undergraduate education were being resolved, there was continuing discussion on medical organization and manpower. The concepts of "need" and "demand" for medical care began to be explored conceptually and analytically, in relation to the supply of service available and the kind of personnel required: indeed, the Commission on Medical Education made these subjects their first item of concern. The movement of physicians away from rural areas into the towns and cities—a result of the lure of hospitals and of increasing specialization—left the rural poor with decreasing opportunities for

45. *AMA Bull.*, 15 (1921), 85–86.
46. In 1929 the federation resolved that the administration of the medical practice act in each state should conform as far as possible to the educational principles of the AAMC; and the following year (1930) the federation revised its bylaws to recognize the AAMC as the standardizing agency for all matters of premedical and predoctoral education. The federation, in turn, described as its proper function the determination of fitness for the practice of medicine and the enforcement of regulatory measures. See Commission on Medical Education, *Final Report*, pp. 166–67.

receiving medical service. Were there still too many doctors, or too few? If there were more, would they solve the problem of the rural areas? Should medical training be lowered in quality to produce rural practitioners? How were practitioners to be taught to compromise in their treatment of patients between what they knew was scientifically desirable and what they knew the patient could afford to pay? How was the personal physician to be retained? And who was to coordinate the care given by the increasing number of specialists? [47] Any professional organization which restricted the supply and cramped the function of specialists and general practitioners would have a bearing on the way in which medicine was organized and on the quality and distribution of the service offered.

The specialty organizations were concentrating on questions of educational content and specialist recognition as if organizational problems in medicine did not exist. The AMA, with an equally narrow focus, was combating supposed political encroachments into the private practice of medicine. The AAMC's Commission on Medical Education in its early reports was expressing the concern of medical education over the evolving system of health services, but university teachers, in the private enclaves of their medical centers, no longer wielded effective power. These activities within the medical profession developed as parallel rather than interdependent efforts. Meanwhile, concern over the rising costs of medical care was leading to other measures. In April 1926 fifteen people who were prominent in medicine, public health, and the social sciences came together to launch a definitive evaluation of the organization and the availability to the public of scientific medicine. Support of prominent citizens was sought; and at a larger conference in Washington in May 1927 the nucleus of the Committee on the Costs of Medical Care was created. Underpinned by the support of eight foundations, the United States Public Health Service, and by supplementary studies by private groups, the committee embarked on an ambitious series of twenty-six fact-finding studies designed to be completed within a five-year period.[48] Three of the members of the Committee on the

47. For expressed concern over these questions, see Mayers and Harrison, pp. vii, 131–33, 151–52, and passim; Commission on Medical Education, *Preliminary Report*, pp. 28–31; William Allan Pusey, "Medical Education and Medical Service," *J. Amer. med. Ass.,* 86 (1926); Allon Peebles, *A Survey of Statistical Data on Medical Facilities in the United States,* pp. 6, 22–24.

48. The committee, chaired by Ray Lyman Wilbur, included 17 physicians and dentists in private practice; 6 representatives from public health; 6 from the social sciences; 10 from institutions and special interests; and 9 members from the public. In all, it produced 28 basic publications, plus other abstracts and contributions, all published between 1928 and 1933. The result was an impressive, comprehensive

Costs of Medical Care were also members of the Commission on Medical Education. The two series of studies thus interlocked: both were well under way by 1929, the year of the Crash; both were the product of public and professional concern designed to reconcile the accelerating progress of scientific medicine in the major centers with the delivery of care to the population; and both committees were to publish their final reports in 1932. By that time the United States was plunging toward depression, and the problems of medical care provision, together with those of medical education and specialist regulation, took on a new light.

As it happened, the depression years tended to crystallize what were basically technological effects into political shadings of the "right" or "left" which got in front of the underlying organizational compulsions of specialized medicine. All through the 1920s the specialty groups had been growing and firming their identities. Some decision was demanded as to how many specialties were to be recognized; otherwise the profession might disintegrate into a kaleidoscope of shapes. The concurrent growth of hospitals and clinics, the maldistribution of resources and the potential costs of specialized medicine testified to other, equally compelling issues of health care policy which were to be reiterated, in a different context, in the 1930s.

---

sweep of existing conditions and of the problems of providing, organizing, and financing medical services of good quality whose scale has not yet been duplicated. See Committee on the Costs of Medical Care, *Medical Care for the American People: The Final Report of the Committee on the Costs of Medical Care,* Publication no. 28 (Chicago, 1932).

PART III: THE SPECIALTIES COME OF AGE, 1930–1950

CHAPTER 9

Medical Specialization and Medical Care

Prospects of Organizational Change

The pressures on the organization of health services and the training of physicians which had been evident in the 1920s were brought to a head in the social turbulence of the early 1930s. In some states in 1933, 40 percent of the people were on relief. The national income was less than half what it had been in 1929, and the rising costs of sickness were coupled with an increasing inability by the population to pay for even part of their medical bills. By 1932, tax funds were meeting 14 percent of the national medical bill, chiefly for hospital care.[1] Nevertheless, voluntary hospitals, under the impact of increasing outpatient visits by people who could not afford to pay and with a decreased use of inpatient beds, faced a financial crisis; there were doubts whether the voluntary hospital could even survive. The interest of the public in medical care was stimulated at the very time that scientific pressures were demanding professional realignments. It seemed likely that there would have to be increasing governmental intervention in health services, as in other aspects of maintaining public welfare.

The critical financial situation of the Depression both emphasized and obscured the preexisting problems of developing an appropriate structure for modern medicine. It became difficult to see the wood for the trees, the wood in this case being the total system of health services and the trees being those parts of the health service which demanded most immediate attention. Continuing, persistent, and necessary concern as to how individuals could pay their medical bills and how the medical institutions themselves could continue to survive threw an emphasis on the *cost* aspect of health services which was to have a long-lasting effect on

1. Committee on the Costs of Medical Care, Final Report, p. 52; and see Michael M. Davis and C. Rufus Rorem, *The Crisis in Hospital Finance* (Chicago, 1932), p. 3 and passim.

American medicine. The provision of shared-risk or third-party payment schemes for medical care became a dominant issue in discussions
for reform. Since one continuing possibility was government sponsorship
of health insurance, either at the state or at the federal level, the cost
aspects of medical care had widespread political ramifications. These
underlying political questions, rather than discussions over bold new
organizational approaches, were the theme of debates within the medical
profession throughout the 1930s (and, indeed, up to the 1970s). Questions of the appropriate role of the hospital, the function of general
practice, and the coordination of specialists—products of intensified
scientific advance—were overwhelmed within the medical profession by
fear of governmental paternalism, "creeping socialism," and other potential external controls.

THE MEDICAL PROFESSION

As a group, physicians fared better than most during the Depression.
The average income in nonsalaried private practice was estimated at
$5,403 in 1929; in 1933 it was down to $3,088 or 57.2 percent of the
1929 level. Industrial wages meanwhile declined to under 42 percent
of the 1929 figures. There was, however, a considerable spread of income among physicians. A survey of net professional incomes in Wisconsin for 1930 showed an income range from under $1,000 to over
$20,000, surgeons and other specialists having consistently higher
incomes than general practitioners.[2] Those at the bottom of the scale
experienced real hardship. There was every incentive for the intern or
resident to stay on in his hospital post, where he at least had board and
lodging, rather than to brave the financial uncertainties of private practice. As a result, the trend toward graduate training in hospitals was
further emphasized.

General practitioners felt the effects of the Depression most severely
in terms of collecting bills; full-time specialists the least. As their incomes
diverged, relationships between general practitioners and specialists,
already strained, became more sensitive. There were also other signs of
tension. The technological desirability of a hospital affiliation for private

2. Comparable proportions for other professions were lawyers, 69.9; dentists, 54.8;
other curative professions, 57.1; consulting engineers, 38.0; clergymen, 74.9. Figures
quoted in American Bar Association's Special Committee on the Economic Condition of the Bar, The Economics of the Legal Profession (Chicago, 1938), pp. 40–42,
44–45. For an analysis of the immediate economic impact of the Depression on
private medical practice, see Falk, Rorem, and Ring, Costs of Medical Care, pp.
195–224.

practitioners, evident in the prosperous 1920s, was matched by important economic advantages in the financial stringency of the early 1930s. Physicians on a hospital staff formed an informal network of influence with respect to the attraction and referral of patients and were thus a source of competition to other physicians. Similarly, other forms of competition, such as group practice, fee splitting, and the development of other types of health personnel, became more potent threats to the solo practitioner as the available supply of fees dwindled. The result was that wide-scale organizational developments in medicine were viewed by the average physician in terms of his own financial survival. Translated into the profession as a whole, this meant reaffirmation of the status quo in terms of the maintenance of general practice, renewed interest in limiting the number of student and immigrant physicians, pressures from organized medicine to open hospitals to all doctors, the establishment of a recognized system of qualifications for specialists, and (by no means least) opposition to any supposed encroachment from government and from other organized collective forms of paying medical fees and of providing medical service.

As in other professions at this time, the concern that too many physicians were being produced was linked with further efforts to upgrade professional education. Arthur Dean Bevan suggested a decrease of about 5 percent in medical students for five years to prevent the alleged menace of professional overcrowding, matched by an elevation of standards in the schools and state boards so as to eliminate the 10 percent or more of "the poorest and least desirable" men entering the profession.[3] The AMA Council on Medical Education and Hospitals had made no complete tours of inspection of the medical schools since just after the Flexner report. Beginning in 1934 a new and painstaking survey of medical schools was made, headed by Dr. Herman G. Weiskotten, then dean of the School of Medicine at Syracuse University. About twenty schools out of seventy-seven were found below the accepted standard; some lost their approval, others were placed on probation, and others were required to make specified changes. One such change was the reduction in the size of classes to produce relatively small schools of high quality. While upgrading standards, the survey also led to a reduction in the number of students; there were fewer medical students in 1940 than there had been ten years before.[4] Thus, to meet the economic demands of the Depression, the Flexner reforms were continued.

3. Arthur Dean Bevan, "The Overcrowding of the Medical Profession," *J. Ass. Amer. med. Coll., 11* (1936), 377–84.
4. The concern as to physician supply and educational standards dapples the pages

Concern about numbers was of course by no means limited to physicians. Whether the number of professional students ought to be restricted was considered in 1934 by the American Council of Education. Lawyers were discussing the concept of a limited bar. The drop in the employment of teachers during the Depression raised the question of a teacher surplus, and there were signs that there were too many engineers. All the issues and the arguments raised by them—the implications of Jacksonian Democracy, whether and how the public is affected by a "surplus," or whether the public ought to trust any group to determine its own numbers—were a direct outcome of Depression conditions. In medicine, however, the question of professional supply was given particular piquancy because of its relevance to interlocking questions of the organization of medical care, the payment for medical service by means other than or in addition to the traditional fee-for-service, and of physician distribution between general and specialist practice. Considerations of these issues coincided. Indeed, each was part of converging social and scientific trends.

Changes in the public's attitude to medicine as a desirable social service could be ascribed to various factors. The increase in public provision of health services was clearly one such factor. School health services, which had developed from the end of the nineteenth century, had become an integral part of the public school system. The experience of organized medical care in military service during World War I and the development of industrial health services had brought organized medical care, though of limited application, into the experience of millions of people. This experience was strengthened by increasing government participation through veterans programs, state and local government hospital services, children's services, and expanding concepts of public health. Medical care was included as an important part of the benefits to recipients under the program of the Federal Emergency Relief Administration (FERA), which provided payment for care in public clinics and in private offices, often to members of the white mid-

of the *Proceedings of the Annual Congress on Medical Education* during the 1930s. See e.g. Raymond Walters, "Should the Number of Professional Students Be Restricted?" and discussion, *Proc. Ann. Cong. Med. Educ.* (1935), pp. 3–9. For a subsequent analysis, see Elton Rayack, *Professional Power and American Medicine: The Economics of the American Medical Association* (Cleveland, 1967), esp. pp. 72–81. A vivid account of the impact of the Weiskotten survey on the weaker schools can be found in Edward J. Van Liere and Gideon S. Dodds, *History of Medical Education in West Virginia* (Morgantown, W. Va., 1965), pp. 42–49; Chapin, pp. 55–59.

dle class who had never had contact with welfare programs before. These interlocking activities could be seen in the early 1930s as a movement crystallizing public opinion in the direction of regarding health as a social right, part of a larger movement toward greater public benefits for all citizens expressed in the development of social services, workmen's compensation, relief programs, and ultimately in the comprehensive Social Security program of 1935. These aspects of public payment for medical care, in some cases the actual provision of medical service under government direction, encouraged discussion of health services as part of developing government maneuvers to counteract poverty in the early years of the New Deal.[5] Health became "political" in the sense that group payment for health services under government programs could be regarded as a politically liberal or leftish position. Private practice, on the other hand, took on the political flavor of conservatism and became identified with a private market system which was supposedly the alternative to governmental control.

But while current social philosophies were being applied to health services, medicine itself continued to change. By the late 1930s, medicine had firmly established its status as a science. The discovery of Salvarsan 606 in 1910 had heralded the modern age of chemotherapy; indeed, the day of antibiotics was not far distant. Hormones, insulin, and vitamins, all twentieth-century discoveries, were being applied in day-to-day living. Blood transfusion had become one of the commonest hospital procedures, together with a variety of X-ray procedures, electrocardiographs, basal metabolism techniques, and other diagnostic and treatment instruments which were transforming medicine from a complex mystery to an increasingly exact skill. In thirty years, public health measures had wiped out wholesale scourges. Diseases such as typhoid fever, dysentery, and diphtheria which previously had engaged much of the attention of physicians were rapidly disappearing. Other diseases, previously unknown, were taking their place: allergies, diabetes, arthritis,

5. See e.g. James H. Bossard, "A Sociologist Looks at Doctors," and other papers in American Academy of Political and Social Science, *The Medical Profession and the Public: Currents and Counter-Currents* (Philadelphia, 1934), pp. 1–10 and passim. On the FERA medical program (set up in 1933), in which doctors agreed to provide relief recipients with the same type of service which would be rendered to a private patient, see Edith Abbott, *Public Assistance,* vol. 1, *American Principles and Policies* (Chicago, 1940), pp. 452–77. An excellent review of the converging social and scientific trends is given by Bernhard J. Stern, *American Medical Practice in the Perspectives of a Century* (New York, 1945), pp. 1–44. And see David Riesman, *Medicine in Modern Society* (Princeton, 1938), esp. pp. 37–72, 146–49.

and diseases of the peripheral blood vessels. And with the new diseases came new specialists.

The rising cost of medical care in the 1930s (and since) was thus the sum of various trends. In part it was the result of rising medical potential, in part of rising social expectations for care, in part of increasing specialist manpower in medical and paramedical fields, and in part of expensive drugs and equipment. Even the same condition cost much more to treat. The diabetic patient of World War I fell into a coma and died; diabetes in the 1930s was controlled with insulin, an expensive process. Amputation of a toe in the modern operating room, with surgeons, anesthetists, laboratory workers, X-ray technicians, and a host of other personnel naturally cost more than the same procedure done by a general practitioner on the patient's kitchen table. The patient seldom had a choice; he could not choose an inexpensive over an expensive method, since the inexpensive methods rapidly withered away. It was less expensive to hire a midwife for a delivery than a physician; but the 40,000 or 50,000 midwives who still existed in the early 1930s were regarded by the medical profession as only a temporary stopgap until all patients could be delivered by physicians; midwifery laws were gradually legislating them out of existence. Another added expense in obstetrics was the trend toward hospital delivery over delivery at home; by 1935, 60–75 percent of the deliveries in most large cities were already institutional, and there was no sign of any abatement.[6] In the face of such costs, the provision of health services raised questions of social ethics which had not existed twenty or thirty years before, when medicine was far less effective. It was one thing to accept that a person could not afford to call in the average practitioner of 1915; it was quite another in 1935 to deny insulin to a diabetic.

But even disregarding questions of patient costs, which raised the possibility of group cushioning of medical bills through insurance, prepayment or other collectively organized schemes, single-handed medical practice (domain of the general practitioner) was rapidly giving way to coordinated medical endeavors. Of 145,000 active physicians in 1931, nearly 25,000 (17 percent) were in full-time specialist practice, the majority being surgeons. The Depression may have slowed the growth, but it did not reverse the trend: by 1940, 23 percent of active physicians were full-time specialists and many other physicians cultivated part-time specialist interests (see table 2). The specialists were concentrated in the

6. George W. Kosmak, "The Training of Medical Students in Obstetrics," *Proc. Ann. Cong. med. Educ.* (1936), pp. 15–18. On midwifery, see Louis S. Reed, *Midwives, Chiropodists, and Optometrists,* pp. 2–6 and passim.

Table 2. Type of Specialty of Physicians in Active Practice,
U.S., Selected Years, 1931–1969[1]

	A. Number					
	1931[2]	1940[2]	1949[2]	1960[3]	1963[3]	1969[3]
Total	145,225	156,970	173,129	199,846	223,212	251,150
Part-time specialists and gen. practitioners	120,399	120,090	110,441	85,268	77,229	57,522
Full-time specialists	24,826	36,880	62,688	114,578	145,983	193,628
Medical	6,674	10,459	19,467	36,892	47,677	59,061
Surgical[4]	14,450	19,890	30,884	52,756	65,023	76,020
Psychiatry; neurology	1,401	2,400	4,720	10,543	14,619	20,649
Other	2,301	4,131	7,617	14,387	18,664	37,898
	B. Percent					
Total	100.0	100.0	100.0	100.0	100.0	100.0
Part-time specialists and gen. practitioners	82.9	76.5	63.8	42.7	34.6	22.9
Full-time specialists	17.1	23.5	36.2	57.3	65.4	77.0
Medical	4.6	6.7	11.2	18.5	21.4	23.5
Surgical	10.0	12.7	17.8	26.4	29.1	30.3
Psychiatry; neurology	1.0	1.5	2.7	5.3	6.5	8.2
Other	1.6	2.6	4.4	7.2	8.4	15.1
	C. Ratio per 100,000 Population					
Total	117.0	118.8	116.0	109.0	117.0	124.7
Part-time specialists and gen. practitioners	97.0	90.9	74.0	46.5	40.5	28.6
Full-time specialists	20.0	27.9	42.0	62.5	76.5	96.1
Medical	5.4	7.9	13.0	20.1	25.0	29.3
Surgical	11.6	15.1	20.7	28.8	34.1	37.7
Psychiatry; neurology	1.1	1.8	3.2	5.8	7.7	10.3
Other	1.9	3.1	5.1	7.8	9.7	18.8

1. Excludes interns, residents, fellows, and those retired, not in practice. Includes those in private and nonprivate practice, both federal and non-federal.
2. Excludes possessions.
3. Includes possessions.
4. Includes anesthesiology.

Source: *Health Manpower Source Book*, sec. 14, Medical Specialists, tables 3, 5; sec. 18, *Manpower in the 1960s*, table 12; American Medical Association, *Distribution of Physicians in the U.S. 1963*, vol. 1, table A; ibid., *1969*, tables 1, 10.

major cities and towns. Questions of costs, which were emphasized during the Depression, were thus juxtaposed with questions of coordination and distribution of services which had been evident before 1929 but which were each year becoming more acute.

THE CASE FOR COOPERATIVE MEDICINE

One means of coordination of the specialists was the hospital. A study in the late 1920s reported that in New York State 99 percent of the specialists had hospital appointments, compared with only 40 percent of the general practitioners.[7] Hospital-based group practice was thus one potent organizational possibility, at least for specialists. Most patients, however, did not seek out hospitals when they were sick, but went directly to a practitioner's private office. Thus the hospital, at least under practice arrangements which existed then, had only limited application as a coordinating agency. Another means of coordination was the channeling of patients to specialists through a general or family practitioner, who would thus act as the hub of a specialist system; this was the British model. But for this model to be effective, the role and the numerical proportion of general practice would have to be sustained, and at the same time both patients and specialists would have to be restrained from bypassing the system. This could be done through change in the behavior of the medical profession so that specialists would refuse to see patients not referred to them by general practitioners; but such a suggestion was only made by a handful of idealists.[8] It also could be encouraged through the operation of a widespread payment scheme such as health insurance, or people might be persuaded to change their use of physicians. As yet, however, there were no such restraints; indeed, the number of physicians in general practice actually declined between 1931 and 1940.[9] A third means of coordination continued to be group practice outside hospitals by specialists in different special fields, but, with notable exceptions, group practice remained largely ignored.

The transformation or revival of the family doctor in a new guise continued to be discussed in the medical press and had some emotive appeal. In 1930 the New England Medical Center in Boston raised nearly $1,000,000 by public subscription under the slogan "Restore the family doctor."[10] But both the public and young physicians had become used to a system of medical specialists. If the trend toward specialism were to be reversed, trenchant measures would be required. Control of specialist education and qualification offered one channel for future restraint. New patterns of medical care delivery might offer others, either through

7. Noted by Peebles, *A Study of Statistical Data on Medical Facilities in the United States*, p. 28.
8. See e.g. J. J. Nutt, "General Practitioners and Specialists," *AMA Bull.*, 21 (1931), 81.
9. From 120,399 to 120,090. See table 2.
10. Joseph H. Pratt, "Better Rural Medicine," *AMA Bull.*, 27 (1932), 122.

organized payment schemes, which would only reimburse specialists where diagnosis or treatment was made at a generalist's referral, or through an organized practice scheme whereby specialists themselves would voluntarily limit their role to consultation. Clearly the strongest method would be for all three restraining devices to operate. If in addition hospitals were included, the various channels of communication and coordination among patients, generalists, and specialists would be further rationalized.

Such rationalizations were at the core of the final reports of the Committee on the Costs of Medical Care[11] and of the Commission on Medical Education,[12] both of which reported in 1932. Both these committees had been set up before the Depression, and in large part they attacked conditions which were already evident in the 1920s but which the Depression had made more acute.

The final report of the Committee on the Costs of Medical Care, together with twenty-seven more detailed reports published by the committee, set before the public a comprehensive survey of health facilities, a vivid description of the unequal provision of care to the population, and an analysis of the results of providing services on the basis of consumer demands rather than consumer needs. In a survey of over 8,500 white families it was found that nearly half of those in the lowest income group (under $1,200) received no medical, dental, or eye care in twelve consecutive months in the period 1928–31.[13] Medical costs were also unequally distributed: less than 4 percent of families incurred 80 percent of the costs.[14] The report as a whole was based on the implicit philosophy that the full potential of medicine should be made available to the entire population. In short, medicine was assumed to be a necessary social service. It was in the interpretation of what such service meant that the interests of the public and the medical profession diverged.

The majority of the committee recommended that medical personnel should be organized in group medical practices, each including physicians, dentists, nurses, and technical personnel, and each preferably focused on a hospital. Group practice would be supported by an extension and reinforcement of public health services, governmental and private, thus spreading the costs of disease prevention. Individual medical bills would, it was suggested, be protected through the encouragement of group prepayment schemes. Opinion was divided on whether such

11. Committee on the Costs of Medical Care, *Final Report.*
12. Commission on Medical Education, *Final Report of the Commission on Medical Education* (New York, 1932).
13. Committee on the Costs of Medical Care, *Final Report,* p. 9.
14. Ibid., pp. 17–18.

schemes should be financed through a system of private insurance, or of tax, or of both; and whether prepayment schemes should be voluntary or compulsory. The way was thus open in the recommendations to a system of compulsory government-sponsored health insurance; but it was equally open to a spontaneous development of local private schemes with no compulsory element, nor any public subsidy. But while the proposals for financing were vague, the philosophy was clear: some kind of group prepayment scheme, with shared risks, was desirable.

It is of course possible to have coordinated payment schemes without necessarily having a coordinated system of medical service. Indeed, this is largely the system that exists today: a mixture of government prepayment (Medicare), tax (Medicaid), commercial and nonprofit insurance, and other prepayment schemes, which is designed to protect the consumer's pocketbook rather than to reorganize the medical system. But the Committee on the Costs of Medical Care deliberately suggested an integrated scheme whereby the providers as well as the consumers of health services would be brought into cooperative relationships. The two outstanding problems of contemporary medicine—rapidly increasing costs and steadily increasing specialization in equipment and personnel—would be dealt with together. Coordinated group practice arrangements might, the committee considered, bring medical specialists into a useful, beneficial, and economic relation with each other; restore the family physician; effect a balance between the existing disparity of income between general practitioner and specialist, which was encouraging fee splitting and unnecessary medical work; and establish a medical referral system. Some two-thirds of all physicians were already thought to be associated with hospitals and clinics; and in many hospitals physicians maintained offices or office hours for seeing their private patients (nearly 1,000 hospitals were so used by 4,500 physicians). [15] The suggestions of the majority of the Committee on the Costs of Medical Care would have expanded this trend, by including all physicians—general practitioners as well as specialists—on hospital staffs and providing them with office space. The staff so formed would become a group practice with community responsibilities, utilizing the hospital and its own subsidiary personnel. Such a model, with its echoes of the army medical groups of World War I, of discussions of medical care in the health insurance movement of 1915–20, and of the successful structure of the Mayo Clinic and other private groups, was evolutionary rather than revolutionary. Its importance lay in the fact that the model was designed not only for reasons of economy but also to tackle a major problem of scientific

15. Ibid., pp. 36, 85.

medicine, the control and efficient utilization of specialists. In the Committee's report, moreover, group practice was linked with the recommendation of prepayment. Instead, then, of a free transaction between one doctor and one patient, each person would purchase an insurance policy or contract for specified services to be given by a health service organization.

The difference between this pattern and the system of primary (generalist) and secondary (specialist) health centers which was advocated in Britain in the 1920s and 1930s—a country, incidentally, which already had national health insurance for its lower-income working population—emphasized the particular relevance of multispecialist group practice as an organizational solution to the egalitarian structure of medicine in the United States. The British medical profession continued to be divided between those who were general practitioners (and as such tended to see patients before the specialists) and those who were specialists, who acted as consultants to GPs and who were in control of the major voluntary hospitals. The lines had become somewhat fuzzy in the 1930s, because the pressures of medical specialization in Britain were no less strong than in the United States. Nevertheless, the British solution was—and still is—to group only the general practitioners into health centers, to which patients would go initially, and to concentrate only the specialists in hospitals.[16] This concept accepted that the general practitioner had a special function as the purveyor of primary medical care, while specialists, at one remove, had a secondary role; organizationally, therefore, generalists and specialists were divided.

The primary care concept has recently appeared, with some force, in American medicine; but it is still little more than a concept, for the valid reason that no special or separate cadre of generalists existed in the United States. Instead, the attempt to recreate a conglomerate "general practice," by pulling together generalists and specialists in one place, was a more logical solution, in the 1930s as later. The traditionally egalitarian structure of American medicine provided no formal channeling of patients from general practitioner to specialist, nor a clear demarcation of function in relation either to the hospital or to the patient. Generalists and specialists competed openly. Physicians expected to have access to hospitals. As a result, the hospital, rather than as in Britain the mechanisms of health insurance and medical professionalism (both of which reinforced the concept of primary medical care), was the organizational hub of medicine.[17] It followed that the hospital might assume some re-

16. See Stevens, pp. 61–64.
17. As far as figures are available, it is probable that one-third of British practi-

sponsibility for community medicine as well as for sophisticated scientific techniques, and that hospital appointments could be an important way of controlling the standards of the majority of physicians. Linking the staff of a hospital with membership of a hospital-based group practice was logical.

But while these suggestions might seem logical, they were by no means politically acceptable to organized medicine. The Committee on the Costs of Medical Care, which had been drawn together from various groups, including private medical practice, professional associations, public health, the social sciences, and members of the public, was itself divided as to how far its recommendations should go. A minority group of nine, which included the AMA representatives, expressed their doubts in terms of the need to restrict "government competition in the practice of medicine" (a threat more readily apparent in the general political environment of the early thirties rather than in the body of the report) and in their opposition to "the corporate practice of medicine." [18] The plan of integrated group practice involving general practitioners and specialists was deemed theoretically attractive, but it was doubted whether, in practice, the general practitioner would be accepted into groups by specialists on equal terms. It was claimed that in a group the general practitioner tends to disappear, that the GP did not need elaborate equipment to conduct his practice and therefore had no need of a group practice center; and it was implied—wrongly—that the majority report ignored the central position of the general practitioner. The minority also opposed both voluntary and compulsory health insurance. It was only too happy, however, to recognize the duty of the state to give complete and adequate care to the indigent, thus freeing private physicians from responsibility for an unprofitable part of their practice. Then, after claiming that it was not opposed to insurance but to its abuses and potential evils, the minority suggested the development of plans for medical care by state or county medical societies. An advantage of this was said to be the removal of the possibility of "unethical competition," since all physicians would be included and fees would be fixed. This plan, if rather vague, could not help but appeal to the majority of the AMA membership. Indeed, it could be seen as a forerunner of later society efforts to establish medical insurance plans through Blue Shield, and (now) through medical society foundations.

tioners had hospital appointments in the 1930s, compared with two-thirds of Americans. See A. Bradford Hill, *J. Roy. Stat. Soc., 114* (1951), 25, 27, 30.
18. Committee on the Costs of Medical Care, *Final Report,* pp. 152–83.

The fact that the majority had not recommended compulsory health insurance became obscured in subsequent debate. In part this can be ascribed to the identification by organized medicine from the 1920s of group, collective, or institutional modes of practice (even if organized privately) with outside or governmental influence. In part, there was to be ready identification of the report with the Roosevelt administration— personified in Edgar Sydenstricker, a member of the committee who was appointed to the technical board of President Roosevelt's Committee on Economic Security, where he did indeed advocate compulsory health insurance.[19] Ironically, Sydenstricker had refused to sign either the majority or minority committee report on the ground that neither dealt with the fundamental economic questions. Nevertheless the belief grew that the Committee on the Costs of Medical Care had proposed some kind of compulsory service which would jeopardize the interests of the medical profession. The rather modest recommendations of the committee were immediately labeled by the AMA as socialist dogma: "There is the question of Americanism versus sovietism for the American people." [20] Its political line hardened in a stubborn, conservative defense of a system of practice which was already, scientifically if not socially, outmoded. The recommendations of the committee were identified with other inroads into solo private, fee-for-service practice: with proposals for federally sponsored health insurance schemes, with increasing hospital power (an important aspect of the "corporate practice of medicine"), or with new types of voluntary prepayment schemes which provided further potential competition.

Thus the recommendations of the Committee on the Costs of Medical Care were left unimplemented by either the private or the public sector. Despite the sweeping reforms of the Roosevelt administration between 1933 and 1935 and the trend toward federal action and control, public intervention in medical care was limited to the poor. A brief possibility in 1934 that a health insurance scheme would be part of the proposed comprehensive scheme of social security was quickly squashed by AMA opposition. The AMA in that year adopted ten principles with regard to insurance; these included control of all features of medical service by the medical profession and the refusal to allow a third party to come between physician and patient in any medical relation. President Roosevelt had spoken confidently of devising a health insurance system, and indeed a discussion of health insurance was included in the 1934 report

19. Editorial, *J. Amer. med. Ass., 103* (1934), 608–09.
20. Editorial, *J. Amer. med. Ass., 99* (1932), 2035.

of the Committee on Economic Security, together with a statement that recommendations would follow.[21] At a special session in February 1935, however, the AMA House of Delegates reiterated its opposition to all forms of compulsory insurance. Following the AMA's action, the administration, anxious not to jeopardize other aspects of Social Security, did nothing. Thus the Social Security Act of 1935 was passed without health insurance provisions.

Without any central provider or purchaser of medical care, there was no national administrative lever to initiate change. The Committee on the Costs of Medical Care had favored local initiative in the formation of group health arrangements. But the constant opposition of the AMA to self-sustaining groups of consumers and providers daunted all but the most determined physicians from establishing or entering such schemes. Dr. Michael A. Shadid, in the fight to establish a cooperative hospital— the first in the United States—at Elk City, Oklahoma, had to take on the state medical association. In 1936 he was summoned before the Board of Medical Examiners to answer charges of advertising, fleecing the public, and soliciting patients.[22] For setting up a group practice, Drs. Donald Ross and H. Clifford Loos were expelled from the Los Angeles County Medical Society. Members of the Group Health Association of Washington, D.C. (started in 1937), and the Group Health Cooperative of Puget Sound, Seattle (1946), brought organized medicine into the courts of law.[23] Medical ethics, designed to ensure mutual trust within the doctor-patient relationship, were being applied to maintain the interests of solo practitioners. It was unfortunate that the types of practice arrangements being condemned by organized medicine were not economic devices alone; they were also organizational adjustments to functional specialism.

PENALTIES OF PROFESSIONAL EGALITARIANISM

That the American Medical Association was the dominant organization of the profession was the result of the egalitarian tradition of American

21. See Arthur J. Altmeyer, *The Formative Years of Social Security* (Madison, 1966), pp. 14–16, 33, 57; AMA, *Digest,* pp. 314–17.
22. Michael A. Shadid, *A Doctor for the People: The Autobiography of the Founder of America's First Cooperative Hospital,* 2d ed. (New York, 1944), p. 189 and passim.
23. See Herman M. Somers and Anne R. Somers, *Doctors, Patients and Health Insurance: The Organization and Financing of Medical Care* (Washington, D.C., 1961), pp. 347–49 and passim; Richard Harris, *A Sacred Trust* (New York, 1966), pp. 8–19; "The American Medical Association: Power, Purpose and Politics in Organized Medicine," *Yale Law Journal, 63* (1954), 980–92.

medicine. Most of the AMA membership were still general practitioners, although the delegates tended to be city specialists.[24] Organized medicine was in effect the spokesman of the private practitioner who had been trained in the pre-Flexner era or the period of post-Flexner reforms. Their medical education had been geared toward a wide-ranging competence coupled with independent authority in diagnosis and practice. Only a minority of the schools of the 1930s included lectures in medical economics or medical organization; indeed, even the teaching of public health was regarded as experimental.[25] Few universities effectively absorbed their medical schools into the intellectual life of the university. The natural conservatism of the profession was enhanced by this educational isolationism as well as by a technology which had outpaced its organizational structures.

Those at the top of a profession, not facing the daily financial headaches of private practice,were free to entertain more progressive or liberal views than those whose livelihoods appeared most threatened, and who had the least time or opportunity to consider the wider ramifications of different policies. But, unlike the Royal Colleges in Britain, the specialist associations and scientific medical leaders inside and outside the universities had no consolidated influence on the profession.

At one time, the American College of Surgeons had offered a real organizational alternative to the professional authority of the AMA. But the stature of the College had declined during the 1920s, and it had not emerged as the force that some had hoped for. The College was still faced with the dilemma of how far it would be willing to go toward providing a standard of surgical competence beyond minimum requirements, and how far it wished to represent all who practiced surgery. It was poised uneasily between autocratic dominance of excellence in surgery and democratic representation of the small-town surgeon. In attempting to standardize surgery, the College had undoubtedly raised average surgical standards. At the same time a rift was developing between the body of surgeons and the emerging surgical leadership in the universities. The university group had become more important with the expansion of medical centers in the 1920s and with the encouragement of full-time university teachers; it seemed evident that the universities would increasingly provide scientific leadership. The stage had not, however, been reached for organizational leadership. There were criticisms of the College's fail-

24. Oliver Garceau, *The Political Life of the American Medical Association* (Cambridge, 1941), pp. 54–57.
25. A 1935 survey had revealed that of 71 schools surveyed, 31 reported some lectures on medical economics, but 27 had given the subject no consideration. Esther Lucile Brown, *Physicians and Medical Care* (New York, 1937), pp. 68–70.

ure to publish a financial statement and complaints that fee spliting continued among fellows and even College regents, that younger men should
be represented at the top, and that standards were too low and fees too
high.[26] The American College of Surgeons was thus at a critical stage in
its development at the very time when it might have left a lasting impression on the organization of medical care.

The AMA therefore continued to attract not only the raw power of
a major union but also the glitter of a more general professional eminence
which might otherwise have found expression in scientifically oriented
medical guilds. Even for men of such eminence as Harvey Cushing, the
presidency of the AMA was a greater prize than leadership in the American College of Surgeons; and the cooperation of the AMA remained
vital in any recommendations of public medical policy. Morris Fishbein
congratulated Cushing for upholding the AMA views in opposition to
compulsory health insurance as a member of President Roosevelt's Committee on Economic Security—and thus Cushing could claim to have had
a large part in the exclusion of health from the Social Security Act of
1935.[27] This desire to uphold ·AMA policy—or at least not openly to
condemn it—may have featured in the actions of more than one eminent
physician of the time.

The American College of Surgeons joined the American Hospital
Association, and disagreed with the AMA, in endorsing voluntary hospital
insurance schemes in 1933. Prepayment for hospital bills—that is, a
scheme whereby contributors pay regular payments in return for specified
hospital benefits whenever these might be required—had been offered by
the Baylor University Hospital of Dallas and the Community Hospital
of Grinnell, Iowa, before the Committee on the Costs of Medical Care
reported. Plans were simultaneously developed in other areas, through
individual hospitals or groups of hospitals in the East and Middle West.
To the low-income patient such group schemes provided a guarantee of
payment for the most expensive—and also the most unforeseen—aspect
of health care. To the hospitals, which had suffered financially in the Depression, the plans also provided a regular and welcome income. The
AMA Bureau of Medical Economics, the Judicial Council, the House of
Delegates, and the AMA *Journal* made repeated statements opposing
group hospitalization schemes.[28] But Franklin Martin, representing the

26. Loyal Davis, *Fellowship of Surgeons*, pp. 290–95.
27. Fishbein, p. 794; Fulton, pp. 649–57.
28. See Michael M. Davis, "Change Comes to the Doctor," in American Academy
of Political and Social Science, *The Medical Profession and the Public*, pp. 63–74;
R. G. Leland, "Group Hospitalization Contracts are Insurance Contracts," *AMA
Bull., 28* (1933), 113–16.

American College of Surgeons, was apparently convinced of President Roosevelt's reluctance to deal further with the AMA. Through its hospital standardization program, the College was more familiar with the financial pressures on the voluntary hospitals than was the AMA, and it was more likely than the AMA to accept hospital insurance as a means of resurrecting hospital finances instead of a threat to private practice. Hence the decision by the College Board of Regents to study methods of organizing medical care, the appointment of its Medical Service Board, and this board's report (accepted by the regents in October 1933) upholding voluntary health insurance under the control of the medical profession and allied services.[29]

At the meeting of the AMA House of Delegates at Cleveland in June 1934 the American College of Surgeons was denounced in terms that echoed past disputes. The College was castigated as a "small group with a specialistic organization," attempting to take over AMA functions, namely to "dominate and control the nature of medical practice." [30] The vehement response of general practitioners, who undoubtedly saw the College action as an attempt to build up hospital services to their exclusion, was fully expressed in the medical journals, and the resulting conflict between the two organizations became widely publicized in the national press. Franklin Martin, who had been in contact with President Roosevelt several times on the subject of health insurance, was however at the end of his long domination over the College. Due to retire from his position of director general in the fall of 1935, he died in the spring of that year, before the College had evolved policies for continuing without his guidance. Thus at a critical time the College was leaderless.

The American College of Physicians, meanwhile, went out of its way not to antagonize the AMA. In a 1934 editorial of the *Annals of Internal Medicine,* J. H. Means, an influential member of the College, advocated that all improved methods of rendering service ought to be tried out—including health insurance, contract practice, group practice, and other measures.[31] But the College generally soft-pedaled economic and political issues. President George M. Piersol, who was with Walter Bierring, Harvey Cushing, and others a member of the Medical Advisory Board to the Committee on Economic Security, stressed that the College should avoid taking an active part in social and economic issues.[32] The College

29. Loyal Davis, *Fellowship of Surgeons,* pp. 305–09; "Principles of Prepayment Plans for Medical and Hospital Service," *Bull. Amer. Coll. Surg., 18* (1934), 3.
30. *Proc. AMA House of Delegates* (June 1934), pp. 42, 49, quoted in AMA, *Digest,* p. 316.
31. Editorial, *Ann. Intern. Med., 8* (1934), 374–75.
32. George M. Piersol, "Presidential Address," ibid., pp. 1–9.

decided not to carry out its earlier intention to publish in the *Annals* a
series of "educational and instructive" articles on medical economics, in
deference to the position then being adopted by the AMA in opposition
to health insurance.[33] Thus, although the American College of Physicians
—again, like the Surgeons—appeared to have a generally more liberal
attitude toward health service policies than did the AMA, it was careful
not to publicize the fact. By 1935 it was reported that the American
College of Physicians was establishing more cordial relations with the
AMA, to which the College then ascribed a "more constructive attitude"
toward medical economic issues.[34] One reason for not embarrassing the
AMA was clearly the overlapping leadership. At the Milwaukee session
in 1933, Dr. Walter Bierring had been elected AMA president and Dr.
John H. Musser vice-president; both were College regents.

Thus the AMA views prevailed. The 1932 report of the Commission
on Medical Education, the product of leading educators, focused to little
avail on the public aspects of medicine, on medical needs of the population, and on the advisability of cooperation among physicians, institutions, and groups.[35] The action in 1935 of the California Medical Association in endorsing voluntary and compulsory health insurance, and the
expression of interest in new types of payment and organizational
schemes both by medical societies and by leading medical individuals,
created ripples but no wide-scale movement. The structure of the profession had not equipped physicians to deal simultaneously with their own
interests and with the public implications of scientific medicine—in terms
of cost, manpower, or organization. When a group of over 400 leading
specialists, medical school deans, and public health physicians finally
came together in the late 1930s to lobby in favor of a national health
policy, they did so through the medium of a new and temporary organization, the Committee of Physicians for the Improvement of Medical Care.
By this time, however, it was doubtful whether, even with a different
organizational structure, the medical profession alone could have un-
raveled the enormous problems of providing medical care.

THE PRICE OF CONSERVATISM

While the views of the AMA were hardening against compulsory health
insurance schemes and the "corporate practice of medicine," the broad
problems of specialized medicine remained. The focus for public action

33. See W. G. Morgan, *American College of Physicians,* pp. 189, 192.
34. "Minutes of the Board of Regents," *Ann. Intern. Med.,* 8 (1935), 1241.
35. Commission on Medical Education, *Final Report,* p. 384 and passim.

during the late 1930s and into the 1940s was largely on how individuals should pay for medical care, rather than how medical care might be organized; but the two were vitally connected. In all its aspects, the organization of health services was of increasing social importance. President Roosevelt stated flatly in January 1939: "The health of the people is a public concern; ill health is a major cause of suffering, economic loss, and dependency; good health is essential to the security and progress of the Nation." [36]

In 1935 the president had set up an Interdepartmental Committee out of which came, in February 1938, the Report on the Health Needs of the Nation. This report not only recommended expansion of public health and maternal and child health services under existing titles of the Social Security Act; it also suggested a new interlocking system of federal grants to states: for hospital construction, for subsidy of state programs for the medically needy, and for state programs of general medical care. Federal action to develop compensation for wage loss due to temporary and permanent disability was suggested at the same time.[37] Thus a federally subsidized and state-organized system of medical care was envisaged—several years before a government paper of similar national application was published in Great Britain. The National Health Conference called by the president (18–20 July, 1938) endorsed these proposals and aroused considerable public interest and support—so much, indeed, that the AMA called a special session of the House of Delegates in September. This special session ensured the continuation of AMA opposition to the establishment of any form of compulsory health insurance. The AMA did, however, with certain qualifications, favor other aspects of the proposals: extension of public health services, expansion of hospital construction, medical care for the medically needy, and income-loss insurance. The AMA also went on record as approving voluntary hospitalization insurance, a concession to an obviously increasing trend.[38]

A bill was introduced in the U.S. House of Representatives in 1938 which would have established compulsory health insurance for lower-

36. U.S., Congress, *Message from the President of the United States to the Congress of the United States,* 76th Cong., 1st sess., Document no. 120, 23 Jan. 1939.
37. The Interdepartmental Committee to Coordinate Health and Welfare Activities began by considering the coordination of existing health activities, but early in 1937 it turned to the broader question of the development of a program for the whole nation—largely through the interests of two members of the committee, Josephine Roche (asst. sec. of the Treasury, and responsible for the U.S. Public Health Service) and Arthur J. Altmeyer (chairman of the Social Security Board). Altmeyer, pp. 93–95.
38. Editorial, *J. Amer. med. Ass., 111* (1938), 1188.

income workers and voluntary insurance for the rest of the population. But this bill died without a hearing.[39] Of serious import to the AMA position, however, was the bill introduced by Sen. Robert F. Wagner of New York at the end of February 1939. This bill incorporated the recommendations of the Interdepartmental Committee and would, if passed, have become the National Health Act of 1939. Besides the less controversial proposals for public health, the Wagner bill suggested maternal and child welfare services, hospital construction and disability insurance, and state-operated medical care programs aided by federal grants to states. Not surprisingly the AMA immediately voiced opposition and began to gird itself for a fight against the bill which was expected to be reported out of the Committee on Education and Labor early in 1940. President Roosevelt, however, appeared to have changed his mind about making a national health program an issue in the 1940 presidential campaign; instead, he proffered a fragment of the Wagner bill, a plan for the construction of small hospitals with federal funds in needy communities. The national health program was thereby sidetracked. At the same time, hospital construction was legislatively separated from other aspects of health service provision—and has so remained; federal grants for hospital construction were finally initiated under the Truman administration through the Hill-Burton legislation of 1946.

One purpose of including hospital construction as part of a national health program was to improve the quality of care by linking all physicians with hospitals. In so doing, cooperative work might be stimulated, general practitioners and specialists be brought together, and the expensive equipment and staff of the hospital be utilized as an extension of the physician's practice.[40] Without such a link there was little organizational impetus to rationalize the increasingly difficult relationship between the generalist and specialist.

The potential of using a payment mechanism to influence an intraprofessional relationship by paying for specialist care only where requested by a primary practitioner was, however, put into operation in the late 1930s in the voluntary White Cross prepayment scheme in Boston. Patients who joined this plan had to have a personal physician; and the

39. For a useful review of the legislative proposals for health provision, see Agnes W. Brewster, *Health Insurance and Related Proposals for Financing Personal Health Services: A Digest of Major Legislation and Proposals for Federal Action 1935–1957* (USDHEW, Social Security Administration, 1958).
40. U.S., Congress, Senate, Subcommittee of the Committee on Education and Labor, *Report and Recommendations on National Health by the Interdepartmental Committee to Coordinate Health and Welfare Activities: Hearings on S. 1620,* 76th Cong., 1st sess., pt. 2, p. 29.

plan paid for referral by these physicians to specialists. Despite complaints of unethical practice made to the Massachusetts Medical Society, on the old grounds of discriminating between the qualifications of one physician and another, most Boston specialists accepted the referrals, and by the outbreak of World War II the plan was providing medical care for about 30,000 people. If it had survived, White Cross would have offered a valuable organizational experiment; but it fell a victim to the disruptions of war. When the war was over, the Massachusetts General Hospital tried to set up its own prepayment scheme (1947), but this was effectively blocked by local physicians. Instead, Blue Cross and Blue Shield programs began their rapid development. Their nature, as was that of the developing commercial insurance schemes, was to shore up preexisting organizational patterns, guaranteeing payment for service, rather than to initiate new delivery forms. It was this lack of experiment with new ways of organizing and providing care which was the real tragedy of medical conservatism in the 1930s.

Meanwhile, specialization of personnel was proceeding rapidly and was increasingly taking on vertical as well as horizontal aspects: that is, in the assignment of specific tasks to new types of personnel as well as the differentiation of physicians above a basic level of training. By 1940, nonmedical health personnel outnumbered physicians by three to one. In some instances, such as medical social work or nursing, the paramedical worker provided a professional function which cut across the specialist divisions in medicine. But in others, such as optometry, laboratory technology, X-ray technology, nurse anesthesiology, physical therapy—the technician's field of competence coincided with the area of a physician's specialization, and even became vital to the successful prosecution of the physician's practice. In 1940, there were less than 1,600 full-time specialists in radiology but as many as 12,000 X-ray technicians; there were under 1,000 full-time medical pathologists, and some 20,000 laboratory technicians; and the fewer than 300 full-time medical anesthesiologists were matched by an estimated 5,000 nurse anesthetists.[41]

The AMA Council on Medical Education and Hospitals in 1934 had begun a program of educational standardization of these ancillary technical services. Included at first were medical laboratory technology and occupational therapy, but the program was later extended to physical therapy, X-ray technology, and medical record technology. Medicine

41. *Health Manpower Source Book*, sec. 18, Manpower in the 1960s (1964), table 10, p. 16; sec. 14, *Medical Specialists* (1962) table 6; U.S. President's Commission on the Health Needs of the Nation, *Building America's Health: A Report to the President* (Washington, D.C., 1952–53), vol. 3, tables 287, 292, 317.

could no longer claim to be the province of the physician alone—or of the physician and nurse, or even the monopoly of particular specialist fields. Accommodations had to be made, and perhaps even the "practice of medicine" had to be redefined, to include or to exclude these groups. But there was still no vehicle, such as national health insurance would have provided, to foster such accommodations.

Meanwhile, for the individual physician there were irresistible urges to specialize. The middle class was used to dealing with specialists, to by-passing the general practitioner, and to "shopping" for specialist care on the basis of self-diagnosis. Although it was impossible to gauge whether, and how far, incomes did in fact affect career choices of physicians, specialists consistently earned more money; the most lucrative field was surgery.[42] Almost all graduates by the early 1930s took at least one year in a hospital internship. After the basic college course, four years of medical training under specialists, and one year in hospital work largely of a specialist nature, the young physician was no longer interested in general practice. In the large towns the pediatrician seemed already to be the last of the general practitioners.[43] General practice was recognized as being a more limited field than previously in that the practitioner was no longer expected to be competent in fields claimed by specialists, but had acquired no new, identifiable skills in their place. The medical schools, true to their scientific inclinations, were not producing the personal physicians that were said to be at the cornerstone of medicine; and there was no recognized graduate training for such a role. All these factors emphasized the changing aspects of medical care. What was a personal physician? And what a specialist? The old patterns were changing; but as yet there was no new model.

An estimate produced by the Committee on the Costs of Medical Care had indicated that general practitioners could care for the great majority

42. For contemporary accounts, see Maurice Leven, *The Incomes of Physicians: An Economic and Statistical Analysis* (Chicago, 1932), pp. 50–54, 96; I. S. Falk, Margaret C. Klem, and Nathan Sinai, *The Incidence of Illness and the Receipt and Costs of the Medical Care among Representative Families,* Committee on the Costs of Medical Care Publication no. 26 (Chicago, 1933), pp. 104–06, 281–82; Commission on Medical Education, *Final Report,* p. 33; E. L. Brown, *Physicians and Medical Care,* p. 143 and passim; "The Incomes of Specialists," *Med. Econ., 21* (1941), 47–51; Seymour E. Harris, *The Economics of American Medicine* (New York, 1964), pp. 154–59.
43. This posed problems for pediatric training as well as for general medical education. Pediatric interns, for example, were not routinely taught to vaccinate a child or to immunize one against diphtheria. Philip Van Ingen, "Whither Are We Bound?," *Trans. Amer. pediat. Soc., 43* (1931), 9–17; and see Herman G. Weis-kotten et al., *Medical Education in the United States, 1934–1939,* p. 202 and passim.

of illnesses without resorting to specialists and without any decrease in quality: a proportion of 82 percent generalists to 18 percent full-time and part-time specialists was suggested.[44] But without large-scale, organizational checks and balances such as those suggested by the Committee on the Costs of Medical Care, without a general system of health insurance, without general recognition of the hospital as the base of community medicine and as the arbiter of quality, and without widespread growth of specialist group practices which could contain both the vertical and horizontal specialist elements, there was no means of testing this in practice. Despite the social upheavals of the Depression, the rapid changes in health manpower, the rises in medical costs, and the publicity generated about health service inequities and deficiencies in the reports of the Committee on the Costs of Medical Care, the organizational system (or nonsystem) of medical care in 1939 was little different from that of ten or twenty years earlier.

It was in this arid political climate that the specialty certifying boards developed.

44. Falk, Rorem, and Ring, *Costs of Medical Care,* p. 223 and passim.

CHAPTER 10

Who Should Control Specialization?

While there was no clear solution in the 1930s to questions of bringing available medical services within the financial reach of all citizens, there was a rapid crystallization of professional organization within the medical profession. The American Medical Association emerged as a unified and powerful political spokesman for the practicing physician. At the same time, in response both to the continuing development of specialist fields and to the economic retrenchments of the Depression, medical specialties became codified and formalized. This process could be seen as a resumption of the interest expressed within different specialty groups in the 1920s for a machinery of formal identification of training and competence for those who wished to be recognized as specialists. On the other hand, Depression conditions undoubtedly accelerated the trend. There were potential financial as well as professional advantages to the well-trained specialist in being able to hold himself out as such, whether through a special diploma, a license, or a degree. General practitioners, likewise, would tend to support the establishment of monopolies based on educational exclusiveness as a means of protecting themselves as well as the public from the competition of pseudospecialists. Just as there were moves to stem the supply of physicians by upgrading standards and limiting the number of students in the medical schools, so the creation of standards for specialists might also be expected to limit their number.

How specialist standards and qualifications should be achieved, for what purposes, and by which professional or public agency were questions, however, to which there were no clearer answers in 1930 than there had been ten years before. Specialist regulation had become a question of interest to various overlapping organizations. The AMA Council on Medical Education and Hospitals was performing functions in the area of curriculum delineation and residency approval; the Association of American Medical Colleges was concerned with the content of graduate study;

and the National Board of Medical Examiners was also considering a role in certifying specialists.[1] State licensure remained a live issue. And new specialty groups were moving to form independent certifying boards. The training and certification of medical specialists was, moreover, closely tied with the concurrent public concern over providing and regulating health services, which led to proposals for compulsory health insurance. In their reports of 1932, both the Committee on the Costs of Medical Care and the Commission on Medical Education recommended standards and formal recognition of specialists.[2] The former put this responsibility on the professional bodies; the latter spoke vaguely of a joint public and professional responsibility and of state specialist registers. Such interest was logical, for if there were to be a national health service or a health insurance system in the United States, it would stand or fall on the structure of the medical profession and the supply of different kinds and levels of physicians.

These various strands tied together. The specialty boards which developed in the 1930s were the outcome of a long intraprofessional movement, which would inter alia reinforce emerging specialty associations and groups. But they were also a response to what seemed the inevitable alternative of licensing of specialists by the states. The boards thus had both a professional and a quasi-public component, and their coordinated development had wide importance. Attempts at such coordination were a major theme of graduate medical education between 1930 and 1933, and in these years the basic structure and interrelationships of the specialty boards were established. The system developed out of no obvious organizational solution but, as with most professional organizations, from compromise among major interest groups.

THE AMERICAN BOARD OF OBSTETRICS AND GYNECOLOGY:
EMERGING IMPLICATIONS OF THE SPECIALTY BOARD

The earlier boards of ophthalmology and otolaryngology, and the American College of Surgeons, besides being expressions of emerging profes-

1. The AAMC Committee on Educational Policies cooperated with the National Board of Medical Examiners in conferring with representatives of the national specialty societies. This committee suggested in 1931 that fundamental requirements for the practice of specialties should include graduation from a recognized medical college, one year of general internship, a residency of unspecified length (or three years of supervised special practice or five years general practice), and at least two years of university-sponsored clinical work, culminating in a university degree. AAMC, "Minutes of the 42nd Annual Meeting," 30 Nov.–1 Dec., 1931, pp. 21–22.
2. Committee on the Costs of Medical Care, *Final Report,* pp. 114–15; Commission on Medical Education, *Final Report,* pp. 125–26, 387.

sional identities, were a response to two pressures on the medical specialties, both of which were of vital concern to aspects of public welfare. The
first was the danger of surgery by untrained hands; the second the growing interest in preventive medicine, particularly in relation to the health
of children. Obstetrics and pediatrics, which grew as specialties during
the 1920s, also had marked public connotations; indeed, they were the
focus of activity of the Sheppard-Towner program for maternal and child
health. The movement for specialty regulation in these fields was part
scientific and part professional, but part also of the maternal and child
welfare movement, a social rather than a professional reform process
which had been gaining momentum from the 1880s and was signposted
by White House Conferences in 1909, 1919, and 1930.[3] Similar concern
over the high rates of maternal and infant mortality was being experienced at the same time in Britain. The establishment in 1929 of the British (now the Royal) College of Obstetricians and Gynecologists, to raise
obstetrical standards, was heralded by leading American specialists as
part of the "forward movement" in that specialty.[4] The following year
American obstetricians and gynecologists created the third medical specialty board.

The encouragement of higher standards of medical obstetrics and
gynecology and the elimination of the untrained GP surgeon in this specialty were obvious incentives for setting up a specialty examining board.
Nearly a third of all major surgical work in general practice was allegedly
gynecological; yet students and interns received little training in the
specialty.[5] Obstetricians were also becoming enthusiastic, sometimes

3. Infant hygiene programs developed from the "clean milk" campaigns—pasteuri-
zation and certification—of the 1890s; by 1920 most large cities had hygiene programs. New York had been the first city to start a division of child hygiene
within the health department in 1908; other cities followed suit. The work of the
American Public Health Association was increasingly involved in child care. The
American Society for the Study and Prevention of Infant Mortality (1910) gave
great impetus to the setting up of registration of infant births and deaths, publicized
problems of infant mortality, and helped bring together various concerned agencies
—governmental, philanthropic, social, and medical. The U.S. Childrens Bureau was
established in 1912. The American Child Hygiene Association (1918) developed
partly as an outcome of the needs revealed by the work of the U.S. Food Administration in World War I. In 1922 a number of children's agencies were merged—
at the instigation of Herbert Hoover—to become the American Child Health
Association. All these programs and agencies fostered increased public and professional interest in maternal and child care as a whole. See G. F. McCleary,
The Early History of the Infant Welfare Movement: and John B. Blake, "Origins of
Maternal and Child Health Programs."
4. *Trans. Amer. Gynec. Soc., 55* (1930), 45; and see Stevens, pp. 43–45.
5. Frank W. Lynch, "The License to Practice Medicine," *Trans. Amer. Gynec. Soc.,
59* (1934), 1–8.

overenthusiastic, surgeons. By 1930, cesarean section was a fashionable method of childbirth, stimulated both by the relative technical ease and safety of this procedure compared with a generation earlier and by the increasing number of patients seeking obstetrical services in hospitals. Between a fifth and a quarter of hospital deliveries studied in New York and Philadelphia in the early 1930s involved operative procedures; the proportions were higher for private patients than for those on the wards, and higher in private hospitals than in municipal hospitals.[6] Since all practitioners could legally perform surgical obstetrics, and since there appeared to be a relationship between operative intervention and maternal mortality, there was cause for concern about both undergraduate and graduate obstetrical training. One major incentive was to restore a balance between the "medical" and "surgical" aspects of obstetrics and gynecology.[7] A second was to link obstetric and gynecological teaching in the medical schools, and thus to draw gynecology away from general surgery; conditions of women would then be taught, if not always practiced, as one interlocking specialty.[8] A third was to discourage the general practitioner from practicing either obstetrics or gynecology. Questions of education, status, and restrictionism were thus intermingled, as indeed was the case in the development of each and every specialty board.

Except in ophthalmology and otology, where the specialty boards were long established, hospitals had no guiding criteria to evaluate the

6. George W. Kosmak, "The Training of Medical Students in Obstetrics," *Proc. Ann. Cong. med. Educ.* (1936), pp. 15–18.
7. See Frank W. Lynch, "The Specialty of Gynecology and Obstetrics," *Trans. AMA Sect. Obstet. Gynec., abdom. Surg.* (1924), p. 21.
8. Obstetricians and gynecologists were already organizationally linked. From 1911, there was a combined AMA Section on Obstetrics and Gynecology. The following year, due to the increasing surgical interests of its members and a jurisdictional battle over the abdomen with the general surgeons, it was retitled Obstetrics, Gynecology and Abdominal Surgery, reverting to Obstetrics and Gynecology alone in 1938. The American Association of Obstetricians and Gynecologists (established in 1888) also linked both aspects of the specialty; and the prestigious American Gynecological Society (formed in 1876) included clinical investigators whose interests ranged over all aspects of female medical care and who were actively concerned with the maternal and child welfare movement. These three organizations were also linked through their association with the American Child Health Association in the Joint Committee on Maternal Welfare. Constructive discussion of maternal welfare in the societies contrasted with the growing vehemence of official AMA opposition to the Sheppard-Towner program. By 1927 the Joint Committee could report accomplishments in stimulating thought and interest among members of the medical profession through the *Journal of Obstetrics and Gynecology* and through letters to state, district, and county branches of the AMA. It was noted as a matter of importance that this had been done without causing any antagonism among the medical profession. Fishbein, pp. 1092–93; and see *Trans. Amer. gynec. Soc., 56* (1931), 45; *55* (1930), 43; *52* (1927), 45–46; *53* (1928), 43.

capabilities of their staff. Among the principal aims of the new board
was to put a "stamp of approval" on qualified practitioners.[9] The American Gynecological Society agreed in 1928, albeit with some doubts, to
set up a committee to cooperate with the American Association of
Obstetricians and Gynecologists and the AMA section to consider a joint
examining board.[10] The American Board of Obstetrics and Gynecology
was established in 1930 with a board of nine members, three from each
society.[11] Franklin Martin, who was a member of the American Gynecological Society, had asked that the American College of Surgeons be
included. This was not done, but an explicit statement was made that
the board would not in any way conflict with or duplicate the work of the
College, or indeed of any other organization. The overt hostility between
the surgeons and the gynecologists which distinguished the birth of the
British College of Obstetricians had been largely avoided.

Gynecology was thus neatly detached from general surgery. It was,
however, much more difficult to link it with the widespread practice of
obstetrics, which was often practiced separately and which was a recognized standby of general practice.[12] While the new board avowed that it
would join together the fields of obstetrics and gynecology as "subjects
which should be inseparably interwoven," [13] from the beginning it was
forced to consider whether it would not be politically expedient to relax
its insistence on a certificate covering both obstetrics and gynecology,

9. Walter T. Dannreuther, "The American Board of Obstetrics and Gynecology:
Its Organization, Function and Objectives," *J. Amer. med. Ass., 96* (1931),
797–98.
10. It was probably encouraged to do so by the recommendation of curriculum
committees of the AMA and Association of American Medical Colleges at this
time that the number of hours allotted to the teaching of obstetrics in the undergraduate curriculum should be reduced—a direct blow to the specialty's status.
The point was also made that if medicine did not regulate specialization, the states
would. *Trans. Amer. gynec. Soc., 53* (1928), 41.
11. Initially, there were three entrance groups. The founders group, in which candidates were accepted on the basis of recognition and prestige, was closed in 1932.
Those with ten years of experience in full-time obstetrics and gynecology took an
examination covering practical, oral, bedside, clinical, and laboratory aspects of the
subjects. Those with three years of acceptable training included in at least five years
of full-time specialist practice also took examinations and had to submit reports
of 50 operations. The board developed a systematic procedure of a written followed
by a practical examination, and clinical examination in a hospital. Fred L. Adair,
Proc. Ann. Cong. med. Educ. (1932), pp. 67–69.
12. In 1929, 2,531 physicians said they were full-time or part-time obstetricians;
1,358 were gynecologists; and 2,164 combined both specialties. Commission on
Graduate Medical Education, *Graduate Medical Education*, p. 261.
13. Certificate of incorporation, quoted by Paul Titus, "The American Board of
Obstetrics and Gynecologists: A Fifteen-Year Review," *Amer. J. Obstet. Gynec.,
53* (1947), 704–08.

and, indeed, the rule was not rigidly enforced until 1940; until then many men trained in and practicing one of the branches were given the regular joint certificate if they could show fundamental knowledge of the other branch. As late as 1951, under the threat of a group of surgeons to found a competing board of gynecological surgery, the board established a moratorium for those with unilateral training and experience, provided they had graduated before 1939. For more recent graduates, the board influenced the unified practice of the two subjects through its specification of training standards and its approval of residency positions. In 1930, there were 167 approved residencies in either or both branches of the specialty; these were increased to 245 in 1935, to 269 in 1940, and numbered 768 in 1946.[14]

Selective appointments to hospital staffs on the basis of board certification provided one means of reducing general practitioner activities in obstetrics and gynecology. By 1936 it was claimed that the medical and the lay public, including hospital directors, had indeed come to use board certification "as a means of discriminating between those who are well grounded as specialists and those who are not." [15] The board also made sure that no part-time specialists would be certified: candidates were required to limit their practice to obstetrics and gynecology exclusively. In the early years, obstetricians caring for infants up to one year were included (they were excluded in 1937) as were gynecologists who did abdominal, urological, or breast surgery in the female. But anyone who accepted male patients for any reason was not regarded by the board as a specialist. By these measures, no general practitioner, however large the proportion of his practice devoted to obstetrics or gynecology and however thorough his training in these fields, might be admitted to examination or considered for a diploma. Quite openly, therefore, the board was not merely certifying a level of competence or quality; it was also attempting to specify who was a specialist and who was not. In so doing, specialist boundaries were defined; and the general practitioner was rejected.

If the board had gone no further, such actions could be regarded as the natural protective devices adopted by any group which wished to establish a concrete identity. The specialty boards claimed, however, a wider public role. The driving force behind the American Board of Obstetrics and Gynecology, Walter Dannreuther, asserted in 1932 that

14. Ibid., p. 707.
15. American Board of Obstetrics and Gynecology, *Yearbook,* 6th ed. This statement was toned down in the 1937 edition to exclude the implication of quasi-mandatory discrimination.

the public had the right to expect the profession to protect it from "the malpractices of mushroom specialists," and that the certificate would offer protection to the hospitals.[16] These statements pointed up roles for specialty boards which were logical if professional certification were to be accepted as an alternative to a public licensing system. The New Jersey licensing bill was, after all, at that time still a live issue, and the development of the new board could not help but have a public as well as a professional connotation; it appeared that the specialists were putting their own house in order. Since the American Gynecological Society decided not to use board certification as a prerequisite to society membership, board certification in obstetrics was not primarily a channel to membership in an exclusive professional group, such as the ophthalmologists and otolaryngologists had in relation to the American Academy of Ophthalmology and Otolaryngology, and the surgeons in relation to the American College of Surgeons. It seemed that the boards in the future might assume the public purpose of guaranteeing—and policing—professional standards.

There was, here, however, an organizational dilemma. As specialty clubs, there was no reason why a number of separate and independent specialty boards should not be welcomed. But if the boards were to become authoritative in the determination of hospital appointments, or in recognition of specialists for public programs, some common policy would be necessary. The three American specialty boards which existed in 1930 were autonomous units. Each drew its members from several specialty associations, including the relevant AMA section. They had no relationship with the AMA Council on Medical Education and Hospitals, which was already engaged in approving residency training programs in these and other specialties, nor with the National Board of Medical Examiners, which had signified its willingness to cooperate in specialty examinations. With the foundation of the American Board of Obstetrics and Gynecology the problems became pressing. A number of other groups were discussing founding their own boards. Once founded, they would be increasingly difficult to coordinate.

ORGANIZATIONAL FRAGMENTATION

With the rapid decline of professional incomes during the Depression, licensing and other forms of registration of specialists had become an

16. Quoted by Clyde L. Randall, "Responsibility for Excellence," *Trans. Amer. Ass. Obstet. Gynec.,* 75 (1964).

engrossing professional topic, and, unless heroic measures were taken, there promised to be a rapid fragmentation into self-regulating specialist organizations. The gynecologist wanted to be recognized as different from the general surgeon. Board certification emphasized this difference —as of course did the board's insistence that its diplomates restrict themselves to 100 percent obstetrical-gynecological practice. Those who did not fulfill the requirements laid down by the board and were therefore not (from the board's view) qualified as specialists would, it was considered, be forced to stay in general practice. The man trained as a genitourinary specialist wanted to attract not only cases needing cystoscopy but also cases of surgery of the prostate and other areas in which the general surgeon, at least of that time, might be equally competent. Again, board certification would help him in his claim. Such competition at the fringe of the specialties was inevitable, since there was not enough specialist practice in a medium-sized community in the early 1930s to make a comfortable living. But even in the depths of the Depression, the financial incentive was not the only, and perhaps not even the primary, reason for carving out carefully delineated specialties.

The specialty boards of ophthalmology and otolaryngology had been applied to fields which were already long established as specialties, had relatively little overlap with other fields, and were easy to define. The new boards of the 1930s were integral to the defining process itself; they helped create their specialty. The continuing importance of this defining process can be seen in recent and current attempts for board certification —and thus specialty recognition—by general practitioners, allergists, and abdominal surgeons. In the early 1930s it was not clear what a specialist was, or should be, let alone how he should be trained. Foreign experience seemed to indicate a general movement toward specialism. Italy, Hungary, Germany, Sweden, Turkey, and Belgium were said to be considering or to have passed specialist regulating powers of one kind or another.[17] Many European countries, however, had well-established systems of national health insurance which could enforce, or at least encourage, professionally codified specialist definitions. The Danish Medical Association, for example, had a special committee which made and kept a list of all recognized specialists. No specialist might advertise without such recognition. Moreover, while the Danish specialist might do general practice, he was not paid for such practice under insurance or municipal practice schemes without the consent of the local medical association. In countries with such programs, divisions between general and specialist

17. E. G. Waters, "Specialists and Specialism," *Penn. med. J., 35* (1932), 492.

practice could be strengthened, as they could not in the United States, through such manipulations of third-party payment schemes.[18]

Since compulsory health insurance was not politically acceptable to the American medical profession in the 1930s, other forms of physician regulation were widely discussed. In 1930 Dr. J. J. Cobb advised the medical societies comprising the New England Medical Council to consider setting up a system of "graduate and registered specialists." [19] Continued interest in state licensure, apparent in 1931 in New Jersey, New York, Michigan, and Iowa, stimulated society interest and in at least the case of Michigan stemmed from the interest of the medical society.[20] There was discussion of state registration of voluntary professional specialist qualifications as an alternative to a license.[21] Frederick Warnshuis, secretary of the Michigan State Board of Examiners and simultaneously the AMA speaker (1922–35) strongly endorsed this approach. Both he and Dr. George Follansbee, chairman of the AMA Judicial Council, urged legal regulation and limitation of specialist privileges to those with a specified training. This restrictive view contrasted curiously with the judicial council's contemporary pronouncements about the dangers of corporate practice and other "artificial schemes," which imposed no such strict or legal sanctions but which were felt to offer more insidious competition to the general practitioner.[22]

18. The Danish association specified training requirements which included six years following graduation. This plan, combining as it did aspects of training, recognition, and demarcation, appealed to Dr. Willard Rappleye, who visited Europe in his capacity as director of the Commission on Medical Education and who was appointed dean of the faculty of medicine at Columbia University in 1931; and this in itself was to have an impact on the specialist structures which evolved in the United States by the end of 1933. See Commission on Medical Education, *Medical Education and Related Problems in Europe,* pp. 116–18.
19. J. J. Cobb, "Education of the Specialist," *New Engl. J. Med., 202* (1930), 21.
20. See Frederick C. Warnshuis, "Who Shall Be Permitted to Continue the Practice of Medicine?" *Proc. ann. Cong. med. Educ.* (1931), pp. 95–96. Henry O. Reik, "Shall the Profession Undertake Control of Specialization in Medicine?" *Delaware med. J., 3* (1931), 217–24; F. J. Kiefer, "Relation of the General Practitioner to the Specialist," *Kentucky med. J., 29* (1931), 240–41. See also *J. Mich. med. Soc., 32* (1933), 456–57; William Jepson, "State Board Examinations," *J. Amer. med. Ass., 96* (1931), 1405.
21. This was, for instance, raised by the AMA Section on Obstetrics and Gynecology when the examining board in that specialty was being discussed; endorsement by the state boards would give legal authority to certification by a voluntary agency. "Section on Obstetrics, Gynecology and Abdominal Surgery," *J. Amer. med. Ass., 95* (1930), 121–22.
22. Follansbee is reported in *Diplomate* (Sept. 1931) 13; see also his article "The Profession and the Public" Ibid. (Dec. 1931) 1–6; and editorial, *AMA Bull., 26* (1931), 2.

While discussion raged on specialist regulation, the formulation of specialist training and identification continued. The New York Academy of Medicine had a committee on medical education studying the problem of specialism and specialist qualifications.[23] The *Journal of the Indiana Medical Society* carried, in its advertising section, a list of members of the society practicing as specialists in each city. The New Jersey Medical Society put its own registration plan into action, thus repeating at the specialist level the much earlier control of professional entry that had been exercised by the medical societies. Although there were those who deprecated the confusion which would result from overlapping medical society recognition and state licensure, from the undoubted spate of legal action that would arise from those not granted specialty status, and from the folly of entering state schemes before considering national qualifying boards, fragmentation of one sort or another seemed foreordained.

Such concern was justified as other specialties followed the obstetricians toward independent examining structures. The American Academy of Pediatrics, formed in 1930, included in its aims the regulation of pediatric practice through the establishment of specialist qualifications, thus providing pediatricians with an action group.[24] Committees were appointed in 1931 by the American Dermatological Association and the AMA Section on Dermatology and Syphilology to explore the possibilities of setting up an examining board; and the following year the American Board of Dermatology was established.[25] Adoph Meyer had outlined in 1928 a diploma system for psychiatry, and in 1931 an American board of examiners was recommended in an editorial in the *American Journal of Psychiatry*.[26] During 1931, the AMA Council on Medical Education and Hospitals joined the ranks of the certifying agencies, by beginning to list qualified medical specialists in pathology, although it did not conduct an examination.[27] Similar arrangements were being made for the listing of radiolo-

23. The academy would approve qualifications in the various specialties and certify those who would be designated fellows in its specialist sections; eventually it was hoped also to include non-academy members and thus to provide a list of recognized specialists for the whole of New York City. John A. Hartwell, "Presidential Address," *Bull. N.Y. Acad. Med., 7* (1931), 135–49; "The Continued Education of the Doctor," ibid., 446–63.
24. Faber and McIntosh, pp. 299–300.
25. See Fred Wise, "The American Board of Dermatology and Syphilology," *Arch. Derm. Syph., 29* (1934), 1–11.
26. Adolph Meyer, "Presidential Address," *Amer. J. Psychiat., 8* (1928), 1; Franklin G. Ebaugh, ibid., *10* (1931), 873. Both cited by Walter Freeman, Franklin G. Ebaugh, and David A. Boyd, Jr., "The Founding of the American Board of Psychiatry and Neurology, Inc.," *Amer. J. Psychiat., 115* (1959), 770.
27. The Essentials for listing as a pathologist included at least three years of gradu-

gists.[28] The chaos in graduate education as a whole was now matched by confusion in the proliferating regulatory structures concerned with specialized medicine.

ATTEMPTED UNIFICATION

It was self-evident that if specialization were to increase, it would be advantageous to have some overall policy on specialist qualifications. When the same question had come up in relation to the basic license, the National Board of Medical Examiners had been instituted—a voluntary organization conducting examinations and granting diplomas which were registrable with state licensing boards. The National Board was now an obvious candidate for specialist coordination, and indeed it had been trying to attract interest in setting up specialist diplomas for a number of years. Early in 1931 the National Board of Medical Examiners decided once more to approach the specialist organizations, with a suggestion for providing cooperative examining arrangements in conjunction with the existing specialty boards. A meeting of specialist groups, called by the National Board to discuss this question in June of that year, at the time of the AMA meeting, expressed broad agreement that further action should be taken to establish specialty boards which would grant certificates with or without examination and which would operate independently or in cooperation with the National Board.[29] The National Board

ate specialization in clinical pathology or other recognized fields of pathology; devotion of the majority of his time to the specialty; and access to or direction of a laboratory undertaking specified types of work. The CME checked basic biographical details of applicants against the AMA biographical files kept on each member and had the services of a committee of over 100 pathologists who acted in an advisory capacity on individual cases. "Physicians Specializing in Pathology," *J. Amer. med. Ass.,* 99 (1932), 1425.

28. "Radiologic Service in the U.S.," *J. Amer. med. Ass.,* 96 (1931), 1784; "Essentials for Admission to List of Physicians Specializing in Radiology," *J. Amer. med. Ass.,* 100 (1933), 414. Radiologists were also required to have three years of special training or exclusive specialist practice for five years. The entry of the Council on Medical Education on their behalf gave pathologists and radiologists an educational lever by which they might hope to force other physicians to recognize their value in specialties which had for long been felt to be beneath professional dignity, or to be the jobs of photographers, amateur electricians, or eccentric researchers in basement laboratories. But the lists also gave the council an expanded function in the specialist field. See e.g. Fred M. Hodges, "Chairman's Address to the Section on Radiology," *J. Amer. med. Ass.,* 95 (1930), 833; Arthur Desjardins, "The Status of Radiology," ibid., 96 (1931), 1749–53; "Should the Radiologist, the Pathologist and the Anesthetist Be Licensed to Practice Medicine?" *Proc. ann. Cong. med. Educ.* (1935), pp. 35–52.

29. Present were representatives of the National Board, AAMC, AMA specialist

expressed its interest in providing a framework for specialty examinations and had the necessary authority in its bylaws to extend into this area; and the assembled group decided unanimously to report to their associations and sections, with a view to taking further action. But enthusiasm rapidly waned; apparently the only organization to take up the idea of affiliation with the National Board with any interest was the AMA Section on Nervous and Mental Diseases.

The AMA was also interested in providing a coordinating framework for specialty boards, and at the AMA meeting which immediately followed the National Board specialty conference, Dr. Carl F. Moll of Michigan asked the AMA, in a long resolution, to assume responsibility for determining specialist standards. He suggested a commission on qualifications for specialists, composed of nine members, which would be appointed by the AMA speaker. Dr. Warnshuis, the speaker, was in favor of this scheme. It was envisaged that the commission would define the various specialties, together with the qualifications and training for each, and, with the assistance of the AMA Council on Medical Education, it would also report to the AMA on the possible enactment of state laws for specialist training.[30] These radical suggestions (which bear some resemblance to recent calls for a commission on graduate medical education) were referred to the Council on Medical Education. But the council proceeded cautiously. The report of the AMA Reference Committee on Medical Education, to which the council was responsible, merely noted at the AMA session the following year (1932) that specialty certification presented a problem of great practical importance, that the Council on Medical Education was studying the question from many angles, and that it was not yet prepared to make recommendations.[31]

The council was at a critical stage in its development. Arthur Dean Bevan, who had dominated the medical reform movement for twenty-four years, had stepped down as council chairman in 1928. The chairman was now the distinguished Ray Lyman Wilbur, who was concurrently a member of the Commission on Medical Education and of the Committee on the Costs of Medical Care, where he and others were exploring broad questions of medical specialization, including the desirable numerical

sections, American College of Surgeons, American Orthopaedic Association, American Academy of Pediatrics, American Neurological Association, and the American Boards of Ophthalmology, Otolaryngology, and Obstetrics and Gynecology. Minutes of the National Board of Medical Examiners, Vol. II, pp. 224, 249–50.

30. "Resolution on Qualifications for Specialists," *AMA Bull.*, 26 (1931), 130.

31. "Report of Reference Committee on Medical Education," *J. Amer. med. Ass.*, 98 (1932), 1893.

balance between generalists and specialists and desirable organizational practice patterns. With his background as dean of the Medical School and then president of Stanford University, Wilbur would be expected to incline toward an educational solution to the question of specialist qualifications, rather than deliberately to duplicate the kind of professional clique represented in the Boards of Ophthalmology and Otolaryngology.

Nevertheless in theory the AMA had a strong case for assuming control over the specialties. Its large financial resources, its influential publications (the AMA *Journal* and the *American Medical Directory*), its established position as the representative of all medical practitioners, and its history of educational upgrading and control made the AMA a natural vehicle for the educational reform movement which was now demanded for the specialists. But in practice the issues were not so simple. Specialty associations had developed outside the AMA; and the existing specialty boards had no desire to be subjected to the Council on Medical Education. Without a system of specialist licensure which it could influence, the council lacked leverage to upgrade graduate educational standards. In 1931 there were only two well-organized, degree-giving graduate medical schools—at the Universities of Minnesota and Pennsylvania. A third major graduate medical center was being developed in New York (the union of the Postgraduate School of Medicine at Columbia with the New York Postgraduate School and Hospital), but there was no general prospect of major university reform for specialist training. Reform of graduate medical education, which was at the core of specialist definition, was increasingly unlikely to follow the pattern so successfully utilized in the era of undergraduate reform. Within the AMA, moreover, the unity of purpose between educators and practitioners which had distinguished the medical college reform movement had broken down—in part a result of the different issues involved in undergraduate and graduate reform, in part a reflection of diverging attitudes among those in private practice and those in salaried university teaching. The leading specialists and teachers of specialists, while represented by the AMA in its increasingly powerful sociopolitical role, were largely independent of the AMA in relation to their educational-professional functions. The development of the specialty boards in the 1930s underlined the shift in focus of the AMA from an educational to a largely political organization.

While, therefore, there was continuing discussion during 1931 and 1932 about the possible delegation of specialist training by state licensing boards to voluntary national organizations and about the needs for an authoritative specialist directory, for a common central, nongovernmental organization of the separate specialty groups, and for common policies and standards, there was no obvious structure to do these things. The strongest contenders were the National Board of Medical Examiners, whose leading spokesmen were Louis B. Wilson and J. Stewart Rodman, and the AMA Council on Medical Education, led by Ray Lyman Wilbur. But neither was able or prepared to assume leadership. The National Board in 1931 and 1932 was willing to be drafted should specialty groups so desire, but it was becoming clear to Dr. Rodman and others that if national coordination of specialism was ever to be achieved, the National Board together with other interested agencies would be well advised to seek a cooperative rather than a dominating role.[32] The AMA Council on Medical Education was becoming increasingly interested in controlling specialty standards, but as yet had no workable plan to do so.

Specialty boards, it seemed, would continue to spring out of the already independent specialist associations, and to assume responsibility for training and examinations in their specialties. Urologists were reportedly discussing a board. A board of certification for specialists in anesthesia was formed in 1932, under the auspices of the International Anesthesia Research Society.[33] During the same year, the American Board of Dermatology was incorporated, and five national radiology societies held a joint meeting to discuss an examining board.[34] The formation of specialty boards could be seen as a remarkably cohesive movement in relation to each specialty. In relation to the whole of medicine, however, each new

32. See Frederick C. Warnshuis, "Who Shall Be Permitted to Continue the Practice of Medicine?" *Proc. ann. Cong. med. Educ.* (1931), p. 96; Louis B. Wilson, "The Function of the Graduate School in the Training of Specialists," ibid. (1932), pp. 62–65; Everett S. Elwood, "State Board and National Board Relations," ibid., pp. 92–95; William H. Wilder, "The Control of Medical Specialties," ibid., pp. 65–66. There were discussions between National Board representatives and the neurologists, public health physicians, and orthopedic surgeons, together with continued consideration of a preliminary examination for specialties under the National Board; and it was suggested that the National Board be enlarged to include a representative of each specialty board. But little came of this. Minutes of the National Board of Medical Examiners, vol. II, pp. 276, 285–86, 295–96.

33. This board is to be distinguished from the American Board of Anesthesiology (1937). It was composed of two representatives each from the Associated Anesthetists of the U.S. and Canada and its four regional societies; and it was empowered to draw up requirements for specialists with a view to forming a list. "Anesthetists Form Board of Certification for Specialists," *J. Amer. med. Ass., 99* (1932), 1662.

34. The American Roentgen Ray Society, the AMA Section on Radiology, the Radiological Society of North America, the American College of Radiology, the American Radium Society. American Board of Radiology, *Booklet of Information* (1966), p. 3.

board represented a fragmentation from existing organizational structures, and another precedent for future organizational rigidity.

THE ADVISORY BOARD FOR MEDICAL SPECIALTIES

But organizations are one thing and people another; and while there was little solidarity of purpose among the professional organizations, there was a small influential and informal group whose interests and affiliations overlapped, and who were to have their own impact on the developing pattern of graduate medical education. Among them were Willard C. Rappleye, then dean of the Columbia University College of Physicians and Surgeons, William Cutter of the American Medical Association, Louis B. Wilson of the Mayo Foundation, and Ray Lyman Wilbur. Dean Rappleye was an influential figure in the Association of American Medical Colleges, becoming its president in 1938; and he in turn was a friend of Walter Bierring, who was an influential member of the American College of Physicians and of the Federation of State Medical Boards. William Cutter, who became secretary of the Council on Medical Education in 1931, had been director of the New York Postgraduate Medical School and was well known to Rappleye and other educators. Louis B. Wilson had been chairman of the specialty committees which reported to the AMA in 1921 and chairman of the committee set up by the National Board; he was also an important force in the AAMC and in the Council on Medical Education.

Outside the universities and professional associations, another powerful group had developed in the American Hospital Association. Its primary spokesman in regard to the specialties was Robin Buerki. These men and others formed an inner circle whose discussions were at least as influential as those of the organization they represented or led, and who, while they did not all endorse similar solutions, were strongly committed to specialty coordination. It was through the individual actions of Wilson, Buerki and Rappleye that the Advisory Board for Medical Specialties was formed, the catalyst being the meeting of the Congress on Medical Education and Hospitals in February 1933.

At this meeting, Ray Lyman Wilbur pressed for a central role in specialty regulation for the AMA Council on Medical Education as a counter to the dangers of self-controlled specialty elites.[35] There was an attempt, led by Walter Bierring, to get the congress to vote in support of council control. But this was foiled by Louis B. Wilson, who had already

35. Ray Lyman Wilbur, "Order in the Specialties," *Proc ann. Cong. med. educ.* (1933), p. 52.

addressed the congress on the desirability of coordination of specialties through the National Board of Medical Examiners, which was considering altering its constitution to include specialty board representation. Dr. Wilson suggested a joint meeting of the various interested parties to discuss the issues; his suggestion was followed. Duly, in June of 1933, representatives of the four then existing specialty boards, the National Board, the Council on Medical Education, the AMA specialty sections, and other organizations came together. The meeting endorsed the formation of new specialty boards, but emphasized that their efficiency would be improved by the formation of an advisory committee or council created by two delegated representatives from each specialty board, together with two from each of the other organizations represented at the meeting.[36] Behind the scenes during 1933 and 1934, Drs. Louis B. Wilson, Rappleye, and Buerki began planning to this end. Out of their actions developed the Advisory Board for Medical Specialties—a coalition between the National Board, the existing specialty boards, and emerging specialist groups. Dr. Wilson was chairman. The Council on Medical Education declined an invitation to accept membership on the Advisory Board, although it agreed to attend its meetings without voting power or responsibility.

At the same time, the AMA retained to itself claims to authority over the specialties. A resolution passed by the AMA House of Delegates at the Milwaukee session of 1933 authorized the Council on Medical Education to express its approval of special examining boards and to formulate standards for such approval; Dr. Morris Fishbein, éminence grise of the AMA in the economic and political fields, appears to have been a decisive factor in this decision. This position was reiterated in an editorial in the AMA *Journal* in August 1933.[37] The Council on Medical Educa-

36. Present at the meeting were representatives from the AAMC, the National Board of Medical Examiners, the American Boards of Ophthalmology, Otolaryngology, Obstetrics and Gynecology, Dermatology and Syphilology, the Federation of State Medical Boards, the several specialty sections of the American Medical Association, the American College of Surgeons, and the Council on Medical Education and Hospitals. Commission on Graduate Medical Education, *Graduate Medical Education,* p. 208.

37. Fishbein was the *Journal*'s editor; editorial, J. Amer. med. Ass., *101* (1933), 714. The resolution from Dr. Samuel J. Kopetzky of New York had suggested that the council be authorized to cooperate with the official specialty boards, the AAMC, the Federation of State Licensing Boards, and the National Board through an advisory council of the kind being suggested by Dr. Louis B. Wilson. Dr. Fishbein represented the AMA Board of Trustees at a meeting of the AMA Reference Committee on Medical Education. The resolution was amended to put total responsibility on the council. "Proceedings of the 84th Annual Session of the AMA," *J. Amer. med. Ass., 101* (1933), 39, 47.

tion was concurrently urging the AMA to reduce the number of physicians and to inform the public "that the profession is already overcrowded." [38] The AMA was also uneasy about the future relation of the
medical profession to hospitals, which, through the American Hospital
Association, had endorsed schemes for hospital insurance and which were
increasingly employing physicians and other nonmedical specialists in
salaried hospital appointments. These and other factors together made
it inevitable that the AMA should wish to control the standards, and
potentially the number, of specialists, and not to delegate this responsibility to outside organizations.

There were thus two supposedly controlling agencies over the specialty
boards, neither as yet with well-defined goals. The newly adopted constitution of the Advisory Board said that it would act to advise organizations seeking such advice "concerning the coordination of the education
and certification of medical specialists." [39] The AMA *Journal* ascribed
to the Advisory Board *nonpolicy* functions concerned with aiding in the
boards' practical operation; and stressed the central role in specialty
regulation of the AMA Council .on Medical Education as the "body
sitting in judgment." [40] It was also expected that the Advisory Board
would be reportable to, and work under the general direction of, the
council. There were however no formal arrangements for any such affiliation, and the respective roles of the two committees remained—and are
today—unclear. Behind the scenes, however, cooperative arrangements
began to be made whereby the Council on Medical Education and the
Advisory Board would adopt common standards for the approval of any
new specialty board. Again, individual relationships were pulling together
formally unwieldy organizations. Under the guidance of Dr. Willard C.

38. Efforts to reduce physician supply were being supplemented by vigorous activity
by the Federation of State Medical Boards (on the council's initiative) to tighten
up the requirements for licensure of American students who had trained abroad
and who thereby undermined the reduction in places in American medical schools.
In 1932–33 there were an estimated 1,911 Americans studying medicine in European schools, many of whom were adjudged to be of poorer caliber than those in
American centers. Interest in restricting the outside supply of physicians switched
later in the 1930s to the regulation of immigrant physicians. One device for doing
so was the introduction by various states of citizenship requirements for the practice
of medicine. Arthur Dean Bevan argued for particular efforts to be made to stem
the supply of Jewish medical students in New York City—not, he emphasized, from
any anti-Semitism but because Jewish applications were increasing steadily and supposedly crowding out other ethnic groups. Arthur Dean Bevan, "The Overcrowding
of the Medical Profession," *J. Ass. Amer. med. Coll., 11* (1936), 377–84; and see
ibid., *8* (1933), 360–66.
39. Advisory Board for Medical Specialties, *J. Amer. med. Ass., 102* (1934), 702;
Article II; *Directory of Medical Specialists, 1* (1939), 8.
40. Editorial, *J. Amer. med. Ass., 102* (1934), 1085.

Rappleye the standards were based on the Danish professional model. These "Essentials for an Approved Special Examining Board" were adopted in virtually identical form by both the Council on Medical Education and the Advisory Board for Medical Specialties on 10 June 1934, immediately before the AMA meeting in Cleveland.[41] A specialty board was to represent "a well-recognized and distinct specialty of medicine"; should include a field of more than 100 specialists; have the support of major specialty organizations and the related AMA section; should be incorporated; and should determine a candidate's training and experience, test his ability, and certify to his competence. The Essentials also outlined the general qualifications and training of board candidates. Three years of training after internship were specified. Candidates were to be scrutinized for moral and ethical standing; they had to be licensed (but not necessarily U.S. citizens); and they had to be members of the AMA or a recognized equivalent.[42]

The Essentials listed twelve specialty fields as appropriate for certification, including those boards already formed. All twelve were in existence by the end of 1937.[43] There was thus a rash of organizational activity from these specialties, and from others which had not been placed on the approved list—notably allergists, gastroenterologists, and anethesiologists. Of these, only the last was successful, becoming the thirteenth field to be recognized in the Essentials. The authority of the new machinery in regulating organizational entry was thus seen to be profound. Boards could be, and have been, set up without the approval of the Council on Medical Education and the Advisory Board; but they faced exclusion from the official directories and the strong pressure of condemnation by organized medicine.

ACHIEVEMENTS AND INADEQUACIES

The formation of the Advisory Board for Medical Specialties brought together the interests of all concerned groups save the AMA Council on

41. "Minutes of Meeting of Council on Medical Education and Hospitals," *J. Amer. med. Ass.,* 103 (1934), 48; *Directory of Medical Specialists, 1* (1940), 6, 10, and passim.
42. The last item was part of the process of strengthening organized medicine, which was a keynote of AMA activities of the early 1930s. It could not be justified on the grounds of quality; membership in specialist societies, which would have a greater claim for such distinction, was specifically excluded. Subsequently the AMA requirement was dropped.
43. Internal Medicine (1936); Surgery (1937); Pediatrics (1933); Obstetrics and Gynecology (1930); Ophthalmology (1917); Otolaryngology (1924); Dermatology and Syphilology (1932); Neurology and Psychology (1934); Urology (1935); Orthopaedic Surgery (1934); Radiology (1934); Pathology (1936).

Medical Education, and the council had already adopted a common set of policies. There was now a framework in which new specialty boards might develop, and this was significant in respect to the initial definition of a "specialty." It would be difficult in the future for specialist pressure groups to gain approval as boards on the basis of numerical strength alone. The existence of standards for approval of new boards restricted the growth of self-styled specialists in scientifically or socially unjustifiably separate fields.

At the same time the new machinery had a basic flaw in its lack of continuing responsibility for specialty boards. Once approved, a specialty board was not subject—in its specification of standards, approval of residencies, and types of examination—to any common or outside control. The Advisory Board and the council acted through their specialty board Essentials as accrediting agencies rather than as educational or manpower associations. It was doubtful whether either committee would be able to extend its function to the broad public issues of the standards, numbers, and distributions of physicians in the specialties and to the increasingly important question of the future of general practice. The structures had evolved out of pressures from self-sustaining medical groups for a unifying or coordinating agent. They were not designed to address the larger issues of the role of medical specialists.

There had been little discussion of the public interest, at least from the economic viewpoint, during the evolution of the new structures. Potential new restrictions on entry and practice within the medical profession were imposed without the public or their elected representatives having any voice on the impact these might have on the provision of service. Much would depend on how many specialists voluntarily took the certification examinations and how such certification was used. If in the future no specialist could make a living or gain prestige without board certification, the existence of the boards might mean a formal restriction in the proportion of specialists to general practitioners, perhaps to the level of 10–15 percent suggested by Arthur Dean Bevan, or the 18 percent suggested by the Committee on the Costs of Medical Care. If so, the specialty boards could be seen as a reinforcement to general practice at the very time it was being threatened. Dr. Walter Bierring was one who considered that the effect of the boards would be to reduce the number of specialists, but that the small group thus created would be of high quality. Thus again, he remarked optimistically (and prematurely) in 1936, "the medical profession has solved another of its important problems." [44]

44. Walter Bierring, "Consistency versus Chaos in Medical Education and Licensure," *J. Amer. med. Ass., 106* (1936), 1097.

But the specialty boards were odd vehicles for such considerations. Though developed under the threat of licensure and though seen by some, including Dr. Bierring, as perhaps leading to endorsement by state licensing boards, the boards were primarily professional groups, not licensing agencies. The creation of the Advisory Board for Medical Specialties encouraged an educational rather than a practitioner-oriented specialty system: it was intended to keep the Advisory Board under the control of university men. But this did not necessarily mean the stimulation of university graduate education or a new coordinating focus through the teaching institutions. The universities as a whole had shown relatively little interest in medical graduates, and the trend was toward diffusion instead of centralization in specialist training.

"Who should control specialization?" was thus only partially answered during the 1930s. It had been tacitly accepted that, once licensing had been recognized as essential for assuring minimum quality control for all physicians, it was not appropriate to allow the market alone to enforce specialist standards. The question was what instruments should be used to aid in the process. So far the answers were mostly negative. No one was allowed primary responsibility—the AMA, the licensing boards, the National Board, the hospitals, or any other preexisting group. Achievements could be seen in the provision of a structure for coordinating specialty board action and for suggesting basic training requirements. But there was still no consideration of specialty certification in terms of the overall organization and delivery of medical care.

CHAPTER 11

Specialties and Specialty Boards

The Defining Process

By 1940, fourteen of the present twenty specialty certifying boards were in existence.[1] Together they had issued some 15,600 certificates, many granted under liberal grandfather clauses; over 40 percent of full-time specialists were board certified.[2] So high a proportion in relatively so short a time was a signal success for the boards. In time the figure might be expected to include the great majority of specialists, so that the boards would fulfill their promise as quasi-licensing agencies. Thus by definition, a specialist and a board-certified specialist would be the same.

Such considerations were one thing, however, as long as specialization was the exceptional form of medical practice rather than the rule, and quite another when the majority of physicians chose to be specialists. While only a minority of physicians specialized—and this was the case through the 1930s—the existence of the boards as professional enclaves of excellence could be held to be to the advantage both of the public and of the majority of physicians. But even in the relatively halcyon phase of specialty board development during the 1930s, problems of specialty stratification were becoming evident as each of fourteen independent specialty groups attempted to carve out the boundaries of its field, to define its content, to describe the function of certification, to establish recommended patterns of training, and—since the boards were professional organizations—to decide on acceptable modes of practice and

1. The specialties of anesthesiology and plastic surgery were added to the 12 areas originally suggested by the Advisory Board for Medical Specialties. For a complete chronological list, see Appendix table A1.
2. The 40 percent is an estimate. In 1940, there were 36,000 full-time specialists in fields then served with certifying boards. Since board certification tended to be restricted to those in full-time specialist practice, it is possible to estimate the numerical impact of certification by comparing the number of diplomas with the number of those full-time specialists. See Appendix table A2.

behavior. Such issues emphasized that the definition of specialties was, at root, a political process, arising from the relative successes of interest groups.

PEDIATRICS: BOARDS AND BOUNDARIES

The specialty of pediatrics, whose certifying board was established in 1933, is a good example of the development and function of the specialty boards as an expression of a relatively narrow professionalism, whose roots lay rather in the evolution of specialist interest in the past, than in any new approach to functional delineations in the profession which would be appropriate to the demands of modern medicine. Pediatrics as a special area of interest has existed since the mid-nineteenth century; Abraham Jacobi had been appointed to the chair of diseases of children at New York Medical College in 1860, and the American Pediatric Society established in 1888. Until the early twentieth century, however, infants and young children were regarded as miniature adults, with similar problems size for size, and there was some question whether pediatrics was a separate "specialty." There was neither a large group of full-time practitioners concerned to raise their status nor an instrumental focus which justified pediatrics on technological lines, and it was only with the increased emphasis on the welfare of mothers and children before and after World War I, providing a social impetus for specialty growth, that pediatrics began to emerge as a professional entity. In 1914, there had been only 138 full-time pediatricians in the United States.[3] By 1921 there were 664; by 1934, the number had increased to 1,734; and in 1938, there were 2,205 full-time pediatricians.[4] But even as late as this, the specialty had a social rather than a scientific rationale.

The lack of a technological focus was reflected in the lack of authoritative professional organizations in pediatrics, compared, for example, with obstetrics. Until the establishment of the American Academy of Pediatrics in 1930, itself generated by the White House Conference of 1929, pediatricians had no generally effective professional group. The American Pediatric Society was small and apolitical. The Association of American Teachers of Diseases of Children, which existed from 1906 to 1928, did much to raise the standards of pediatric teaching and to place pediatricians in teaching positions in medical schools,[5] but it had limited aims

3. Faber and McIntosh, pp. 311–12.
4. Figures from the directories of the AMA, cited by Borden S. Veeder, "Trends of Pediatric Education and Practice," *Amer. J. Dis. Child., 50* (1935), 1–10; and Commission on Graduate Medical Education, *Graduate Medical Education*, p. 261.
5. Harvard had been the first medical school to set up a separate department of

and membership, as did the National Society for Pediatric Research, formed in 1929 by physicians interested in scientific aspects of child care. These societies offered a nucleus of interest in the more esoteric and scientific aspects of child development and childhood disease, but they largely ignored the general pediatrician and the general practitioner with a pediatric interest, who were the bulwark of pediatric practice. It was only with the formation of the academy that the question of the standards of pediatric practice began to be tackled.

The existence of such a group stimulated consideration of the role and future of the specialty. Pediatrics flourished in part because of lack of interest or qualification on the part of general practitioners. It was based on a patient's age rather than his illness or condition, and in this respect it was unlike all the earlier special fields, which were based on instrumentation or special techniques. The teaching of pediatrics in most medical schools was inadequate. Specialty leaders such as Borden Veeder considered that more attention to pediatrics in the undergraduate curriculum would give general practitioners adequate skills for the normal care of children, and that as a result, during the 1930s the number of pediatricians would be reduced.[6] According to this reasoning, the trend to full-time pediatric practice was a temporary phase, filling a vacuum until well-trained general practitioners were able to take over most of the work, side by side with a small group of highly trained pediatric consultants. One question, therefore, was whether pediatrics should be limited to a consultation specialty (as in Britain) or whether it should be extended to all aspects of general practice applied to children.

But this question was soon to be academic. Once established in the United States, the specialty of general pediatrics proved resilient. It was attractive both to a middle class which was becoming accustomed to using medical specialists and to medical graduates looking for a relatively uncomplicated specialty as an alternative to general practice. The American Academy of Pediatrics was created in part to establish specialist qualifications, and the same committee which had studied undergraduate training in pediatrics for the White House Conference began to study graduate

pediatrics—under Thomas Morgan Rotch, who had been the first professor of pediatrics at the University of Pennsylvania (1888) and who was a pioneer of clean milk and infant nutrition, in the care of premature babies, and in physical development from fetus to infant to child. P. W. Beaven, ed., *For the Welfare of Children: Addresses of the First Twenty-five Presidents of the American Academy of Pediatrics* (Springfield, Ill., 1955), p. viii; Faber and McIntosh, pp. 54, 92, 239–40; Garrison, *History of Pediatrics*, p. 141.

6. Borden Veeder, "Trends of Pediatric Education and Practice," *Amer. J. Dis. Child., 50* (1935), 4–5.

training for the academy. In 1932, at the very height of discussion as to which agency should be responsible for specialty regulation, the academy joined the American Pediatric Society and the AMA pediatric section to form a joint examining board focused on general rather than consultant pediatrics. The American Board of Pediatrics was incorporated in 1933 and was approved the following year by the Advisory Board for Medical Specialties and by the AMA's Council on Medical Education.[7] By 1940 the board included nearly 1,500 active diplomates: the equivalent of six of every ten full-time pediatricians.[8] The existence of the specialty board had stimulated the growth of general pediatrics as a specialty. With its specification of training requirements as a prerequisite of candidacy, the board both defined and labeled its field. And its ensured its continuation through the development of new and longer hospital residency programs. Training requirements for the American Board of Pediatrics in 1939 included a year of internship and two years of service in a pediatric center, this being defined as an acceptable hospital or a graduate course which included pediatric inpatient and outpatient service; the candidate had also to have an additional two years of specialized study or practice or both. Although these requirements were not strictly enforced until 1945, by 1939 there were over 200 pediatric residencies of two years or more.[9] These residencies, which were to burgeon after World War II, provided a continually fed pool of new specialists; indeed, Borden Veeder, the first chairman of the Pediatric Board, warned in 1937 against producing more pediatricians than could be assimilated into private practice.[10] Pediatric specialists gravitated more toward full-time than part-time practice not only to maintain their distinction as specialists but also because after so much training they had become unaccustomed to, and possibly uninterested in, dealing with adults.

Pediatrics was thus launched as a specialty in the 1930s, while retaining a primarily generalist function. While the view was still taken in the 1940s that pediatrics was a narrowing field, with inevitable competition both from the better-trained general practitioners and from obstetricians (who had, to the pediatricians' alarm, moved into baby care during the first year of a child's life), to the individual physician making his practice

7. Certification was made a prerequisite of membership in the academy. See "American Board of Pediatrics, Inc.," *J. Amer. med. Ass., 113* (1941), 813; Pease, pp. 64, 110–13; Borden Veeder, "The Relationship of the Hospital Residency to Graduate Education in Pediatrics," *Hospitals, 11* (1937), 91–95.
8. See Appendix table A2.
9. Commission on Graduate Medical Education, *Graduate Medical Education,* p. 263.
10. Borden Veeder, "The Relationship of the Hospital Residency," pp. 91–95.

choice there were financial and prestige incentives to specialize. Pediatrics rose as general practice declined; indeed, there was probably a direct relationship. The number of full-time pediatricians increased from 1,600 in 1931 to 2,400 in 1940, and to 4,300 in 1949; today there are over 17,000.[11] The board-certified and the self-styled pediatrician, rather than the general practitioner, gave innoculations and vaccinations and tended the well-fed, healthy child as well as the sick child in hospital. Whether for most of his work he needed his long specialty training was a question both unanswered and unrecognized. The existence of the specialty board, duly approved by the profession, had given pediatrics professional sanction to exist. Pediatrics was recognized in the board system as different from general practice and parallel to internal medicine and obstetrics. The question, What is a Specialty? could now be answered in terms of whether or not there was a specialty board.

PSYCHIATRY AND NEUROLOGY: ONE SPECIALTY OR TWO?

While the American Board of Pediatrics played its part in carving out a role for the pediatrician, the American Board of Psychiatry and Neurology was at the same time having a formative impact on the combined development of two specialties; its impetus was similar to that of the American Board of Obstetrics and Gynecology, which had also provided an organizational framework to link two previously different fields. In Britain, neurology and psychiatry remained distinct, with neurologists tending to align themselves more nearly with specialists in internal medicine and with neurological surgeons, than with the mental hospital psychiatrists. The late-nineteenth-century American psychiatrists and neurologists had similar functions to their British counterparts: the psychiatrists practiced, more or less in isolation, in outlying hospitals for the insane; the neurologists conducted private practice and held the academic posts. There was almost a professional class difference.[12] During the early twentieth century, however, psychiatry began to be integrated into the rest of medicine. The first university psychopathic hospital for research

11. *Health Manpower Source Book,* sec. 14, table 6; AMA, *Distribution of Physicians, Hospitals, and Hospital Beds in the United States,* 1969, vol. 1 (Chicago, 1970) table 1.
12. The eminent neurologist S. Weir Mitchell castigated the psychiatrists before the American Medical Psychological Association in 1894 for their rural isolationism and their divorce from the intellectual developments of the specialty. "Your hospitals are not our hospitals; your ways are not our ways." Quoted by Deutsch, p. 279.

and education was founded at the University of Michigan in 1901, the first psychopathic treatment ward in a general hospital (at the Albany hospital) in 1902. The mental hygiene movement following Clifford Beers' book *A Mind That Found Itself* (1908) opened mental illness to public view; indeed, the concurrent movements for promoting mental health and for protecting the health of mothers and children ran on similar and parallel lines. During World War I, psychiatry and neurology were brought together in the discovery and treatment of shell shock, or war neurosis, and a combined division of neurology and psychiatry was set up within the surgeon general's office. After the war, increasing efforts were made to classify and analyze mental illness, through the integration of psychiatry and social work and through the establishment of clinics, departments, and research institutes which gave an organizational focus for combined neuropsychiatric development.

By the early 1930s there was some, though often minimal, psychiatry taught in all American medical schools; under the pressure of Dr. Franklin G. Ebaugh and other psychiatric leaders the amount was gradually being increased and formalized.[13] Different forms of treatment were also emerging. Insulin therapy was first used in 1936; electric shock therapy followed. Freudian methods crystallized the link between psychiatry and the remainder of medicine. With Freudians dominant in academic psychiatry from the late 1930s, psychoanalysis began to take organizational root with the opening of the first psychoanalytic institute in New York in 1931; sixteen others were to follow.[14] As a whole, the links between psychiatry and neurology were still fluid, but more physicians practiced neurology and psychiatry as a combined specialty than focused on either separately. In 1938 there were only 197 full-time and part-time neurologists and 1,030 psychiatrists, compared with 1,656 in combined practice.[15] Nevertheless, the three groups were divided organizationally. The leaders of the American Psychiatric Association in the early 1930s were primarily interested in psychiatry from the psychoanalytic point of view; those in the American Neurological Association were primarily organic neurologists; and those in the largest group, the AMA Section on Nervous and Mental Diseases, tended to practice in the general field of neuropsychiatry. Although there were vast differences in the scientific approach to the various aspects of neurology and psychiatry—some, for example,

13. E. L. Brown, *Physicians and Medical Care,* pp. 52–55.
14. See Hall, Bunker, and Zilboorg, pp. 318–19, 481, 487; F. G. Alexander and S. T. Selesnick, *The History of Psychiatry* (New York, 1966), pp. 410–12.
15. Commission on Graduate Medical Education, *Graduate Medical Education,* table 9, p. 261.

coming to neuropsychiatry through neuroanatomy, others emphasizing psychological aspects—there was a general feeling that the two belonged together.[16] Numerically, moreover, they were well advised to combine, if only to ward off outside threats. Clinical psychiatrists were bitter about invasions of their field by lay practitioners and by the numerous self-styled specialists who set themselves up with little training. All specialists in these fields were concerned about the inadequacy of undergraduate medical education. It was also known that the Council on Medical Education was trying to avoid overlapping (i.e. competing) specialty boards, and that the chances for approval as an examining board would be greatly enhanced by combining the neurological and psychiatric fields.

Psychiatrists discussed a specialty board as early as 1931, but the discussion on specialty certification only became focused in 1933 when the American Psychiatric Association set up a board of five examiners to determine classes of membership in that organization and to prepare a plan for specialist certification. This move was prompted by the desire to forestall possible action by the AMA, the National Board, or any other organization: "If you sit idly by and do nothing, the next annual meeting may be too late." [17] The AMA Section on Nervous and Mental Diseases had already showed interest in possible certification of specialists by the National Board of Medical Examiners; it decided to cooperate in this revised plan. Since the section included neurology as well as psychiatry, the American Neurological Association was also invited to participate. Representatives of all three groups met in New York in December 1933, and organization was completed in October 1934.

Professional union in the American Board of Psychiatry and Neurology did not, however, mean automatic harmony between the professional groups, which coexisted on a separate-but-equal basis. The board comprised four members each from the psychiatric and the neurological association, together with two psychiatrists and two neurologists from the AMA section; there were separate examinations and certificates for neurology and psychiatry. Disputes arose as to which specialty should come first in the title, and there was an angry exchange over whether there should be double fees for the dual certification of neuropsychiatrists, the single fee being adopted. Once these issues were resolved, however, the two groups, which at the first meeting "got along like a couple of strange

16. See Henry R. Viets, "Neurology: Past and Present," *J. Amer. med. Ass., 109* (1937), 399; Walter Freeman, Franklin G. Ebaugh, and David A. Boyd, Jr., "The Founding of the American Board of Psychiatry and Neurology, Inc.," *Amer. J. Psychiat., 115* (1959), 773–74.

17. Statement by William A. White, in "Proceedings 89th Annual Meeting, the American Psychiatric Association," *Amer. J. Psychiat., 13* (1933), 387.

bulldogs," [18] began to meld into an effective unit. Under the rules adopted, those who wished to be considered neuropsychiatrists had to take both examinations offered. The general practitioner of the specialties would thus be more highly recognized than the full-time neurologist or psychiatrist—a reversal of the situation then in existence. In so doing, the board helped to crystallize the differences as well as the similarities between the two specialties. The number of self-defined neuropsychiatrists appears to have increased during the 1940s and then, with the rapid increase in the number of psychiatrists, suffered a severe decline.[19]

While under the same rubric, therefore, neurology and psychiatry remained separate. Indeed the differences were to be compounded by the polarization among psychiatrists between those who viewed mental illness as an organic disease and those who had a primarily psychological approach. The existence of one examining board for these fields, which after all diagnosed and treated one range of conditions in patients, did at least prevent the offshoot of other specialist examining groups, and thus the development of further organizational rigidity. At the same time, there was a tendency to think of psychiatry and neurology as one specialty when in fact the views and methods of exponents within the group varied widely.

RADIOLOGY AND PATHOLOGY: SEARCH FOR STATUS

Radiology and pathology were also specialties which, even in the 1930s, covered fields which contained a wide variety of practice and interests, and in which there were both general and specialist exponents: the general radiologist who was interested in both diagnostic and therapeutic radiology, and the general pathologist who was responsible for the general hospital laboratory, for postmortem examinations, and for clinical work. But radiologists and pathologists were, with anesthesiologists (and later, specialists in physical medicine), in a special situation as medical specialists. They were hospital based, providing necessary services to other physicians as a back-up or second-line function, particularly to patients within the hospital. The product of nineteenth- and twentieth-century discoveries, these specialties did not fit into the prevailing concept of the physician as a frontline private practitioner. They were vulnerable to

18. Dr. Louis Casamajor, quoted by Freeman, Ebaugh, and Boyd, "Founding American Board of Psychiatry," p. 775.
19. In 1949, 2,408 physicians stated an interest in both fields; the number was down to 1,676 in 1961. During the same period the number of psychiatrists increased from 2,210 to 9,059, neurologists from 102 to 625. *Health Manpower Source Book,* sec. 14, table 6.

criticism as "technicians." As a result, in the 1930s, and later, they were particularly concerned with creating for themselves increased status and prestige.

A crucial question for practitioners in these fields was not whether they were specialists, but whether they were medical specialists. The ophthalmologists had been forced to fight the optometrists over a similar issue many years before; and they still competed with each other in the area of refraction. Competition in optics was, however, at the level of attracting patients; there was not effective competition as to which should be consulted by other physicians. Indeed, the ophthalmologists had received great benefits from the AMA in the use of ethical sanctions to restrain physicians from contact with optometrists; and these sanctions were also brought to play on the behalf of psychiatrists in the physician-psychologist relationship. Significantly, they were not however fully utilized in protecting the interests of the medical pathologist, the radiologist or anesthesiologist from direct contact between other physicians and the nonmedical technicians in these specialties. The internist liked to be able to direct laboratory and X-ray technicians; the surgeon welcomed the nurse anesthetist. The medical specialists concerned therefore felt the need to assert their authority in defense of control over their respective specialties.

The mechanical aspects of X-rays, laboratory tests, and simple anesthesia could be, and were, carried out by technicians, nurses, and other aides. Without such aides, the special services would have collapsed. In 1933, there were 4,677 hospitals with X-ray departments and 4,324 hospital laboratories, but there were only 1,170 full-time medical radiologists in the country and 650 full-time specialists in pathology and bacteriology, and not all of these were working in hospitals. Even allowing for a physician supervising more than one department, there were clearly not enough specialists to go around. AMA figures suggested that a fourth of the X-ray departments and a third of the laboratories were not directed by a physician; and many of the others may have been directed by a physician whose primary interest was not in the relevant specialty.[20] Not unnaturally, both pathologists and radiologists were engaged in a struggle for recognition as clinical specialists. More materially, it was claimed that the nonprofessionals were siphoning off medical incomes. Both wanted to be the consultants of other physicians, not merely photographers or workers at the laboratory bench, and there were numerous articles and comments in the medical press about the relative standing of medical and nonmedi-

20. "Hospital Service in the United States," *J. Amer. med. Ass.*, *102* (1934), 1014; Commission on Graduate Medical Education, *Graduate Medical Education*, p. 261.

cal specialists.[21] But both specialties, with their equipment, departments, and auxiliary staffs, had become integral parts of hospitals. They depended on hospital rather than on individual office practice, and they were regarded by the clinicians who used them as part of the hospital's service rather than as a medical consultation service.

In Britain, where parallel scientific developments had raised similar issues about the status of these specialties, the ultimate badge of prestige was a full appointment of such specialists to the staff of a major voluntary hospital, on equal terms with other specialists. Since hospitals traditionally had a relatively small, closed staff the specialist group formed an identifiable elite. In the United States, however, hospitals were still largely on an open-staff system. Thus the radiologist or pathologist, often employed on a salary by the hospital and with little or no private practice, was in a different professional category from other, more prestigious physicians. The major status question in America was also an attempt to approximate the hospital specialties, however inappropriately, to the conditions of private practice; but here the symbol was monetary. How these physicians received their income—by salary, contract, fee-for-service, or other means—became a burning issue in the battle by pathologists, radiologists, anesthesiologists, and physiatrists to enhance their own prestige in relation to other medical specialties. This movement received dramatic emphasis with the increase in voluntary hospital insurance schemes which tended to assume, not unnaturally, that the services of these medical specialties were an integral part of hospital care (and thus different from private medical practice). In its battles against compulsory health insurance, the AMA had hallowed the fee-for-service system as a vital element of independent practice. By the late 1930s, the demands of the hospital-based specialists to be reimbursed by hospitals on a fee basis instead of a salary or proportion of the department income had become crucial activities of the professional associations in these specialties. Some agreement was finally reached between radiologists and the hospitals in 1937; a similar statement of principles of the relationship between anesthesiologists and hospitals was reached the following year; and negotiations were proceeding in pathology and physiatry.[22] The professional

21. See, for instance, Fred M. Hodges, "Chairman's Address to the Section on Radiology," *J. Amer. med. Ass.*, 95 (1930), 833; Arthur Desjardins, "The Status of Radiology," ibid., 96 (1931), 1749–53; "Should the Radiologist, the Pathologist, and the Anesthetist Be Licensed to Practice Medicine?" *Proc. ann. Cong. med. Education* (1935), pp. 35–52.
22. *Trans. Amer. Hosp. Ass.*, 40 (1938), 51, 62; and see editorial, "The Roentgenologist, the Pathologist, and the Anesthetist under Hospital Insurance Plans," *J. Amer. med. Ass.*, 111 (1938), 158–59.

view was summarized at the AMA meeting in San Francisco in 1938; hospitals are corporations; the practice of medicine by a corporation by hiring physicians is undesirable, particularly where it results in a profit to the corporation by selling the services of physicians. Instead of including medical services in the hospital bill, each person insured for hospital care should receive separate benefits for physician care, so that he be free to purchase medical services at his own volition. In broad outline, these policies have remained. But the bitter feelings and protracted negotiations which were a feature of hospital-specialist relations in the 1930s left their mark. Contemporary insistence, by the professional groups under Medicare, on the importance of maintaining the elements of private practice for the hospital-based specialties as a gauge of professional independence, is part and parcel of the same movement. In short, what were basically professional and status questions were crystallized in terms of fiduciary relationships.

The development of specialty boards in the hospital specialties have to be appreciated in this context. Radiologists and pathologists and anesthesiologists were deeply concerned in the early 1930s with carving out boundary lines and in achieving full recognition. The AMA Council on Medical Education and Hospitals was already listing approved radiologists and pathologists, and providing one status gauge. Indeed, one of the council's primary functions in these two specialties was insistence on their *medical* aspects; physicians employed by laboratories which were under lay control were not listed. But, with other specialties moving toward specialty boards, a mere list was not enough.

The American Board of Radiology grew from a meeting of five national radiological societies in 1932, following discussion at the meetings of the AMA and the American College of Radiology on the establishment of a board to replace the AMA council's list.[23] The combined committee met during the AMA Milwaukee meeting in June 1933, and it was unanimously agreed to form a board. The first meeting was held in May 1934, and the American Board of Radiology duly became a member of the Advisory Board for Medical Specialties.[24] The board stated as its first

23. Committees were appointed by the College of Radiology and the AMA section. The council suggested that the question also be brought to the attention of the American Roentgen Ray Society, the Radiological Society of North America, and the American Radium Society—each of which also appointed a committee. Hence the involvement of five societies. "The American Board of Radiology," *J. Amer. med. Ass., 102* (1934), 641.

24. The Council on Medical Education and Hospitals did not, however, officially extend its recognition to the board until December 1935, after which the council's own list of radiologists was dropped. "Current Comment," *J. Amer. med. Ass., 106* (1936), 630.

purpose the elevation of standards and advancement of the cause of radiology. Like the existing boards, it proposed to test qualifications through examinations, to issue certificates, and to maintain a list of diplomates. Some of the societies in other specialties used board certification as a condition of society membership. The radiology board, in contrast, required its candidates to be members of at least one of the societies which appointed members to the board. Radiologists were thereby brought together into organizational affinity in order to press for other prestige-enhancing claims. After the appearance of the Essentials, which specifically disapproved the stipulation of specialist society membership, this requirement was formally dropped.[25] However, specialist society membership continued to be stressed by this and other boards as an important factor in the appraisal of a candidate's suitability for certification. Thus the political and the educational aspects of the specialty were linked.

The establishment of a board was heralded as a vital measure in raising radiologists once and for all above the level of basic technical competence, and in recognizing radiology as a strictly medical field. Besides providing a criterion for lay and professional groups for judging and selecting radiologists, it was expected that hospitals and other organizations would gradually establish rules limiting service on their staffs to those certified; that specialization would be limited to those qualified to practice in the specialty; and that specialist societies would restrict their membership to diplomates.[26] At the same time radiologists were strengthening their control over nonmedical radiological training. There had been a registry of radiographers since 1922, under the auspices of medical and nonmedical radiological societies, but only 470 technicians had been so certified by 1927. In 1933, the registry began a list of accredited training schools with radiologists as instructors; and within a year there was a total of 1,165 certified technicians. The registry was incorporated in 1936, with the title of *X-ray Technician*, more clearly to distinguish its diplomates from medical radiologists in the minds of other professions and the public.[27] An article of 1933 described how a young nonmedical

25. In the first complete listing of board requirements in 1939, the American Board of Radiology required AMA or equivalent membership, but no specialist society membership.
26. "Current Comment," *J. Amer. med. Ass., 102* (1934), 621; "The American Board of Radiology," ibid., p. 641; Henry K. Pancoast, "The Future of Radiology as a Medical Specialty," *Amer. J. Roentgenol., 30* (1933), 716; E. P. Pendergrass, "The Situation of Radiology in Medical Education in the U.S. and Canada," *Radiology, 30* (1938), 338–40.
27. The *American Registry of Radiographers* (1922), changed to *X-Ray Technicians* (1936), and to *Radiologic Technologists* (1962), was sponsored by the Radiological Society of North America and the American Society of X-Ray Techni-

man who had obtained training as a technician had set up in private practice in Philadelphia, received the appointment as roentgenologist in the local hospital, and even attempted gastrointestinal diagnoses; by 1940, such practices had been virtually eradicated.[28] Radiological technicians, as a result of these moves, gradually came to recognize, as optometrists did not, a primary allegiance to physicians in their specialty. With the establishment of a specialty board for physicians, with effective agitation against salaried hospital practice, and with control over nonmedical technicians, radiology achieved standing as a specialty.

Pathologists followed a similar route in their search for recognition. The salaried hospital pathologist was, it was claimed in 1935, "often treated in a patronizing manner by clinicians often his inferiors in the fundamental knowledge of disease," and was "denied his proper place as a consultant, to the detriment of the highest type of practice of scientific work being undertaken in university teaching centers." [29] Both the American Society of Clinical Pathologists, founded in 1922 to improve both the scientific status as well as the prestige of the specialty, and the AMA Section on Pathology and Physiology set up committees in June 1935 to act jointly in the establishment of a medical specialty board. Agreement was unanimous. By May 1936, the two groups had set up bylaws and authorized four members from each group to act as members of the board; organization was completed in July 1936.[30] The board was "to encourage

cians; it was also sponsored by the American Roentgen Ray Society. One reason for its establishment was to reduce lay interference in the practice of radiology and to formulate ethical relationships between physician and technician. In 1944 the Radiological Society of North America withdrew its sponsorship in favor of the American College of Radiology, in order to provide more representative participation by radiologists. At the same time, the AMA Council on Medical Education assumed responsibility for inspecting and approving technician schools.

28. Pancoast, "Future of Radiology," p. 716; and see Homer P. Sanger, "Cooperation between Organized Radiology and the American Medical Association," *Amer. Coll. Radiol. Bull., 3* (1936), 10; Arthur W. Erskine, "Organized Roentgenology in America," *Radiology, 45* (1945), 549–50.

29. J. P. Simonds, "The Point of View of the Pathologist," *Proc. ann. Cong. med. Educ.* (1935), pp. 40–41.

30. The board as originally formed did not include a cross section of specialist societies in pathology. This was rectified in 1959, when the organization was changed, to include on the board representation from three other organizations: the College of American Pathology (formed in 1946 and including as major objectives the socioeconomic and scientific improvement in pathologists' status), the American Association of Pathologists and Bacteriologists (formed in 1901 as an offshoot of the Association of American Physicians), and the American Society for Experimental Pathology (1913). Esmond R. Long, *A History of American Pathology* (Springfield, Ill., 1962), p. 205 and passim; "American Board of Pathology, Inc.," *J. Amer. med. Ass., 113* (1939), 812–13.

the study and promote the practice of pathology," to elevate its standards, and advance its cause. The certificate was to be used as a voluntary and unofficial vehicle to distinguish the thoroughly qualified. Examinations were to be based on the broad principles of pathology, with emphasis on diagnosis and interpretation; applicants could choose to be certified in either pathologic anatomy or clinical pathology or both. These arrangements were similar in form to those of the Board of Psychiatry and Neurology; in effect the new board recognized pathology as two specialties rather than one.

Meanwhile the American Society of Clinical Pathologists was also taking steps to establish control over nonmedical practitioners. A registry of medical technologists was formed in 1928, administered by the society in conjunction with the American College of Surgeons; and continuous study was made of the curricula of schools for laboratory technicians. The Council on Medical Education was also concerned with laboratory personnel, as a result of its surveys of hospitals and its listing of approved laboratories. In 1936, the council set up Essentials for approved schools for laboratory technicians. The desire to ensure the supervision and absolute control of the medical profession over laboratory technicians was a basic reason for their being adopted.[31] Laboratory technology, like X-ray technology, had little chance to develop outside the overall guidance of the medical profession.

INTERNAL MEDICINE: THE ROLE OF THE COLLEGE
AND LURE OF THE BOARD

Specialty self-interest might have been reduced if the American College of Physicians and the American College of Surgeons had been organized as centrifugal organizations. That the American Colleges did not provide the cohesive influence such as that of the Royal Colleges in Britain in maintaining a unified profession was partly a result of their late development as potential medical guilds, itself the product of the basic egalitarianism of American medicine. But it was also partly a question of outlook and of timing. The American College of Physicians was in no position to assume leadership of the specialist movement for the nonsurgical specialties. George Piersol, who was secretary-general of the College from 1926 to 1932 and again from 1937, campaigned with others

31. *Proc. AMA House of Delegates* (May 1936), pp. 40–41, 45, 46, in AMA, *Digest,* p. 442. A similar case was made for controlling physical therapists. Ibid., p. 467.

for entry by merit instead of the previous bases of influence and personal contact.[32] But such a move came too late to influence any specialties other than those most intimately connected with internal medicine. Psychiatrists, pediatricians, radiologists, and pathologists had long had their own specialist associations, and now had separate, independent certifying boards. The College therefore continued to reflect the special field of "internal medicine," and not the broad area of general medicine.

At the meeting of specialty board representatives in June 1933 which led to the setting up of the Advisory Board for Medical Specialties, there had been a feeling that the Advisory Board should concern itself with specialist qualifications in a more strict sense than the Colleges, which were therefore excluded from this new and potentially highly influential organization. The Board of Regents of the American College of Physicians meanwhile was considering setting up a College system of examinations for the purpose both of admitting its own fellows, and for certification of specialists in internal medicine and its related specialties. The College was thus intimately concerned with the establishment of qualifications in internal medicine and was not initially interested in endorsing an independent national certifying board. Indeed, the view was expressed by Dr. Walter Bierring, the College's spokesman for specialist qualifications, that internal medicine was not a specialty in the sense of narrowly defined special areas such as ophthalmology and otolaryngology.[33] The pediatricians, however, had decided that pediatrics was a specialty, even though it was a holistic area; and, with the increasing interest in qualifying mechanisms, it was doubtful whether such an argument could prevail. Meanwhile there were obvious advantages to the College's meeting demands for specialty recognition through a written examination held for membership in the College; and favorable discussion by the board of regents along these lines continued through 1934. One possibility was to have an open admittance of interested internists as College associates, and then offer an examination for transfer from associate to fellowship. This plan had the advantages of putting no curb on College membership as a whole, while at the same time establishing as objectively as possible a recognized fellowship elite. By this time, how-

32. James Alexander Miller, in W. G. Morgan, *American College of Physicians,* p. 117. In 1928 the College had 1,290 fellows and 521 associates; but few professional leaders were included in this number. From the late 1920s, successful efforts were made to transform the College into an increasingly academic organization. By 1940, the fellowship had increased to 3,210, and there were 1,269 associates; few leaders were now missing.
33. "Abstract of Minutes of the Board of Regents," *Ann. intern. Med.,* 7 (1934), 1564–65.

ever, the Advisory Board for Medical Specialties had been formed and had developed its Essentials for independent specialist examining boards. The proposed boards included internal medicine. The Essentials included an organizational requirement of representation from the AMA section as well as from the independent specialist groups. It therefore appeared wise for the internists to unite with the AMA in creating a group which would have a controlling voice in determining certification in their specialty. If not, the College might be bypassed, either by the AMA or by public licensing mechanisms. These latter arguments were used with some force by Dr. Maurice Pincoffs in an editorial of the *Annals of Internal Medicine* in March 1935;[34] they became the new, modified view of the College.

In April 1935, the Board of Regents of the American College of Physicians assumed leadership in the certification of internists by approaching the AMA section. A joint examining board was suggested, but with a controlling College interest. It was agreed that College fellowship should eventually be contingent on certification from this board. It was also resolved that the Association of American Physicians, which had come to represent academic physicians, be asked to cooperate in the plan; but the association declined. Privately, certain leading internists were opposed to a certifying board. Thomas R. Boggs of Johns Hopkins, then the president of the Association of American Physicians, saw the specialty boards as a regimentation in medicine that he considered unnecessary and threatening. But the association took no official action.[35] The AMA Section on the Practice of Medicine had no such compunctions. In June it resolved to cooperate with the College, and in so doing it chose a committee with strong College affiliations. The new board was approved by the AMA Council on Medical Education and the Advisory Board for Medical Specialties during 1936. It included five representatives of the American College of Physicians and four of the AMA section; the College thus had the casting vote.[36] At least three of the College members and two of the section members were to be of professorial rank in approved medical schools of the United States or Canada.

The structure of the American Board of Internal Medicine, whose first chairman was Walter Bierring, made it much more of a creature of the American College of Physicians than a separate examining structure, and gave it a strong university rather than practitioner flavor. The new board was organizationally independent and autonomous, as were the other spe-

34. Editorial, *Ann. intern. Med.,* 8 (1935), 1163–64.
35. James H. Means, *The Association of American Physicians: Its First 75 Years* (New York, 1961), pp. 193–94.
36. Representation is now seven from the American College of Physicians, five from the AMA section.

cialty examining boards. But with only two participating organizations, with the close connections between College and section leadership, and with the numerical advantage of College representatives on the board itself, this board proved to be a more flexible organization than boards which report back to three or five separate specialist societies. There was, moreover, some disagreement among the early members of the board as to how internal medicine should be classified and what certification was for. Some members held that certification should only be granted to those who could qualify as consultants, but this view was overruled, one board member remarking that under the standards proposed only three physicians in the United States would qualify. As in pediatrics, therefore, board certification was geared toward the well-trained general internist. It was, however, decided that educational requirements in internal medicine would be made very flexible and that the test of quality would be set by the level of the examinations.[37] Parenthetically, it should be noted that the American Board of Internal Medicine has continued to remain outstanding among the specialty boards for its refusal to apply rigid rules as to where and how training should be obtained.

The new board was not to provide a focus for all nonsurgical specialties, but its formation was sufficiently timely for it to be able to retain the emerging subspecialties of internal medicine—gastroenterology, cardiology, metabolic diseases, tuberculosis, and allergy. While the so-called American Board of Gastroenterology and the American Board of Tuberculosis existed in embryonic form in 1938, they could not prosper without endorsement by the Advisory Board for Medical Specialties and the Council on Medical Education of the AMA, and this was not forthcoming. Quite apart from the professional respectability thereby gained, such endorsement was increasingly necessary to persuade hospitals to establish residency programs in a specialty. The American Board of Internal Medicine had decided right from the beginning to offer subspecialty certificates, but the machinery was not put into effect until 1941. At that time allergy, cardiovascular diseases, gastroenterology, and tuberculosis were incorporated into the framework of the board. All candidates for the subspecialties had to pass the written examination in general internal medicine, a practical examination consisting of a long case and an examination in the subspecialty, and an examination in particular techniques of the subspecialty.[38] In the medical specialties there was now both hori-

37. An invaluable account of the founding of the board is Walter L. Bierring's "The American Board of Internal Medicine," in W. G. Morgan, *The American College of Physicians,* pp. 88–102, from which much of the material here is drawn.
38. "Subspecialties of Internal Medicine," *J. Amer. med. Ass., 116* (1941),

zontal and vertical stratification. A pediatrician was recognized as practicing in a different branch of medicine from a specialist in internal
medicine, or a psychiatrist. The internist interested in cardiology went on
to qualify in the subspecialty; the pediatrician also interested in cardiology
would however have to seek eventual subspecialty certification under the
pediatric board. Where would this lead? The prospects were confusing
and likely to become more so as overlapping continued, and as emerging
interests cut across the established pattern of the boards. The American
Board of Internal Medicine had, however, checked the progress of further
division in its related specialites, and this augured well for future overall,
structural coordination.

SURGERY: ONE BRANCH OR MANY?

In the surgical specialties organizational fragmentation was already quite
far advanced before the American Board of Surgery was founded. The
establishment of the American Board of Orthopaedic Surgery in 1934
ended any hope of grouping all surgical specialties under one general
surgical umbrella.[39] Ophthalmology, otolaryngology, and obstetrics-gynecology, which already had specialty boards in surgical fields, while surgically based, were topical specialties, relating to specific regions of the
anatomy. Orthopedic surgery was more closely related to general surgery;
it was itself general in that it was especially concerned with the skeletal
system and related structures, thus crossing through areas in part assigned
to other specialties. For reasons both of raising standards and increasing
prestige, the American Board of Orthopaedic Surgery endeavored, like the
other boards, to restrict its examinations to those predominantly practicing the specialty and expected that hospitals and other institutions would
limit their staffs to diplomates, so that the practice of orthopedic surgery
would eventually be limited to those "properly qualified." Orthopedic
surgery was thus recognized as fundamentally different from general surgery, as well as organizationally independent.

In 1935 the American Board of Urology was incorporated.[40] Urology

1979. On the background of the subspecialties, I am indebted to Dr. Victor Logan,
personal communication.
39. The American Board of Orthopaedic Surgery was established with the joint
action of the American Orthopaedic Association, the AMA Section on Orthopaedic Surgery, and the American Academy of Orthopaedic Surgeons. Both the
American Orthopaedic Association and the Academy of Orthopaedic Surgeons
restricted their membership to board diplomates. Advisory Board, *Directory of
Medical Specialists, 2* (1942), 767.
40. At a meeting of the American Association of Genito-Urinary Surgeons in May
1932 Dr. William F. Braasch called the attention of urologists to the various spe-

had developed as a separate specialty only after World War I, arising quickly around instrumentation and with developments in chemotherapy and endocrinology. The practitioner in this specialty could claim more scientific exactness than any other medical worker, and by 1934 there were thought to be nearly 2,400 full-time or part-time urologists in the country.[41] Urology was sufficiently important to be included in the AMA's first list of appropriate fields for specialty boards. Indeed, so many practitioners were there—more than the number of radiologists, pathologists, ophthalmologists, and many other specialties—that the establishment of the board had implications both in raising standards and in reducing numbers. There were fears from its critics that the board would develop into an exclusive, undemocratic group; but those who supported it considered that eventually all those primarily interested in urology would be board certified. A grandfather clause was useful in this board as in others as an attraction to eminent members in the field; and by 1936 there were 151 foundation members.[42] The process of formalization was barely complete, however, by the outbreak of World War II. In 1940, only 39 percent of the 1,700 full-time urologists were board certified.[43]

The emergence of the boards for orthopedic surgery and urology raised problems as to what was "general surgery"—problems, moreover, which continue. Generalism in medicine was increasingly assuming negative tones. The man who did a great deal of obstetrics, coupled with orthopedics, was eligible neither for the American Board of Obstetrics and Gynecology nor for the American Board of Orthopaedic Surgery; he was ipso facto a general surgeon. At the same time general surgery, like general practice, was diminishing in qualitative emphasis. A full-time ortho-

---

cialty boards then being established, and he made the first official request for an examining board in urology. A committee was appointed to report on the subject the following year. The American Urological Association independently appointed a similar committee in 1933; and a third committee was appointed by the AMA Section of Urology at the AMA Milwaukee session. These committees merged later in 1933 and decided that a board should be incorporated to protect patients from unprepared practitioners and to raise standards of education in urology. After their early start in establishing a specialty board, urologists lost ground while ratification was sought from the component societies. A temporary board was formed in 1933; organization was developed during 1934, with three members from each of the three societies; and incorporation was finally achieved in May 1935. The first examinations were the following year. William Niles Wishard, Jr., "Your American Board of Urology, Incorporated," *J. Urol., 82* (1959), 178.

41. Commission on Graduate Medical Education, *Graduate Medical Education,* p. 261.
42. Wishard, "Your American Board of Urology," p. 178.
43. See Appendix table A2.

pedic surgeon, with his board diploma, might be assumed to be more competent in that specialty than the general surgeon. With the eye, ear, gynecological, and urological surgery removed from his primary jurisdiction, the general surgeon was to be pushed into a position of defending his monopoly of what remained in the abdomen. Organizationally, too, general surgery was fast implying the practice of this relatively limited specialty. The American College of Surgeons was faced with a dilemma of purpose much like that of the American College of Physicians. Men such as Evarts Graham of the Surgeons, and Charles Martin of the Physicians, were bringing young academic blood into the Colleges at the very time when the specialty boards were being discussed, but too late to control their overall development.

The two aspects of College reorganization and specialist recognition merged. There was a growing rift between the old guard of practitioners who donated their time to teach medical students and the new brand of full-time clinical teachers. Samuel Harvey, professor of surgery at Yale and one of the Young Turks of university-led surgical reform, was made chairman of a committee on graduate teaching in surgery appointed by the American College of Surgeons in October 1934—after the Advisory Board for Medical Specialties was established. The American Surgical Association and the AMA surgical section were also discussing graduate training. Edward W. Archibald used his presidential address to the American Surgical Association in the spring of 1935 to make a detailed analysis of the problems which had arisen in the wake of the rise of small-town hospitals throughout the country, when "Fingers replace brains, and handicraft outruns science." [44] The American College of Surgeons had its own foundation in response to such criticisms of operations which were technically possible but scientifically or individually undesirable, but the College was felt to have failed; it was said to be ineffective, with low standards, and with an inadequate test for the fellowship. [45] The Essentials for specialty boards included a proposal for a board in surgery, and this proposal became the springboard for the reform movement led by the younger, university surgeons. A committee of the American Surgical Association to study training and qualifications, chaired by Evarts Graham, started with acknowledgment of the desirability of an examining board outside the American College of Surgeons. Its first action was to

44. Edward W. Archibald, "Higher Degrees in the Profession of Surgery," *Ann. Surg.*, *102* (1935), 481–95.
45. There was no examination in the basic sciences or in surgical pathology; at no time was the candidate seen by his examiners; and the training requirements were minimal—one year of internship and two years' surgical apprenticeship. The fellow was admitted chiefly on presentation of case reports.

propose a joint national committee to elevate standards in surgery which would have only minority representation from the College. This committee of twenty-four met in October 1935 at College headquarters in Chicago: six representatives each from the College, the AMA, and the American Surgical Association; and two each from regional surgical groups—the Western, Southern, and the Pacific Coast surgical associations. Discussion was reportedly bitter at times, with College representatives taking the view that a national committee was unnecessary. But the majority favored the proposal for a board, and all organizations agreed to appoint representatives to attend the first meeting of the national committee in February 1936. The organization of the American Board of Surgery was thus under way.[46] Professor Harvey's committee advised the American College of Surgeons to cooperate in its foundation. While some doubt was expressed in the board of regents that such a move might weaken College authority, there was little the College could do; and it accepted its part gracefully. The American Board of Surgery held its first organizational meeting in January 1937 and was officially approved later that year. Evarts Graham was elected chairman, with Allen O. Whipple as vice-chairman and J. Stewart Rodman as secretary-treasurer.[47] The board decided, as had the College before it, to take a definite stand against fee splitting:[48] from the start, evidently, it was to take an active role in influencing ethical as well as technical standards. There was also an immediate interest in the relationship between the American Board of Surgery and the surgical specialties still without their own certifying agencies.

SURGICALLY RELATED SPECIALTIES

Anesthesiology had developed in the United States as an adjunct of surgery; it could thus be claimed as a surgical affiliate if not as a surgical subspecialty. Before World War I, when the procedure was still relatively

46. Loyal Davis, *Fellowship of Surgeons,* pp. 336–37; J. Stewart Rodman, *History of the American Board of Surgery, 1937–1952,* pp. 2–4.
47. Rodman, p. 11; "Announcement," *J. Amer. med. Ass., 108* (1937), 1723. The original board was of 13 members—3 each from the American Surgical Association, the American College of Surgeons, and the AMA Section on Surgery, and 1 each from the 4 approved regional associations. Stress would be on the basic sciences in part 1 of its examination; part 2 would be clinical.
48. "The Board, believing that the practice of fee-splitting is pernicious, leading as it does to traffic in human life, will reserve the right to inquire particularly into any candidate's practice in regard to this question." First *Booklet of Information,* quoted by Rodman, p. 13

simple, the surgical intern or an operating nurse had often administered the anesthetic. Although medical interest was rising, it was only with the general use of nitrous oxide and oxygen, stimulated during World War I, and with further developments in the 1920s of gas anesthesia together with local anesthesia and spinal anesthesia, that the trained physician anesthetist came into his own. By this time, however, the nurse anesthetist was well established as a protégée of the surgeon, and was often better trained than the average physician. Indeed, many of the medical anesthesiologists of the 1930s were introduced to anesthesia during their internship by nurse anesthetists.[49] The relationships between surgeons and nurse anesthetists were strong; the nurses were much more efficient technicians than the average intern; and the physician anesthetist scarcely appeared necessary. While, therefore, the medical anesthesiologist felt to the nurse anesthetist much of what the ophthalmologist felt toward the optometrist (who had also become established in his specialty before the appearance of the medical specialist), the surgeon stood in the way; there was an uneasy triangle of surgeon, nurse anesthetist, and medical anesthesiologist.[50] The situation in the 1930s was thus one of increasing activity, on the one hand on the part of the nurse anesthetists (who formed their national association in 1932) supported by the surgeons, and on the other, new organizational activity by the much smaller number

49. The Mayos had given the anesthetic function to Edith Graham and (in 1893) to Alice Magaw; and, with the Mayos' increasing impact on surgery, the practice of nurse anesthetics had rapidly spread throughout the Middle West. By 1911, an estimated one-fourth of American hospitals employed nurse anesthetists, and by 1936 the nurse anesthetist was well established. Agatha Hodgins, who was the leader of the professionalism of the nurse anesthetist in the early 1930s, had been trained in 1908 by George Crile of Cleveland—a leading member of the American College of Surgeons. A. S. McCormick, "Some Observations on Anesthesia as a Specialty and the Anesthetist as a Specialist," *Am. J. Surg. Suppl., 33* (1919), 66–68; and I. C. Herb, "The Staff Anesthetist," ibid., pp. 1168–71; G. P. Muller, "The Changing Status of Anaesthetics," *Ann. Surg., 86* (1927), 244–50; Virginia S. Thatcher, *History of Anesthesia with Emphasis on the Nurse Specialist* (Philadelphia, 1953), pp. 52–64, 87.

50. The Medical Society of Washington, D.C., passed a resolution in 1920 for the limitation of anesthesia to licensed physicians, surgeons, and dentists, with graduate nurses involved only in the cases of emergency; in Ohio, the state medical society prohibited nurse anesthesia after a major legal battle. In 1923, however, the American College of Surgeons came out against any legal restrictions which would prohibit trained nurses from giving anesthetics. By the late 1940s it was generally accepted that the nurse anesthetist might legally administer anesthetics as an agent of a qualified physician (i.e. a surgeon) and that to administer anesthetics one had to be trained in the field—whether a nurse or a physician. Emmanuel and Lillian Hayt, *Law of Hospitals, Physician, and Patient* (New York, 1947), pp. 194–96.

of medical anesthesiologists, who founded the American Society of Anesthetists in 1935.[51] The AMA took the view that only physicians and dentists should provide anesthesia; but at the same time it was noted that enforcement was inexpedient.[52] The anesthesiologists, frustrated, were forced into a desperate position, in which they felt they had rapidly to develop their professional image. Perhaps because of the success of the nurse anesthetist, perhaps the result of difficulties by women in establishing private practices, anesthesiology was also an attractive specialty for women physicians. The University of California course pioneered in 1919 was reportedly entirely under the control of a group of San Francisco women. Thus the up-and-coming scientific anesthesiologist had to contend with the female image as well as with the difficult task—common to anesthesiologists in all countries of a similar stage of development—of presenting his specialty as a real focus of medical expertise.[53]

Like the pathologists and radiologists, the anesthesiologists sought to enhance their prestige with financial, ethical, and educational arguments. Salaried hospital practice by anesthesiologists became suspect and was to be openly criticized in the 1940s.[54] At the same time educational standards for physician anesthesiologists were set. Committees were appointed in 1931 and again in 1933 to consider board certification, but not until 1937 was the Board of Anesthesiology finally founded. The existence of the board, and the recognition of standards which rivaled those of other specialties, enabled anesthesiologists, like pathologists and radiologists, to prescribe the boundaries of the specialty and to assert both its status and

51. The name was changed to the American Society of Anesthesiologists in 1945. In 1940 there were 285 full-time medical anesthesiologists in the U.S. compared with some 2,500 members of the American Association of Nurse Anesthetists.
52. See e.g. editorial, *J. Amer. med. Ass.*, *108* (1937), 2218.
53. See Editorial, *Am. J. Surg. Suppl.*, *33* (1919), 29; and Agatha Hodgins, "The Nurse Anesthetist," *Am. J. Nurs.*, *30* (1930), 865. The director of the Laboratory of Applied Physiology at Yale, tired of watching dramatic operating scenes in movies when the only evidence of the anesthesiologist was in pictures of filling rubber bags and of jingling valves, suggested changing the image through a campaign of propaganda, including radio programs, magazines, and books in which the anesthesiologist appeared as a central figure. Howard W. Haggard, "The Place of the Anesthetist," *Anesthesiology, 1* (1940), 1–12. See also Ralph M. Waters, Hubert R. Hathaway, and William H. Cassels, "The Relation of Anesthesiology to Medical Education," *Proc. ann. Cong. med. Educ.* (1939), pp. 37–42.
54. See e.g. James Raglan Miller, "Relation of the Anesthesiologist to the Hospital," *J. Amer. med. Ass.*, *139* (1947), 9–11; "Report of Committee to Study Special Services, Council of Massachusetts Medical Society," *New Engl. J. Med.*, *237* (1947), 874. In 1951 the American College of Anesthesiologists decreed it unethical for any anesthesiologist to be employed on a salary if the hospital offered his services for a fee. Radiologists and pathologists followed with stronger statements in 1958.

monopoly potential.[55] Meanwhile nurse anesthesia continued as a separate and rival profession. The nurses, seeking their own program of
certification, made overtures to the American Board of Anesthesiology in
1938 which might have enabled the two movements to combine and the
anesthesiologists to take on responsibility for the nurses' training. But the
attitude of hostility was already set, and the nurses were summarily rejected; indeed, there was anxiety (probably not unfounded at the time)
that if the board approved training schools for nurse anesthetists, surgeons would feel they had a carte blanche to replace their medical
anesthesiologists with nurses.[56] In so doing the board missed a golden
opportunity, for nurse anesthetists were increasingly demanded by the
hospitals. Indeed in hospitals which did not have sufficient anesthesia for
a full day's work, the duties of nurse anesthetists were combined with
administration, charge of supply room, record librarian, x-ray technician,
and charge of a ward.[57] The nurse anesthetist had become a familiar and
essential figure in the hospital routine. To the surgeon, the physician and
the nurse anesthetist were still alternatives; and to the anesthesiologists
the nurse was thus a continuing source of competition. By the early 1940s
physician anesthesia had become technologically essential to many surgical procedures.[58] Meanwhile a great deal of harm had been done to inter-
professional and intraprofessional relations, and only recently, with
general recognition of a shortage of manpower in anesthesiology have the
two groups begun to come together.

In this context of professional aspiration and material struggle, it was
unlikely that the anesthesiologists would be content with any junior board

55. The board's requirements of 100 percent limitation by diplomates to the practice of anesthesiology and its imposition after World War II of a two-year residency
training forced the American Society of Anesthesiologists to form a second organization—the American College of Anesthesiologists, established in 1947—to admit
anesthesiologists to membership in that organization; the College requirements were
set at 51 percent anesthesiology and one year of training. *Scientific and Technical
Societies of the United States and Canada* (Washington, D.C., 1961), p. 42; and see
Paul M. Wood, "Functions of the American Board of Anesthesiology," *J. Amer.
med. Ass., 139* (1947), 11–12.
56. The board appointed a study committee to review possible relations with the
nurse anesthetists. This committee remained inactive on the books until 1954. Minutes of the American Board of Anesthesiology.
57. *Trans. Amer. Hosp. Ass., 42* (1940), 1029–30. The American Hospital Association (and not the anesthesiologists) cooperated with the nurse anesthetists between 1933 and 1940 in reviewing their examining and accrediting system; indeed,
the AHA gave the American Association of Nurse Anesthetists space in its building.
Thatcher, pp. 9–11.
58. See I. S. Ravdin, "A Surgeon Comments on the Specialty of Anesthesiology,"
Anesthesiology, 2 (1941), 207.

status. While, therefore, the Board of Anesthesiology was approved in 1938 by the Advisory Board for Medical Specialties and the AMA Council on Medical Education as an "affiliate" of the American Board of Surgery,[59] the Board of Plastic Surgery being approved as a subsidiary at the same time,[60] these links did not last long; both of the new specialty boards were granted independent status in 1941.

The American Board of Surgery was thus rapidly losing control over the surgical specialties. Neurological surgery was already developing independently; a board was established in this specialty in 1940. Even the small specialty of colon and rectal surgery, accepted as a subspecialty in 1939, was to break its links with the American Board of Surgery ten years later.[61] A correlation could be drawn between the desire for prestige and the desire for a board. Of all the surgical specialties only thoracic surgery, which had no need for any organizational structure to enhance its glamour, made no move at that time toward separatism. The Board of Thoracic Surgery was approved as an affiliate of the surgical board in 1949, and remains so to this day.[62] It was doubtful if the Board of Sur-

59. The sponsors were the Section on Surgery of the AMA (there being as yet no section for anesthesiologists), the American Society of Anesthetists, and the American Society of Regional Anesthesia. The founders group included professors and associate professors in U.S. medical schools, those of 15 years standing in the specialty, and those with the certificate of fellowship in the ASA. The examination was in two parts, a written exam and an oral-practical. "Announcement," *J. Amer. med. Ass., 110* (1938), 1761.
60. What was meant by "subsidiary" was not very clear. The plastic surgeons had a separate examination system from the American Board of Surgery and retained the responsibility of certifying applicants. The American Board of Surgery, however, had the power to veto any individual accepted by the subsidiary board, subject to the latter's acceptance or to a joint conference. "Announcement," *J. Amer. med. Ass., 111* (1938), 635.
61. The proctologists had organized their board in 1934 and incorporated the following year, but had not been granted official approval as an independent board. In 1939 the American Board of Surgery agreed to accept proctologists as a subspecialty and set up a central certifying committee in proctology for this purpose. The successful candidate was certified by the Board of Surgery as qualified in general surgery with special reference to the field of proctology. Rodman, pp. 26–27; American Board of Colon and Rectal Surgery, *General Information* (Nov. 1966), p. 3; "Announcement," *J. Amer. med. Ass., 116* (1941), 2707.
62. Certification of thoracic surgeons was discussed by the American Association for Thoracic Surgery in 1936, and a committee appointed; but this committee decided that there was no need for separate certification. In 1945, the same committee reopened the question; and in 1946 a board of thoracic surgery was recommended as an affiliate of the American Board of Surgery. A three-year general surgical training was then followed by a two-year program in thoracic surgery; candidates would pass *both* the ABS examinations and an examination in their specialty. The new board was officially approved by the AMA Council on Medical Education and the Advisory Board in 1949 and incorporated in 1950. Advisory Board, *Directory of Medical Specialists, 11* (1964), 23, 1860; Rodman, pp. 78–79.

gery would ever be able to establish a dominating role; surgery was established organizationally as many branches rather than one.

Indeed, in general the branches of medicine were being firmly established. There was medicine; and there was also pediatrics, psychiatry and neurology, and dermatology. There was surgery; but there was also obstetrics and gynecology, ophthalmology, otolaryngology, and other fields which had relationships with surgery, but were not necessarily regarded as surgical subspecialties. And there were specialties such as pathology and radiology which were not "clinical" specialties in the sense of the other groups and were related to neither medicine nor surgery alone. How many branches of medicine were there? The original suggestion had been for twelve specialty boards; but arrangements by the Boards of Obstetrics and Gynecology, Psychology and Neurology, and Pathology for more than one kind of specialty certificate added to the fragmentation; and other groups would undoubtedly be added. Medicine itself was changing rapidly. It might be supposed that in the future constant readjustments and cross-alignments would have to be made in the educational structure of physicians. That the boards were being used as part of a dynamic professional process of status recognition—most acutely evident in the hospital specialties but present in all the boards—tied the specialist structures of the 1930s into a system of virtually immutable vested interests.

CHAPTER 12

The Boards As a System

The specialty boards were and were not a system; they had developed independently, but they were also loosely federated. The AMA Council on Medical Education on the one hand, and the joint Advisory Board for Medical Specialties on the other, had assumed responsibility for accrediting each new examining board as it arose. Louis B. Wilson, Willard C. Rappleye, and others had urged that specialist training be supervised by university teachers, such as themselves; the Advisory Board was designed with this intent. Of the 147 members of the 13 boards listed in the *Directory of Medical Specialists* in 1940, at least 100 held academic or clinical appointments as professor, associate professor, or assistant professor. On this evidence it might be assumed that the specialty boards were primarily educational agencies. But the nature and functions of the specialty boards remained unclear. Sponsored by specialist societies, with responsibility both for educational approval of residencies and for specialist certification, and with implications for the future development of specialist numbers, the boards had a peculiar, mixed heritage.

With the development of the voluntary certifying boards within the medical profession, discussion of licensing specialists had died. Formal public responsibility for medical standards, reflected in the general medical license in each state, remained in the 1930s (as now) at an educational level which, for the increasing segment of the profession who chose to be specialists, no longer reflected a "safe" or reasonable level of skill. The license to practice medicine was granted after the M.D. degree or after the M.D. plus a year of internship, depending on the state. Professional standards, reflected by 1940 in the educational requirements of the different specialty boards, required for specialists much more than this. The Boards of Anesthesiology, Pediatrics, and Otolaryngology required the least further training in specifying less than three years of formal graduate training following the internship; two boards (surgery and plastic surgery) demanded five years, the other nine boards three years. Besides the specification of formal training, moreover, eleven boards prescribed additional time—usually another two years—to be spent in practice before certification. As much time was being spent after licensure in preparation for the boards as was required for licensure itself. If it were accepted that the standards of the specialty boards were reasonable gauges of the training needed to produce a fit and competent specialist, basic qualifications for a sizable minority of physicians were being prescribed by professional associations rather than through a public licensing mechanism. Whether the individual specialty boards wished it to be the case or not, the boards had public as well as professional implications. Brought together as a coordinated organization, the specialty boards might develop as a potent force in supervising graduate medical education and in influencing medical manpower trends. Left alone, there was danger of their becoming introverted guilds. The important questions in the 1930s—as now—were how the boards operated; how far they were coordinated and what coordination might be expected to achieve; and how the certificates were in fact used. What, in short, was the power of these new agencies? And was this power appropriately housed?

THE BOARDS AS PROFESSIONAL ORGANIZATIONS

Structurally, each of the specialty certifying boards was a conjoint examining board on the lines originally suggested by Edward Jackson for the American Board of Ophthalmology. In each case one of the sponsoring societies was the appropriate scientific section of the AMA. The number of other sponsoring societies ranged from one, as in the case of the American Board of Internal Medicine, to six, as in the case of the American Board of Surgery. But the overall design was similar. Each board included a specified number of members nominated or appointed from each sponsoring group; each conducted examinations—some with written and oral examinations, some with oral and practical examinations alone; each set certain prerequisites of training, experience, and other qualifications; and each issued a certificate.

The Advisory Board for Medical Specialties offered an umbrella organization, including representatives of each approved board, together with representatives from certain other bodies; it specified standards for the approval of new boards in relation to their organization, and the general and professional qualifications to be expected of candidates. These standards or "Essentials," which were endorsed by the AMA Council on Medical Education, recommended that every candidate for board certification be a member of the AMA (a requirement that was later dropped), that he be graduated from a medical school approved by the AMA Council on Medical Education and have completed an internship in a hospital approved by the council, and that he should have completed a period of special study of at least three years after internship.[1] There was, however, nothing to stop already approved boards from diverging from these standards, improving upon or embellishing them for reasons of educational or professional advancement, since neither the Advisory Board nor the council had continuing supervisory power. A number of variations and discrepancies therefore arose, and there was a real danger, expressed by Ray Lyman Wilbur as early as 1935, of "shut-out" organizations developing, similar to fraternities and some of the existing specialist societies: "Those who have arrived are often human enough to set up unfair and even personal obstacles to prevent competitors from getting in." [2]

The boards tended to restrict candidacy for their examinations to those who agreed to limit their practice—or the great majority of their practice—to that specialty. By 1940, five boards specified that 100 percent of the applicant's practice should be devoted to the specialty, as defined by the board; three demanded at least 70 percent concentration; the other six boards had no rigid requirement.[3] While limitation of practice had certain advantages in maintaining a high overall level of standards among those already certified (it being presumed that the surgeon whose entire practice was in surgery was likely to be more competent, or at least more experienced, than his colleague who was a surgeon only 30 or 40 percent of the time), the requirement raised questions of public policy and was likely to antagonize general practitioners. One of the major medical care issues of the 1930s was the provision of medical care to rural areas. Yet the 100 percent restriction was a disincentive for the well-trained specialist to attempt to set up in practice in any but a large city. General practice was supposedly worth conserving as the cornerstone of health services, yet the standards prescribed by the boards virtually excluded the general practitioner. Moreover, the definition of specialist practice was not always clear-cut; if

1. The "Essentials for Approved Special Examining Boards" are given in the various editions of the *Directory of Medical Specialists,* first published in 1940.
2. Ray Lyman Wilbur, "Report of the Council on Medical Education and Hospital," *Proc. ann. Cong. med. Educ.* (1935), pp. 1–3. One outstanding obstacle was race. As late as 1947 there were only 93 black physicians in the United States who were board-certified (Morais, p. 97). Other professionally "disadvantaged" groups of the 1930s included Jewish immigrants and women.
3. B. R. Kirklin, "Summary of Eligibility Requirements of Certifying Boards," *J. Amer. med. Ass., 116* (1941), 2616.

it were, it ran the risk of being classified as arbitrary. The obstetrician-gynecologist, for example, was supposedly confined to the female reproductive system. In practice, however, a line could not easily be drawn between the reproductive organs and the other contents of the abdominal cavity. Gynecologists were allowed even breast surgery in the female, but not reproductive surgery in the male. General surgery was defined as including diagnosis and preoperative and postoperative care, but not normal obstetrics or general practice. The surgeon was thus by definition one who cut, rather than one who prevented or conserved. The American Board of Anesthesiology had to decide whether to enforce its 100 percent restriction rule in the case of anesthesiologists who occasionally engaged in obstetrics, were on general medical call to a baseball team, could not make a living in their area without some outside practice, or acted as a part-time medical administrator.[4] Much of the time of the boards in these early years was spent on deliberations of what might be included as the practice of each specialty, and what denied. There were echoes in this process of earlier attempts by the medical profession at large to define, in fighting competition by nonphysicians, what was meant by "practice of medicine." Only this time the process was at one remove, being exercised by jostling groups within the profession.

Decisions on specialist practice were vital to the effective delineation of specialist boundaries, which in turn reflected the relative success of each professional segment in proclaiming a unique mission or identity. They could be justified in terms of raising professional competence and quality. But at the same time, in deciding not only on a level of training and skill but also on the type of practice of specialists, the boards ran the very real danger of a carry-over of quasi-political interests into the certification field. This was reinforced in the links between the boards and the specialist societies whose interests were more clearly functional or ethical. At a time, for example, when the pathologists and radiologists were fighting the practice of salaried employment in hospitals, it was unlikely that physicians who accepted such terms would be thought fitted for professional endorsement by either the specialist societies or the relevant specialty boards. Professional associations have traditionally been concerned with conduct, or behavior, as well as with a level of knowledge; indeed, the guarantee to the public of a level of known integrity, incorporated into an ethical code, has long been the distinguishing mark of a profession, as against the practice of a trade. The boards'

4. Minutes of the American Board of Anesthesiology, 24 May 1938; 29–30 Mar. 1941.

problem was one of degree: how far recognition of conduct should be part of certification and by whom (and for what purposes) such recognition should be made. The AMA *Journal* warned in 1941 that the boards' conduct should never be such as to cause them to be regarded as a means of creating a monopoly or of protecting specialists from competition, came out firmly against the requirement of 100 percent limitation of practice as restrictive, and asked the boards to limit themselves to defining merely the ability and integrity of their candidates.[5] But the question hinged on the purpose and meaning of certification. Professional advancement of the specialty and the protection of the public's interest were beginning to conflict.

Until the end of World War II the number of candidates examined each year by most of the boards was still relatively small. Through the specialist societies and through established diplomates, applicants to the boards were often personally known, or known at second hand, to those sitting in judgment upon their qualifications for practice. Admission to candidature was thus in some ways like admission to a club. It was possible to take into account (and these are actual examples) the fact that one applicant's child was sick at the time he sat for the examination or that another was unduly tense, and thus did not do his best. The young man might be evaluated differently from the old, and the man from the small rural town, with poor facilities, might be treated more gently than the candidate from a large Eastern center. Whether the candidate's hospital required him to have a board certificate was another factor to be taken into account, since the impact of failure on one individual could be so much greater than on another. A review of the minutes of one board reveals great efforts by the board members to be fair in making these and similar decisions.[6] It was, however, a fairness seen in intraprofessional terms rather than through the eyes of a quasi-licensing agency.

A member of the American Board of Surgery proudly claimed that in no instance did that board reach any decision save on merit.[7] One could not, however, be certified by the American Board of Surgery, or indeed by any of the boards save pediatrics, unless a member in good standing of the AMA. Thus dismissal from the AMA, exclusion for whatever reason (such as lack of the requisite social attributes, race, etc.), or unwillingness to join because of conflicting views on the cor-

5. Editorial, *J. Amer. med. Ass., 117* (1941), 789.
6. Minutes of the American Board of Anesthesiology, 21 July 1939; 6–7 June 1942; 9 June 1944.
7. Fred Rankin, "The Responsibility of Medicine in Wartime," *J. Amer. med. Ass., 119* (1942), 539.

porate practice of medicine or on attitudes to compulsory health insurance had a direct bearing on the definition of specialist "merit." Each of the boards examined the candidate's ethical and moral standing, and each interpreted this in the light of its own expectations as to what ethical practice might be. This was in line with the stated purpose of the specialty boards, that they were to test "fitness" for practice rather than technical ability alone. The Boards of Obstetrics and Gynecology, Pathology, Radiology, and Urology stated that they intended to "elevate the standards and advance the cause" of their respective specialties. Radiologists noted that their certificate might be competed for by any radiologist who was practicing "honorably and efficiently." [8] The American Board of Psychiatry was not alone in conducting "investigations" as well as examinations of candidates. The American Board of Obstetrics put on its examiners the duty of investigating credentials and making a survey of the candidate's character; and the American Board of Anesthesiology developed a special local system of observing not only the candidate's work but his relations with other staff members as well. Ophthalmologists were also compelled to accept the standards of ethical practice of each local community, since they could forfeit their board certification if expelled from any recognized medical society; nor were they allowed to accept commissions from opticians, druggists, or appliance makers. Radiologists' certificates were likely to be revoked if the diplomate was expelled from a recognized radiological society. Surgeons were not allowed to split fees. Psychiatrists, while not forced to limit their practice to psychiatry or neurology, were not accepted by the specialty board if they were already certified by another board. [9]

None of the boards made public the names of those passing its examinations, and each reserved the responsibility for granting a certificate in the way it saw fit, giving balance to character and practice as well as to performance in the examination. [10] Indeed, several boards required candidates to sign a waiver of legal rights in case of refusal to grant a certificate. Only the American Boards of Obstetrics and Gynecology and of

8. The Boards of Dermatology, Anesthesiology, Ophthalmology, Otolaryngology, Psychiatry and Neurology spoke of "fitness"; Obstetrics, Pathology, Pediatrics, and Urology mentioned the definition of "competence" as their goal. Internal Medicine spoke merely of "qualification," and Orthopaedic Surgery of providing a criterion for the public. Announcement, "Approved Examining Boards in Medical Specialties," *J. Amer. med. Ass., 113* (1939), 817.
9. *Directory of Medical Specialists 1* (1940), 20, 254; III 1946, pp. 801, 855, 867.
10. E.g. the American Board of Orthopaedic Surgery, art. 7, sec. 3: "Each applicant shall be examined and his qualifications determined by the Board in such matter as it may designate, and his record shall be reviewed by the Board in the light of all assembled information." *J. Amer. med. Ass., 113* (1939), 810.

Otolaryngology published regular figures in the AMA *Journal* comparing the number of candidates examined with the number passed or failed.[11] A general aura of mystery thus surrounded board activities. The boards could also revoke certificates at their discretion. Only four boards (dermatology, psychiatry, radiology, and urology) listed in their official notices specific causes for which revocation might be demanded.[12] The question of *continued* competence was raised, a problem not yet tackled by the licensing bodies, and certainly not by the universities in granting the M.D. degree.

All this was in line with the operation of a private voluntary professional group granting its own fellowship or diplomas. The gray area of qualitative evaluation made certification a private rather than a public process. Board certification certainly meant acknowledged integrity and competence, but within professionally prescribed boundaries which all were not allowed to enter. Besides questions of ethics (which included the attitude of the ophthalmologist to the optometrist, the anesthesiologist to the nurse anesthetist, and the radiologist to salaried hospital practice) and practice limitation, six boards also required United States or Canadian citizenship. Indeed, the Boards of Obstetrics and Surgery insisted that foreign-born candidates, however well qualified medically, should have held U.S. citizenship for at least three years. Such conditions were plainly restrictive, as was the rigidity with which curriculum and experience requirements were usually prescribed. The boards were becoming guilds. In their functions they could be seen potentially as providing what the Royal Colleges had long offered in Britain: the designation of a carefully selected, self-perpetuating elite. By 1940, however, the process was still incomplete.

The profession was faced with the implications of this movement if the specialty boards were to become the sole arbiters of specialist rank. Indeed, board members themselves were concerned with their possible expansion to autocracy, if and when certification achieved of-

11. The pass rate for the American Board of Otolaryngology during the 1930s varied from 72 to 92 percent. The American Board of Obstetrics had an overall pass rate of 83 percent of those examined from 1930 to 1942. Announcement, *J. Amer. med. Ass., 112* (1939), 68 and passim; Walter T. Dannreuther, "The Educational Objectives of the American Board of Obstetrics and Gynecology," *J. Amer. med. Ass., 120* (1942), 169.

12. Dermatology gave as cause for revocation (a) where certification had been contrary to any provision in the board bylaws; (b) where the physician was in fact ineligible to receive the certificate; (c) where he had made a misstatement of fact; (d) conviction in a court of a felony or misdemeanor involving moral turpitude; (e) license revoked or disciplined or censored as a physician by a court or other body having proper jurisdiction or authority. *J. Amer. med. Ass., 113* (1939), 805.

ficial acceptance through a system of public registration (the equivalent of a license) or through public medical programs.[13] Not least concerned was the general practitioner; and it was no accident that in 1941 the AMA House of Delegates deemed that it would be unwise for any specialist group to be given the right to display any special insignia.[14]

INSTITUTIONAL RECOGNITION

Despite, then, the creation of specialty certifying boards, the philosophy of specialist recognition remained in doubt. Had the time come when formal qualitative and functional distinctions within the profession would have to be made? The answer was contingent on developments in graduate medical education and in the coordinated structure of practice itself. Even assuming that some identification of a well-qualified specialist was necessary, certification by a national professional group was not the only possibility. The specialist could be recognized on the basis of educational attainment without an examination or possession of a university degree or through his institutional affiliation. In Britain, for example, the specialist on the staff of a prestigious voluntary hospital was known to have attained a level of distinction. In the United States, either hospitals or group practices (or both) could have a similar distinguishing role. Such a system—recommended by those who distrusted the parochial specialist interests of the specialty boards, or who saw greater merit in local review than in the issuing of national professional certificates—would work, however, only where the hospitals assumed responsibility for selectivity, or stratification, of their staffs. This in turn implied a community orientation of the hospital, or at least of the hospital medical staff, toward evaluating physicians—which even now has not materialized.

For a time in the 1930s, however, hospital endorsement of specialists seemed possible, either with or without the recognition of specialty board certification. Appointment to a hospital staff was already an important aspect of professional practice. The hope that hospital directors would be influenced by board certification in choosing between those who were well fitted and those who were not appeared regularly in the outlines of purpose and value which the boards included in their

13. See B. R. Kirklin, "Summary of Eligibility Requirements," *J. Amer. med. Ass., 116* (1941), 2618; Howard T. Karsner, "A Pathologist Scrutinizes the Specialty Boards," *J. Amer. med. Ass., 117* (1941), 1–4; Rankin, "The Responsibility of Medicine in Wartime," pp. 539–60; "Minutes of the Sections," *J. Amer. med. Ass., 116* (1946), 2867.
14. AMA, *Digest,* p. 678.

public pronouncements in the late 1930s. The American Board of Orthopaedic Surgery, for example, stated its expectation that hospitals and other organizations would establish rules limiting service on their permanent staff in that specialty to those who were certified, thus gradually limiting the practice of orthopedic surgery to those "properly" qualified.[15] The American Board of Ophthalmology noted with satisfaction that already promotion in many hospitals could not be obtained without board certification; the same was true, to a greater or lesser extent, in all the specialties.[16] In its hospital standardization surveys, the American College of Surgeons was already trying to encourage hospitals to select as heads of departments only recognized specialists, those for example with board certification or membership in the American College of Surgeons.[17] This encouragement could be extended to all hospital medical appointments. But this would mean the adoption by hospitals of a more restricted type of staff, tending toward a closed-staff rather than an open-staff system, and would open hospitals to criticism that they were acting as a monopoly.

If the recommendations of the Committee on the Costs of Medical Care had been followed, the hospital would have become the pivot for all aspects of medical care, and the open-staff or closed-staff issue would not have applied. Presumably distinctions would have been made in the type of hospital privileges offered to each physician, but at least all physicians would have had a basic hospital affiliation. One reason for AMA opposition to the committee's majority report was the fear by general practitioners that such a system would create a medical hierarchy in which the distinctions between general practitioners and specialists would be administratively refined.[18] But any such refinement would at least have been in a coordinated group practice setting. In contrast, a closed-staff hospital structure limited to specialists posed many more difficulties. The most obvious was the danger that the general practitioner would be excluded from any kind of hospital affiliation—as in Britain.

15. Advisory Board, *Directory of Medical Specialists, 1* (1940), 466.
16. Ibid., p. 346. See also pp. 34 (dermatology), 529 (otolaryngology), 833 (pathology), 994 (radiology); W. H. Crisp, "Standards and Licensure in Ophthalmology," *J. Amer. med. Ass., 101* (1933), 849; Frank W. Lynch, "The License to Practice Medicine," *Trans. Amer. gynec. Soc., 59* (1934), 1–8; Sanford R. Gifford, "The Function of Special Boards of Examiners," *Proc. ann. Cong. med. Educ.* (1933), p. 47.
17. Malcolm T. MacEachern, "Discussions on Regulation of Medical Specialists," *Proc. ann. Cong. med. Educ.* (1932), p. 71.
18. See "Minority Report Number One," in Committee on the Costs of Medical Care, *Final Report,* p. 155.

Others, however, continued to see advantages to general practice in making the specialties formally distinct, whether through hospital appointments or through public registration or licensing. Dr. Willard Rappleye, then president of the Advisory Board for Medical Specialties and a continued advocate of legal registration of specialty diplomas in the states, was one who saw advantages to the general practitioners in such a clarification of specialist function; for the fewer the specialists, the greater the number of general practitioners.[19] Discussions on the possibility of using board certification as a specialist license were held up to 1940 between representatives of the specialty boards and the state licensing boards. As with many other aspects of professional development, however, interest in specialist licensing decreased with World War II.

The question of delineating which physicians should have access to hospital appointments continued unabated. In New York, where in the early 1930s scarcely more than 50 percent of licensed physicians held a hospital appointment, the medical profession began to press for legislation to give all licensed physicians the right to have membership on the staff of government hospitals.[20] There followed a profusion of litigation, in which the crucial issue was the right of the hospital to select its staff versus the right of physicians to have automatic access to an increasingly necessary medical workshop. The hospitals won. Although in the late 1930s most voluntary hospitals still had an open-staff system, many had adopted bylaws or rules governing eligibility to practice in a hospital; and such rules had been legally upheld. A decision in the New York State Court of Appeals also put responsibility on the hospital for aiding and abetting in the practice of any unqualified physician or layman in that hospital; there was thus a direct incentive for hospitals to ensure that their medical staff was good.[21] How far hospitals would, or should, go above this basic level and insist on board certification or other evidence of advanced graduate skills remained a hotly debated point.

Hospitals had arisen and were expanding in profusion without any common definitions as to what kinds of medical staff appointments were

19. Willard C. Rappleye, "The Functions of the Special Examining Boards," *Proc. ann. Cong. med. Educ.* (1938).
20. Michael M. Davis, "Do Corporations Practice Medicine?" *Proc. ann. Cong. med. Educ.* (1932), p. 89.
21. See *Harris* v. *Thomas,* 217 S.W. 1068; *Hendrickson* v. *Hodkin,* 276 N.Y. 252, 11 NE (2d) 899; both cited in editorial, "The Right of Hospitals to Admit Physicians and Choose Staff," *Hospitals 13* (1939), 74–75.

available; the term "attending staff" had different meanings from one hospital to another. Both the American College of Surgeons (by means of its hospital standardization program) and the American Hospital Association (representative of the hospitals themselves) were trying to bring order out of chaos. Thus the surgeons' standardization program required approved hospitals to have an organized medical staff with specified functions and duties, without making any pronouncements as to whether the staff should be open or closed.[22] The American Hospital Association was openly interested in the potential of specialty certification as a standard of hospital appointment. This interest appeared in the report of the association's Committee on Nomenclature in Uniform Staff Organization in 1935. If the classification used by specialty boards could be applied to a system of grading hospital staffs, a national uniformity might be achieved. "No longer would a physician's proper social standing with a particular trustee be the sole means of gaining professional prestige and position in a hospital, nor would it be the foundation upon which to build a successful medical career with a rapid rise to local medical fame." [23] The AHA committee recommended a national board of standards in staff organization, composed of representatives of the AMA, the American College of Surgeons, the American College of Hospital Administrators, the American Hospital Association, and the specialty boards. This board would, it was thought, launch a program to certify all physicians connected with hospitals; it followed that it would also exclude all noncertified physicians from hospital staffs.

The AHA adopted this report unanimously. But there was not an enthusiastic reception to the idea from all the other organizations, and in 1936 the committee backed down, stressing that it had no intention of creating any new organization, but of merely combining existing forces. It now recommended that the three organizations with the most powerful influence on hospital standards (the AHA, AMA, and American College of Surgeons) form a joint committee to collaborate with other organizations to coordinate and standardize hospital staffing requirements, and to form a list of prerequsites for promotion from one hospital rank to another.[24] Nothing, however, was done. In 1937 the Committee

22. See Malcolm T. MacEachern, "Medical Staff Organization," *Hospitals 17* (943), 87–95.
23. "Report of the Committee on Nomenclature in Uniform Staff Organization," *Trans. Amer. Hosp. Ass.,* 37 (1935), 143.
24. The ranks suggested were chief or attending physician, associate, adjunct, assistant, clinical assistant, in consecutive descending order. *Trans. Amer. Hosp. Ass., 38* (1936), 173–75.

on Nomenclature suggested its own dissolution, in favor of a more general (i.e. vaguer) committee on personnel relations in hospitals; the attempt to provide a uniform gauge of hospital ranks had failed.[25] Indeed, hospital staff appointments are still made under diverse titles for similar responsibilities, or identical titles for differing duties; and except for interns and residents, the public remains unable to gauge from a physician's hospital title what his professional standing is, or what level he has reached in his career.

The American Hospital Association did however encourage hospitals to use specialist certificates even without uniform staffing procedures. In 1936, the association's president was Robin Buerki, a foundation member of the Advisory Board for Medical Specialties and a strong advocate of specialty regulation. The hospitals now had a yardstick of competence; Buerki's intention was that they should use it.[26] During 1936, each institutional member of the AHA was sent a letter recommending that in future, when hospitals made staff appointments, only those with specialty certificates (or eligible for certification by virtue of other qualifications) should be considered for appointment to specialist services. It became common practice for hospitals to expect specialists to hold a specialty board diploma or to explain why they did not have one, and as a result the standards of training and experience set down by each board were given a quasi-official sanction. Nor was such use confined to hospitals. The University of Vermont College of Medicine, for example, required that no person be appointed as professor or head of department in any subject until he had received certification by the relevant American board,[27] and, at least in ophthalmology, instructors and more senior teaching staff at Northwestern University were formally expected to be board certified.[28] It appeared that the specialty boards were fast becoming professional monopolies, as indeed, had largely been their intent.

It was precisely the monopoly aspects which caused alarm. Yet at the same time, specialization in medicine seemed to call for some overall

25. *Trans. Amer. Hosp. Ass., 39* (1937), 143–46.
26. Robin C. Buerki, "Presidential Address," *Trans. Amer. Hosp. Ass., 38* (1936), 303. The journal *Hospitals* also advocated this position. See editorial, "Diplomates for Staff Positions," *Hospitals 14* (1940), 69–70.
27. If no board existed in his field, he was to have attained membership in one or more of the most prominent societies in his subject. This recommendation was part of the conclusions by the Committee on Reorganization of the University of Vermont College of Medicine, May 1937. Chapin, p. 58.
28. Sanford R. Gifford, "The Function of Special Boards of Examiners," *Proc. ann. Cong. med. Educ.* (1933), p. 47.

labeling or planning so that appropriate numbers and kinds of physicians would be produced. The establishment of the specialty boards had been a tacit acceptance by the specialty groups that the public could not look to the market system alone in medicine for assurance of reasonable specialist standards. There was also a question whether the distribution of specialists, by specialty, could be left to the market mechanism.

The Committee on the Costs of Medical Care had made a major attempt to assess the existing and the desirable supply of physicians, and had concluded that to give optimal services the medical profession would be divided into 82 percent general practitioners, with 18 percent as full-time or part-time specialists.[29] President Roosevelt's Committee on Economic Security (1934) had in its discussions of federally supported health insurance raised questions of defining family medical care and of providing specialist services.[30] Had comprehensive national health insurance legislation been passed in the 1935 Social Security Act, some further numerical, as well as qualitative, crystallization of specialists and specialties would undoubtedly have been necessary. Sen. Robert Wagner's proposed national health act of 1939, which would have established state-operated medical care programs aided by federal grants to the states, included provisions for establishing standards of medical and institutional care and would probably have led to reassessments of the needed proportions of specialists and generalists in medicine. But such legislation was not passed, and there was little attempt through the public sector to decide what were appropriate manpower trends. The Children's Bureau, responsible for administering federal grants to states for maternal and infant care under the 1935 Social Security Act, encouraged the use of board certification in the selection of staff appointed to state administrations receiving federal funds and in the appointment of consultants to whom children should be sent for treatment. State workmen's compensation programs also favored the use of specialty examining boards, together with other forms of specialty definition, in paying specialist fees, despite a running battle between the medical profession and the various legislatures during the 1930s over "free choice" of physician by the employee, rather than assignment of physician by the employer or insurance carrier.[31] Until World War II, however, public endorsement of specialists was slow.

29. Falk, Rorem, and Ring, *Costs of Medical Care*, p. 223.
30. Edgar Sydenstricker and I. S. Falk, "Public Provisions Against the Economic Risks Arising out of Ill Health." Staff Report to the Committee on Economic Security, Sept. 1934, Appendix D (National Archives).
31. In New York, for example, under a 1935 amendment the injured employee had the right to select a physician from a list made up by the compensation administra-

In the absence of large-scale organized medical services, hospitals and other institutions were in a strategic position to make decisions about the relative ability of physicians. They developed as local foci of medical care and had a well-organized, stratified staffing structure. In a scathing article on the certifying boards, Alan M. Chesney, dean of the Johns Hopkins Medical School, made a strong argument for this view: "Continued membership of the staff of a hospital where appointments and reappointments are carefully scrutinized each year by the head of the service will be a cachet of competency, and will have the virtue of being at least a recent endorsement, instead of one, ten or twenty, or thirty years old." [32] There were many conditions to be met, however, before hospitals could assume any such role, not the least being the reluctance of hospitals to come in conflict with local medical societies. The specialty certifying boards came to prominence because of just such failures on the part of other groups, because of the lack of viable alternatives to defining standards or relative roles. The boards were willy-nilly becoming important policy-making instruments and at the same time increasingly important to the individual practitioner who wished to be recognized as a specialist.

In the interest of the public, there was a need to compromise between the machinery of professionalism and the expectations of licensure. The first leaned toward a highly subjective evaluation of the specialist as an individual, of his contributions to the profession, and of his general professional behavior; these were, after all, recognized bases of acceptance to the specialist societies. The second required clinical objectivity in relation to competence, and also judgments about the numbers and proportions of physicians in each specialty. The first was a personal, and to the outsider often a mysterious, process. The second succeeded only by its openness; however bad the system, it had to be seen as fair. Reconciliation of these approaches was not easy. The peculiar relationship between the Advisory Board for Medical Specialties and the boards and the virtual independence of the specialty boards themselves gave the individual physician without certification no channel of recourse; yet increasingly, appointment to a hospital position or to a medical faculty depended on the possession of a board certificate.

tion in cooperation with county medical societies. Although all licensed physicians had the right to be included, the medical societies determined what types of injuries each might treat. Marshall Dawson, *Problems of Workmen's Compensation Administration,* U.S. Department of Labor, Bureau of Labor Statistics, Bulletin no. 672, 1940, pp. 101, 103. And see Stern, *Medical Services by Government,* p. 126.
32. Alan M. Chesney, "Should Medical Administrative Officers Be Certified? A 1938 Fantasy," *J. Amer. med. Coll., 14* (1939), 1–8.

THE SYSTEM OF GRADUATE MEDICAL EDUCATION

The specialty boards were not, however, just certifying agencies; they were also deeply involved with specialist training. While therefore board certification was having an impact on individual acceptance or rejection for hospital appointment, the existence of the boards was affecting the development of hospital residency programs. This too could be seen as an extension of the boards' purely "professional" role. The number of residencies doubled between 1934 and 1940, and the acceleration was to continue after World War II.[33] By 1945 the number of residencies available exceeded the number of internships for the first time. The length of the residency was also increasing. In 1934 the AMA classified 331 residency programs which were designed for three years or more; in 1939, there were 1,791.[34] By 1942, twelve specialty boards required three or more years of graduate training. Early training requirements by the boards had included apprenticeship to established practitioners. By the late 1940s, these old preceptorships were being phased out.[35] Under the pressure of specialty board requirements, the residency was steadily being modified from a period of academic learning, individually oriented, into a generally acknowledged hospital training system.

The type of residency developed at Johns Hopkins and the Mayo Clinic had been designed to produce an exceptional minority of teachers, scholars, researchers, and practitioners; indeed, the residency program at the Brady Urological Institute at Johns Hopkins in the late 1930s, as set up by Hugh Young, could stretch over six years. The new residencies were frequently in hospitals without educational directors, and often without a graded system of training and responsibility. Despite the lengthening of the average program, well over half of the residency programs offered in 1938–39 were of two years or less,[36] and few hospitals could offer adequate facilities for training in the basic sciences. The specialty boards could provide a stimulus to improving residencies if the pressure of their requirements led individuals to seek residencies at

33. For 1934 figures: *J. Amer. med. Ass., 165* (1957), 61; for figures from 1940–59: *Health Manpower Source Book*, Section 13, Table 6.
34. Commission on Graduate Medical Education, *Graduate Medical Education*, pp. 15, 259.
35. Not allowable by five boards, and most of the other boards imposed careful limitations on recognition of individual preceptors and on the maximum credit allowed. Only five boards allowed *any* certified board member to be recognized as a preceptor; only one board (dermatology) was reported as having a list of preceptors for the benefit of students. AMA, "Medical Education," *J. Amer. med. Ass., 134* (1947), 1395.
36. "Announcement," *J. Amer. med. Ass., 110* (1938), 668.

the hospitals with the better programs. In the meantime there was still considerable nepotism by hospitals and competition among interns in seeking residency places, and there were no adequate common educational standards.

Unless this burden were shouldered by someone else, the specialty boards had acquired an implicit responsibility for specialist training. Each specialty board reviewed each candidate's training, and some boards began attempts to standardize the curriculum. The American Board of Ophthalmology established in 1938 a "preparatory group" of prospective candidates for its examination, provided a syllabus, a leaflet of instructions, the rental of slides, and a list of residencies graded into A, B, or C categories. The American Board of Dermatology considered numerous drafts of a syllabus for graduate training in that specialty from the mid-1930s, culminating in the publication of an agreed syllabus in 1939. Other boards were considering training in conjunction with the AMA Council on Medical Education, which had set up its own residency inspection system in the late 1920s and which was trying in the late 1930s to strengthen its residency approval system, following endorsement by the AMA House of Delegates that "cooperative relations" for specialist training be explored with the examining boards and specialist societies. The Boards of Radiology, Pathology, and Anesthesiology expressed interest in cooperating with the council in inspecting residencies early in 1939. By March 1940 the council was developing cooperative arrangements with ten of the certifying boards, as well as with the American College of Physicians. But these arrangements were not crystallized before World War II. A joint conference committee in internal medicine (of the council, the American Board of Internal Medicine, and the American College of Physicians), which held its first organizational meeting in 1940, was also interrupted by the war, and a fully codified joint system of residency review was not to be effected until the 1950s.[37] There was thus no effective standardization movement such as had, in regulating the proprietary medical schools earlier in the century, intermeshed the interests of educators and the AMA. The residency remained unstandardized: each hospital developed its own training program, which in some cases was barely a program at all; each specialty board looked at residencies in its own field, and there was no incentive for joint pursuit of educational policies.

37. Only the American Board of Ophthalmology actually joined in the plan suggested in 1939, and in doing so limited itself to supplying information. See E. L. Turner, "Background and Development of Residency Review and Conference Committees," *J. Amer. med. Ass., 165* (1957), 61–64.

The Advisory Board for Medical Specialties was a potential central structure in specialist certification and in graduate medical education. Aided by foundation grants, it attempted from the late 1930s some coordinated activities. In June 1937, the Advisory Board decided to launch a study of graduate medical education, which would focus on the problems common to all specialty boards. The Commission on Graduate Medical Education was organized later the same year, and reported in 1940.[38] Dr. Willard C. Rappleye of the Advisory Board was chairman; Dr. Robin Buerki acted as director of study, and the membership was in large part a reshuffling into a new pattern of the dominant figures in graduate medical education and in organized specialist groups. The commission ranged over the whole of graduate education, including discussion of the problems of the internship (which, with the growth of residency training, was in an increasingly ambivalent position in relation to medical education as a whole), the residency, and postgraduate training. In addition, the Advisory Board began preparations in 1939 for its own *Directory of Medical Specialists,* distinct from the AMA listing process. The first edition of the directory was published in 1940.

The Advisory Board had, however, no real authority over the independent specialty boards; this could emerge only if the boards were seriously interested in subordinating their own interests in favor of general goals. The Commission on Graduate Medical Education set out such goals but in large part they were not followed. It recommended the encouragement of a general (rather than a specialist) internship in a hospital with an educational structure, preferably affiliated with a medical school. The internship would thus prepare either for the general practice of medicine or for beginning advanced specialist training; it would still in effect be the fifth year of basic training. The residency was advocated as the most satisfactory form of specialty training. It was, however, stressed that the residency should be organized as a real educational experience, and be a joint responsibility of universities and hospitals. If the specialty boards had come together in the Advisory Board and supported the policies suggested in the Commission on Graduate Medical Education for the specialties as a whole, there might indeed have developed a closely meshed specialist educational system. But they did not. Nor were the university medical schools in any position to take on the additional responsibility that would be implied in their acceptance of graduate training.

In the financial crisis facing the universities in the 1930s, some medical schools were already being looked at as expensive luxuries. It was no

38. Commission on Graduate Medical Education, *Graduate Medical Education.*

time for them to be contemplating additional, and not strictly necessary, expense. Medical school deans were alarmed at the logistic problems of acquiring responsibility even for the internship; and there was a reluctance to face the inevitable political problems of university medical schools, traditionally conservative and isolationist, to seek to supervise graduate training in local community hospitals. A commission appointed by representatives of the specialty boards had, then, recommended enhanced university responsibility for training, but the universities were loath to rise to the challenge—as they had been previously and as they have been since.[39] University reluctance to take responsibility for graduate medical education was to have a lasting effect on medical education. As a result, the individual specialty boards and the AMA Council on Medical Education—all professional organizations, and each acting individually—were left with the responsibility for training as well as certifying specialists. There was neither a commission on specialist qualifications (as had been suggested in 1932) nor a permanent commission on graduate medical education. Some such centralized focus, or foci, became more desirable as graduate medical education became both more important as the period for learning vocational skills and increasingly diffuse and fragmented.

Both internships and residencies were inspected, approved, and listed by the AMA Council on Medical Education. In the absense of university leadership or a strong Advisory Board for Medical Specialties, the council was in a strong position to provide a unifying force for the specialties. C. G. Heyd, a leading educator and AMA president in 1937, attempted to encourage this role, which would in effect have made the council the arbiter of all aspects of vocational training: certification of competence, the listing of training facilities, and the education of the public (and public institutions) on the value of specialist certification.

39. Dr. Rappleye, as the chief spokesman of the Advisory Board for Medical Specialties, was a firm believer in removing responsibility for medical education from medical societies and returning it to the medical schools. All but 3 of the 14 specialty boards listed in the first *Directory of Medical Specialists* included men then on the Mayo Clinic staff. The influence of this Rochester group may be presumed to have been profound on the general development of specialty boards, and to have encouraged the university training ideal. Each of the specialty boards, moreover, included a majority of university professors; and it might be supposed that they would not have been opposed to university expansion into specialist training. Willard C. Rappleye, "The Internship," *J. Ass. Amer. med. Coll., 16* (1941), 1–4; *Directory of Medical Specialists, 1* (1940); Lucy Wilder, *The Mayo Clinic* (New York, 1939). For contemporary discussion of the deans' point of view see Dean William Pepper of the University of Pennsylvania, "Discussion on Paper by Robin C. Buerki," *J. Ass. Amer. med. Coll., 15* (1940), 16; and "Discussion on Paper by Willard C. Rappleye," *J. Ass. Amer. med. Coll., 16* (1941), 11–17.

Heyd foresaw a centralization of medical resources in the hospitals and the rapid extinction of the ill-trained specialist.[40]

Changes in the method of choosing its members had the effect of removing the Council on Medical Education from at least some of the political pressure of the AMA House of Delegates.[41] These changes by no means obscured the fact that in the last resort the council was still part of the AMA machine, but they tended to open the council to the more liberal views of the educators in place of the more traditional views of the body of AMA membership.[42] The Essentials for Approved Specialty Examining Boards were also revised in 1939, to provide that all applications for new specialty boards would be first processed by the council, rather than primary endorsement by the Advisory Board for Medical Specialties. The new Essentials also inter alia liberalized requirements for board certification by dropping the requirement that diplomates be members of the AMA; membership was merely "recommended." [43] Taken together with the council's increasing efforts with the specialty boards to control standards of residency training, the council's expanding sphere of interest became clear. But these developments alone could not give the council dominance; distrust of the AMA amongst the specialty groups made such a solution to the problems of standardization politically impracticable.

On another front, Willard Rappleye in 1935 had suggested a national council on medical care, which might have provided another focus for specialty development. This council was suggested as a means of providing—outside the prevailing conservatism of the AMA—professional leadership to attempt to grapple in a statesmanlike way with what ap-

40. C. G. Heyd, "Relation of AMA to Certification of Specialists," *J. Amer. med. Ass., 108* (1937), 1017–19.
41. In 1939, the method of choosing council members was changed from selection by the house of delegates for nomination by the AMA president to nomination by the board of trustees to the house of delegates. The following year this was changed again to provide for seven members, each serving for seven years, with election on the nomination of the AMA president. Fishbein, p. 448; AMA, *Digest,* pp. 463–64.
42. E.g. Heyd himself had noted the need to think of graduate education in terms of its relation to programs of social betterment, including old-age pensions, sickness insurance, and other public programs. Ray Lyman Wilbur, in his report for the council in 1936, recognized that "More and more, the physician is becoming the agent of society," and that "Health and education proceed together, and welfare is not far behind." Charles Gordon Heyd, "Trends in Graduate Teaching," *Proc. ann. Cong. med. Educ.* (1935), p. 60; Ray Lyman Wilbur, "Report of the Council on Medical Education and Hospitals," *Proc. ann. Cong. med. Educ.* (1936), pp. 1–2.
43. "Advisory Board for Medical Specialties," *J. Amer. med. Ass., 115* (1940), 750.

peared in the mid-1930s to be the coming social changes: collectivism, cooperative enterprise, and increasing governmental control.[44] While this proposal came to nothing, a modified version in 1938 providing for a coordinating body for medical education, licensure, and hospitals was productive. It was envisaged that the new organization would study the major educational needs of American medicine, formulate standards, and advise the regulatory bodies and government agencies; primarily, it would provide a clearing house of information for the profession, the universities, the hospitals, licensing bodies, and for the future the health programs of the entire country. Given such a coordinated council of the various organizations concerned with education, the medical profession would have a great opportunity for leadership in public policy. Dr. Rappleye, moreover, was in a strong position for suggesting such an organization. He was concurrently president of the AAMC (1938–39), president of the Advisory Board for Medical Specialties (1937–44), and president of the Commission on Graduate Medical Education. He also had the support of other educators.

AMA representatives could not, however, be expected to see the new organization in the same light. Dr. Morris Fishbein, at the Annual Conference on Medical Education in February 1938, attacked the "rumors as to new types of bodies and super-bodies" by identifying the proposed national council with undesirable federal governmental influence.[45] And with the strong opposition from Fishbein it was unlikely that the national council could in fact assume any dominant position. Perhaps to avoid allegations of such control, and after Dr. Rappleye had canvassed the professional, educational, and hospital organizations, the new body was named the Advisory Council on Medical Education, Licensure, and Hospitals. It was now stressed that the council would be purely advisory and would function without any governmental association or support. On this basis the joint council was established. Dr. Rappleye became the president, and Dr. Robin Buerki secretary-treasurer. It was announced that the council would set up committees to study the internship, specialist training, and other aspects of medical education and licensure.

Ray Lyman Wilbur and his colleagues on the Council on Medical Education and Hospitals had the difficult political decision of accepting or rejecting membership in Dr. Rappleye's council in the light of Dr.

44. Willard C. Rappleye, "The Larger Social Aspects of Medical Education," *Proc. ann. Cong. med. Educ.* (1935), p. 17.
45. Discussion, *Proc. ann. Cong. med. Educ.* (1938), pp. 37–38; and see "Council on Medical Education, Licensure and Hospitals," *Ann. Surg., 108* (1938), 489–97.

Fishbein's opposition. They carefully referred the decision to the AMA House of Delegates, with a recommendation that membership be approved.[46] But meanwhile the AMA Board of Trustees authorized an adverse editorial on the Advisory Council in the AMA *Journal* (of which Dr. Fishbein was editor) and attempted to strengthen its own position by meeting with the hospital associations.[47] The AMA was in effect consolidating its opposition to an organization that might threaten its own authority, and the suggestion of AMA membership on the new Advisory Council was disapproved.[48] Without AMA participation, the Advisory Council on Medical Education was doomed from the start to add to the confusion caused by overlapping educational agencies rather than to provide a long-term focus for the problems of graduate education; for without AMA support the Advisory Council had no power. It was finally dissolved in 1944. There was still no central, responsible organization for all aspects of graduate training.

Dr. Rappleye's council was, however, important in stimulating other types of liaison among medical organizations, a process accelerated by the shadow of war. The AMA Council on Medical Education established cordial relations with the American Hospital Association in 1939 and held discussions with the American Colleges of Physicians and Surgeons. The council had ceased meeting with the AAMC in 1923; better relations now began, and a liaison committee of the two organizations was formed in 1942. This liaison, however, concentrated on the undergraduate and internship phases of education.[49] It was not intended to consider the broader aspects of licensure, hospital relationships, specialty boards,

46. "Report of the Council on Medical Education and Hospitals," *J. Amer. med. Ass., 112* (1939), 1385.
47. "Abstract of Minutes of Board of Trustees," *J. Amer. med. Ass., 112* (1939), 1167; editorial, *J. Amer. med. Ass., 112* (1939), 734.
48. "Report of the Reference Committee on Medical Education," *J. Amer. med. Ass., 112* (1939), 2170; AMA, *Digest,* pp. 463, 678.
49. In 1943 a joint committee of the AAMC, the AMA Council on Medical Education, and the AHA was set up to study intern problems in the emergency. In 1945 the AAMC suggested a new plan for a uniform date for the appointment of interns; this was adopted by the AAMC in 1947, endorsed by the CME and by the hospital associations, and put into effect in 1949. Thus was born the National Intern Matching Program. Finally, in 1954, a joint internship review committee was established, to review the reports of the CME inspectors on individual programs and to suggest to the CME any action that should be taken on programs and any changes in policies or requirements. The Internship Review Committee includes representatives of the CME, AAMC, AHA, Federation of State Medical Boards of the United States, and the American Academy of General Practice. Weiskotten and Johnson, *History,* pp. 16, 23; *Trans. Amer. Hosp. Ass., 45* (1943), 10; "Announcement," *J. Ass. Amer. med. Coll., 23* (1948), 267–69.

university responsibility for specialist education, and other aspects of
health services which had been proposed for the Advisory Council on
Medical Education. Yet the need to formalize the residency training and
to relate the internship and residency as one interlocking graduate program was self-evident. By the early 1940s the intern was being regarded
by hospitals more as a "quasi hospital servant" than as a graduate student; the resident was often an unwelcome intruder. Medical schools
had some influence over hospital residencies; hospitals had some interest in organized educational programs. But their efforts and interests
were not coordinated. Nor were the medical specialist groups effectively
interlocked. The specialty boards were still relatively new organizations,
groping for their appropriate function. Young men were reportedly at
sea as to what the requirements of those boards might be.[50] There was
a remarkable amount of confusion. The Advisory Board for Medical
Specialties provided a forum for discussion of common standards and
ideals of board certification, such as whether an individual should be
allowed to hold certification from more than one board, whether society
membership should be expected, and whether the requirements of particular boards were unduly stringent. In this respect the boards did see
themselves as a "system."

Yet the important connections were not made. If the boards were a
system, rather than individual and separate expressions of isolated scientific groups, they would invariably be pushed to define their collective
impact on medical care. What were specialty boards actually for? Would
all specialists be certified in a matter of time? If they were, was it not
appropriate for general practitioners also to have graduate recognition?
How was a broad generalist outlook to be maintained in an increasingly
specialist environment? Could the general practioner survive? In what
specific ways was medical education and training related to quality of
medical care? And what kind of organization should supervise graduate
education and training? The problems were no longer merely of what
kind of specialist regulation was most apt, but also of manpower distributions, of the organization of medical care ideally to be encouraged,
and of assigning relative responsibility for education and training. Specialty certification was a reality before the purpose of such clarification
was fully ascertained. There had, moreover, been a shift of emphasis
during the 1930s as to the function of specialist regulation. The earlier
restrictionist, quasi-licensure approach—applicable to a situation of a
minority of specialists and a majority of general practitioners—had begun

50. Burt R. Shurly, "Discussion," *Proc. ann. Cong. med. Educ.* (1937), p. 26.

to give way to concern as to the boards' monopoly functions, applicable to a situation in which the predominant pattern of professionalism was an increasing desire to specialize.

The appearance of the first edition of the *Directory of Medical Specialists* in 1940 was the culmination of a long phase of specialist development. There now was a readily identifiable technological elite; the medical profession could be divided into those who were certified specialists and those who were not. Hospitals were already using board certification as a qualification for hospital staff membership; and it was reasonable to suppose that the boards would on the outbreak of war be used to classify physicians in the armed services. But the process was not complete. The specialty boards could not presume to claim the sole privilege of identifying who was and who was not a specialist as a formal licensure system would indeed have done.

A professional coordinating agent, such as Dr. Rappleye's joint Advisory Council, might have been able to come to grips with the compelling problems involved in increasing medical specialism, but with the opposition of the AMA the council quietly failed. University responsibility for specialist training had been advocated again and again from the early part of the century, but the universities had done little. Nor had the Advisory Board for Medical Specialties or the Council on Medical Education welded the specialty boards into an effective force.

An idiosyncratic professional system had emerged out of the melting pot of the 1920s and 1930s. Undergraduate medical education was the responsibility of university medical schools. There followed for virtually all physicians a year of internship in a hospital accredited for this purpose by the AMA Council on Medical Education. At this point the student sat for the state licensing examination. He might then go into private practice or continue his training in a hospital. If he wished to specialize, he was well advised to read the specifications for training set out by the appropriate specialty certifying board and to proceed to a residency in a hospital approved by that board; however there was nothing to prevent any physician from calling himself a specialist. The specialty boards themselves were professional clubs rather than objective appraisers of the competence needed for giving the public adequate medical care.

The general organizational confusion in medicine was provoking criticism even before World War II. With the outbreak of war, and the subsequent acceleration of specialization, problems of both medical education and service became acute.

CHAPTER 13

Medical Care in the 1940s

The specialty boards had developed as professional responses to a scientific movement. This same movement, in changing the very content and value of medicine, was simultaneously stimulating public interest in developing a more appropriate economic and administrative structure in which to provide modern medical care. The internal professional issues and the external social issues arising out of increasing medical specialization thus developed side by side and placed a double stress on the medical organizations. The general practitioner, in particular, found himself embattled against both professional and social movements: against the expanding cadre of medical specialists on the one hand, and against governmental inroads into practice on the other.

A more Machiavellian profession might have seized the opportunities inherent in the disruptions of World War II to rebuild general practice, to redefine generalist-specialist relations, to examine the emerging role of the hospital: in short, to dominate evolving practice patterns from the position of strength which would naturally flow to organized medicine in any national health service system. But medical advance had outstripped the mental agility of the profession. Those physicians in their late fifties or older at the time of serious proposals for a national health service between 1939 and 1950 had entered medical school before the Flexner report. In the intervening years they had made enormous readjustments to the developing content of medicine; in their own careers they had seen the development and expansion of auxiliary professions, the enlargement and changing function of the hospital, and the development of the specialty boards. They remembered all too clearly the issues of group practice as defined in the 1920s, their own personal privations of the 1930s, the suppression of the suggestions of the Committee on the Costs of Medical Care, and the exclusion of health insurance from the Social Security Act of 1935. The projected image of medical practice was still that of the trusted bedside physician, as so nobly portrayed in the famous portrait by Sir Luke Fildes (used effectively by organized medicine in the anti-health-insurance campaigns of the late 1940s), and the older physicians at least continued to interpret their functions in terms which were fast becoming obsolete.

SOCIAL PROVISIONS FOR THE NATION'S HEALTH

At the time of American entry into World War II, the future structure of public medical care was in limbo. The Depression had, of dire necessity, legitimized a federal role in providing medical relief, that is in paying for medical care for those who were destitute as part of their assistance benefits. The massive Federal Emergency Relief program did not survive the worst years of the Depression. But the states' public assistance programs, stimulated by federal grants under the 1935 Social Security Act, provided a growing base for the development of health care for the indigent. During World War II, the governmental role also increased with respect to various population groups. By 1944 the War Food Administration was responsible for health centers or clinics in about 250 areas where agricultural labor was concentrated.[1] And between 1943 and 1949 the Children's Bureau organized a comprehensive program of emergency maternity and infant care for the dependents of servicemen (EMIC). Meanwhile 12 million servicemen were offered complete medical care in the expanding system of hospitals and health centers organized by the armed services; after the war, they became eligible for a greatly increased program of health benefits under the Veterans Administration. The farm and EMIC programs ceased during the 1940s, but the case for expanding health services to the indigent remained part of the AMA's legislative policy. The battleground in the 1940s, as in the 1930s (and as in the much earlier debates over "hospital abuse"), was not in denial of all or any governmental intervention into health services, but in limiting such intervention to those who were demonstrably and acutely in financial need. At issue was the provision of medical care for the middle class, who were still receiving their medical services through the traditional private

1. The Farm Security Administration had begun to establish medical care program in 1936 as part of a program of income security for farm workers; the service was extended to meet the needs of migrant workers. By 1944, when the program was transferred to the temporary War Food Administration, there were organizations for migratory farm workers in all states. The War Food Administration was dissolved in 1945, its work being incorporated into the Department of Agriculture. Franz Goldmann, "Medical Care for Farmers," *Medical Care, 3* (1943), 19–35; Stern, *Medical Services by Government,* pp. 156–58.

practice system, with direct fee-for-service payments between patient and physician.

A second legacy of the Depression years was the deteriorating financial situation of voluntary hospitals. Government subsidy of hospital construction had been part of the unsuccessful national health bill of 1939. It was a part, however, which appealed both to the struggling hospitals and to the medical profession, whose members depended on adequate hospital facilities for the successful and effective practice of medicine. President Roosevelt called for a program of federal hospital construction in rural areas in 1940, but subsequent legislation failed. The Hill-Burton Act was finally passed under President Truman in 1946, becoming the most important piece of health legislation in the postwar decade.[2] Meanwhile, the other elements of a national health program remained uncertain.

The concept of a national health insurance scheme which would cover the whole population, not merely the indigent, had little chance of being endorsed by the medical profession. Instead, the AMA relaxed its views on voluntary hospitalization insurance and encouraged the establishment of medical society prepayment plans for covering physician bills.[3] In so doing the association accepted the need for organized prepayment or insurance plans for the financing of health services. But its acceptance was grudging and limited. Approval of hospital insurance schemes made a virtue of necessity. The hospitals needed the guaranteed income such schemes could provide; it was no accident that the nonprofit Blue Cross schemes, which developed rapidly in the 1940s, were created by the hos-

2. "A Recommendation for the Construction by the Federal Government of Small Hospitals in Needy Areas of the Country Presently without Such Facilities," 30 Jan. 1940, *The Public Papers and Addresses of Franklin D. Roosevelt, 1940* (New York, 1941), p. 65. A hospital construction bill, based on this message, was introduced by Senators Wagner and George, and in the Senate it received bipartisan support. It was, however, defeated in the House. Altmeyer, p. 146. For the AMA's views see Nathan B. Van Etten, "An American Health Program," *Proc. ann. Cong. med. Educ.* (1940), pp. 65–67; AMA, *Digest,* p. 370. Sen. Lister Hill and Harold H. Burton introduced their bill in January 1945 calling for federal grants to the states and to local nonprofit agencies for hospital construction; in November President Truman also called for a hospital grant program. The Hill-Burton Act, endorsed inter alia by the AMA's Council on Medical Education (whose full title was still the Council on Medical Education and Hospitals) and the American Hospital Association, authorized one-third matching grants to states and nonprofit groups for hospital construction and funds for surveys of state hospital needs. *Congress and the Nation, 1945–1964,* pp. 1130–31.
3. The role of the AMA in the endorsement and sponsorship of voluntary health insurance is documented in detail in a number of sources. See especially Burrow, pp. 201–04, 288; "The American Medical Association: Power, Purpose, and Politics in Organized Medicine," *Yale Law Journal, 63* (1954), 1007 et seq.; Elton Rayack, "The American Medical Association and the Development of Voluntary Insurance," *Social and Economic Administration, 1* (Apr. 1967), 3–25; *1* (July 1967), 29–55.

pital associations. Both hospital insurance and Hill-Burton were necessary if voluntary hospitals were to survive. Survival was also, at least in part, at issue in the concurrent development of Blue Shield prepayment plans for medical bills, under medical society sponsorship. The first full-fledged example of the latter was the California Physicians Service, which was started in 1939; by the end of 1946, this plan had over 419,000 subscribers. The later Michigan plan already had over 840,000 and Massachusetts over 460,000.[4] In parallel, insurance company plans for medical care were also expanding, and other types of independent organizational plans—consumer prepayment groups, employer-union organizations, or private group clinics—were developing.

In endorsing hospital insurance and in actively developing medical service plans, the medical profession committed itself to private health insurance as the means for spreading the financial risks of sickness for the majority of the population. To Blue Cross, Blue Shield, and to insurance companies' health plans were attached the label of "voluntary" health insurance, as opposed to the continuing proposals for compulsory health insurance advocated by those who sought automatic coverage of the population for medical care under a publicly organized system. Voluntary health insurance joined private fee-for-service practice as a desirable and defendable feature of the evolving health system as seen from the medical profession's point of view. One concept reinforced the other. At issue was not merely whether an insurance system should be ventured into at individual volition (voluntary insurance) or through the force of legislation (compulsory insurance), but how far medical payment schemes would, and should, become an organized force in shaping the development of medical care. Welfare medical programs were grafted onto preexisting professional modes of practice, and accepted them. Private health insurance, purchased from a variety of sources to meet a variety of hospital and medical benefits, also enabled money to be injected into the health network without a deliberate effort to control its standards or change its structure. In contrast, organizational change would almost inevitably follow the introduction of national health insurance or any other form of national health service system since the responsibility for providing adequate service and the power to provide service through appropriate financing would be concentrated in one national agency. There was thus a potent factor of control. At issue was not merely a social philosophy of private enterprise versus government responsibility but also the continuing professional independence of the

4. J. F. Follmann, Jr., *Medical Care and Health Insurance* (Homewood, Ill., 1963) pp. 107–11; Burrow, p. 289.

physician in a scientific environment which was demanding increasing institutionalism, group payments, and the provision of service through specialists and teams. The terms voluntary and compulsory polarized the fears of physicians as to how long they themselves could survive as independent entrepreneurs. Private health insurance shored up the physicians' independence, as it shored up the independence of the voluntary hospitals.

At this crucial time, the movement toward voluntary hospital insurance was stimulated, by one of the vagaries of history, through the wage stabilization policies which were put into effect during World War II. Before the war there had been both labor and employer interest in health services, but benefits rarely appeared as part of the process of collective bargaining. During and immediately after the war wage increases were restricted, but as a result, fringe benefits acquired a new importance. After a series of administrative rulings and court decisions, pensions and insurance were placed within the scope of collective bargaining. By the end of 1949, voluntary health insurance through collective bargaining was surging through the vast steel and automobile industries; already 3 million workers were covered, and the tide was barely under way.[5] This impressive movement provided a major stimulus to the growth of private health insurance after World War II. In 1940 only 9 percent of the civilian population was covered for some kind of hospital benefits, 4 percent for surgical benefits and 2 percent for in-hospital medical benefits. Comparable estimates for 1950 were 51 percent, 36 percent, and 14 percent; and for 1966, 81 percent, 74 percent, and 60 percent.[6] The health insurance industry (including the nonprofit Blue Cross and Blue Shield plans) could congratulate itself on one of the most spectacular selling achievements of modern times. But while these figures were sufficiently dramatic to sustain the concept of voluntary health insurance as a valid approach to the problems of financing medical care, they by no means provided the whole answer. Health insurance, as it evolved, only paid part of the medical

5. The crucial moment for acceptance of fringe benefits was the Inland Steel case, 1948, which found that welfare bargaining was covered in the phrase "other conditions of employment" on which management had to negotiate. The unions had already negotiated health and welfare plans but it was only after 1948 that the massive rise of voluntary health insurance began. The settlement of a major steel strike in 1949 further clarified the issue. Within three months of the settlement there were 236 contracts in the steel industry providing for group insurance and pensions, and by the summer of 1950 all major auto companies had negotiated health insurance plans. Raymond Munts, *Bargaining for Health: Labor Unions, Health Insurance, and Medical Care* (Madison, 1967), pp. 9–11, 250, 262.
6. Louis S. Reed, "Private Health Insurance: Coverage and Financial Experience, 1940–1966," *Social Security Bull., 38* (Nov. 1967), 12–13.

bills and was directed primarily toward hospital and surgical care, was applicable only when the person was sick (it was not a mechanism to keep him well), and was dependent on existing facilities and services. Even today private health insurance covers less than one-fourth of expenditures for personal medical care.[7] Moreover, as a predominantly middle-class phenomenon, voluntary health insurance did not meet the expenses of those in direst medical need.

NATIONAL HEALTH INSURANCE

Nonetheless organized medicine was able to use the enormous growth of voluntary health insurance as an effective argument for opposing the introduction of a national health insurance program which would cover the whole population, a program proposed repeatedly through the 1940s. Bill after bill died in Congress on the subject of government subsidy, provision, or organization of a socially inclusive national prepayment plan, which would bring the middle class and the poor under one risk-sharing umbrella and which would inter alia influence the organizational development of the health care system. The 1939 Wagner bill had been based on a state-regulated medical system. The first Wagner-Murray-Dingell bill (1943) advocated a national (i.e. federal) compulsory system of health insurance, financed from payroll taxes and providing comprehensive health and medical benefits through entitlement to specified medical service (service benefits) rather than through money payments (cash indemnity). The plan would have had to comply with listed provisions in the legislation and be approved by a national insurance board. The Eliot and Green bills (1942–45) proposed federally operated insurance programs under the Social Security Act. Other suggestions were limited to specific population groups, such as the Lodge proposal for medical care for the unemployed (1939–40), or the Capper bills (1939–41), which suggested a state-operated compulsory plan for low-income workers. No health insurance provisions came near enactment.[8]

President Roosevelt spoke in his State of the Union message January 1945 of the right to good medical care, but he pressed for no specific recommendations. To the surprise of many, President Truman took a

7. Dorothy Rice and Barbara Cooper, "National Health Expenditures, 1929–1970," ibid., *34* (Jan. 1971), 13.
8. Indeed, it was not until 1946 that hearings were held. U.S., Congress, Senate, Committee on Education and Labor, *National Health Program: Hearing on S. 1606,* 79th Cong., pts. 1–5. The only earlier hearings were in 1939. Details of legislation proposed in this period are usefully summarized in Brewster, *Health Insurance.*

strong position in advocating national health insurance. In November 1945, against a background of rising AMA opposition, he sent a message on health legislation to Congress which outlined a comprehensive prepaid medical insurance plan for all age groups, to be financed through a 4 percent raise in the Social Security tax; needy persons not covered by Social Security could be covered by payments from general federal revenues.[9] The resulting bill, the national health bill of 1945, would have produced a compulsory comprehensive national health insurance system. Labeled by the AMA as "regimentation" and "totalitarianism" [10] and by Sen. Robert A. Taft of Ohio (and others) as "the most socialistic measure that this Congress has ever had before it," [11] the bill had little chance of passage. Individual, fee-for-service private practice had taken to itself the label of free enterprise. Truman's insistence that "socialized medicine means that all doctors work as employees of the government," [12] which would not at all be the case in an insurance scheme which merely reimbursed physicians for services rendered to those insured, fell on deaf ears. Republicans had control of both chambers of Congress. The AMA, in turn, sponsored Senator Taft's alternative proposals of federal grants to states for aiding only the medically needy.[13]

When the Eighty-first Congress convened in 1949, with the president reelected and Democratic majorities in both Senate and Congress, there was renewed hope by its advocates that compulsory national health insurance would finally be enacted. Truman called for health insurance in his State of the Union message in January 1949. He did so again in a special health message in April, and on other occasions.[14] But hearings on the legislation were marked by bitter debate, wide-scale publicity, and renewed allegations by the AMA of socialized medicine; there was

9. "Special Message to Congress Recommending a Comprehensive Health Program," 19 Nov. 1945, *Public Papers of the President of the United States: Harry S. Truman* (Washington, D.C., 1961), p. 475.
10. Editorial, *J. Amer. med. Ass., 128* (1945), 883.
11. Quoted in *Congress and the Nation, 1945–1964,* p. 1152.
12. Ibid.; see also Burrow, pp. 329–35.
13. The Taft bill, S. 2143, would have authorized grants to states to pay for medical care for those unable to afford it, i.e. the indigent. There was also a provision that states could pay part of the private health insurance premiums for those above the poverty level. The focus of the bill was thus two-pronged: it favored government financing of medical care for the needy, as a natural extension of the states' public assistance programs, but at the same time encouraged the nonindigent to use private health insurance—both of which were aims shared by the AMA.
14. "Annual Message to the Congress on the State of the Union," 5 Jan. 1949; "Special Message to the Congress on the Nation's Health Needs," 22 Apr. 1949; "Remarks and Address in St. Paul as Part of Minnesota's Truman Day Celebration," 3 Nov. 1949; *Public Papers of the President of the United States: Harry S. Truman 1949* (Washington, D.C., 1964), pp. 1, 226, 547.

also opposition from the drug and insurance industries. Truman repeated his request the following year,[15] but again no action was taken. The movement for a national health program through a compulsory insurance system was moribund. In 1951, on the advice of Oscar Ewing, then federal security administrator, President Truman's administration withdrew from its position. Instead of pressing for national health insurance for the whole population, it decided now to favor more limited goals, with respect both to the population to be covered and to which services would be provided.[16] Between 1951 and 1965 (when the present Medicare program was passed) health insurance proposals initiated by both Republicans and Democrats focused on health programs only for the aged; and even for this group comprehensive care—general practitioner care, specialist services, home care, and hospitalization—was replaced by the relatively modest provision for hospital benefits.

Instead, then, of World War II providing the opportunity for a structural realignment of health services, and for constructive debates within the medical profession, it had the reverse effect. Public medical programs were introduced in the exigencies of war and in the immediate postwar years, but they approached health services piecemeal. There was the Children's Bureau's program of maternity and infant care for the dependents of servicemen, and the farm workers' program. The Lanham Act of 1941 authorized a special grant program for rapid treatment centers for venereal disease. Vocational rehabilitation programs were set up for servicemen and for civilians, and a federal government nurse-training program was authorized. The Hill-Burton Act enabled federal

15. See, for instance, U.S., Congress, Senate, Committee on Labor and Public Welfare, *National Health Program: Hearings on S. 1106, S. 1456, S. 1581, and S. 1679,* 81st Cong., 1st sess., 1949, pts. 1–2; "Annual Budget Message to the Congress: Fiscal Year 1951," 9 Jan. 1950, *Public Papers of the President of the United States: Harry S. Truman 1950* (Washington, D.C., 1965), p. 44.

16. The Social Security amendments of 1950, P.L. 81–734, had meanwhile boosted programs of medical care for the indigent (in four categories of assistance programs) by allowing federal matching grants to states for payments made by the state to hospitals, doctors, and other providers of medical care to public assistance recipients. Previously, federal grants had been given with respect only to payments made directly to welfare recipients. The new "vendor payments" to medical personnel and facilities encouraged states to provide expanded medical care. Vendor medical payments for public assistance (federal, state, and local) rose from $51 million in 1949–50, to $212 million in 1954–55, to $493 million in 1959–60, and an estimated $1620 million in 1965–66. They also shored up the idea of expanded federal subsidy of health services to the indigent as an alternative to governmental health insurance. For a valuable account of the administration's change of policy in 1951, see R. Harris, *A Sacred Trust,* chap. 10. See also Altmeyer, p. 279 and passim; Ida C. Merriam, "Social Welfare Expenditures 1965–66," *Social Security Bull., 29* (Dec. 1966), table 1.

subsidies to be made for hospital construction through recognized state agencies. It offered a potential base—but only in some dim and distant future—for a well-organized national hospital system. On another front, federal funding began to pour into biomedical research, as one after another the present National Institutes of Health appeared.[17] But taken together these did not make a health service. Indeed the social and professional responses to changes during and after World War II were similar to those of World War I. Again, there was detailed discussion of health insurance—only this time under federal rather than state jurisdiction. Again, there were expectations that the experience by numerous physicians of the highly organized medical services in the military would have an impact on the structure of civilian medical services after the war. Again, the end of the war was followed by a period of prevailing conservatism, marked by increasing opposition by organized medicine to government intervention into medicine, whether through stimulating new forms of medical practice, through health insurance, or through educational and training programs.

Yet the implications of specialized medicine were more urgent in the 1940s than they had been in 1918. Social Security programs had become part of the American way of life. So had public education. The lack of socially guaranteed programs for health services was a prominent gap both in the individual's financial protection and in his potential qualitative development. As many as 40 percent of the 22 million men of draft age in the mid-1940s could not meet the medical requirements of general military service.[18] The technological advances of scientific medicine were not being transmitted to the general population. Medical services continued to be maldistributed both in terms of income (the richer members of society receiving more service; the poorer, less) and of geography (some areas being far better served than others with hospitals, doctors and other personnel). With greater specialization of facilities and personnel, such inequities were becoming more acute. The affluent family in a large city had available to it an array of specialists and superspecialists with appropriate support facilities in the specialized departments of a large hospital. Small towns and villages could not support the services of specialists, even if they could lure specialists away from the intellectual

17. The National Institute of Health, originally founded in 1887 to undertake bacteriological studies for the U.S. Public Health Service, continued research by its own personnel in its facilities until 1937. In that year, Congress set up the National Cancer Institute, with power both to do intramural research and to make grants to outside institutions and individuals. The other specialized institutes followed after World War II, each with its own grants program.
18. See Burrow, p. 298 and passim.

attraction of the major urban centers. As a result, the difference between urban and rural health services, which had been a source of anxiety as early as the 1920s, became even more marked.[19]

The Hill-Burton Act was an attempt to rectify the balance by subsidizing the building of hospitals in rural areas. But buildings were only part of the problem. The greater the degree of specialization, the larger the group of people required to guarantee the full spectrum of services to be made available to offer optimal medical care in case of need. In medicine alone, the number of full-time specialists increased from under 37,000 in 1940 to over 62,000 in 1949; concurrently the number of general practitioners declined.[20] To spread the services of this new-style medical profession over the population was not merely a matter of scattering them evenly over a population map, but of ensuring appropriate clusters of specialist services which would provide medical care for the population of an area or region. Specialization in the medical profession (and concurrently in the continuing development of health professions) thus had implications in relation not only to increasing the value and the costs of services but also to distributing the appropriate professionals and facilities on a regional or areawide basis so that services were in fact available to those in need.

The proposals for a national health system in the 1940s included these structural as well as financial elements. President Truman put stress in his special congressional messages on the right of the individual to adequate protection from the economic fears of sickness. But in the programs he endorsed, compulsory health insurance for medical bills and protection against wage loss during sickness were only two items of a more general program which was designed also to encourage the expansion of medical education; to establish community health centers, diagnostic clinics, and specialist group practices; to improve disease prevention and control programs; and to further continued improvements in biomedical research. Strong opposition by the AMA to the financial elements of the program, and to any element (including loans to establish group practices) which threatened the status quo of practice, killed the

19. A comprehensive statistical and narrative review of the status of health and of health facilities and personnel in the late 1940s and early 1950s is given in *Building America's Health*. A Report to the President by the President's Commission on the Health Needs of the Nation, volumes I–V (Washington, D.C., 1952, 1953). This Commission, appointed by President Truman in December 1951, stated that access to health care was a basic human right and came out in favor of a federal-state health insurance system, group practice, and regional organization of health services. But the recommendations came only a few weeks before Mr. Truman left office. They were not picked up by the Eisenhower administration.
20. See table 2, p. 181.

development of a comprehensive design toward health services. Biomedical research programs were encouraged—indeed, the federally financed research effort after World War II was to result in a massive fiscal program which has to this day affected the development and structure of the nation's medical schools—while the means to transfer the knowledge so gained to the general population was largely ignored.

The combined impact of voluntary health insurance, public medical assistance, and, later, Medicare reinforced existing patterns of medical organization and medical care. The legislation that was passed stifled rather than innovated. That which failed took with it the potential of recognition, through the organization of health services or through prepayment plans, of the comparative functions and competencies of physicians. In the United States decisions on these matters continued to be left to the medical profession. In other advanced countries, in contrast, plans were being developed which linked the producing and functioning of health professionals to estimates of national and regional manpower needs.

Instead, then, of a national policy for medical manpower which would have been reflected in the structure of the profession and the development of specialist training programs for an organized health service, recognition of different specialists and functions continued to be a private, professional responsibility. Yet the interactions between the public and the private sectors of medicine were too important to be ignored. The political power of organized medicine, so effectively exercised against national health insurance in the 1940s, brought the medical profession firmly into the public domain; the doctors were now fair game for public criticism. But, quite apart from this overt political activity, the structures of the profession were being adopted into those public medical programs which did exist in the 1940s. Specialty certification, developed as a private intraprofessional process in the 1930s, became locked into the regulations of official services—of the military and of some civilian health programs. From all points of view the vast and rapid changes in medicine were breaking down distinctions between "professional" and "public" responsibilities.

RECOGNITION OF SPECIALISTS BY THE MILITARY

In World War I there had been relatively little official classification of medical officers into position categories corresponding with an assessed degree of proficiency. The armed forces of World War II, however, were served by a highly sophisticated specialist medical service, and appropriate assignments by types of skill were of importance. Although the Army Medical Department had reportedly made repeated attempts to introduce an effective, detailed classification system, no such system had been introduced by the time the Mobilization Regulations were issued in September 1939. These regulations required medical assignments to be designated beforehand and to be based on both individual qualifications and the requirements of the situation.[21] Action was thus required on a large scale to set up a system of slots and definitions not only for physicians already in the army but for all physicians in the country who might be called into service. The Department of War ordered a classification scheme for the Army Medical Reserve in 1940. Each individual was given a symbol which marked both his general level of skill (e.g. general surgeon, orthopedic surgeon) and his performance in that level (superior, excellent, satisfactory, unsatisfactory) as rated by his commanding officer. But this system, which was outside the specialty boards, was barely started when mobilization began.

Meanwhile the AMA, at the request of the surgeon general of the army, appointed its own Committee on Medical Preparedness in 1940.[22] The AMA Bureau of Economics, in behalf of the new committee, mailed questionnaires to the physicians listed in the AMA directory, including questions on professional qualifications. By June 1942, the AMA held records and punchcards on more than 181,500 physicians. The Committee on Medical Preparedness successfully canvassed for the establishment of an official procurement and assignment agency for recruiting and distributing physicians for the army, navy, U.S. Public Health Service, and other services. The committee thereafter worked closely with the new agency, with specific subcommittees, and with the joint use of AMA records. In addition, early in 1942 the staff of the *Directory of Medical Specialists,* the publication of the Advisory Board for Medical Specialties, established for the Department of War a secret "control file" of about 10,000 names of applicants for certification as a means of identifying specialists who were not yet certified, so they could be either disqualified or given better ranking assignments. Names on the file, of which the surgeon general had a copy, were marked "cleared" (board eligible, in respect to training and other qualifications) or "not cleared" (not yet accepted for examination, failure to pass examination requiring complete reapplication, and certificate revoked). By this method the spe-

21. U.S. Army Medical Service, *Personnel in World War II* (Washington, D.C., 1963), pp. 267–70. And see Fred W. Rankin, "The Responsibility of Medicine in Wartime," *J. Amer. med. Ass., 119* (1942), 539.
22. "Report of the Committee on Medical Preparedness," *J. Amer. med. Ass., 119* (1942), 653 and passim, from which material in this section is largely drawn.

cialty boards were able to give the surgeon general of the army information on 28,000 specialists (18,000 in the Advisory Board's Directory and
10,000 in the central file). In some cases the specialty boards submitted
suggested proficiency grades, together with other information which
enabled the army to classify its specialists. Through the use of such information, efforts were made to promote board diplomates from the
grade of lieutenant within six months, The surgeon general could also
make direct requests to the boards for additional information about particular physicians. Possession of a board diploma thus had immediate
advantages. The specialty boards joined the AMA—opponent of socialized medicine—to become, in the exigencies of war, agents of the federal
government.

The general practitioner, with no board or qualifying society, together
with the self-styled specialist who could not give evidence of his skills
through the listed criteria, was generally made a first lieutenant; the
certified specialist might find himself a captain.[23] There was clearly in
these rankings an incentive to specialize and to take specialty board
examinations, or at least to fulfill the eligibility requirements for the board
examination. There was also an incentive for groups of specialists which
did not yet have boards—for example, specialists in physical medicine
or aviation medicine—to press for them after the war. The surgeon general of the army asserted constantly that the lack of a board diploma
would not in itself place an individual in a lower category if he had
demonstrated a high professional capacity in other ways; but there were
undoubtedly cases in which it did. If for no other reason, specialty board
diplomates fared better than others simply because they were easier to
identify. If the officer were board certified, it was taken for granted that
he was qualified in his field. If he were not certified, but was qualified, it
was much more difficult to evaluate him.[24]

23. The policy governing grades for those entering the Army Medical Corps was
officially announced in May 1942. As a basic appointment a physician might be
recommended as a first lieutenant; but those aged 37–45 might be classified as cap-
tains, by reason of previous commissions, or on account of their general unclassified
medical training and experience. Those below the age of 37 might, it was stated,
also qualify for the rank of captain if they held certification by an American specialty board (or equivalent formal training), fellowship in the American College of
Surgeons or American College of Physicians, membership in another national recognized quality society or association, or some other training recognized as appropriate to the recommended corps assignment. Those whose additional training and
experience justified initial assignment as chief of service or senior office in a large
military hospital might be appointed as majors. "Procurement and Assignment
Service for Physicians, Dentists and Veterinarians," *J. Amer. med. Ass., 119*
(1942), 33–34; editorial, ibid., pp. 30–31.
24. George F. Lull, Col., U.S. Army Medical Corps, "Medicine and the War," *J.*

During 1943 the Office of the Surgeon General renewed its efforts to develop uniform standards for each of four degrees of proficiency within each specialty; these included a place for the board diplomate, or the equivalent in medical training.[25] By mid-1945 the classification process in the Army Medical Corps was well organized and fairly standard throughout all units. The rating and classification of over 26,000 specialists had been undertaken, some half of all full-time specialists in the country. Less than 20 percent of the 26,000 had been rated in categories A or B.[26] The men responsible for advising on policy and doing the classifications were often the leaders of the peacetime specialties and members of the specialty boards—men such as Elliot C. Cutler, an examiner for the American Board of Surgery, who was chief consultant to the European Theater for Surgery of the U.S. forces, or Byrl R. Kirklin of the American Board of Radiology, who was consultant in radiology to the Office of the Surgeon General. The good relations established between the specialty groups and the Department of War were probably strengthened by the appointments of Fred W. Rankin of the American Board of Surgery and then a brigadier general as AMA president for 1942–43 and of James E. Paullin, a member of the Committee on Procurement and Assignment, for the following year. While the military classifications themselves were not transferred into civilian life, it might be expected that those who came out of the service after the war would have a healthy respect for the value of board certificates and other readily identifiable labels, and at the same time a healthy criticism of how these certificates were awarded.

CIVILIAN MEDICAL PROGRAMS

Despite the failure of a national health insurance system, public specification of physician standards was becoming a feature of a number of civilian as well as military programs. The Children's Bureau was labeling and identifying specialists in its expanding programs of medical care

---

Amer. med. Ass., 121 (1943), 639. The Department of War announced in May 1943 that the Office of the Air Surgeon had placed in accordance with their professional fields 98.8 percent of all Army Air Force medical officers who were qualified as specialists through a specialty board or college; and most of the remaining 1.2 percent were on administrative duty—as executive officers and commanding officers of hospitals—because of special talents in that direction. "Announcement," *J. Amer. med. Ass., 122* (1943), 447.
25. A fairly complete standard classification over all war zones and theaters was not, however, accomplished until June 1945. U.S. Army Medical Service, *Personnel in World War II,* pp. 277–78, 284.
26. Ibid., p. 417.

through federal grants to states for maternal and child care under the Social Security Act of 1935. It was stipulated under this act that all personnel under state plans which received federal support must be employed on a merit basis, and selection for most employees was based either on the state civil service systems or under a merit system plan established by state executive action.[27] This opened up for physicians the potential use of the standards of the specialty examining boards as qualifications in the choice of members of the state staff and of consultants to whom children would be sent for treatment; and, indeed, federal grants were used in this way to influence the personnel policy of the states—a matter of controversy among those who argued that the Constitution did not give the federal government such jurisdiction.[28] The Children's Bureau, however, interested in assuring minimum standards, continued to insist where possible on attaching qualification standards in its grant provisions.[29] There was an unresolved dilemma in how professional standards were to be assured to the public, and whether any such assurance could be achieved without resort to national norms.

Besides dealing with obstetricians and pediatricians, the Children's Bureau also dealt indirectly through the Crippled Children program with orthopedic and plastic surgeons and other specialists. This program (part of the various Social Security Acts) provided for medical, surgical, corrective, and other services for children suffering from poliomyelitis, rheumatic fever, and other crippling conditions; and again state plans had to be approved by the bureau. There was a potential under this program to use board certification as an eventual gauge for recognizing quality. Meanwhile, there was growing speculation in the profession as to whether

27. The U.S. Public Health Service attempted to make the same stipulation, but merit provisions in that case were not included in the legislation itself so the Public Health Service lacked power and generally approached the question of employee standards with greater timidity than did the Children's Bureau.
28. See Stern, *Medical Services by Government,* p. 126.
29. For example, Johns Hopkins Medical School was asked by the Maryland State Department of Health to provide a consultant and training service in obstetrics in the counties of Maryland, under its maternity and child health program. The plan for the work, to be done by two full-time members of the medical school faculty, was agreed upon by the university and the state, but then had to go for approval to the Children's Bureau. Here a clause was inserted that Johns Hopkins should agree that professional personnel engaged in the plan should be diplomates of the American Board of Obstetrics and Gynecology, or eligible for such certification. The university refused to sign on these terms, even though the staff members under consideration were board certified, on the grounds that the institution should have the right of free selection of its personnel; and eventually the plan was brought into effect without the university having to yield. Alan M. Chesney, "Some Impacts of the Specialty Board Movement on Medical Education," *J. Ass. Amer. med. Coll.,* 23 (1948), 86.

the boards measured quality at all, and if they did, whether they should
be given a monopoly.

The large emergency maternity and infant care program (EMIC)
which the Children's Bureau organized under existing legislative provisions in 1943 emphasized the dilemma of prescribing standards. EMIC, a
national program administered through the states, provided medical care
to the wives and infants of servicemen in the four low-pay grades of the
armed forces, and of aviation cadets. By 1945 the program was in force
in all states and territories, had cared for nearly 850,000 maternity cases
and 110,000 infants, and was estimated to have been used by 75–85 percent of wives qualified to receive it.[30] The Children's Bureau specified the
standards for physician services, for maternity care and for sick infants,
and for hospital care.[31] In so doing the bureau retained considerable
authority, in wartime circumstances and to fulfill wartime needs, in
specifying who would and who would not be recognized as a specialist.
As early as 1942 (before the first special appropriation for the EMIC
program) the Children's Bureau suggested to states that board-certified
or board-eligible obstetricians and pediatricians should be appointed as
consultants by the state health departments, and wherever possible should
be made available for consultation with general practitioners participating
in plans for maternity and child care for the wives and infants of servicemen.[32] The first policies issued by the bureau under EMIC itself included
a statement that board-certified specialists might receive approximately
one-fourth to one-third higher fees than general practitioners; and other
specialist services and schedules were also to be submitted to the Children's Bureau by the state health agency.[33] Those who were board cer-

30. Stern, *Medical Services by Government*, p. 129.
31. The Children's Bureau, supported by Congress and strongly opposed by the
AMA, provided service benefits to recipients of care, with direct payments to physicians, hospitals and nurses. Physicians had to agree not to accept payment from the
patient or the patient's family and were paid according to fixed amounts determined by the states but below a national maximum. The AMA wanted cash grants
to be made to recipients and the establishment of negotiations between individual
doctors and patients as to the fee to be charged, on the traditional sliding-scale
basis. The bureau held out against any imposition of a means test; the surgeons
general of the army and navy testified to the morale-building effect of the program
(the purpose for which it was established). The AMA continued to demand that
full control and regulation of the EMIC program should be placed in the hands of
state health departments, which the state medical societies could more easily control. Ibid., pp. 131–36; AMA, *Digest*, p. 93. And see "Report of the Special Committee on the EMIC Program," *J. Pediatrics, 25* (1944), 92–96.
32. Sinai and Anderson, pp. 57–58.
33. When the appropriation bill for 1944 was passed (in July 1943), the state
health departments were informed that the Children's Bureau was prohibited under
this appropriation from establishing standards which would discriminate between

tified undoubtedly tended to favor such policies. Those with less training might be recognized, but only as assistant consultants and without a differential rate of pay.[34]

These standards were, however, only applicable where states wished to identify specialists, and this raised the question of what the standards were for, and for whose benefit. States with few board-certified surgeons and large rural populations had obvious difficulties in defining the qualification for surgeons; in such cases, rather than pay more to those board certified, it was more important to motivate the general practitioner at least to consult with experts before himself performing a surgical operation. By no means all physicians were in favor of board certification, and there were many specialists with experience and training which did not exactly fit the eligibility requirements of the boards.[35] Sinai and Anderson, reviewing the program in 1948, noted that the imposition by state medical advisory committees of standards in obstetrics or pediatrics comparable to those of the specialty boards would have resulted in a "quick and adverse response from many members of the profession." [36] As a result, the states chose *not* to include differential fees for specialists (with the exception of Nebraska, where the few qualified specialists, concentrated in Omaha and Lincoln, were isolated from the mass of rural practitioners). EMIC, then, provided a clear case of the simplicity of prescribing board certification as a defining criterion and the reluctance of the profession to accept it as such.

Physical and occupational rehabilitation programs raised similar questions concerning the method of payment for specialist services. By 1943, all states except Louisiana were awarding medical benefits under workmen's compensation laws, and some states (Ohio, for example) employed medical staff for this purpose on a full-time or part-time or fee-for-service basis. In that year it was estimated that $140 million was being spent

---

persons licensed under state law to practice obstetrics (i.e. all licensed physicians). But the states could still establish differential rates of pay between GPs and specialists, and the Children's Bureau stated that if this were to be done, those designated specialists should have to show themselves to have superior training. It was suggested in the official policies that states should designate as specialists for this purpose only those certified by or qualified for a specialty board. Ibid., pp. xxxx, 62–65.
34. Ibid., pp. 71–72; p. xxxxi. The standard for an assistant consultant was one year of training in an AMA-approved residency and one year in practice.
35. By 1949 there were 2,595 board-certified obstetricians out of a total full-time pool of over 5,000; there were 2,923 certified pediatricians of 4,315 full-time specialists (see Appendix table A3). But there were also many more part-time practitioners in these particular fields who felt themselves to be, and in many cases probably were, competent to provide specialty care.
36. Sinai and Anderson, p. 132.

on medical benefits under workmen's compensation laws.[37] The long and heated debates over the commercialization of workmen's compensation and its abuse, and the insistence by the AMA during the 1930s that free choice of doctor be maintained, were still in progress.[38] But relatively few had unlimited free choice of physician, and in some states there were compensation panels of physicians, where specialists were only allowed to treat patients in their area of competence; physicians were selected for panels by the medical advisers of industrial commissioners or by the county medical societies on the basis of minimum requirements.[39] Workmen's compensation was therefore another public program in which specialists were widely used and in which, again, board certification might be used as a selecting agent.

Closely linked with workmen's compensation was provision for the vocational rehabilitation of workers. The federal government had been aiding state rehabilitation programs since 1920, but although all states were cooperating in the state-federal program in 1942, the emphasis until 1943 was on vocational education, not on medical care.[40] However, the impact of a long campaign waged by the National Rehabilitation Association and others and the focus on war production by civilians combined in the early 1940s to create a demand for a physical as well as an educational program of rehabilitation for injured workers. The movement reached its peak in a bill introduced by Senator LaFollette and Representative Barden in 1942, which would have provided a federal program of comprehensive rehabilitation for all the injured—not only in civilian life but also in the armed forces. But these radical proposals aroused opposition both from those who opposed a federal takeover of existing state programs and also from the powerful veterans groups, which were sponsoring a separate plan for the rehabilitation of veterans. In a decisive move, the veterans bill reached the floor, was passed, and was signed by the president in March 1943,[41] while the combination bill was standing. The two rehabilitation programs were thus to remain separate. The new

37. *Social Security Yearbook 1943*, cited by Bernhard J. Stern, *Medicine in Industry*, p. 175.
38. See Walter F. Dodd, *Administration of Workmen's Compensation* (New York, 1936); Somers and Somers, *Workmen's Compensation*, p. 175 and passim.
39. Even where there were panels, however, as in New York, physicians were found to be bill padding and accepting kickbacks, even though the latter was not only against the ethics of the AMA, the American College of Surgeons, and the American Board of Surgery but also against the rules of all approved hospitals. Stern, *Medicine in Industry*, pp. 178, 183.
40. C. Esco Oberman, *A History of Vocational Rehabilitation in America* (Minneapolis, 1965), pp. 273–74 and passim.
41. P.L. 78–16. There had been a vocational program for those injured in World War I, but this had lapsed in 1928. *Congress and the Nation, 1945–1964*, p. 1339.

law for civilians opened up the potential for federally subsidized state programs for physical restoration as a legal and integral part of the whole rehabilitation process,[42] and another public service area where specialist skills were in demand. Under the legislation the federal government was authorized to establish basic standards, administered through a new office of vocational rehabilitation.[43] Professional advisory committees were set up at federal and state levels, including medical and other specialists involved in the program, to fix rates of pay and to make general recommendations.

It was the reorganized and expanded Veterans Administration, established by an act of 1946, which provided the culmination of the public use of specialty board certificates.[44] The legislation provided that no one be rated a medical, surgical, or dental specialist unless he was certified by an American specialty board; and if no board existed the specialist would be examined by a board of qualified specialists from the Department of Medicine and Surgery. Those rated specialists were to receive a 25 percent addition to their basic rate of pay, up to a specified ceiling.[45] This was a direct incentive to attract young board-certified specialists into the VA system and to encourage those in the system to take the examinations. Here, if nowhere else, the boards had finally established themselves as independent monopolies within the medical monopoly.

IMPACTS: PROFESSIONALISM AND PUBLIC PROGRAMS

The increasing complexity of emerging public programs and the extended influence of the specialty boards were not coincidental. Both sprang from

42. In 1942, however, four states (Connecticut, Michigan, New York, Wisconsin) had been allowed under existing legislation to undertake limited physical rehabilitation programs. Oberman, p. 289.
43. Originally in the Federal Security Agency; now the Vocational Rehabilitation Administration in the Department of Health, Education, and Welfare.
44. Paul R. Hawley, who was chief surgeon of the European Theater in World War II, was appointed chief medical director of a new department of medicine and surgery in the Veterans Administration, with its own system of operations and pay. Hawley immediately began to build up the VA hospital system by coördinating the hospitals with medical schools and by removing physicians from civil service restrictions.
45. The only stated exception to this rule was for cases where there was a shortage of board-certified or equivalent personnel. P.L. 79–293, sec. 8 (b). The 25 percent increment for certification was to continue until 1958, when it was reduced to 15 percent (with a raised ceiling of $17,200). In 1962 the wheel turned full circle by attaching physicians to the Civil Service General Schedule. The automatic percentage was then dropped, and a system of grading was adopted, placing physicians in five progressive ranks with applicable pay increments within each rank; but credit continues to be given for board certification. P.L. 85–462; sec. 4108 of title 38, U.S. Code; P.L. 87–793.

radical changes in medicine which demanded specialization of personnel, fragmentation of function, and increasing expertise. Before World War II it was still possible to consider the medical specialist in terms of a technocratic elite. The specialty boards remained the direct descendants of prewar professional attitudes. Born in the depths of the Depression and sired by exclusive professional groups, the specialty boards were rapidly overtaken by events. With the recognition of specialty board certificates by the armed services and by certain public medical programs, a cycle of professional development was complete. There had been one cycle of development from emerging specialization to demands for formal recognition of medical specialties; this cycle had extended from the early part of this century to the early 1930s, culminating in suggestions for specialist licensure. The period immediately following World War II marked the end of a second cycle, from the establishment of the specialty boards as a system in the 1930s to their formal acceptance, however limited in scope, by the public. But at the same time a third cycle was beginning, with the movement toward some eventual and further rationalization of specialist services, which would be linked both with the specification and supervision of graduate education and training for all medical practitioners and with publicly and professionally articulated manpower needs.

Strong outside pressures, such as the enactment of legislation for national health insurance or for any other form of developing a national health service, would have forced the specialty structures to reform. In this context, it is interesting to examine the proposals for defining generalist and specialist physicians which were written into the documentation surrounding the Wagner-Murray-Dingell bills of the 1940s. Under the 1943 Wagner-Murray bill and later manifestations of the same principles, all licensed physicians would have been entitled to engage in basic (general practitioner) health insurance work; but the surgeon general would have the responsibility for determining which physicians from the general list would qualify as specialists for particular aspects of the service. Distinctions were thus made between those who were general practitioners and those who were specialists, and their functions were quite clearly separated. The act would have set up a referral system from general practitioner to specialist, with the focus of health care being placed on the general practitioner. The patient would not have the right to select a specialist unless referred by his general practitioner; otherwise he would have to bear the cost himself.[46] The system suggested was similar to that introduced in Britain under the National Health Service Act of

46. S. 1161, sec. 905; and see Earl E. Muntz, *Social Security: An Analysis of the Wagner-Murray Bill* (New York, 1944), pp. 56–58.

1946, although the proposed method of financing (through a social insurance mechanism rather than through general taxation) was different. The designation of "specialist" was to be made in accordance with standards developed in consultation with a new National Advisory Medical and Hospital Council; but it was expected that wherever possible standards and certificates developed by appropriate professional groups would be used. Such proposals were designed to balance the supposed desirability of each person having a general or family practitioner, who would act as the point of access to the medical care system and as a diagnostician and general health adviser, with the need for a rational selection of specialist medical care.

Later documents on the Wagner-Murray-Dingell proposals reiterated and clarified the provisions for the generalist and specialist. A report prepared by the Social Security Administration for the hearings on the 1945 bill defined the scope of free choice of doctor. Free choice there would be, but only within recognized limits; only licensed physicians would be included under the scheme. Similarly, only qualified specialists would be acceptable under the payment plan, and the patient would have access to such specialists (for benefits, under the plan) only through his general practitioner.[47] The new provisions, it was argued, were not intended to be restrictionist but to ensure that free choice be exercised wisely and efficiently. Thus a proposed national public program came to conclusions on the desirability of a recognized system of stratification for physicians similar to those reached before World War II by the specialist medical societies in the formulation of the specialty boards.

The use of existing certifying machinery and the standards of certain professional associations, it was thought, would produce 25,000–35,000 fully qualified specialists.[48] In addition, there would be others who might qualify for limited purposes under the act. It was made clear that it was not intended to produce an absolute division of the profession into specialists and general practitioners; but the use of certification and other professional procedures, and the provision in the Wagner-Murray-Dingell bill for differential types of payment to generalists and specialists, might well have had just this impact, as did the National Health Service Act in

47. The report also noted that already there were limitations on free choice because of the availability of physicians in a particular community, because of financial and racial barriers, because of the patient load the individual physician wished to carry, and because of his right to accept or reject any patient. U.S., Congress, Senate, Committee on Education and Labor, *Medical Care Insurance: A Social Insurance Program for Personal Health Services,* Report from the Bureau of Research and Statistics, Social Security Board, 79th Cong., 2d sess., 8 July 1946, Senate Committee Print no. 5, pp. 33, 38, 40–41.
48. Ibid., pp. 33–40.

Britain. Some 25,000 specialty board diplomas had been issued by 1945—a number which, while the component specialties may have been unevenly distributed in relation to optimal patient care, bore a close relationship to the number of specialists eligible for qualification under the Wagner-Murray-Dingell proposals.

These measures would have reinforced the specialty boards as quasi-licensing agencies and as the professional conduits and arbiters of public health programs, and forced them to reevaluate their role. Board certification was already recognized in various fragmented and limited public programs. But in none of these cases did the boards themselves receive the public scrutiny or power implied by appointment as professional intermediaries in a national health program. The public was accustomed in the state licensing boards (still largely influenced by state medical societies) to delegating the setting and supervision of basic professional standards to the medical profession. But above the basic level there was as yet no widespread publicly endorsed system for specialist choice. The inept or inexpert physician could, as always, be sued for negligence before the courts of law. Both the medical profession and the proposed legislation, however, implied that this was not enough.

Meanwhile, even the limited official recognition of board diplomas during the 1940s added a new dimension to the structure of the medical profession. Government-sponsored health insurance might be seen as a political proposal, while the growth of specialty boards was of purely professional concern. But as time went by, the internal organization of the medical profession could not be indefinitely divorced from the type of environment in which future medicine would be given.

Why was there the divorce within the medical profession between the organizational and the educational implications of specialized medicine? Such a divorce there certainly was by the 1940s. The specialties had come of age educationally, as the burgeoning process of residencies and specialist certification testified. Yet specialization was still being discussed as if new forms of organization and financing were irrelevant. The identification of national health insurance with other New Deal welfare programs was clearly one prevailing factor; health care financing moved into the congressional limelight, while specialist regulation did not. Professional self-interest was another factor. Individually, physicians would be subject to government control and regulation under national health insurance; their incomes and freedom to practice where they wanted and in which specialty might be curtailed. More broadly, there was the question of a profession's responsibility for self-regulation. It was not clear in the growing confusion of health services of the 1930s and 1940s how far professional dicta should also govern the way which medical practice is organized; this was to be an increasingly important issue in the 1950s and 1960s.

But perhaps above all other factors was the continuing speed of change in specialized medicine, with all its attending and confusing complexities. Through the technological advances of a previous generation the practitioner had learned that the hospital (rather than the community) was the doctor's natural workshop; yet access was being restricted by specialist hospital departments. It was increasingly important to specialize, yet the specialty boards were providing another potential restriction on freedom to practice. Prepaid groups, lists of physicians for workmen's compensation programs, organization in the armed services and in civilian programs, had an undoubted cumulative effect on the building of professional resistance to other forms of public intervention. Opposition to national health insurance was on the whole emotional rather than reasoned, the product of past tensions, not future needs.

Thus the specialties came of age, but the implications of specialization in medicine remained in early adolescence. On the one hand were the continuing questions of how the medical profession itself should be organized—the role of general practice, the structure and purpose of specialty regulation, the development of medical schools, the control of graduate medical education. All of these were to be under increasing stress after 1950. On the other hand were the equally important questions of how medical services should be financed and distributed. The old questions of Who Should Control Specialization? were still valid. But they had taken on a different meaning. In a medical system geared to produce specialists and superspecialists, with its attendant institutions, paramedical personnel, and costs, "specialization" implied not merely one profession but the regulation of an industry. It is out of this mixed heritage that the professional and social issues of medicine in the last quarter century, to the present, have been generated.

PART IV: PROFESSIONAL STRUCTURES REEXAMINED

CHAPTER 14

Specialization and the General Practitioner

The role of the generalist in medicine has been, and remains, the most important single issue in modern medicine, for the structure of the medical profession hinges on whether—and how—general practice is recognized. The defeat of the Wagner-Murray-Dingell bills in the 1940s sounded the death knell for the possible public support of the general practitioner through a health service payment scheme. Given such support the decline in the number of general practitioners might have been stemmed, as it was under the National Health Service in Britain.[1] The problems of general practitioners as a group would not automatically have been solved, for these problems ran deep. But the organized financial support of generalists in such a plan would at least have provided a potential financial inducement to physicians to become a generalist rather than a specialist, as well as a base for practical discussion of the structures of practice and of the problems of providing individual or personal medical care in terms broader than professional education, status, and demarcation disputes.

As it was, the general practitioner was in a perplexing position. The old-style generalist, with less training than the specialist and with a wide field of practice, was with some justification withering away. Those who remained were fighting an uphill, ultimately a losing, battle to retain their professional standing in comparison with the specialist. At the same time, the need to reconstitute a generalist role in medicine through rational organization of physician services was pointing toward an increasing emphasis in the future on the idea of primary medical care—that is, the encouragement of a stable and continuing relationship between each

1. General practitioners in Britain have had their own acute problems of position and status, but they begin with the solid advantage of a vital function in the National Health Service as doctors of first contact. The acceptance of this function by the public and by specialists gives a base for further discussion of the future of the GP; it is this very base that is lacking in the U.S. See Stevens, p. 357 and passim.

person and a particular physician, who would act as the general manager and coordinator of the patient's care. Such a physician would not be a general practitioner, in the sense of being willing to treat patients over the whole range of medicine, including areas preempted by specialists. Rather, he would be a generalist by virtue of his function as the selector, initiator, orchestrator, and interpreter of the services of specialists. As patients flocked to pediatricians, internists, obstetricians, and psychiatrists, the general practitioner could not claim this role. He was left with a shrinking span of competence and an uncertain future in competition with the specialists.

If a national health service had been introduced in the 1940s, before the number of general practitioners had declined too far, the general practitioner might have been able to move at one jump from the past to the future. Without the formal consultation or referral structure which a national health service promised to provide, general practitioners were left to fend for themselves. Seeking to enhance their position in the years following World War II, they sought to justify the continued existence of general practice in terms of professional status rather than health service organization. It is an interesting observation on the professionally dominated medical care system of the United States that the raison d'etre of the whole operation—the patient—was rarely consulted; nor, indeed, following the failure of national health insurance, did he show much interest.

GENERALIST AND SPECIALIST: CHANGING EXPECTATIONS

The professional problems of general practitioners arose because specialization was superimposed on a profession which was designed to produce one general physician. From the time of the Flexner report until the 1960s, generalism was conceived as a foundation—the base of a pyramid —on which specialist experience would be built. As the span of medical knowledge grew, the general educational base had been expanded to include a general internship. As late as 1940, the Commission on Graduate Education reinforced the general practitioner concept by suggesting: "There should be no fundamental difference between the internship offered to the man going into general practice and the internship for the man who plans to take a residency in order to prepare himself for one of the specialties." [2] Thus the physician was still in theory first a generalist and then a specialist. This theory had important implications for medical

2. Commission on Graduate Medical Education, *Graduate Medical Education,* p. 39.

education, and thus for the structure and internal balance of the profession, for it assumed that the generalist required less training, and was thus implicitly less important than the specialist. Since the specialty boards had been created, a practitioner wrote in 1940, medical students had increasingly obtained the impression that general practice was "what the specialists discarded." [3] The dilemma of the general practitioner was not merely a question of the changing content of his practice; it was also a social process, part of the ever present political processes of professionalism.

In terms of what physicians were actually doing, all physicians in the 1940s were limiting their practice in one way or another; the dichotomy in medical practice between those who were specialists and those who were not was largely disappearing. Yet the labels of "general practitioner" and "specialist" lingered. If the American general practitioner had had a formally defined function, so that patients used him as the physician of first call and specialists would scrupulously only accept patients on referral (as was, largely, the European system), the division of the medical profession into generalists and specialists would have had some organizational justification, and the generalist a well-defined professional identity. Instead, as the number of general practitioners declined, the mantle of primary medical care was also necessarily assumed by pediatricians, internists, obstetricians, and other specialists. What, then, was the distinction between the generalist and specialist? If specialization meant the pursuit of excellence, then the pediatrician was a better general practitioner for the care of children than was the self-styled general practitioner. In relation to adults, the general practitioner might be seen as an incompletely trained internist. In this process the general practitioner's morale was unlikely to be raised, and he became concerned with guarding his own interests. This concern, crystallized after World War II, took three major forms: action to stop the encroaching activities of the specialty boards; action to develop curricula for a new specialty of family medicine; and action to compete professionally with other recognized groups in the formation of a specialty certifying board. All these actions emphasized the legitimate role of the general practitioner at the *graduate* level, and medicine as a multitude of disciplines, each of which was entered after a common medical education that could no longer pretend to produce a safe practitioner. The generalist was claiming equal training and equal rank.

Even before World War II there were movements in this direction.

3. Wilburt C. Davison, "Opportunities in the Practice of Medicine," *J. Amer. med. Ass., 115* (1940), 2230.

General practice was not included in the lists for potential specialty boards developed in the 1930s by the Advisory Board for Medical Specialties and by the AMA Council on Medical Education and Hospitals, for the simple reason that it was not regarded as a specialty. There were, however, alternative proposals for recognizing well-trained generalists. Certification by state medical societies had been argued persuasively by Nathan Sinai and F. C. Warnshuis in a report on the education of the general practitioner for the Michigan State Medical Society in 1934.[4] Such certification was to be based on the completion of specified postgraduate courses, and it was thus tied in with the state society's interest in sponsoring short courses for practitioners as a form of continuing education.

There were also serious proposals by Dr. Robin Buerki and Dr. Louis B. Wilson in 1939 that the National Board of Medical Examiners establish a higher qualification for general practitioners, who would be known as "Fellows of the National Board." Not only would this have had the virtue of consolidating in the National Board all questions of general medicine, and enabling decisions to be made as to what subjects were appropriate to the generalist·at the undergraduate and graduate levels; it would also have endorsed the position of the generalist in the postwar world. The proposal was to examine and certify general practitioners ten years after graduation, taking into account their record of work, postgraduate education, and testimonials by their colleagues; it was emphasized that recognition should not be solely based on an examination. In the next two years extensive discussion was given to this possibility by the executive committee, and early in 1941 a committee to consider certification of general practitioners was set up. During 1941, however, the committee began to have second thoughts. Committee members became alarmed by the complexity of setting up the system, and it was feared that the other work of the National Board would suffer if general practitioner certification were included; the arguments were similar to those used earlier by the National Board for avoiding a major responsibility for specialty examinations. A conference between the National

4. The study was designed to survey the facilities for postgraduate education of physicians and their impact on the general practitioner. The survey showed only a few general practitioners taking postgraduate courses even when such courses were available. State medical society control was suggested for general practitioners instead of a national board because of differing conditions and requirements in general practice in various parts of the country. Presumably it was felt that GP standards ought to be allowed to vary geographically, whereas specialist standards ought not. Michigan State Medical Society, *Postgraduate Medical Education and the Needs of the General Practitioner* (1934).

Board and the AMA Council on Medical Education was planned for February 1942, but Pearl Harbor intervened; certification of general practitioners by these agencies was postponed indefinitely.[5]

In the wisdom of hindsight, a logical solution then as now would have been for the specialty certifying boards to come together, pool their resources, and offer a structure for graduate education and certification in all fields and branches of medicine, including general practice. Logic, however, had little to do with the case. Lone voices suggested that the American Board of Internal Medicine, many of whose diplomates were in effect practicing primary medical care, should absorb general practitioners, so that in the future the general practitioner would be replaced by a new-style clinical specialist who was an expert diagnostician. But this suggestion had little appeal to the existing crop of general practitioners, who had not fulfilled the training requirements specified by the Board of Internal Medicine and would not therefore qualify for certification. Nor—at least at that time—was it likely to appeal to the internists, who continued to define their field as a consultative or referral specialty, and who saw general medicine in terms of the wards of university hospitals rather than in terms of the city streets.

THE IMPETUS TO SPECIALIZE

World War II both encouraged the rise of specialization and enhanced the attractiveness of board certification for all physicians. General practice was at low ebb. In 1940, there were 36,880 full-time specialists, compared with 120,090 part-time specialists and general practitioners; by 1949 the number of full-time specialists had risen to 62,688 (half of whom were board certified), but there were still only 110,441 general practitioners and part-time specialists.[6] Excluding physicians in training programs, but including all other physicians in active practice or retired, board diplomates represented between 15 and 20 percent of the profession; and it seemed probable that this percentage would rise. General

5. Dr. William Cutter, the secretary of the AMA Council on Medical Education, who was greatly interested in general practitioner certification, had died in December 1941, and no one came forward after the war to take up the theme. Minutes of the National Board of Medical Examiners, Oct. 1939–Feb. 1942.

6. In 1940 board diplomates constituted 42.3 percent of all full-time specialists, being particularly strong in radiology (88.4 percent), pathology (71.5 percent), ophthalmology and otolaryngology (61.6 percent), pediatrics (60.8 percent), and orthopedic surgery (60.5 percent). By 1949 the number of board-certified diplomates had risen to include 52.1 percent of all specialists. See Appendix tables A2–A4.

practitioners had no certifying machinery and not even an AMA section. The pressure for both of these symbolized the search for a new self-image for general practice as a separate field of interest rather than a base from which specialization developed.

At the AMA session in Cleveland in June 1941, Dr. Henry A. Luce of Michigan presented a resolution calling for the establishment of a section for general practice. The plea was disapproved. Instead, the AMA House of Delegates approved an experimental session for general practitioners within the Section on Miscellaneous Topics. But this could hardly appeal to those who saw general practice as a specialty. At the same meeting, Dr. George Dillinger of Indiana presented a resolution calling for a study on the means of developing certification for general practitioners, "in recognition of special training, experience and fitness, and special qualifications for general practice." [7] In addition Dr. L. B. Christian of Michigan asked for a resolution from the AMA to prevent government agencies from using the specialty board diplomas as a requirement for government service. The effective mobilization of the generalist had begun. Although none of these measures was successful, the scene had been set for further bids to upgrade the status of the generalist. At the same time such resolutions sounded a warning note to the future authority of the specialty certifying boards. It was by no means coincidental that it was also in 1941 that the AMA House of Delegates upheld the opinion of the AMA Judicial Council that no insignia should be allowed for specialists.

Meanwhile, the future of the general practitioners remained in doubt. Wartime classification schemes put a premium on specialists. Professional leaders might look forward to the "wide open opportunities" in postwar America for the good general practitioner because the specialties were said to be overcrowded, and general practice sometimes to be better paid.[8] But this was an unrealistic view. Not only were there concurrent statements that there was actually a general shortage of physicians,[9] a situation unlikely to push physicians into general practice from economic

7. "Resolution on Certification in Recognition of Special Qualifications for General Practice," *J. Amer. med. Ass., 116* (1941), 2790.
8. See e.g. Wilburt C. Davison, "Readjustments of Returning Medical Officers," *J. Amer. med. Ass., 124* (1944), 818–19.
9. The Ewing report of 1948 considered that the overall supply of physicians fell short by nearly 20 percent. *The Nation's Health: A Ten-Year Program,* Report to the President by Oscar R. Ewing, Federal Security Administrator (Washington, D.C., 1948), p. 37. The Magnuson report concluded in 1952 that, partly because of the increase in military requirements for physicians in the Korean War, there were then fewer physicians in relation to the civilian population than there had been in 1940. U.S. President's Commission, *Building America's Health,* vol. 1, p. 12.

reasons alone; there were also positive pressures toward increasing specialism, both during the war and immediately afterward.

Leading specialists looked with enthusiasm at the well-defined specialist groups which had developed in the armed forces. In orthopedics, for example, each certified surgeon was assisted during the war by three or more partly trained surgeons. A large new group of men—about 900—had thereby been brought into contact with this specialty, and might themselves be expected to aspire to full-time specialization. The number of full-time orthopedic surgeons in fact doubled between 1940 and 1949 and had virtually tripled by 1955. Evidence collected by the AMA bore out the trend toward specialism. It was expected in 1945 that over 13,000 returning medical officers would seek specialty certification. The military experience thus had a profound effect on medical practice in the postwar world. Indeed, the Army Specialized Training Program and the Navy V-12 program absorbed some 90 percent of the medical class of 1945, and less than one-fifth of this group went into general practice.[10] At the same time it was probable that the expanded specialist supply would be more than met by the expanded demand for specialist care generated by those who had served in the war.

The trend toward specialism was, moreover, actively encouraged through public subsidy of graduate medical education under the GI bill (Servicemens Readjustment Act) of 1944, which was unprecedented in the scope of benefits offered to veterans of World War II. Undergraduate medical education clearly fell within the terms of tuition and living allowances for returning veterans. It was logical that graduate medical education—if, indeed, this was education rather than experience offered through an apprenticeship—should also do so. The AMA raised the question with the Veterans Administration late in 1945. In an answer which was to affect the pattern of specialty training in the late 1940s and early 1950s, the Veterans Administration ruled that payment of tuition and living allowances could be made to hospitals and to physicians taking graduate training in acceptable hospitals. This ruling had some instant effects. The returning physician was offered a subsidized residency train-

10. Guy Caldwell, "The Postwar Challenge to Orthopedic Surgery," *J. Amer. med. Ass., 126* (1946), 270; Harold C. Lueth, "Results of Pilot Questionnaire to Physicians in Service," *J. Amer. med. Ass., 125* (1944), 558; Harold C. Lueth, "Postgraduate Wishes of Medical Officers," *J. Amer. med. Ass., 127* (1945), 759; Victor Johnson, Harold C. Lueth, and F. H. Arestad, "Educational Facilities for Physician Veterans," *J. Amer. med. Ass., 129* (1945), 28; V. Johnson, "45th Annual Report on Medical Education," *J. Amer. med. Ass., 129* (1945), 39–71; Herman G. Weiskotten, Walter S. Wiggins, Marion E. Altenderfer, Marjorie Gooch, and Anne Tipner, "Trends in Medical Practice: An Analysis of the Distribution and Characteristics of Medical College Graduates, 1915–1950," *J. med. Educ., 35* (1960), 1080.

ing of up to four years with a living allowance which was generous in comparison with prewar residency programs. Hospitals, too, were able to claim a subsidy for offering residency programs to GIs at the very time that there was an increasing demand by hospitals for house staffs. The ruling made no distinction between residencies in hospitals affiliated with medical schools and those without such affiliation. As a result, there was an outpouring of interest from hospitals as well as from individual physicians greatly to increase the number of residencies. The AMA Council on Medical Service went on record in favor of stimulating as great a number of veterans as possible to go into residencies, and the Council on Medical Education was deluged with requests for information from GIs and from hospitals, in turn encouraging the latter to set up new programs.[11]

So it was, at a time of great emphasis on the general practitioner, that both the federal government and the AMA were busily endorsing a rapid shift toward specialty training. In 1940, 5,233 approved residency positions had been offered; in 1944 the number was inflated to 7,666 and by 1946 there were over 12,000.[12] The biggest proportional increases were in the specialties of anesthesiology, neurological surgery, physical medicine, and plastic surgery. But it was in the large specialties that the changes would have most effect. The number of residencies in general surgery shifted from only 808 in 1940 to more than 4,000 in 1950.[13] This shift has had a continuing effect on the existence in American medicine, compared with other countries, of a relatively very large proportion of surgeons. While, therefore, the GI bill had as its underlying political assumption the rewarding of veterans for service to their country, not a plan for the health manpower needs of the United States in the 1950s, it had nevertheless a substantial effect on patterns of medical education and practice. The AMA Council on Medical Education apparently thought that the acute demand for residency training would drop off once demobilization was complete. But the inflated number of residencies, once created, did not decline; in 1952 over 22,000 residencies were offered, by 1957 there were over 30,000 and by 1970, over 45,000. So great was the initial response to the expansion of residency programs that the council field staff was unable to survey all new programs. Instead,

11. "Hospital Residencies under the GI Bill," *J. Amer. med. Ass., 130* (1946), 214, 216–17; "Report of the Committee on Postwar Medical Service," ibid., pp. 220–21.
12. *Health Manpower Source Book,* sec. 13, table 6; "Annual Report on Graduate Medical Education in the United States," in AMA, *Directory of Approved Internships and Residencies* (1969–70), table 14.
13. For a more comprehensive picture of the increase in the number of residencies by specialty see below table 9, p. 395.

temporary approval had to be given on the basis of paper applications, in some cases authorizing totally inadequate teaching programs.

In theory it would have been possible for the Council on Medical Education to design its system of residency approval to match some system of estimates of the kinds of medical manpower which would be most relevant to the postwar world—particularly, estimates of the numerical role of general practice in relation to the growing army of specialists. Victor Johnson, secretary of the AMA Council on Medical Education and Hospitals, stated in 1947—on the basis of a survey of the opinions of members of the American medical specialty boards—that the then existing specialist population of about 51,000 (including those board certified and those not) approached the optimum number for the best medical care.[14] But the political climate was against any attempt to put a constraint on the physician's freedom of choice in choosing a specialty. Once again there was a clash between populist and elitist views in the profession. Actions by various specialty boards in the late 1940s to upgrade their requirements for eligibility (and thus to limit the number of diplomates) were regarded as the exercise of an undesirable exclusiveness. A massive effort might have been launched by the specialty boards, by the Council on Medical Education, or even by the Veterans Administration through the operation of the GI bill, to provide outstanding training opportunities for general practice. General practitioner training, however, fitted neither the increasing specialist departmentalism of hospitals nor the inclinations of physicians. Of 12,000 residencies offered in 1947, less than 800 were described as giving general or "mixed" training.[15] The relationship between the internship and residency was irrevocably changed; there were now more residencies than internships; a period of residency was becoming a common part of medical training for the majority of physicians. Yet there remained no large-scale training program for the general practitioner. Once again he was left outside the scope of specialty provisions. Once again the GP was identifiable by what he lacked, rather than by what he had.

GENERAL PRACTICE AS A PROFESSIONAL IDENTITY

Organizational representation of general practitioners was tied up in, and to some extent thwarted by, the continuing difficulty of coming to grips

14. Victor Johnson, "Implications of Current Trends toward Specialization," in Mahlon Ashford, ed. *Trends in Medical Education,* pp. 173–78.
15. "Report of the Council on Medical Education and Hospitals," *J. Amer. med. Ass.,* 134 (1947), 1320.

with "general practice." Was it a field, a function, or a specialty? Historically, general practitioners had looked to the AMA to represent their
interests. As the balance of general and specialist practice changed, the
average physician became a specialist and the AMA would no longer
represent general practitioners as a distinctive group. Indeed, Oliver
Garceau's study of the AMA published in 1941 showed that already
those most influential in the AMA were the specialists.[16] While the house
and the committees of the AMA might continue to feel the importance
of general practice as the cornerstone of medicine, or a basic educational
building block for subsequent specialization, the AMA itself could not
offer general practitioners the sense of organizational identity which
would enable them to examine their status, education, and function in
comparison with the specialties. Specialties had grown around specialist
societies and had derived their organizational and professional strength
from such associations. General practitioners were faced with the reverse
process; they were in existence long before they were separately organized. As a result, at a critical stage in medical development—critical both
in the sense of internal professional politics and of the emerging structures of health services—the specialists were highly organized, while
general practitioner representation was disorganized and diffuse.

Organizational cohesiveness of the GP was, however, gradually improving. In 1945, a section on general practice was approved by the
AMA House of Delegates, and in the same year a proposal for a certifying board for general practice was submitted by the Council on Medical
Education to the Advisory Board for Medical Specialties. Both of these
actions were efforts by general practitioners themselves to redefine general practice in terms of a recognized function or specialty, instead of
maintaining it as the cornerstone on which the remainder of medicine
was built. The Advisory Board turned down the application, pending
presentation of "more concrete objectives" by an organized general practitioner group;[17] like the council, it refused to accept responsibility for the
most vital manpower issue in postwar medical care. But the professional
importance of a certifying board continued. Board certification alone
might not stimulate general practitioners to keep themselves up to date,
but it would (as other boards had done) help to define the generalist's
field; and there would be invaluable by-products in the opportunity to

16. Garceau, pp. 54–57.
17. "Resolutions on Creation of Board of General Practice," *J. Amer. med. Ass.,*
125 (1944), 584; "Report of Reference Committee on Medical Education," ibid., p.
641; AMA, *Digest,* p. 295; "Board of General Practice," *J. Amer. med. Ass., 129*
(1945), 464.

raise the general practitioner's status and prestige and to proclaim his legitimate right to be included on the attending staffs of hospitals.

In October 1946, the AMA delegated the issue of a certification board for general practitioners to a subcommittee of its Committee on Postwar Medical Service. Two of the three members of the subcommittee, both of whom were also members of the Advisory Board for Medical Specialties, initially supported the concept of certification. The third member pointed out that creaming off 10,000 or so general practitioners through certification would not solve the overall problem of general practitioner access to hospitals nor the restrictive use by the Veterans Administration of certification in defining a specialist.[18] Indeed, the definition of an elite within general practice might aggravate rather than reduce the general practitioners' problems, which were material as well as educational. Concurrent AMA recommendations for including general practitioner services in hospitals and general practice sections in state and county medical associations were already tackling one set of problems. Educationally, there was also some feeling that the general practitioners' major problem was in keeping up to date rather than proving competence at one point in time. None of the existing specialty boards had provisions for periodic reexamination, nor for requiring evidence of continuing study. There was thus no such clear-cut argument for a certifying board in general practice as there had been for the specialty groups, and general practitioners themselves were divided over the ultimate desirability of certification.

Nevertheless, by the summer of 1947 the general practitioner movement was in full swing. The AMA section had begun to function actively, giving general practitioners one professional base. Another base of crucial long-term importance was the American Academy of General Practice, established by a group of physicians during the AMA meeting at Atlantic City in June 1947. The Academy quickly took hold, as state and county chapters developed all over the country; by 1950 it had over 10,000 members; by 1970 the figure was over 31,000.[19] So rapid was the academy's growth that a bare six months after its foundation, the question was being raised within the AMA of the Academy's conflict—or competition—with the basic aims of the AMA.[20] The reaction was similar

18. "Report of Subcommittee on Specialty Board for General Practitioners," *J. Amer. med. Ass., 134* (1947), 377; and see *133* (1947), 942–43, and *135* (1947), 518.
19. American Academy of General Practice, personal communication.
20. "Report of Subcommittee on Specialty Board for General Practitioners," *J. Amer. med. Ass., 136* (1948), 778.

to that of the AMA to the growth of specialty societies in the late nineteenth century. Organizationally, general practitioners had arrived. They now had national vehicles to express their problems—the American Academy of General Practice and the AMA section. Through these, effective demands could be made for the next process of formal specialization: the establishment of a certifying board.

On this question, however, the professional leaders themselves continued to be divided. The Academy was in a rather similar position to that which had faced the American College of Surgeons on its foundation. Was it more important to "standardize" (i.e. upgrade) general practice as a whole, or to establish a level of recognized fitness or excellence to which all might aspire but not all achieve? The College of Surgeons never really resolved this issue, but had developed on the first principle; the second principle was adopted in the separate organization of a specialty certifying board in surgery. The Academy of General Practice followed along similar lines. The Academy decided in the 1940s not to press for a certifying board in general practice, on the grounds that this was both undesirable and unnecessary. Alone of the medical societies, the Academy requires its members to maintain a regular level of postgraduate education, and it was claimed that this corresponded to specialty certification; general practice would be defined through continuing education rather than through a specified residency program. The question of a board therefore dropped into the background, not to be revived until the 1960s.

Instead of pressing for a board, which would have split the ranks of general practitioners, the Academy attempted to unite general practitioners through emphasizing the generalist's central role as an upholder of voluntary or nongovernmental forms of medical practice, upgrading continuing education, and pushing for general practitioner appointments in hospitals. These aims were stated in the "basic tenets" adopted by the Academy,[21] and were furthered in its own sponsorship of courses and in its *Manual on the Establishment and Operation of a Department of General Practice in Hospitals*. The journal *GP,* started by the Academy in 1950, provided a forum in which GPs could rediscover their own values. It exhorted general practitioners to preserve general practice "for

21. The academy established five basic tenets: (1) voluntarism in medical practice (no government control); (2) general practice is the foundation of medical practice; (3) medical practice is a public trust; (4) every competent physician should have access to hospital staff membership; (5) there should be postgraduate studies for all physicians on a continuing basis. *GP, 2* (1950), 95.

ourselves, our children, and the American public." [22] With such organizations the GP could work toward creating definitions of his specialty.

THE GENERAL PRACTITIONER AND THE HOSPITAL

The American Academy of General Practice attempted to provide general practitioners with an inclusive base. At the same time parallel efforts were made to include all general practitioners on the staffs of hospitals. But here there were other problems of professional egalitarianism versus a qualitative elite; for the role of the hospital in medical care was (and remains) in transition.

Two compelling but conflicting arguments could be advanced in relation to the kind of access hospitals should give to local practitioners. An open-staff system, favored by general practitioners, acknowledges the place of the hospital as the necessary scientific nucleus for all physicians, as a community practice center, and as a place for professional cross-fertilization. The hospital thus becomes the potential center for medical care. The widespread adoption of hospital-based group practice, as advocated by the Committee on the Costs of Medical Care, would have endorsed this approach, by pulling the physicians together in one place. Such practices were, however, still rare in the 1940s; the average practitioner continued in solo private practice, or at most in small convenience partnerships. As medicine flowered into a series of distinctive disciplines, the hospital could not afford to take on trust the level of skills of all local practitioners in relation to all aspects of inpatient care. Herein lay the dilemma—which remains. Unless hospital staff privileges are carefully defined in relation to skills, and unless adequate review of performance is maintained (both difficult if not impracticable aims), the standard of inpatient care may be uneven, and even in some cases dangerous, for example where an inexperienced surgeon attempts major surgery. A closed-staff system, on the other hand, may ensure high medical standards for patients undergoing care in the hospital—the university teaching hospital provides a good example—but it also implies a professional monopoly that may be disadvantageous to out-of-hospital medical care. Moreover the closed-staff system is repugnant to a profession whose traditions have demanded equal recognition for all. This latter situation has represented the general approach in the United States.

At their extremes the one system assumes that medical care is a spectrum from physician's office to hospital bed and back, with an individual

22. A. E. Ritt, "A Tradition Well Worth Preserving," ibid., p. 123.

physician and patient involved at each stage; from the physician's point
of view, his hospital work is part of his private practice. The other system
assumes a cadre of physicians whose work is predominantly or entirely in
the hospital and a second cadre whose work is primarily outside the
hospital; in this model the hospital is at the fringe of medical care, and
the hospitalized sick are seen as requiring unusual and acute forms of
diagnosis and treatment. The role of the hospital thus depends in large
part on the predominant patterns of physician distribution, in terms of
function, economics, and prestige. Where both those with and those without hospital appointments compete in private practice for the same
patients—the American situation—denial of a hospital appointment is
not merely a matter of standards but of livelihood. This was the situation
facing American general practitioners in the 1940s, and since. The perceptions of hospitals and general practitioners were inevitably different.

By the 1940s, general practitioners were clamoring for hospital attach-
ments. The combined impact of immigration, post-war demobilization,
and hospital staffing policies had created a pool of physicians who had
no hospital access of any kind; nearly 2,500 physicians in New York City
had no hospital appointment in 1948, and there was an increasing (and
not unnatural) tendency for hospitals to demand specialty certification.[23]
But board certification for hospital staff appointments, which had been
actively encouraged by the American Hospital Association and tacitly
assumed by the specialty boards in the 1930s, was by then recognized as
a guild system in action. Indeed, the movement to encourage the appointment of generalists in hospitals was in large part an effort to reduce the
restrictive impact of the specialty boards. The AMA House of Delegates
resolved in 1946 that hospitals should be encouraged to develop general
practitioner services and that the criterion of whether a physician may
be a member of a hospital staff should not be dependent on certification
by the various specialty boards or membership in special societies. Copies
of this resolution were sent to the American College of Surgeons, the
American College of Physicians, the major hospital associations, and
every hospital in the country. The following year it became official AMA
policy that hospitals should have no rule barring physicians from staff
privileges because they did not possess a board diploma or membership
in a special society.[24] These policies remain in force today.

There were pressures other than general practitioner self-interest operating in these pronouncements. The question of whether, and how far,

23. Herbert E. Klarman, *Hospital Care in New York City*, p. 14.
24. AMA, *Digest*, p. 295; editorial, *J. Amer. med. Ass., 134* (1947), 1484.

hospitals could (and should) restrict the physicians on their staffs through demanding professional memberships had been a bitter issue in the battle between the AMA and the Group Health Association of Washington, D.C., which was started as a health cooperative in 1937 and which became a target of vehement opposition for organized medicine. Physicians in the cooperative were excluded from AMA-affiliated medical societies (on grounds that they were unethically participating in a closed-panel prepayment scheme) and subjected to exclusion from hospital staffs—the latter reinforced through alleged pressures on the hospitals by threats of withdrawal of AMA approval of internships and residencies if the hospitals did not comply. In 1943, after four years of litigation, the Supreme Court of the United States found the AMA and the Medical Society of the District of Columbia guilty of restraint of trade under the Sherman Act.[25] A question central to the whole issue was how far hospitals should restrict physicians on their staffs through requiring membership in the local medical society or through other arbitrary qualifications. The AMA defeat and subsequent action in relation to other prepaid plans caused both hospitals and specialty boards to take a second look at the use of board certification as a possibly illegal restrictive device.

The new line was quickly followed. In a special report on the prestige of general practitioners, in 1947, the AMA Council on Medical Education disclaimed any responsibility for encouraging specialty board certification or any type of medical society membership as an important credential for hospital staff appointments in its approval of internship and residency programs. The council did concede, however, that hospitals might have interpreted the Essentials in just this way.[26] Since the residencies were

25. The Group Health Association (GHA) was organized by employees of the Federal Home Owners Loan Corporation living in Washington, D.C. It set up a clinic, employed physicians on a salary, and established a system of financing through monthly membership contributions. The District of Columbia Medical Society objected to both the insurance and the closed-panel arrangements, which together were viewed as the undesirable "corporate practice of medicine." The society did not expel physicians; it persuaded nearly all the hospitals in the District to deny staff privileges and bed space to GHA physicians, using as one weapon a resolution adopted by the AMA in 1934 that all members of the staff of hospitals approved for internship, residency, and nurse training be members of a component medical society. Further battles along similar lines between organized medicine and the Group Health Association of Puget Sound (established in 1946) and the Health Insurance Plan of Greater New York (which began operating in 1947), both of which the "plans" ultimately won, emphasized the legal limitations of professional restrictionism. See "American Medical Association: Power, Purpose and Politics in Organized Medicine," *Yale Law Journal* (May 1954), 990–96.

26. "Supplementary Report of Council on Medical Education and Hospitals," *J. Amer. med. Ass., 134* (1947), 711; Donald G. Anderson, in "Report of Subcom-

primarily geared to the requirements set out by the specialty boards, it was only natural that the hospitals should have done so; indeed, the council still makes a point of recording the number of diplomates on the staff of each hospital seeking residency approval. The council also attempted in 1949 to survey the degree to which specialty certification was actually used by hospitals in appointments. In reply to the question of whether certification was required, only 270 hospitals were bold enough to answer yes; 2,135 said no, and 2,184 did not reply.[27] The legal position of hospitals in relation to medical staff appointments was still not sufficiently defined for such requirements to be disclosed in public, and less formal documentation did indicate that board certification was being generally used as a measure for hospital staff appointment.[28] In law the hospitals had the responsibility of exercising reasonable care in the choice of attending physicians; they might also require evidence of specific skills and restrict staff to defined privileges. The GHA case had shown the requirement of medical society membership to be illegal. It was not, however, clear at the time whether this meant that no defined professional criteria could be used.

Meanwhile the specialty boards, themselves alarmed at charges of exclusiveness and also with an eye to possible antitrust action, were disclaiming any intention of being agents of restrictionism. The American Board of Surgery stated in February 1947 that it was not concerned with special privileges for its members, including the definition of hospital appointment.[29] This statement was quickly adopted by the Advisory Board for Medical Specialties and by several of the specialty boards. The implication that the specialty boards had never intended to be used as dis-

---

mittee on Specialty Board for General Practitioners," *J. Amer. med. Ass., 136* (1948), 778.

27. "Hospital Service in the United States," *J. Amer. med. Ass., 140* (1949), 34.

28. The serious degree of weight actually given by hospitals to board certification as a criterion for staff appointment—the sole criterion available for the hospital administrator and lay boards of trustees in evaluating specialists, in the absence of as yet well organized hospital medical staffs—was, for example, stressed by several speakers at an invitational meeting of the Advisory Board for Medical Specialties in February 1949. Advisory Board for Medical Specialties, "Annual Meetings and Conference, February 6, 1949," mimeographed.

29. "It is neither the intent nor has it been the purpose of the board to define requirements for membership on the staffs of hospitals. The prime object of the board is to pass judgment on the education and training of broadly competent and responsible surgeons—not who shall or shall not perform surgical operations. The board specifically disclaims interest in or recognition of differential emoluments that may be based on certification." "American Board of Surgery," *J. Amer. med. Ass., 133* (1947), 337.

criminating agents might be thought hard to swallow in the light of the boards' own prewar statements, but the boards were bending with the changing times. It was not, however, evident that in their response to an immediate crisis, they were bending in an ultimately constructive direction, for as a result board certification took on a limited and ambiguous meaning.

Meanwhile, in their strivings for recognition by hospitals, general practitioners achieved some success. The Council on Medical Education endorsed the resolution from the American Board of Surgery; revised its "Essentials of a Registered Hospital" to include general practice as a hospital section; and extended its "Essentials of Approved Residencies and Fellowships" to exclude any implication that the medical staff of a hospital approved for training should be certified, as well as excluding .statements that most residency programs were designed toward specialty board certification and that GP residencies normally carried no such training credit. These measures would, in the council's view, obviate the need for a separate GP certification board.[30] A survey by the AMA in 1951 indicated that as many as one of three general hospitals had general practice sections, concentrated in the small and medium-size hospitals.[31] Hospitals by then paid lip service to their impartiality in medical staff selection by not using certification as the sole measure of quality, even though some evidence of quality was increasingly required.

In 1948 the AMA Council on Medical Education established a new category of hospital residency training in general practice, and the following year a gratifying response was noted to the new program. But the program was not well thought through. In the early 1950s the Section on General Practice requested *fewer* GP residencies except in hospitals fully associated with medical schools; but the medical schools themselves were becoming less qualified each year to teach medical generalists. Only 40 percent of GP residencies were filled in 1952; there were then approved GP residency programs in ninety-three hospitals.[32] The council itself was not then prepared, nor has it been since, to take any mandatory measures to restrict the supply of residencies by category, thus forcing physicians into GP programs. This suggestion was made, as was another disapproved

30. The council did not however go as far as one 1948 resolution to the AMA which would have the council disapprove hospitals which made certification a necessary qualification for promotion or appointment. AMA, *Digest,* pp. 298–99.
31. "Hospital Service in the United States," *J. Amer. med. Ass., 149* (1952), 163.
32. John C. Nunemaker, "The Present Status of Graduate Education for Family Practice," *Second Regional Conference on Graduate Medical Education in General and Family Practice* (1965), p. 3.

AMA resolution that half of the specialist residencies be allotted to applicants who had served five years as GPs in smaller communities.[33] The residency was thus not manipulated to encourage the development of particular skills. While there were continuing calls for *more* general practitioners in the 1950s, there was still no responsible manpower machinery with which to follow through. In retrospect, the general practitioners would have been best served by an early endorsement of hospital-based group practice, in which both their role and numbers might have been sustained.

THE EDUCATIONAL MILIEU

Instead, out in practice, patients could—and did—bypass the general practitioners at any time in favor of specialist medical care. The GP still had not only to win over his peers (including an increasing number of medical students) but also to sell his value to the general public. This task was formidable; in a continuing system of solo private practice, it was probably impossible. Except in their pressures for hospital appointments, general practitioners did not openly acknowledge that their problems derived more from the way medical practice was organized than from the way general practitioners were trained. Instead, the focus of general practitioner reform in the 1950s and early 1960s was almost entirely on the educational content of primary medical care. In his wish to see himself as an equal to other specialists, the generalist tended to gloss over the framework in which he intended to fulfill his ideal role.

There were numerous attempts during the 1950s to require some general practice of all specialists. A Texas resolution to the AMA in 1952 called for a mandatory period of general practice before specialization. But this suggestion was logical only if general practice were to be regarded as the foundation of practice for all physicians; and in the 1950s this could no longer be claimed. The AMA House of Delegates resolved that one of the requirements for entering a specialty should be a year or more of general practice; it was suggested that there should be conferences to discuss such a proposal with the Advisory Board for Medical Specialties, with a view to increasing the number of general practitioners. But the specialty boards remained uninterested. The AMA in 1952 appointed a committee on general practice prior to specialization. After five years of deliberation, this committee eventually issued its report. It had not been able to reach a unanimous opinion, but it was generally agreed that an individual should be free to go into general practice prior to

33. See AMA, *Digest,* pp. 301, 680.

specializing, but that he should not be required to do so. There was also general agreement that all graduates have at least two years' hospital experience in a well-rounded teaching program. But there was no force in these proposals. The committee avoided the question of defining general practice in functional terms by accepting a very broad definition: general practice was described as any form of diagnosis and treatment commensurate with the physician's competence, and assuming a total continuing responsibility for the health of the individual or the family as a unit. There was no indication how this was to be achieved. Nor did the committee see any future in mutual discussions with the specialty boards. The AMA, it was felt, should dictate neither to specialty boards nor to individuals: "The distribution of physicians is following a natural pattern that is in the best public interest." [34] This "natural pattern" pointed to the generalist's ultimate disappearance. No one was willing to seize the initiative.

Following these somewhat unsatisfactory recommendations, in 1957 the AMA set up a joint committee of representatives of the Council on Medical Education, the AAMC, and the American Academy of General Practice to restudy general practice. Again the emphasis was on training rather than on structure of practice, but this time the training emphasis was geared to provide a definition of general practice as a distinct specialty, "family practice." The report of this committee, "Final Report on Preparation for Family Practice" (1959), recommended new two-year pilot programs of graduate medical education in hospitals, designed around internal medicine and pediatric training.[35] The two-year program was to be in effect a two-year mixed internship, but designed not with the purpose of rounding out the physician's general education but of creating a special proficiency. In form, therefore, general practice was at last to be recognized as equivalent to other specialties.

But the suggested curriculum did not include surgery, and this was to be an immediate cause of complaint from existing general practitioners who still felt that general practice should be interpreted literally as encompassing both medicine and surgery. At least eight resolutions of protest were introduced at the AMA meeting in 1960, directing the Council on Medical Education to consider other two-year programs which would include surgery and obstetrics. These resolutions were passed by a House of Delegates attuned to the wishes of the majority, and became AMA policy. Confusion was evident between those who sought a new role for

34. AMA, *Digest,* pp. 682–86.
35. The "Final Report on Preparation for Family Practice" is printed in AMA, *Directory of Approved Internships and Residencies* (1961), pp. 19–22.

the generalist in family practice—the application of internal medicine and pediatrics, with elements of other specialties, to the diagnosis and general supervision of a family's medical care—and those fighting a rearguard action to maintain the old general practitioner's status quo. The latter viewed the recommendation not as the development of a new and strengthened role but as the attenuation of their own importance.

Following the AMA resolutions 20 two-year graduate training programs were introduced. Since they included elements of surgery and obstetrics the council termed them "general practice" instead of "family practice." There was thus now a small number of residencies for general practitioners who had completed an internship and an even smaller number of the two-year pilot programs; neither could be claimed as a success. By 1966, there were only 17 active two-year pilot programs, offering positions for 89 trainees; only 49 were filled. There were 146 residency training programs in general practice, offering 824 positions; only 132 of these were filled by American or Canadian graduates.[36] The number of general practitioners continued to decline.

The American Academy of General Practice had seen itself as an alternative to a specialty board. It had not, however, been able to stem the tide of general practitioner decline either in numbers or in prestige. In 1940, three of every four physicians had thought of themselves as generalists; by 1966, the proportion was less than one out of three. As the problems mounted, and prompted by the more militant AMA Section on General Practice, pressure began to build within the academy for the establishment of a specialty board. The question was raised annually at academy meetings from 1958; each year the opposition, which included the academy leadership, lost some ground. There was the organizational danger, namely that if the academy did not act, an independent board would move into action.[37] To be board certified was to appear as the specialist's equal. The pressures built up in parallel with an increasing number of articles on the problematical future of family practice in the medical press; and with concern as to the general problems of graduate education.

In 1963 the AMA appointed John Millis, president of Western Re-

---

36. AMA, *Directory of Approved Internships and Residencies* (1967–68), pp. 2, 8.
37. According to the AMA *Proceedings,* the AMA Board of Trustees met with representatives of an "American Board of Family Practice" in September 1963. The AMA's view at this time was that a board should await studies of general practice, and that the application should in any event be made to the Advisory Board for Medical Specialties rather than to the AMA. *Proc. AMA House of Delegates,* Nov.–Dec. 1964, p. 23.

serve University, to chair a commission to study the whole area of graduate medical education, and the following year the AMA created yet another committee (the Willard committee) to study general practice preparation; both reported in 1966, and both endorsed board certification of primary or family practitioners.[38] Meanwhile, in the spring of 1965, the American Academy of General Practice decided after all to endorse, and to press for, a certifying board. It was decided that the new board would include two radical innovations: it would have no grandfather clause, and it would, as did the academy itself, require periodic recertification. The following June a series of resolutions to the AMA urged approval of a board of family practice, and these were referred to the Council on Medical Education. The certifying board was finally approved in 1969. Meanwhile, the academy set up its own committee to develop detailed requirements for certification of the family physician. This committee emphasized the place of family medicine as a specialty, defined as "comprehensive medical care in which the physician accepts continuing responsibility regardless of the age of the patient." The new family physician would, it was reported, be an expert in the physician-patient relationship and put emphasis on sociological as well as strictly scientific skills.[39]

In the summer of 1967 a committee of the Academy of General Practice began working with the staff of the National Board of Medical Examiners to develop the new board's first examination, which was given in the spring of 1970, a rigorous six hours of written tests, followed by a second day of examination based on visual materials, including charts, graphs of diagnostic data, and motion pictures for analysis of patient management problems. Thus, thirty years after the previous, unsuccessful proposals that the National Board certify general practitioners, it found itself as an expert to, and agent of, the American Board of Family Practice. It has been claimed that the carefully constructed examination, based on the National Board's substantial experience in its own examinations and research, is among the most advanced medical testing devices in the world. The family practice board has meanwhile specified a graduate educational period of three years, with retesting of diplomates every six years. Future board diplomates in family medicine will be justly recognized as at least the equals of their specialist peers.

38. Citizens Commission on Graduate Medical Education, *The Graduate Education of Physicians*; AMA, Ad Hoc Committee on Education for Family Practice, *Meeting the Challenge of Family Practice*.
39. American Academy of General Practice, Committee on Requirements for Certification, *The Core Content of Family Medicine*, 1966.

Nor—such is the reversal of fortune—is this type of certification the only channel now open to the aspiring family physician. In a rapid (if belated) sequence of events following the academy's change of heart toward a certifying board, the American Boards of Internal Medicine and Pediatrics modified their own requirements to encompass a type of personal or family care. Through an agreement reached between the two boards in 1967, physicians may be eligible for certification by both boards with four years of graduate medical education (two years in each specialty, of which one year may be a straight internship). Alternatively, the physician will be able to take advantage of changes in the examinations of the American Board of Internal Medicine, scheduled for 1972. Under the new arrangements candidates may take the certifying examination (a written examination) in general internal medicine in the final month of the third postdoctoral year of training. The time needed for board certification will thus be substantially reduced, although those wishing subspecialty training will be offered additional programs and certification in nine narrower areas: the four existing subspecialties, endocrinology and metabolism, hematology, infectious disease, nephrology, and rheumatology.

From the indeterminate professional status of the generalist in the 1950s to such recognition in the 1970s is a professional triumph indeed. Educationally, the generalist may claim equality to the specialist. If anything, the future family physician may be overeducated for the functions he is expected to perform. But such a comment ignores the compelling pressures of professionalization, toward higher educational standards and peer recognition.

THE SOCIAL MILIEU

With this commitment to professional equality for general or family practice, the educational question was firmly settled; family practice was recognized as equal to other specialties. An important professional status had been won; the family practitioners had defined and were regulating their specialty. This action alone did not, however, necessarily solve the social and functional problems of general practice. There is no guarantee, even with a specialty board, that family medicine will become the cornerstone of medical practice. While the movement for professional status was gathering strength, a dwindling number of people were using the general practitioner as a purveyor of family or primary medical care. Changing the generalist's education and title does not of itself promise to reverse this trend; a change in consumer behavior is also necessary. At the same time, to assure the availability of family care by qualified practitioners to all or most of the population would require a revolution in physician career choices. The battle for recognition of family practice thus has some Alice in Wonderland qualities.

Other problems also remained unsolved. While the great majority of general practitioners now hold some hospital appointment, there is still no common specification as to what family practitioners may do in hospitals which are normally organized as a series of specialist inpatient departments and outpatient clinics under designated specialist chiefs. Where there are GP sections, these often have no actual clinical responsibilities. Few general practitioners teach regularly in the medical schools; nor do they take regular responsibility in the hospitals (or in their own practices) for undergraduate or graduate medical education. In the increasingly research-conscious schools of the 1950s and 1960s—a critical time for the development of the family physician—all the pressures were toward specialization. Not only were students taught by specialists in the classroom; they modeled themselves on the specialist teachers in clinical training.[40] Nor can students have been impressed by the few studies of general practitioners at work. The Peterson study of general practice in North Carolina in the early 1950s[41] and a later study by Clute in Canada[42] showed an appalling range of practice and standards—from good to bad—among existing general practitioners.

As general practitioners sought to maintain their practices and positions in an unfavorable competitive situation, without the benefit of professional and organizational constraints which would have consolidated the family practice role, unethical practices continued. An AMA report of 1954 described conflicts between general practitioners and surgeons over who would undertake surgery, the widespread prevalence of fee splitting, and the existence of "ghost" surgery; the report concluded that the supervision of organized medicine over ethical standards of physicians was not adequate to protect the public or the good name of the profes-

40. Patricia Kendall's study of medical students in three schools in the 1950s documented a striking difference in career expectations during the course of medical education. In one school, 60 percent of the first year class said they were going into general practice; by the fourth year the proportion was down to 16 percent. This tendency was probably true of most schools at the time, and there is no reason to suppose that it has changed. Patricia L. Kendall and Hanan C. Selvin, "Tendencies Toward Specialization in Medical Training," in Robert K. Merton, George G. Reader, and Patricia L. Kendall, eds., *The Student-Physician* (Cambridge, Mass., 1957), pp. 153–74.
41. O. L. Peterson et al., "An Analytical Study of North Carolina General Practice," *J. med. Educ., 31* (1956), no. 12, pt. 2.
42. Kenneth F. Clute, *The General Practitioner: A Study of Medical Education and Practice in Ontario and Nova Scotia* (Toronto, 1963).

sion.[43] In this environment, it was not surprising that young medical students should choose to specialize. But perhaps the most important factor was that a specialist field is clear-cut. It was relatively straightforward to grasp and define at a time when even the general practitioners were having difficulty in delineating their function and specialty. The scientifically oriented students of the 1950s and 1960s, selected according to their intellectual abilities, naturally gravitated to fields which promised to engage their mental interests.[44] The premise was, of course, that medicine is indeed an intellectual field, all of whose branches would give intellectual gratification rather than the emotional rewards which many of the older general practitioners undoubtedly received in supporting and sustaining their patients. Intellectualism was, after all, the heritage of the Flexner reforms. The generalist was stuck with a virtually impossible definition.

The general practitioners' own efforts to achieve their continuance and enhancement through the professional route, culminating in the foundation of a specialty board, won the battle but not the war. It would be unrealistic to expect board certification to change professional attitudes overnight. What it will do, is to define the new family physician as distinct from the old general practitioners—rather as the board of ophthalmology, when it was set up, distinguished the well-trained ophthalmologist from the "six-week specialist." The major issues still remain. If the new family physician is to stand at the gateway to the patient's medical care, acting as his primary and continuing source of contact with the medical specialties—as seems to be envisaged in the Academy's description of his role—he will require either strong public recognition of this function so that patients choose to use him as a family physician, or the development of appropriate professional or organizational referral structures. Implicit in the success of board certification are thus issues of health care organization, policies, and financing. If present trends continue, and the family physician virtually vanishes, replaced on the one hand by physicians in other specialties and on the other perhaps by nurse-practitioners and physician assistants acting in a similar role, certification will have seemed unnecessary.

So far the traditional professional milieu has not been able to encom-

43. "Report to the Board of Trustees of the American Medical Association of the Committee on Medical Practices, November, 1954," *Northw. Med. (Seattle), 54* (1955), 844–59. This report is said to have been suppressed by the AMA Board of Trustees and did not appear in the AMA *Journal.*
44. On the importance of intellectual interest as a factor influencing specialty choice, see Fremont J. Lyden, H. Jack Geiger, and Osler L. Peterson, *The Training of Good Physicians* (Cambridge, 1968) pp. 49–54 and passim.

pass such questions. The general practitioners, like their colleagues in other fields, have sought professional justifications and solutions for problems of medical practice which demand readjustments in the organization of medical services and a much wider view of the nature of health services than traditional professional structures have provided.

CHAPTER 15

Pressures for New Specialty Boards

A Process of Fragmentation

The decline in the number of general practitioners and the concurrent movement to recognize family practice as a specialty threw into new emphasis the way in which the medical profession was developing. Questions of the availability of health services to the population of the 1940s, as of the 1970s, demanded increasing—not decreasing—generalism in medicine, so that patients could be assured of basic, coordinated medical care when and where they needed it. The specialty certifying boards were established with laudable but quite different aims. Each was predicated on a goal of technological excellence in a defined specialty area, rather than as one component of a manpower plan for adequate service. As the specialty groups came to dominate graduate medical education (and thus the stratification of the medical profession) in the decades following World War II, a curiously structured profession developed. Medicine became a variety of disciplines exercised by specialists of exceptional competence, compared with most other countries of the world. In this the specialty boards could claim great success. Yet these specialists were practicing in the old isolation of solo or small partnership private practice. There was no guarantee that the sum of specializations was adequate service. The specialty boards were on the horns of a dilemma; indeed they largely precipitated it.

Between 1942 and 1952 the total number of active diplomates of the medical specialty boards increased from less than 20,000 to more than 48,000, and by 1969 there were 131,517 (see table 3). By 1950, at least 50 percent of all full-time specialists were board certified, either by examination or through the boards' generous grandfather clauses;[1]

1. It is impossible to distinguish from the available figures the proportion of the total number of active diplomates qualified under grandfather clauses. By 1940, the American Board of Internal Medicine had issued 2,158 certificates, of which only

the proportion is little different today.[2] These changes exerted pressures on the specialty boards for a variety of reasons and from a variety of sources. Their parochial organization—typically with one or two clerks or secretaries working out of an office located in the area where the board president or secretary-treasurer happens to live—was an inappropriate base for a coordinated national examining organization. Their differing requirements and independent assessments of residencies posed problems not only for candidates but also for the hospitals as teaching institutions. Residency services in the hospitals were classified under the rubric of one board or another—whether or not the gynecologist might have benefited from some training in general surgery, or the internist, dermatologist, and neurologist from having their training closely coordinated. Whether the boards should be involved in educational matters at all deserved reexamination. What was to be their purpose—both within organized medicine and on behalf of the public—in a medical profession which was becoming totally stratified into specialties?

THE BOARDS AS PROFESSIONAL ASSOCIATIONS

The autonomy of each board without question stimulated advances in average standards in the specialties. But the boards' pervading influence over almost all residency training, and over certificates which appeared to have an increasing material value, drew sharp criticism from the 1940s. The general practitioners were by no means the only physicians after World War II concerned about the role of specialty certification. Rumors circulated that the boards intended to make it difficult for ex-serv-

358 were by examination; the American Board of Surgery had issued 1,152 certificates under grandfather clauses. W. G. Morgan, *American College of Physicians,* p. 265; Rodman, pp. 6, 28, 47.

2. As previously indicated (see chap. 14, n. 6), the number of board-certified diplomates, after rising dramatically during the 1940s, tapered off and stabilized through the 1950s and 1960s. A study published in 1960 in the *Journal of Medical Education* showed that while 40.6 percent of the class of 1940 were board certified, this percentage had increased to 46.2 percent for the class of 1945. However, in the case of the class of 1950, only 46.6 percent had achieved board certification. Weiskotten et al., "Trends in Medical Education," *J. med. Educ., 35* (1960), 1107. Further evidence of this situation can be seen by examining class trends over a series of five-year periods. Of those physicians graduating from medical school from 1935 to 1939, 41.4 percent were board diplomates. For graduates from 1940 to 1944 the figure was 49.4 percent. From 1945 to 1949 it had reached a high of 56.6 percent, and with the classes of 1950–54 it had begun to decline to 49.8 percent, where it would seem to have stabilized. "Distribution of Physicians by Year of Graduation," *J. Amer. med. Ass., 206* (1968), 2075. See also Appendix tables A2–A4.

Table 3. Annual Specialty Board Certification, 1942–1969[1]

Year	No. of boards in existence	No. certified	Cumulative totals
1942	15	1,756	19,694
1943	15	2,172	21,866
1944	15	1,578	23,444
1945	15	1,308	24,752
1946	15	1,320	26,072
1947	15	2,424	28,496
1948	16	3,002	31,498
1949	19[2]	4,479	35,977
1950	19	3,827	39,804
1951	19	4,552	44,346
1952	19	4,118	48,464
1953	19	4,022	52,486
1954	19	4,133	56,619
1955	19	3,843	60,644
1956	19	3,083	63,727
1957	19	5,424	69,151
1958	19	3,970	73,121
1959	19	4,306	77,427
1960	19	3,985	81,408
1961	19	4,234	85,642
1962	19	4,826	90,468
1963	19	5,376	95,844
1964	19	5,598	101,442
1965	19	5,386	106,827
1966	19	5,852	112,679
1967	19	5,848	118,527
1968	19	6,555	125,221
1969	20	6,296	131,517

1. Figures for 1942 to 1949, inclusive, are for year ended March 31; other years for year ended June 30.
2. One board, the American Board of Proctology, did not certify any candidates during this period.

Source: American Medical Association, *Directory of Approved Internships and Residencies*, selected years.

icemen to attain certification. These were aggravated by the variations among the boards in the credit allowed toward certification for training and experience in the service. There were proposals that the specialty boards be abolished, that they be centralized, and that their relationship to the regulation of medical standards be investigated. The boards, it was claimed, "sit harpie-like with Molotovian veto on progress. . . ." [3]

3. William Bennett Bean, "A Testament of Duty: Some Strictures on Moral Responsibilities in Clinical Research," *J. Lab. clin. Med., 39* (1952), 5–7.

Criticism was stimulated by the continuing intermeshing of the self-interest of specialty associations—including parochial "ethical" questions such as the relationship between anesthesiologist and nurse anesthetists—with educational matters.[4] There was equal dissatisfaction engendered by the lack of unity in educational policy and programs among specialty boards in contiguous fields and by the lack of a strong policy-making group which could evaluate the purpose of graduate education in terms of the evolving demands of medical care.

Members of the boards, with some notable exceptions, appear to have been curiously oblivious to the impact of their certification machinery on graduate medical education, and thus, increasingly, on the emerging structure of the medical profession. A senior member of the American Board of Internal Medicine noted that the board "has never touched the field of medical education directly, either undergraduate or graduate."[5] That board could indeed claim continuous flexibility in its requirements. Yet clearly the stereotyped hospital residencies which had developed by the 1950s, with their rather rigid emphasis on blocks of time to be spent on different activities, were almost entirely the result of specialty board specifications. Even the medical schools found it difficult to develop new types of residencies in their affiliated hospitals without penalizing individuals seeking to conform with the requirements of the boards.[6] In this sense, it was claimed, the specialty boards had usurped the function of the universities. But as yet the universities themselves had shown little interest in regulating graduate medical education. A vicious circle had developed. For a successful and satisfying private practice, the specialist needed privileges at a good hospital. While the hospitals were increasingly careful not to include certification as a prerequisite of appointment, the diplomate had a clear-cut advantage over the nondiplomate, and the man who was not eligible for certification might well be penalized. The situation in civilian medicine in the 1950s was similar to that in the armed forces in World War II.

The continuing discrepancies in the noneducational requirements of the different boards in the early 1950s could not be upheld in this near-monopoly situation. The American Board of Otolaryngology required

4. The minutes of the American Board of Anesthesiology, for example, reveal acute concern by candidates in the 1940s and early 1950s over the attitude of the American Society of Anesthesiologists (to which candidates had at that time to belong) toward the relationship between anesthesiologist and nurse anesthetist, and the acceptability of the physician in salaried hospital practice.
5. Truman G. Schnabel, "The American Board of Internal Medicine," *J. Amer. med. Ass., 152* (1953), 1591.
6. See John E. Deitrick and Robert C. Berson, *Medical Schools in the United States at Mid-Century* (New York, 1953), pp. 278–79 and passim.

candidates to have been U.S. citizens for three years before taking the examination; the American Board of Anesthesiology required candidates to be members of the American Society of Anesthesiologists; the American Board of Obstetrics and Gynecology stated that it would revoke a certificate if the diplomate were expelled from the AMA or any state or county society affiliated with the AMA.[7] None of these requirements had anything to do with technical competence, and little to do with professional integrity.

Most of the obviously irrelevant requirements were to be dropped by the mid-1960s, although five boards still specify citizenship (see Appendix table A5). But there remained a reluctance by the boards to relinquish the privilege of assessing professional behavior. Individual specialty boards are still faced with decisions, based on information through the grapevine of their own members, about whether to admit a particular candidate who is under psychiatric treatment, has a mistress, is suspected of drug addiction, thought to engage in questionable monetary transactions such as fee splitting or bill padding, known to let residents perform operations in his absence without the knowledge of the patient, or (in one reported case) to be a successful publisher of pornography. Such assessments of ethical behavior are not made by the National Board of Medical Examiners, which has a rather similar professional regulatory function to that of specialty certifying boards. Nor is there any logical reason why the specialty boards, as examiners of technical competence, should duplicate responsibilities for adjudicating behavior which are vested in the state examining boards on behalf of the public, and in the county medical societies and AMA Judicial Council on behalf of the medical profession. The problem in the 1950s (and, still, to some extent) was that the specialty boards viewed themselves as extensions of organizations whose purpose was to upgrade the professional status of the specialty, rather than as quasi-public agencies. It was in this "professional" context that requirements such as citizenship were discounted by some senior members of the boards as of minor concern and legitimate interest.[8] The disadvantages of having board mem-

---

7. Robert A. Moore, "Variations on a Theme," *J. Amer. med. Ass., 154* (1954), 1217–18.
8. See, for instance, George M. Lewis, "Evolution, Revolution, and Board Certification," *J. Amer. med. Ass., 156* (1954), 115. For a sampling of other contemporary views on the functioning of the boards, chiefly focusing on their educational inflexibility and professional parochialism, see A. M. Chesney, "Some Impacts of the Specialty Board Movement on Medical Education," *J. Ass. Amer. med. Coll., 23* (1948), 83; Henry A. Christian, "Present Day Undesirable Trends in the Training of Physicians and of Teachers of Internal Medicine," *Ann. intern. Med., 33* (1950), 533–43; H. G. Weiskotten, "Responsibility of a Profession for the Promo-

bership drawn from parent specialist societies were evident. Each board continued to have more in common with the societies in its own specialty than with any of the other boards; the narrow view of each specialty held by each board, each with its requirements, its own examinations, its own residencies overshadowed broader considerations.

While the boards were being criticized both by academic physicians and by candidates who felt their regulations or examinations were unfair, the board members—individual physicians striving to improve conditions in their specialties—had no clear idea of what their role should be.[9] The universities were still showing no inclination to develop their own graduate training programs;[10] nor did the hospitals, greedy for resi-

tion of Educational Standards," *J. Amer. med. Ass., 142* (1950), 1119; William S. Middleton, editorial, "The Value of Specialty Boards," *Minn. Med.* (March 1955); Byrl R. Kirklin, "The Specialty Boards," *J. Amer. med. Ass., 160* (1956), 1327–29; Russell Meyers, "A Critical Look at Medical Education in the United States with Comments on the Role of the Specialty Boards," *Perspect. Biol. Med., 1* (1957–58), 48–68; John McK. Mitchell, "Medical Education and American Specialty Boards," *J. med. Educ., 34* (1959), 555–60; Herman E. Pearse, "The Effect of Specialization on Graduate Education in Surgery," *J. Amer. med. Ass., 170* (1959), 301–09; Robin Buerki, editorial, *J. med. Educ., 35* (1960), 369.

9. A review of the minutes of the American Board of Anesthesiology during the years 1940–50 shows that the idealistic intentions of board members, who gave up hours of their time to grade papers and discuss candidates from the point of view of behavior as well as competence, led to charges of discrimination by candidates, who gave vent to general feelings of frustration and helplessness at autocratic decisions from which they had no appeal. In addition there were criticisms in the national press and hostility from surgical groups. In particular there was criticism of the stand then being made by organized anesthesiology against the nurse anesthetists and against salaried or contract work by anesthesiologists for hospitals. While the board itself did not take a formal position on these issues, it did discuss them at its meetings. When evaluating candidates, the board put emphasis on personal references and reports from local anesthesiologists, seeking information not only on the physician's background but also on the hospital's attitude to anesthesia, the payment arrangements, the anesthetist's standing in the hospital, the surgeon's attitude toward anesthesia and the anesthetist, and the attitudes of other hospital medical staff. The board also asked its local surveyors whether the candidate complied with the ethical standards set out by the American Society of Anesthesiologists and whether his method of remuneration conflicted with that of other anesthesiologists in the area. Besides the competitive element, it was presumed that a salaried anesthesiologist was willing to regard himself as a technician. From 1949 to 1953, prospective diplomates were also required to be members of the ASA. These were all the normal exercises of guild exclusiveness; nor were they by any means restricted to this board. By the late 1940s, however, guildlike restrictionism was an inappropriate organizational form for the exercise of influence over the physician's education. Criticisms of the boards' functions would disappear only when they were able to limit their role to the administration of objective tests of skill. Minutes of the American Board of Anesthesiology, 1944–54.

10. One of the consequences of separate specialty board development was that no accurate statistics were available in the early 1950s as to where all the residencies were located. By 1960, when statistics were available, the majority of residencies

dency staff to man their services, show any promise of stimulating alternative developments in graduate education. There remained therefore no presently existing alternative to the boards. Criticism of their authority, while not unfounded, could not be effective without professional or public guarantees of standards of specialist care. And such assurances were not forthcoming. Thus the boards were in large part insulated against their critics. Feeling misunderstood, each board continued the practices which were deemed by many to be monopolistic and unfair but which the boards themselves considered the normal exercise of professional discretion; there was a continuing breakdown in communication between the boards and the physicians they supposedly served.

ATTEMPTS TO PREVENT FURTHER FRAGMENTATION

A stronger Advisory Board for Medical Specialties might have been able to standardize and rule on ethical questions for all the boards, as well as on educational specifications and (not least) their manpower implications. There was discussion (but only discussion) at the meetings of the Advisory Board in 1942 and 1943 on problems of the distribution and supply of medical specialists and of the possibility of the Advisory Board's initiating a system of long-term specialist manpower planning. But the Advisory Board, while attempting on various occasions to strengthen its central role, had no power over the independent specialty boards; its influence rested on the provision of a forum for debate. And unfortunately many of the debates, rather than stimulating action and cooperation, appear to have had a cathartic effect on the participants.

In 1945, the Advisory Board considered a suggestion by the National Board of Medical Examiners that the boards should have a common basic science examination, under the latter's direction. At the same time, the American Board of Surgery made strenuous but unsuccessful efforts to develop a common examination in surgery for the surgical specialty boards. But the various boards' feeling of independence was too strong. Dr. Rappleye's Advisory Council on Medical Education, which met twice a year between 1939 and 1944 to discuss problems of medical education, considered launching a postwar study of medical education. But at the very time it was most needed, the committee, opposed by the AMA and by the hospitals and lacking its own budget and even office facilities,

---

were in hospitals affiliated with medical schools (17,866, as compared with 12,272 residencies in nonaffiliated hospitals). Medical school affiliation did not, however, mean that the medical school accepted graduate education as an integral university function, and the pattern of training was still that suggested by the specialty boards.

fizzled out; and such projects disappeared with it.[11] Discussion of graduate education continued; but there was no effective structure in which
the outcome of such discussions could be translated into reality.

Unable to achieve unification of the existing specialty boards, the Advisory Board for Medical Specialties announced in 1942 that it would
approve no more certifying boards; further specialty groups would, it
was suggested, be provided for as far as possible within the Boards of
Internal Medicine and Surgery.[12] But the action came rather late. There
were already nine surgical boards: in ophthalmology (incorporated in
1917), otolaryngology (1924), obstetrics and gynecology (1930), orthopedic surgery (1934), urology (1935), surgery (1937), plastic surgery
(1937), anesthesiology (1937), and neurological surgery (1940). There
was also a board of colon and rectal surgery (1935), but this had not yet
received approval by the Council on Medical Education and the Advisory
Board for Medical Specialties. On the medical side, there were six boards;
dermatology (1932), pediatrics (1933), psychiatry and neurology
(1934), radiology (1934), internal medicine (1936), and pathology
(1936). General practitioners were also discussing a board in that area.
Nevertheless, the action of the Advisory Board did prevent yet more
primary stratification. While the American Board of Surgery was unable
to bring under its aegis the surgical specialties which already had autonomous and officially accepted boards, it did create in 1949 a lasting
relationship with the Board of Thoracic Surgery, its acknowledged affiliate.[13] Internists had no authority over the dermatologists or the pediatricians, but the cardiologists, allergists, gastroenterologists, and chest
physicians were firmly annexed in 1941 as subspecialties by the American Board of Internal Medicine. The subspecialty, then, became a convenient device for fitting new groups into the prevailing pattern of the
specialties. In addition to the subspecialties of internal medicine, subspecialties were later to be recognized in pediatric allergy and pediatric
cardiology (the American Board of Pediatrics) and in child psychiatry
(the American Board of Psychiatry and Neurology).[14]

11. Willard G. Rappleye, personal communication.
12. Advisory Board, *Directory of Medical Specialists, 2* (1942), p. 9.
13. In practical terms, affiliate status meant that candidates had to be previously
certified by the parent body and after a specified interval go on to examinations for
the further certification. Affiliate status was dropped in 1970.
14. By 1960, however, the American Board of Internal Medicine was attempting to
reverse the formal fragmentation into subspecialties by discontinuing its own custom of identifying particular residencies for training in allergy, cardiology, and
gastroenterology. By recognizing separate residencies, there were dangers that the
subspecialties would themselves soon feel able to flower as full specialties. Meanwhile separate residencies were identified in pediatric cardiology, pediatric allergy,

The development of subspecialties was by no means painless. The American Board of Internal Medicine had proceeded in 1940 by signing agreements with selected specialist associations for membership on the subspecialty boards (originally called advisory boards) and by using lists provided by these associations of those who were already board certified in internal medicine, a prerequisite of subspecialty certification, to identify those who would enter under grandfather clauses. During the 1940s there were struggles over representation on the subspecialty boards from associations which felt unjustifiably excluded; indignation over whether the board or the subspecialty group had jurisdiction over membership in the subspecialty boards (the former won); and periodic demands from subspecialties for independent board status. The American College of Chest Surgeons pressed for a separate board in that specialty in 1947; the struggle by the allergists for a board continues to this day. The American Diabetes Association applied to the American Board of Internal Medicine in 1943 on the grounds that diabetes had as much right to a subspecialty as did tuberculosis or allergy; but it was turned down by the board the following year. In the wake of so much activity and agitation, in the early 1950s there were serious suggestions in the American Board of Internal Medicine of divesting the board of subspecialty certification and of reforming the board from a specialty board with subspecialties to a board whose interests would range comprehensively over general medicine. These suggestions fell on deaf ears at the time, but were partially achieved in revised board requirements in 1969. In the revision, in full circle, advanced training in general internal medicine was made the equivalent, and not the prerequisite, of training in a subspecialty.[15] Meanwhile, pediatricians, dermatologists, and neurologists continued to be educated along separate specialist tracks, with no common grounding in general medicine. It was still not evident what internal medicine signified and what its relationship to the rest of medicine should be; too many precedents had been set.

The question of precedent was important to specialist groups which had been strengthened during World War II, and in some cases—for example, abdominal surgery and allergy—formally recognized in the services. The existence of autonomous boards was implicit recognition of equality. Urology and orthopedic surgery were recognized as parallel to

and child psychiatry. See editorial, "Roads to Rome," *J. Amer. med. Ass., 174* (1960), 572; and Alexander Nadas, "Pediatric Cardiology and the Sub-Boards," *Pediatrics, 32* (1963), 159–60.

15. For information in the development of subspecialty boards, Dr. Victor Logan generously allowed me to review an early draft of his history of the American Board of Internal Medicine.

general surgery. Why not then, as their protagonists argued, separate treatment for hand surgery, abdominal surgery, or trauma? Dermatology had been recognized as equal to internal medicine; but if dermatology, why not allergy? The existing specialty boards had succeeded because of their struggles to establish a special social and professional identity; the new specialty movements were no different. Despite the policy of the Advisory Board for Medical Specialties to approve new specialties only within the boards of internal medicine and surgery, three further specialty boards were recognized before 1950. Joined by the American Board of Family Practice in 1969, the total number of specialty boards has reached twenty.

THE NEW BOARDS: PROCTOLOGY, PHYSIATRY, AND PREVENTIVE MEDICINE

The new boards were successful on the same grounds as the old, because of their ability to maneuver successfully in relation to other specialty groups. Proctology (now called colon and rectal surgery) had been accepted by the American Board of Surgery as a subspecialty. But the American Board of Surgery closed the founders group in proctology as of January 1944 and after this, candidates had to meet the requirements of both general surgery and proctology. As a result, the would-be proctologist had to undergo five or six years of training. The urologist, on the other hand, certified by a separate board, was required to take only three years of residency training (a subject of some obvious jests). The proctologists, practicing in a neighboring and related field, had no wish to claim any greater skills that such additional training might imply; to them the training system was unfair. Since there seemed to be little likelihood of a reversal of policy within the Board of Surgery, which was committed to a philosophy of general surgical education as a base for the surgical specialties, the only apparent way to shorten the training period was to establish an independent organization.

In 1946 a group of leading proctologists contacted Dr. Byrl Kirklin, then the secretary of the Advisory Board for Medical Specialties, to press for their specialty's independence. The Advisory Board duly discussed proctology at its meeting in February 1947. It was concluded that those interested in practicing proctology alone should not be required to pass the whole examination of the American Board of Surgery, and that those who aimed to do both proctology and colon surgery should be examined in abdominal (rather than general) surgery. The American Board of Surgery did not feel able to comply with these suggestions, which in effect meant a breakdown of the board certificate in surgery at the very time that the board was trying to strengthen its certificate's central position. But there was sympathy for the proctologists from the other surgical specialty boards, who were bent on maintaining their own independence. After the meeting of the Advisory Board in February 1948, Dr. Kirklin (a radiologist) resorted to stronger tactics, informing the American Board of Surgery that the Advisory Board was prepared to give proctologists an independent board if the surgeons would not change their requirements. But this threat had no effect, and in the following year the proctologists were granted separate status. The smallest board (in terms of numbers) had been born virtually by default.[16] One incidental but by no means coincidental factor in the board's success was leadership in colon and rectal surgery at the Mayo Clinic, where Dr. Kirklin and other specialty board leaders were located.

Hand surgery, another surgical specialty for which there were requests for a board in 1948, received no such recognition. Nor did industrial surgery. Nor did traumatic surgery—which was successfully opposed by both the American Board of Surgery and the American Board of Orthopaedic Surgery, each of which considered trauma to be part of its own domain. On at least two occasions trauma was suggested as a possible joint subspecialty of these two boards, but the American Board of Surgery rejected the suggestion,[17] in this instance successfully.

Meanwhile, the orthopedic surgeons were vulnerable to the growing claims of specialists in physical medicine, the physiatrists. Physical medicine provided a bridge between the operating room and complete physical restoration. As the field developed, and under the stimulus of World War II, more physicians began to concentrate on physiatry. By 1949, 234 physicians reported full-time specialist interest in this field;[18] today there are 1,140. While this number was small in relation to the number of hospital departments of physical medicine, it was large enough for the specialists to feel a common interest and to move toward public recognition as an established medical field. Since the nonmedical physical therapists working in hospitals without physiatrists often came under the jurisdiction of the department of orthopedic surgery, there was an obvious conflict of interest among the specialists.

Louis B. Wilson had proposed the establishment of a certifying board

16. By June 1969, the American Board of Colon and Rectal Surgery had awarded over its history only 97 certificates. AMA, *Directory of Approved Internships and Residencies* (1969), p. 340. For the development of the board, see Rodman, pp. 45, 62–63, and passim.
17. Rodman, p. 49.
18. *Health Manpower Source Book, 14,* table 6.

in physical medicine as early as 1936, when he was president of the Advisory Board for Medical Specialties. One of his colleagues at the Mayo Clinic, Frank H. Krusen, had set up the first department of physical medicine there the year before; and the two men had begun negotiations on setting up a specialty board.[19] But Wilson died before any concrete action was taken, and leadership of the Advisory Board moved away from the Mayo Clinic, to return there in the early 1940s when Dr. Kirklin became Advisory Board secretary. By the time Dr. Krusen made a definite request to Dr. Kirklin for a specialty board, the Advisory Board had resolved that new boards were to be placed within the existing board structure. Since physical medicine did not fall neatly into internal medicine or surgery, the Advisory Board set up in 1942 a special committee of three, comprising members respectively of the American Board of Surgery, the American Board of Internal Medicine, and the American Board of Orthopaedic Surgery, to decide on alternatives. This committee, chaired by an orthopedic surgeon, delayed action on an American Board of Physical Medicine for five years. Action was resumed in 1947, when the American Board of Internal Medicine decided to move unilaterally to certify physiatrists, but at the last minute changed its mind. Instead, presumably in reparation for jilting the physiatrists, the internists recommended to the Advisory Board, at its meeting which was held just before the AMA meeting in Atlantic City, that there should be a separate board of physical medicine. Although it was loath to breach its principle of no more independent boards, the Advisory Board concurred; a compromise was reached. The Board of Physical Medicine was set up in that same year with a unique (but short-lived) form, as a subsidiary of the Advisory Board's own Committee on Standards and Examinations; it was not formally independent, but neither was it responsible to any existing board.

The gradual formation of this board in physical medicine was concurrent with the separate development of rehabilitation of the war-wounded. In terms of techniques and personnel, the two fields largely overlapped. But the two terms were not synonymous. There were certain parts of "physical medicine" which were not "rehabilitation", such as application of heat, massage, or exercise to an acutely sprained ankle. There were also parts of rehabilitation which were not physical medicine, such as training for the blind. In general, those who practiced the former worked with physical therapists in general hospitals while those in the latter saw rehabilitation as a new entity, drawing from a wide variety of disciplines and using facilities, such as Howard Rusk's center in New

19. Dr. Frank H. Krusen, personal communication.

York, which existed independently of the hospital. The question was whether these were two specialty fields or one. A request to the AMA Council on Medical Education that it approve a new residency program in medical rehabilitation brought the question to a head. Since the proposed courses were so close to those being offered in the residency program in physical medicine at several medical centers, the council suggested that they should be united in a combined certifying board of physical medicine and rehabilitation. The Advisory Board for Medical Specialties approved the naming of this board in 1948. The following year the American Board of Physical Medicine and Rehabilitation became officially autonomous.[20]

The third specialty board to be approved in the 1940s raised similar questions as to how a medical specialty should be defined. For preventive medicine, like rehabilitation—to which prevention was closely related in the whole cycle from health to sickness and back to health—was not really a specialty at all. As a term, preventive medicine was used as a catchall phrase for the field of interest of physicians in public health agencies, industry, and other areas not closely identified with private practice or hospital residency programs. Since no other group had a lien on the phrase (prevention apparently being far less interesting than cure), there was little opposition to the new board. The area was of low status in comparison with private practice in general and accepted specialties in particular; the movement for a board would encourage numerical gain and raise prestige for a group of physicians who had little share of the professional limelight—and who had, inter alia, suffered during World War II from a lack of specialist identification.

The American Public Health Association and the AMA Section on Preventive and Industrial Medicine were brought together to form the American Board of Preventive Medicine and Public Health in 1948; recognition from the Advisory Board and the AMA Council on Medical Education came in 1949. The original concern of the board was the certification of properly qualified specialists in public health. Quite rapidly, however, specialization developed. The term "and Public Health" was dropped from the board's title in 1952. The following year aviation medicine, a field developed through special courses of instruction dur-

20. One requirement for a board was a national specialist society of at least 100 members. The existing American Congress of Physical Medicine was composed of MDs in *all* fields. A new society exclusively for physicians specializing in physical medicine was thus required—and the American Society of Physical Medicine was formed. With the change in name of the board, this society (renamed "academy") added "and Rehabilitation" to its name.

ing World War II, was added to the certification process; the inclusion of this field for certification coincided with the AMA presidency of Louis H. Bauer, former commandant of the U.S. Air Force aeromedicine school and a leading exponent of the field. Industrial physicians had also been pressing for the establishment of a board, the American Association of Industrial Physicians and Surgeons having begun negotiations with the AMA Section on Preventive and Industrial Medicine for the establishment of a board in 1941. But they lacked a sufficiently powerful lobby. Their request was deferred by the Advisory Board for Medical Specialties, and in 1955 the industrial physicians (specialists in occupational medicine) were included in the American Board of Preventive Medicine. Finally, in 1960, the category of general preventive medicine was added.[21] Thus the American Board of Preventive Medicine developed four parallel specialty tracks. Since there were no residency programs in public health, it became necessary to develop them, often by designating existing positions as "residencies." These were not primarily in hospitals, but in health agencies of various kinds, and the whole system developed with a different focus from the hospital-based training and examining programs on which medical residencies were traditionally based. The close relationship between a specialty board and increasing specialty prestige was never more evident.

The specialty boards had developed as a professional alternative to the political control over specialism which might have emerged through a system of specialist licensure. But, as each of these three new boards had shown, they were themselves part of a dynamic "political" process. There was no guarantee in the establishment of the boards that proctology, physical medicine, and public health, as services, would be better in terms of quality, quantity, or distribution. Acceptance or rejection of new specialty boards was based on the opinion of interested groups. From the public's point of view, it is not clear that orthopedic surgeons should take a major part in deciding whether trauma should be encouraged as a specialty; nor that existing specialty boards should have the power of adjudicating the fate of new specialties, including the long-rejected family practice. Meanwhile, for new professional groups which

21. On the development of this board, see John C. Hume, "Development of Residency Training in Preventive Medicine," *J. Amer. med. Ass., 198* (1966), 271; "Aeromedicine: A New Specialty," *J. Amer. med. Ass., 151* (1953), 1016; T. F. Whayne, "Preventive Medicine in Medical Schools," *Arch. environm. Hlth., 3* (1961), 308–14; "Report of the Education Committee of the American Academy of Occupational Medicine: Board Certification in Occupational Medicine," ibid., *11* (1965), 272–95.

did not fall neatly into any of the established categories, there were incentives for seeking recognition by exerting their own pressures for political separatism.

Within individual boards, too, professional politics operated. The American Board of Ophthalmology, concerned about the low standards of eye surgery, appointed a committee in 1954 to examine the possibility of setting up a new surgical certificate. Two years later, the committee suggested that ophthalmic surgery should be recognized by the board as a subspecialty, following certification in ophthalmology and specified additional experience. But this plan was greeted with vehement opposition by ophthalmologists—including the majority of those board certified, who might have found themselves excluded from hospital surgery in favor of those with the new subspecialty certificate. The plan was dropped, and there is still no public mark of who is and who is not a competent ophthalmic surgeon.

A rather similar situation existed in the American Board of Radiology in relation to radiotherapy. The board recognizes therapeutic radiology as a separate field for certification after a three-year special training in that field plus an additional year of further training or practice; it may be assumed that this is a reasonable level of competence. Yet it continues to offer certification in general radiology, which requires a minimum of only twelve months of therapeutic radiology in a three-year training. Of 10,606 certificates granted by the American Board of Radiology through June 1969, only 344 have been in therapeutics alone. A hospital may thus set up a radiotherapy department with radiologists who, while they may be board certified, are not adequately trained by the board's own standards for radiotherapy. It may be argued that the specialty boards are merely providing opportunities for certification, and that it is the responsibility of hospitals and individuals to examine each physician on his own record, on the principle of caveat emptor. The corollary to this position would however be to allow specialty groups a wide flexibility to examine and issue certificates as they think fit, to give the buyers an effective choice. For example, recognizing an existing situation, the American Board of Surgery might be encouraged to issue two-year, three-year, and four-year certificates to fledgling surgeons whose services, while of less quality than those with a five- or six-year training, might be recognized by hospitals for limited procedures, and by patients because of lower fees.

The position has been generally taken by the boards that they act as qualitative arbitrators in their specialties, and thus implicitly as guardians of the public interest. It was here that there was a conflict between professionalism and patient care in the 1950s and 1960s.

THE POLITICS OF FAILURE: ABDOMINAL SURGERY

The dilemma of reconciling the public and professional implications of specialist certification, apparent in successful boards, is even more apparent in those which have been unsuccessful; abdominal surgery is a major example. Abdominal surgeons made up a substantial group who felt they did not fit into the prevailing pattern. In the armed services abdominal surgery had been organized as a specialty section, and those so assigned regarded their field as parallel to other specialties. There existed, however, no civilian structure which would automatically accept them. The American Board of Surgery examined in general surgery; it refused to bend its standards for those without the required five-year residency training.[22] Like the proctologists, during the 1950s the potentially much more numerous abdominal surgeons saw the formation of a separate specialty board as the obvious course of action.

The driving force behind the new organization was Dr. Blaise Alfano, who received his M.D. degree in 1950, finished his residency in 1954, and went into private surgical practice in Massachusetts. In 1957 he wrote to eighteen chiefs of service of hospitals with residency programs in surgery suggesting the foundation of a board for abdominal surgery, and he received ten favorable replies.[23] These men promptly organized themselves as the Board of Governors of an American Board of Abdominal Surgery, with Dr. Alfano as the secretary. Strong opposition from the American Board of Surgery, the Advisory Board, and possibly other surgical specialties, was inevitable.

The new group set standards for qualification which followed the "essentials" for approved boards, and suggested as acceptable training for foundation members four years of residency or three years of formal training and two years of practice or sixteen years of acceptable practice. Such standards provided a convenient means of certification for many

22. Qualifications for the American Board of Surgery by 1946 included at least five years of special training in surgery following a year's internship. Three of the five years had to be in general surgery, and two years might be spent in specified related fields. One year of credit was given for the first year of service with the armed forces, and further credit was possible when merited by army medical experience. Advisory Board, *Directory of Medical Specialists, 3* (1946), 876–77.
23. Unless otherwise stated, information on the abdominal surgeons is from Dr. Blaise Alfano, personal communications.

surgeons who had missed the foundation group of the American Board of Surgery (which had been closed in 1941) and who did not qualify for the examinations of that board but who might well be reasonably trained. As foundation standards, they were not out of line with the previous grandfather clauses of the boards already in existence, and the immediate response to the new board was outstanding.[24] By September 1959, 4,300 applications had been received; and by 30 June 1960, when the founders group was closed, there had been 5,383. The Board of Abdominal Surgery had begun to represent a real threat to established institutions.

Within four months of the founders' letter going out, all ten members of the original board of governors (whose names were prominent on the letterhead) had resigned. These surgeons had found themselves in a peculiar position. The new board had not sprung from the mutual effort of established societies and had not been authenticated by the usual authorities—a fact emphasized in a prominent, black-bordered statement in the *Bulletin of the American College of Surgeons*.[25] Fellows of the College were urged not to lend their support to the board before its official professional approval. The College was particularly sensitive to the issue, for only a few years earlier it had been fighting another potential contestant, the International College of Surgeons, which had also attempted to found a specialty board in surgery. This board had been abolished in 1952 after opposition from the American College of Surgery and the American Medical Association, both of which maintained that there could be no justification for more than one certifying board in the same professional field.[26] Thus in the fall of 1958, Dr. Alfano had no board of governors, the opposition of the major professional organizations in surgery, and a desk piled high with applications for board membership. There were two urgent needs: first, the creation of a new board of governors, and second, an adequate mechanism to handle the applications. The two interlocked. Dr. Alfano's board of trustees (himself, his brother, and a judge of the Superior Court of Massachusetts)

24. These conditions may be compared with the grandfather clause of the American Board of Surgery, as set out in 1936. That board automatically included all members of certain surgical societies together with all full, associate, and assistant professors in class A medical schools, and allowed a 2-year grace period during which those who had limited their practice to surgery for the previous 15 years could apply and be certified without examination. The American Board of Surgery ultimately included 1,152 founders without examination; the number was equaled by diplomates by examination in 1943. Davis, *Fellowship of Surgeons*, pp. 343–44; Rodman, pp. 28, 47.
25. *Bull. Amer. Coll. Surg., 43* (1958), 244.
26. L. Davis, *Fellowship of Surgeons*, pp. 408, 411, 502–03.

selected surgeons in each state, some 300 in all, as state credentials committees to review applications in accordance with the standards already set out. These men collectively formed the new board of governors. The new board held its first meeting in Atlantic City in September 1959. Meanwhile the board's long quest for official approval began.

The requirements for professional approval—since revised, as a direct outcome of the abdominal surgeons' quest—included official sponsorship of the board by the relevant national societies and the appropriate AMA section, and subsequent approval by both the AMA Council on Medical Education and the Advisory Board for Medical Specialties. The Advisory Board's decision that any new special groups should be provided for, so far as possible, within the Boards of Medicine and Surgery was strengthened in 1950 (after the approval of the proctologists, physiatrists, and public health physicians) by agreement with the Council on Medical Education that the greatest discretion should be exercised in approving any new boards. Other requirements included recognition of the new group as a "distinct specialty of medicine" and a membership in the special field of at least one hundred members. Except for the last, these were formidable requirements, but the abdominal surgeons were undaunted. In February 1959 the journal *Abdominal Surgery* was launched, and a series of editorials exhorted readers to consider the formation of the board. Efforts were being made meanwhile to win the approval of the AMA Section on Surgery.[27] This last was a vital preliminary in the political process of board approval. But the officers of the section were not in favor of any such endorsement. Bitter fighting developed between the section and the abdominal surgeons from October 1958, when the first application was made, until June 1961, when the abdominal surgeons gained a majority at the annual meeting of the section, passed a resolution in approval of a board of abdominal surgery, and elected their own representatives as the new section officers. The AMA House of Delegates reportedly attempted to reverse the section proposals, but this action was disallowed on administrative and consti-

27. Its full name, somewhat irritatingly to those who opposed the abdominal surgeons, was the "Section on Surgery, General and Abdominal." This title was a legacy of infighting before World War I, when both gynecologists and general surgeons claimed priority in the abdomen. It could now be used to indicate that "general" and "abdominal" surgery were somehow different. At the section meeting during the AMA meeting at Atlantic City in June 1959, the chairman took as his theme the section's name, purpose, and history. He argued for a return to generalism in surgery, particularly in teaching medical students; and he urged, in reviewing its history, modification of the section name. This latter was duly done, and the section became the Section on General Surgery. See John H. Mulholland, "Surgery, General and Abdominal, 1859–1959," *J. Amer. med. Ass., 171* (1959), 550–53.

tutional grounds by the AMA Law Department. During the same period, to meet the objection that there was as yet no specialist society representing the group, the American Society of Abdominal Surgeons was formed; and the first Clinical Congress of Abdominal Surgeons was held in 1960.

The representatives of organized medicine and surgery had chosen to fight abdominal surgeons through the formal organizational machinery for establishing specialty boards, rather than by opening up for discussion the future of general and abdominal surgery or the possible limitations of the existing certification system in terms of specialization or fragmentation. This opposition had backfired. By taking over the AMA section machinery, and with the backing of a large specialist group, the abdominal surgeons had both a prima facie case for board approval and the large numbers which made their pressure politically strong. By 1961 the founders group alone numbered 2,266. Those opposing the new board were interested in revealing exactly who these members were. In 1962, therefore, the AMA Council on Medical Education, intending to bring the now protracted dispute concerning the board to a conclusion, held a unique hearing, attended by representatives of both the American Board of Abdominal Surgery and the American Board of Surgery. The very fact that such a hearing was held, reporting the views of both sides to members of the AMA House of Delegates, drew attention to the factors which had become the basis for specialty board approval. Following the hearing, the Council on Medical Education rejected the claims of the abdominal surgeons.[28]

In essence the council rejected abdominal surgery as a legitimate spe-

---

28. First, it was stated that abdominal surgery as defined ("surgery pertaining to the contents of the abdominal cavity, its walls and orifices") was the sum of components already recognized in the American Boards of Surgery, Obstetrics and Gynecology, and Colon and Rectal Surgery. Thus the new board did not meet the requirement of the Essentials that it represent a "recognized and distinct specialty or well-defined field of medicine." Second, and perhaps on more shaky ground, a distinction was made between specialties which were based on different organ systems, or differing modalities of diagnosis or therapy, and specialties which were circumscribed on a primarily anatomical basis, such as abdominal surgery; existing approved specialties, it was claimed, essentially reflected a functional and methodological approach. But while these statements were generally true, it was not entirely so. Colon and rectal surgeons covered an area already included by the American Board of Surgery; thoracic surgery included an anatomic area bisecting several organ systems; gynecological surgeons did not always restrict themselves to surgery of the female reproductive system. The case of the abdominal surgeons seemed destined to run into questions of semantics and to shed more light on the artificiality of other specialty demarcations than on the future of surgery. "Supplementary Report of the Council on Medical Education and Hospitals," *Proc. AMA House of Delegates* (June 1962), pp. 63–73.

cialty of medicine. Abdominal surgery, it was claimed, brought no new tool or technique as a focus for specialism. No residency programs had been set up in abdominal surgery; the board's structure was criticized; and the council took the view that the educational standards of a new board should be higher, not lower, than those of the American Board of Surgery, something the politics of the upstart board militated against. In short, abdominal surgery was to remain a refinement or subspecialty of general surgery. The onus for training surgeons to operate in the abdomen was put squarely on the American Board of Surgery, which indeed was already devoting a major part of residency training to abdominal surgery and a large part of its board examination to the abdomen, and whose diplomates were in effect primarily abdominal surgeons.

But if this were so, it was logical to ask why the American Board of Surgery was not an acceptable base for those seeking an identity in abdominal surgery. A study by the AMA of a sample of the abdominal surgeons' founders group had indicated that these on the whole were full-time surgical specialists; nearly 60 percent of the sample were already certified by one of the approved specialty boards. Nearly half the sample, however, including some of those already certified under the approved boards' generous grandfather clauses, had no more than two years' residency training; in terms of the requirements of the American Board of Surgery, they were less than half-trained.[29] Even in its own terms, the Board was guilty of admitting as founders some surgeons of much lower training than might be expected of its diplomates by examination. The surgical board—which had, after all, been founded in the 1930s as the basis for surgical excellence rather than an all-inclusive badge of merit for the small-town surgeon—thus had a prima facie case for excluding them. But whatever the merits of the case, a new board would encroach on established professional patterns, to which a natural reaction was opposition rather than cooperation. No suggestions were made at the time for taking a new look at the patterns themselves, the

29. The AMA ran a 20 percent sample of the 2,266. They were shown to be a heterogeneous group. Of the 453 members sampled, 75 percent were members of the American College of Surgeons, and 24 percent members of the International College of Surgeons. Ninety-four percent were stated to be full-time specialists, and 97 percent said their primary interest was in surgery. The group was thus not primarily of general practitioners and clearly contained a large number of surgeons whose competence was already attested from other sources. Length of residency was thus their principal weak point. However it was entirely possible that a similar survey of other specialty boards, some of which had also had large foundation groups, would have had similar results. The sample was thus a sample without reference to any control; and no subsequent studies have yet been done to make comparison possible. Ibid., p. 71.

nature of training in surgery as a whole, and the desirable educational process for the production of surgeons. No overtures appear to have been made by the American Board of Surgery to the abdominal surgeons, or vice versa, to see what their objections were, and whether they had any validity in terms of surgical standards. Nor was it evident that if the abdominal surgeons failed, the American Board of Surgery would be able to fill the gap. On the other hand there was ample evidence that, from the patient's point of view, the existence of the board in general surgery, with its high standards, had neither limited the number of self-styled surgeons nor restricted surgery to the better-qualified. Either the board needed to exert its position as a potential monopoly on surgical practice, to protect the public, or it would remain vulnerable to charges that its standards were too high for the average surgeon.

It was possible that the abdominal surgeons, if not approved, would attempt to exist as a maverick group, offering a second-class examination for those who failed the Board of Surgery. The actions of the established surgical organizations and the AMA had demonstrated that this was against the profession's interest. Yet in the public interest, it might have been desirable to provide an alternative channel for physicians to achieve recognized surgical training or to insist that all surgeons take the higher training. But there was as yet no machinery to do so. Meanwhile 2,500 surgeons continued to think they were practicing a specialty when organized medicine considered they were not. While a pronouncement had been made on the inadmissibility of abdominal surgery as a medical field, it was still steadily progressing as a self-recognized professional force. By 1967 the American Society of Abdominal Surgeons included more than 9,000 members. Pressures for a specialty board continued to be felt within the AMA surgical section.[30] Meanwhile there have been continued attempts to redefine the foundation membership of the board through imposing higher eligibility requirements. Here, temporarily, the matter

30. The abdominal surgeons retained control of the AMA Section on Surgery for 1962–63, with Dr. Alfano as its secretary through 1962–65. But, encouraged by the American College of Surgeons, the general surgeons rallied, and at the California meeting of 1964 the abdominal surgeons lost office; they were defeated again in June 1965 at the New York AMA meeting. In 1967, at a meeting in which charges of "packing" and of "unethical" practices were made by those deposed, the abdominal surgeons once again regained control. "Abdominal Surgeons Win AMA Section Leadership," *Medical Tribune,* 3 July 1967; "AMA Delegates Defy Abdominal Surgeons Actions," ibid., 6 July 1967. The power conflict between the two groups was resolved by modifying the membership of the Section Council to include representatives of various interests, including two representatives from the Society for Abdominal Surgeons.

rests: a threat to the fabric of the specialty boards, and a continued question mark as to the future regulation of surgery.

The confrontations of the abdominal and the regular surgeons, who themselves do mostly abdominal surgery, offer fascinating insights into the political infrastructure of modern medicine. There is something remarkably odd in a system which, in delineating in the name of the public what is a useful and proper area for specified graduate training and specialty regulation of physicians, relies on the number of partisans each side can muster. The jockeying of various groups and persons for positions on the Advisory Board for Medical Specialties had succeeded in the case of the colon and rectal surgeons, physiatrists, and specialists in public health; but it was in the last resort a crude means of making decisions that had impacts on the structure of specialist medical care. In the struggles of the abdominal surgeons the duality of defining a specialty was once again brought out. Somehow the scientific, professional, and social elements inherent in specialty demarcations needed to be synchronized.

OTHER SPECIALTIES

The shifting nature of scientific and social demands means that the medical specialties are in a constant process of flux, battering against the rigid demarcations of the profession. The would-be allergist, for example, may still obtain certification in his field only by first taking the examinations of the American Board of Internal Medicine and then its subspecialty examination in allergy. The board-certified dermatologist has no direct route to certification as an allergist, nor does the board-certified psychiatrist; yet both dermatologists and psychiatrists have legitimate interests in the field. Of 902 full-time and part-time allergists in 1961, only 154, or 17 percent, were board certified, a much lower proportion than in most other specialties.[31] Allergists have claimed that the increasing complexity of their field demands special training programs and separate specialist certification, that there is no case for separating allergy of adults and allergy of children (pediatric allergists receiving their training through the American Board of Pediatrics), and that the existing certifying boards are not interested in the field.[32] Unlike the abdominal

31. *Health Manpower Source Book,* sec. 14, table 9; and see Appendix table 1.
32. See "Report of an Ad Hoc Committee of Section on Allergy of the American Medical Association, Presented to the Section June 27, 1966," *Ann. Allergy, 24* (1966), 511–13.

surgeons, however, the ranks of the allergists have been divided, in part because of a difference in views between those who regard themselves as allergists and those who are immunologists. Just as the AMA Section on Allergy was deciding in 1966 to approach the Advisory Board for Medical Specialties to ask for an independent board, an unapproved board was set up by a new specialist organization, the American Association of Clinical Immunology and Allergy—an action group to counter stalement between the other allergy organizations.[33] The American Board of Clinical Immunology and Allergy, with its own training and certification mechanism, stands outside the Advisory Board structure ,in a rather similar relation to the "approved" boards as that of the Board of Abdominal Surgery. Thus the questions remain: whether allergy has reached the stage of being a full-fledged "specialty" and what organizational responses are most appropriate to meet the expressed needs of those with interests which cross established specialty lines.

Another example of increasing specialist overlap is endocrinology, a valuable adjunct of medicine, surgery, and gynecology. A third is nuclear medicine, which is now a part of surgery, internal medicine, pediatrics, pathology, and other specialties, rather than strictly a subspecialty of radiology. And there are others. The stresses on the structure of the specialty boards have been particularly severe where a new group seeks a relationship between two specialties, each of which already has a board, as for example between pediatrics and neurology, pediatrics and radiology, pediatrics and surgery. Pediatric cardiology, on the other hand, was approved as a subspecialty of pediatrics and child psychiatry as a subspecialty of psychiatry in 1960.

A field still in dispute as a recognized subspecialty is pediatric surgery, which emerged after World War II as a specialist interest supported by pediatricians rather than by the general surgeons.[34] Indeed, the first

33. S. H. Jaros, "The Totem Pole and Clinical Immunology," *Ann. Allergy, 24* (1966), 508–09; Dr. Clifton Brooks, personal communication.
34. Surgeons had concentrated before this on the surgery of children in children's hospitals. Dr. William E. Ladd began to teach pediatric surgery in Boston in 1908 as a member of the visiting staff of Boston Children's Hospital, where he remained for 20 years. Many of today's leaders in pediatric surgery were trained under him. Generally, however, the specialty developed as surgical pediatrics—a surgical interest—rather than as a new specialty. In the late 1940s Dr. Herbert Coe of Seattle entered into negotiations with the American Academy of Pediatrics to establish a section of pediatric surgery, and the pressure for separate recognition began. See Herbert E. Coe, "Pediatric Surgery in North America: A Review of Its Development and Progress," Paper delivered at International Congress of Paediatrics, 22 July 1959, Montreal, mimeographed. For information on the development of pediatric surgery and its attempts to acquire board approval, I am indebted to

request to the American Board of Surgery for special recognition of pediatric surgery (made in 1955) was through the American Academy of Pediatrics. In 1956 the American Board of Surgery agreed to establish a mechanism for certification in pediatric surgery, but this proposal was blocked in the Advisory Board for Medical Specialties; pediatric surgery, after all, cut across specialties other than general surgery, including urology and orthopedics, and its acceptance by the other surgical specialty boards might entail a threat to the integrity of their own fields. In this horizontal aspect, pediatric surgery bore professional dangers similar to those of the specialty of trauma, which was brought up again at the same time. The American Board of Surgery withdrew its support of pediatric surgery in 1957, but again the debate has continued.

As in the earlier development of specialties, new areas of interest could not be neatly categorized. In the 1930s, the struggle for a certifying board was part of each specialty's defining process. The struggle for recognition from the 1950s to the present has been equally concerned with describing each field. At the scientific level there are questions of building a cadre of talent for the future, so that current developments in the special field will in fact be translated into practice, teaching, and new research. And these questions shade into other interests, such as the establishment of departments in the specialty in major university medical centers and large hospitals, the provision of separate, earmarked training grants from the National Institutes of Health, and the expectation that there would be a gradual increase in the referral of patients. By now, however, the field is crowded with the claims and constraints of the older organizations. New special interests such as pediatric anesthesiology or pediatric urology (and, for that matter, pediatric radiology and pediatric neurology) could be classed with pediatric surgery and child psychiatry as attempts to focus the traditional specialty groupings around the needs of the child. On the other hand, there are specialty boards in each of the sectional areas, and the definition of a specialty division by age group does not hold up outside pediatrics; there is still, for example, no specialty board for gerontology. A growing interest in nephrology—the study of kidney conditions—could be classified schematically as being similar in emphasis to cardiology, both focusing on particular organ systems and being offshoots of internal medicine. But fetology, the study of the human fetus, could be seen both as a subspecialty of obstetrics and as an extension back into the embryo of pediatrics. Hand surgery, whose

Prof. Lawrence Pickett of Yale University Medical School, chairman of AAP Section on Surgery.

exponents still have no separate certification, is like head and neck surgery or abdominal surgery in its application of surgical techniques to a specific part of the body, and could be seen as an adjunct of general surgery. Yet groups such as otolaryngologists and the colon and rectal surgeons had long-established precedents for a regionally defined surgical focus. Other new specialties are arising around new machinery, just as, over a hundred years ago, ophthalmology developed around the ophthalmosocope, and over sixty years ago, radiology around the X-ray machine. The laser, the hyperbaric chamber, and the increasing use of electronic devices are their modern equivalents.

Ideally the framework of medicine would be sufficiently flexible to allow for specialization in any potentially beneficial direction. Professional structures had not met the need. By the 1960s it was only too clear that the uncoordinated framework of the specialty boards allowed little open discussion of the development of medical fields in terms of their potential value in rendering health care to the public and that its rigidity was an increasingly unsatisfactory response to the dynamic process of specialization. Medicine became a variety of skills, tied to definitions of "specialties" which were developed in the 1920s and 1930s.

THE BOARDS IN TRANSITION

The juxtaposition of the older structures for specialty regulation with the demands for new specialties produced a byzantine web of specialist training programs and examinations. Together, the twenty approved boards in existence in 1970 offered certification in forty-five specialty and subspecialty areas; in addition, five boards give separate certificates to foreign graduates (see Appendix table A5). In some boards, alternative certificates proliferated; the American Board of Pathology offers seven types of certification in virtually distinct specialties and the American Board of Radiology, ten. Yet there are still demands from unrecognized groups for further demarcations. The specialty boards had begun modestly in the years before World War II, when their purpose was to provide a limited cadre of experts; they were overtaken by events. Responsible for the shape, length, and standards of 42,000 hospital residencies, the specialty boards assumed a responsibility for medical education (or had it thrust upon them) which is as great as that of the universities.

Other professions have split apart, or recognized specialties, under the impact of an enlarged body of knowledge; there are, for example, tax lawyers, corporation lawyers, labor lawyers, and other specialists in the finer points of law. But in no other profession has there been the necessity for such a complete and sudden stratification of skills as in medicine in the post-World War II decades. Onto the earlier process of standardizing medical practice into one profession, with high-caliber medical schools, is superimposed a new mode of professional fragmentation, with new (and shifting) responsibilities. In their development, the specialty boards emphasized the narrowness of response within the medical professional to what was nothing less than a technological revolution.

The blend of oligarchy and jostling for a place in the sun which distinguished the development of the various specialty boards is clearly inappropriate for a situation in which all physicians are to be recognized as specialists. Thus the boards are now in a period of transition to new (but as yet unspecified) forms and purposes. During the 1950s and much of the 1960s the older specialty boards claimed immunity from criticism because of their purely educational function, just as general practitioners viewed their development in terms of education and certification rather than of the necessary redefinition of the role of a generalist or of generalism in a highly stratified health service system. But already the tide was changing. One impetus for change was the development of examining techniques that made it possible for the boards to depend more heavily on assessment of candidates at one point in time and less on other individual assessments, including educational experience and colleague references. A second was the belated emergence, from the mid-1960s, of university interest in graduate medical education; a third, the potential need for some certification of specialty status (if not quality) in any future health service system.

The mood of the specialty board examination itself began to change, at least in the more progressive boards, in the 1950s. One secretary of the Board of Psychiatry, describing the organization of that board's unscreened oral examination in the 1950s (which disorganized the work of a hospital for a week) reported, "Candidates arrive in panic, and the secretary's first duty is to have a period of group psychotherapy." [35] In the 1960s this board followed others in initiating a first-stage written examination, a move facilitated by the general acceptance of multiple-choice examining techniques. With this latter development it was possible for the specialty boards to move quite rapidly from subjective ap-

35. Francis J. Braceland and David A. Boyd, "Secretary of the Board: Apologia Pro Vita Sua," *J. Amer. med. Ass., 148* (1952), 711.

praisals of "fitness" to objective, computerized tests, a leader of which was the National Board for Medical Examiners, which incorporated multiple-choice tests into its own examination in the early 1950s. The American Board of Pediatrics set up the first formal arrangement with the National Board for assistance in its written examination in 1961. Eight of the twenty specialty boards were drawing on the expertise of the National Board by the spring of 1970, including the Board of Family Practice. There was no intention in this process of technical assistance of subjugating the function of the specialty boards to the National Board of Medical Examiners. Nevertheless, through these activities, and through a continuing series of evaluations of physician performance and training programs, the National Board is becoming an important focus and resource of testing competence in specialized medicine. Having lost the opportunity to coordinate specialist qualifications in the early 1930s, the National Board now has a new potential as the future coordinating and technical agency for specialty certification.

Most boards now require a written examination, followed after a specified length of time by an oral examination. Eligibility for the oral examination of most boards occurs after at least one year of practice following specified training; specified residency training ranges from two years (pediatrics) to five years (surgery), following a one-year internship. The American Board of Internal Medicine may be leading a trend, however, in allowing its examinations to be taken immediately after the residency. Indeed, the specialty boards and their related specialist associations are going through a period of ferment that began in the 1960s and has been generated by knowledge and the need for knowledge in evaluating competence. The American Board of Orthopaedic Surgery has been involved in research to define the specialty as a result of which the board examinations have been modified. The Boards of Neurological Surgery and of Obstetrics and Gynecology have set up in-training tests for the evaluation of residents. And several boards are following the example of the American College of Physicians, which developed in 1967 informal, voluntary self-assessment examinations as a form of continuing education.

One development of particular importance was the decision of the American Board of Internal Medicine to set up a general qualifying examination after two years of residency; this was followed by the present proposals for full certification in general internal medicine after three years of graduate (post M.D.) education. Meanwhile, at the meeting of the Advisory Board of Medical Specialties in February 1970, a surgical council was finally organized to set up a common basic surgical examination, again to be taken by surgical specialists after three years of training; it is intended to begin the examination in 1972. A third major development is the decision by the American Board of Family Practice, followed by a similar announcement from the American Board of Internal Medicine, that they will require periodic recertification; a certificate will only be valid for a stated number of years (six years for family practitioners). These moves extend the range of the specialty boards back into the residency and forward into the testing of practicing physicians. Again, many of these new developments are being conducted in cooperation with the National Board for Medical Examiners.

Finally, after 37 years of indeterminate function and status, the Advisory Board of Medical Specialties voted to strengthen its organization. At the same meeting which voted for a common surgical examination that would tie together at least the basic science elements of the separate surgical specialty boards, the Advisory Board agreed to change its name to the potentially stronger American Board of Medical Specialties. The future functions of the new organization have been described. Besides the old functions of approving new specialty boards as they arise (through the Liaison Committee for Specialty Boards), issuing the Directory of Medical Specialists, and providing a forum for discussion among specialty board representatives, the reconstituted Board has specific authority to generate both educational and manpower studies, including studies of the "proportionate production of medical specialists" and "their relationships with members of allied health professions." [36] With the motto, *Animis Opibusque Parati* (Prepared in Knowledge and Resources) pointing toward an expanded service as well as educational role, and standing as a representative organization for all specialties, including family practice, the American Board of Medical Specialties could develop into an important focus for medical specialty policies and development.

All these activities strengthen the role of the specialty certifying boards as independent voluntary examining agencies, akin, in the graduate period, to the role of the National Board in testing physicians in and after medical school, but scattered in twenty different places. But there remain the continuing and less certain roles of the boards as fragmented and introverted professional organizations, governed by representatives from component specialist societies; as educational agencies, still heavily involved in graduate medical education; and as quasi-licensing agencies, with a substantial if by no means complete influence on the specialist distributions of physicians.

36. *The American Board of Medical Specialties,* leaflet, February 1971.

The establishment of the American Board of Medical Specialties does not necessarily herald a greater cohesion among the boards in the future than in the past; nor the resolution of the various directions and purposes of board certification. The same impetus for independence in each specialty, the guarding of each specialty's boundaries, exists now as it did on the other occasions when a cohesive policy for specialty development has been suggested. Nevertheless the auguries are more hopeful now than in earlier periods. The history of the specialty boards, like that of other organizations, has shown that changes arise not out of committees or other structures but from a combination of personal leadership and outstanding pressures. In an almost cyclical development, the new American Board has as its president the director of the National Board of Medical Examiners, Dr. John P. Hubbard. This tying together of the two sets of examining structures is of particular importance; for the National Board itself as the primary external evaluator of medical students is also facing a reevaluation of the goals and purposes of medical education. The retirement of Dr. Louis A. Buie, Sr., after many years as executive director of the Advisory Board for Medical Specialties also provided the opportunity to move the organization from Rochester, Minnesota (and, incidentally, the long, if tenuous relationship between the specialty board structures and the Mayo Clinic), to the Chicago area. The American Board was incorporated in April 1970; the central office was set up in July in Evanston, Illinois. Geographically, the Board is thus well-sited in relation to other educational organizations, notably the AMA. At the same time Dr. John C. Nunemaker was made executive director of the American Board. His previous role as director of graduate medical education for the Council of Medical Education of the AMA adds another dimension to future cooperation among the professional agencies.

But while these and other personal links are significant factors in the developing role of the specialty certifying organizations, eclipsing them in importance are the growing outside pressures for change in the educational and regulatory structures of medicine. Who is to be responsible for deciding whether there should be fewer or more family practitioners? Which organization will ultimately adjudicate how far the move by abdominal surgeons for a specialty board is a reflection of broader manpower issues—for example, that there are now too many surgeons? The specialty boards have not taken responsibility for these kinds of decisions, and are perhaps not the appropriate organizations to do so. The need for such decisions, however, will force some organization (governmental, private, or mixed) to assume regulatory authority over specialty manpower development. If it does not move quickly into this sphere, the American Board (and thus the specialty boards) will find itself bypassed. The future of the American Board is thus poised between a situation on the one hand of statesmanlike authority for adjudicating, or at least assisting in the development of, policies in such areas as the appropriate numerical production of physicians by specialty, the impact of certification on American and foreign-trained physicians, or the desirability of new coordinated forms of conjoint examining boards for physicians in overlapping specialties (such as allergy or nuclear radiology); and on the other hand, of attenuated functions in providing only a qualifying test (similar to the Medical Colleges Admissions Test or the National Board examinations) for externally determined specialties.

Which way—and how quickly—the specialty boards will develop is an important question for the 1970s. The boards now have the opportunity for rapid, coordinated action, but there is as yet little evidence that they will seize it. Meanwhile, a series of simultaneous and connected developments in the medical schools and in graduate medical education in teaching hospitals are creating further pressures on the structure and regulation of specialized medicine. As national health insurance approaches, all of these professional systems are in rapid transition.

CHAPTER 16

Professionalism and the Medical School

A hundred years ago the physician was trained largely by apprentice-ship, supplemented by didactic teaching in small proprietary schools. Teaching was closely linked with practice, and vice versa. There was a marked absence of licensing laws, or other restraints on medical educa-tion; and it was customary for medical students to enter a three-year preceptorship with only a common-school education. In short, except for those who went abroad after a college education, medical education was parochial, clinical, and socially open, drawing its students from a diversity of economic backgrounds. The medical schools themselves were didactic institutions, designed to supplement but not offer clinical teach-ing; and thus many of these remained until the educational reform move-ment, epitomized by the Flexner report, swept them away or expanded them into the clinical-research models of the major Eastern medical schools. In the post-Flexner reforms the medical schools largely ignored the training of the medical specialist. Instead, hospital residency pro-grams developed under the aegis of the profession and became the major focus for practitioner training. Undergraduate medical education became a preprofessional process, and the universities lost the vocational purpose which had been the dominant theme of the Flexner report; only now are the medical schools beginning seriously to reevaluate their role in gradu-ate (vocational) medical education.

But while the Flexner reforms were far-reaching and pervasive, with echoes reverberating to the present day, the medical schools were soon under pressures for further reforms. By the 1940s medicine could no longer be regarded as one scientific discipline. It was, rather, a federation of diverse disciplines, founded on anatomy, physiology, bio-chemistry, microbiology, and other scientific areas which in themselves were rapidly expanding and blossoming into a series of clinical and research specialties. These scientific developments radically changed the character of medical education during the 1950s, emphasizing the production of the physician as a high-grade scientific specialist. During the 1950s, moreover, the federal government assumed and expanded the role which in the 1920s and 1930s had been that of private foundations, namely the subsidization of scientific medical research. By 1960, the medical school was in large part a federally dominated research institution whose purpose was only partially to educate student physicians. In 1969, over 272,000 students who were not medical students in the traditional sense received some instruction in medical schools. They included graduate physicians, research scientists, nurses, public health students, and a variety of other health personnel. Even in terms of full-time student equivalents, non-M.D. students outnumbered student physicians by about three to two.[1] In the 1960s, too, medical schools became involved in the operation of mental health centers, neighborhood health centers, regional medical programs, prepaid group practice schemes, and other innovative service programs, which promise to increase in emphasis in the 1970s. Many of these activities were also undertaken under the primary stimulus of federal funding, arising out of the medical care legislation of the Eighty-eighth and Eighty-ninth Congresses, and through a rising sense of awareness within the universities of community responsibility and social action.

Today's medical school, with its sprawling complex of departments, teaching programs, research units and service facilities, its sheer size, its dependence on public support, bears little resemblance to the schools which emerged from World War II, whose mission was primarily to educate physicians. As a result of these rapid and continuing changes, the medical schools are faced not merely with crucial questions of medical student education, in terms of educational standards, student numbers, and curricula; they are concurrently grappling with their own future as institutions.

MEDICAL PROFESSIONALISM AND THE NEW PROPRIETOR

The most striking and far-reaching change in medical school development since World War II has been in its sources of financing, and thus in the long run in control. Abraham Flexner long ago remarked, "Practically the medical school is a public service corporation." [2] At a time

1. The AMA estimated that the 272,000 students represented teaching equivalents of about 55,000, compared with nearly 36,000 undergraduate medical students. "Medical Education in the United States and Canada," *J. Amer. med. Ass., 210* (1969), 1476–78.
2. Flexner report, p. 154.

when medical education was almost entirely financed from private funds, his argument was based on the accountability of medical schools to society for the production of professionals. In the past two decades, however, what was always the medical schools' public accountability in moral terms has become public accountability in fact. At least 50 percent, and perhaps as high as 75 percent, of current medical school expenditures—taking the private and state medical schools together— is derived from the federal government.[3] Most of this money is, more-over, tied to sponsored research and teaching programs whose con-tinuation and direction are determined outside the medical schools. Tak-ing federal and nonfederal money together, as much as 58 percent of the teaching and research budgets in medical schools is dependent on outside, earmarked support.[4] The day of the independent medical school is over. The federal government has become the medical school's new proprietor.

This dramatic change in fiscal control—accompanied by a very rapid expansion of medical school activity—is a relatively recent development, representing in large part the mushroom growth of public expenditure for biomedical research after World War II. The change has been most evident in the private medical schools, which traditionally relied for their income on tuition fees, endowments, gifts, and other private sources. A survey of thirty-seven of the forty privately supported schools which existed in 1950–51 showed an increase in the proportion of fed-eral income of from under 3 percent in the academic year 1940–41 to over 30 percent ten years later.[5] The increasing proportion represented a massive infusion of additional income into the medical schools. Taking

3. The AMA's report on medical school expenditures for fully operating schools for 1967–68 shows federal funds of $614.7 million out of a total budget for 89 schools of $1,175.4 million. These figures are, however, admittedly rough; nor do they include capital outlays. Figures from the National Institutes of Health esti-mated that federal funds comprised 60 percent of total medical school expenditures for fiscal year 1967. Another estimate (Allen) put the proportion for fiscal year 1968 as high as 75 percent. More precise estimates await the completion of de-tailed cost studies which are being undertaken by the Association of American Medical Colleges. Whatever the exact proportion, the amounts are considerable. In fiscal year 1968 the Department of Health, Education, and Welfare poured $686 million into the 89 operating and 13 developing medical schools—an average of $6.7 million per institution. See "Medical Education in the United States and Canada," *J. Amer. med. Ass.*, 210 (1969), 1485–89; U.S. Department of Health, Education, and Welfare, National Institutes of Health, *DHEW Obligations to Medical Schools Fiscal Year 1967*, p. 1; *Fiscal Year 1968*, p. 3 and passim; Ernest M. Allen, "Fiscal Relations between the Medical Schools and the Federal Govern-ment," *J. med. Educ.*, 43 (1968), 698.
4. "Medical Education in the United States and Canada," *J. Amer. med. Ass.*, 214 (1970), 1521.
5. Deitrick and Berson, p. 95 and passim.

public and private medical schools together, the average income per school rose threefold during the 1940s, from less than $0.5 million in 1940–41 to nearly $1.5 million in 1950–51.[6] Subsequent expansions were even more rapid, through the heyday of federal research support of the 1950s and early 1960s. The average medical school had an estimated total income of $3.7 million in 1958–59; the average rose to $15.0 million by 1968–69,[7] a more than fourfold increase. In twenty-eight years medical school budgets had swollen to an average of thirty times their former size.

With the changing budget—changing, that is, both in terms of size and in terms of fiscal control—came a change in purpose within the medical schools; indeed, the one was largely predicated on the other. The medical schools emerged from World War II not only with depleted faculties and straitened budgets but also with a teaching mission toward the education of undergraduate medical students which followed in direct line the mission of the medical schools of the 1920s and 1930s. Indeed, the medical schools were still completing the long process of professional reform which had followed the Flexner report of some forty years earlier. As before, the movement was one of standardizing medical education at the highest possible level, while keeping the number of physicians relatively small. The Flexner legacy was the recognition of medicine as one scientific discipline, and the educational effort of the medical schools continued in the 1940s and 1950s to move toward this goal, through improved scientific and clinical facilities. It was typical of the growth of medical schools as scientific enclaves in this period that biology and chemistry continued to be developed in medical schools as "basic medical sciences" separately from the development of these fields elsewhere in the university. Constantly fed by grants for research, the medical school became a scientific and research complex which, both ideologically and financially, was largely independent of the university which sheltered it.

The American Medical Association supported federal funding of biomedical research in the schools, while opposing federal aid to teaching by the same faculties. As a result, much teaching in medical schools came to be hidden in research budgets. In this way the federal scientific establishment came to be the "proprietor" not only of the medical school researcher but also of the medical school teacher whose salary was often paid on the representation that he was a full-time or nearly full-time

6. Calculated from ibid., p. 92.
7. See "Medical Education in the United States and Canada," *J. Amer. med. Ass.,* *214* (1970), 1519–23.

researcher. The shift in favor of increasing research emphasis and against emphasis in teaching could not have been greater. But while the prevailing professional attitudes toward financing medical schools might seem contradictory, in terms of professional ideology they were not inconsistent. Both followed the apparent messages of the Flexner report to raise medicine's scientific standards. The medical profession as a profession was not threatened by governmental subsidy of research; rather the reverse. All professions have an interest in advancing their fields through research; the more research which is done, the greater the possibilities for expanding human knowledge and professional excellence. Moreover, research support did not imply an inroad by an outside agency into the cherished domain of private practice. Millions of dollars could be spent on basic cancer research without any necessary change in the detection and treatment of cancer in practice; and even when changed scientific methods were indicated (for example, through encouraging better detection of cancer of the cervix through widespread use of the Pap smear), they did not challenge the physician to change the financing or organization of his practice. In contrast, implicit in governmental subsidy of medical education were questions of potential governmental control over an area which was at the core of the concept of professionalism: the freedom to describe, to choose, to regulate new entrants to the profession.

Control of access goes back to old concepts of professions as self-sustaining guilds. The American medical profession had an added motivation in resisting governmental intervention in medical education in the 1950s, in that the prevailing professional and governmental philosophies toward medical education were radically different. As a heritage of the phenomenal earlier success of pre- and post-Flexner medical reforms, raising the standards of medical education through professional action, while carefully controlling the number of physicians, had gained a momentum of its own. The Council on Medical Education of the American Medical Association had dropped its rating of medical schools into three classes (A, B, and C) as early as 1930, by which time the number of schools had been reduced to 76 (from 131 schools in 1910); there were only 78 schools in 1949. But the council continued to keep a close watch both on standards and on the number of students in the individual schools. Each year the educational number of the AMA *Journal* continued to produce statistical assessments of educational progress, designed to raise medical education to the status of a full graduate degree. Three-quarters of a century after the establishment of the Johns Hopkins Medical School, the movement continued to standardize medical education to the Hopkins model. By 1953 the council was able to insist, in its requirements for accrediting schools, on three years of college before medical school. Of the entering class of 1954–55 no one was admitted with only two years of college education, and 71 percent had baccalaureate degrees. By 1959, the proportion of freshmen with four years of college or a college degree had risen to 81 percent. The latest available figures, for the entering class of 1969, show 89 percent of students with four years of college and 90 percent with an earned degree.[8] Sixty years ago it was possible to earn an M.D. degree in three years from grade or secondary school; with few exceptions, it now takes eight (although the future trend may be to shorten the period to seven years, or six).

The constant raising of the intellectual standards and content of medical education fostered the concept of the physician as scientist, and in turn encouraged the trend toward specialization. The M.D. degree had risen from its early status as basic vocational training to the equivalent of a Ph.D. The schools were becoming better and better at producing highly educated scientists, while both public reports and the annual meetings of the AMA deplored the lack of general practitioners. The profession's support of federal funding for research in the medical schools, while opposing aid for education, only increased the emphasis.

QUALITY AND QUANTITY IN MEDICAL EDUCATION

The question of standards and content of medical education was one side of the coin. That of the number of physicians was the other. At a time of declining professional incomes it had been natural to attempt to restrict physician supply in the cause of raising educational standards, as the AMA did during the 1930s, and these attitudes survived World War II. The old arguments in relation to the "oversupply" of physicians, the accelerated three-year medical curricula and increased production of physicians during the war (as a result of which some 7,000 additional medical students had been graduated),[9] and the reappearance into civilian life of thousands of physician veterans seemed to indicate a need for continuing caution. As the medical schools relaxed back into their four-year peacetime curricula, the AMA established its policy of no major expansion in the number of medical students. The Council on

8. "Medical Education in the United States," *J. Amer. med. Ass., 159* (1955), 587; ibid., *174* (1960), 1451; ibid., *210* (1970), 1514.
9. Fishbein, p. 917.

Medical Education stated in 1946 that the "normal annual number of graduates from existing schools is adequate for the peacetime needs of the country, granted distribution is equitable." [10]

This statement was followed by a series of studies by the AMA's Bureau of Medical Economic Research reviewing the number and distribution of physicians. The AMA publications argued that physician productivity had been phenomenally expanded as a result of technological programs in medical care, that changes in distribution of physicians from rural to urban areas was not confined to doctors but was a feature of all occupations, that additional investment in education was more crucial in other professions, and that mortality rates and other health indices did not indicate a breakdown in medical care. Indeed, it was notable that during World War II, with 40 percent of physicians abroad, the health of the civilian population apparently improved. It was concluded that the distribution of physicians to population had been improving in the 1940s to the point of excellence, and that there was, if anything, not a physician shortage but a potential physician surplus.[11] Whether one ranged on the side of a doctor surplus or a doctor shortage was a matter of opinion. There was, and is, no concrete or objective criterion as to how many doctors are enough. But whatever the merits or deficiencies in the argument, the AMA views achieved reality. The number of graduates from the medical schools fell from a high of nearly 6,400 in 1947 to just over 5,000 in 1949—almost exactly the same number of graduates as in 1940. In the year 1949 there were 135 physicians for every 100,000 population, just one more than in 1942. From 1949 to 1959, moreover, the physician-population ratio actually declined; there were 133 MDs per 100,000 in 1959.[12]

There were more than three applicants for each place in medical schools between 1948 and 1950; thereafter the ratio slowly fell.[13] The Council on Medical Education urged the medical schools to use the opportunity of the increased competition to cream off those with the

10. Quoted by Rayack, pp. 81–82.
11. F. G. Dickinson and C. E. Bradley, *Comparisons of State Physician-Population Ratios for 1938 and 1948,* Bureau of Medical Economic Research, Bulletin no. 78 (Chicago, 1950); F. G. Dickinson, "Supply of Physicians Services," *J. Amer. med. Ass., 145* (1951), 1260–64, and "How Bad Is the Distribution of Physicians?" ibid., *154* (1954), 1209–11.
12. "Medical Education in the United States and Canada," *J. Amer. med. Ass., 210* (1969), 1484, table 23; Rayack, p. 71.
13. The ratio of applicants to those accepted fell to 1.7 in 1960 and 1961; that is, there were less than two applicants for every available place. Thereafter the tide began to turn. Between 1964 and 1969 there were on average more than two applicants per place. *J. Amer. med. Ass., 214* (1970), 1512.

highest academic ratings. Students with less than a B average in their undergraduate years must, it was stressed, "present other outstanding qualities of character, personality, aptitude, and motivation that compensate for their relatively low academic standing." [14] By 1954, 17 percent of freshmen medical students had A averages in their college records. But unlike other phases of the standardization movement, this level of upgrading did not continue; for as medicine itself became more scientifically motivated, medical schools competed increasingly with the growing demand in the 1950s for scientists in other fields. By 1959, the proportion of A students in the first year of medical schools had dropped to 15 percent, and medical school deans were reporting difficulties in filling their first year classes with acceptable students.[15] Acceptable in this context meant those with relatively high scientific abilities who could afford the cost of graduate study for four years in medical school. If this were the criterion for admission to the medical profession—and the canons of previous professional development had so indicated—there was a good case for not attempting to expand the number of physicians.

Increasingly, however, the "if" was being questioned. Medicine in the pre-Flexner period, for all its defects of inadequate night schools, poor preparation, short courses, and low standards, had offered opportunities to the poor boy to become a physician. (And incidentally, the surfeit of physicians had at least provided physicians, albeit the less qualified, in the poorer areas.) As standards rose, and as the costs and length of education expanded, medicine became staunchly middle-class. The unmarried student could expect expenses of $10,000 or $11,000 for the four-year degree, followed by an ill-paid internship, and a two- or three-year residency; a 1963 study noted that over 80 percent of the average medical student's expenses came from his own earnings and savings and from those of his family.[16] The relatively arduous economic process of gaining a medical education, coupled with a delay in professional and economic gratification through internship, residency, and perhaps the lean years of practice, brought to medicine a new spirit of mercantilism. The physician was tempted to feel that, for demanding a spartan youth, society owed him a rich

14. "Medical Education in the United States and Canada" *J. Amer. med. Ass., 144* (1950), 125.
15. The proportion dropped to 12 percent in 1961, but began rising again from 1964. In 1969, in contrast, approximately 18 percent of first year medical students had A averages. Ibid., *159* (1955), 588; *214* (1970), 1514; Bane report, pp. 24–25.
16. Marion E. Altenderfer and Margaret D. West, *How Medical Students Finance Their Education*, USDHEW, Public Health Service, 1965, pp. 70–71.

return. And, indeed, to become a practicing physician was to enter the most highly paid of all occupations.[17] This economic by-product of professionalism was not lost on a public which was becoming attuned to the increasing gap between medicine as practiced in the scientific medical centers and medicine as seen by poorer members of the population.

The medical school stood between the professional expectation of quality above quantity in medical education and concurrent statements of the need for *increased* medical manpower which were emanating from governmental, congressional, and other groups. The apparent difficulty the medical schools would have in producing an expanded number of physicians was given widespread public emphasis in 1948 in a report by the federal security administrator, Oscar Ewing.[18] This was followed by proposals for direct federal aid for medical education (as well as education of dentists and other health professionals) in a number of bills before Congress in 1949, including the Wagner-Murray-Dingell proposals for a national health program.[19] Up to 1950, the AMA successfully opposed all forms of federal aid to medical education, while the spokesman for the Association of American Medical Colleges urged federal financing of teaching to shore up and expand the teaching budgets of the medical schools. Once again the American Medical Association found itself in disagreement over educational policy with the independent medical schools. Indeed, the association took a position toward federal aid to medical education which was rather similar to its position toward national health insurance, Medicare, and other proposals designed to expand and streamline the health service system. There were denials that a problem existed, claims that governmental intervention would cause a deterioration in standards, and a trusting belief in the

17. There is little available or reliable information on physician incomes. A study of 1959 incomes as reported on tax returns showed the median earnings of physicians, including interns and residents, at $14,651, a figure which exceeded that of all other professions. Next in line came dentists ($11,858); and third, lawyers and judges ($10,587). Louis S. Reed, *Studies of the Incomes of Physicians and Dentists,* USDHEW, Social Security Administration, Office of Research and Statistics, 1968.
18. Oscar R. Ewing, *The Nation's Health: A Ten Year Program,* Report to the President (Washington, D.C., 1948).
19. The bill would have authorized payments to schools for the costs of instruction, including support of faculty salaries and operating facilities, grants for construction and equipment of schools, and federal subsidy of scholarships. The argument made for such support, at this time as later, was one of shortage of qualified professionals. U.S., Congress, Senate, A bill to provide national health insurance and public health and to assist in increasing the number of adequately trained professional and other health personnel, and for other purposes, 81st Cong., 1st sess., S. 1679, title I. Other bills incorporating similar proposals were S. 1106, S. 1456, S. 1581, H.R. 3894, H.R. 4312, and H.R. 4313.

efficacy of the proven professional attitudes of earlier generations. It was pointed out that it was the medical profession—not a few medical school deans—who had taken the leadership in raising the standards of medical education in 1905, and it was capable of doing so again.[20] The AMA was giving an old answer; unfortunately it was directed to an irrelevant question. The issue was no longer one of professional standards, which were recognizably high, but of professional service; and here the Congress demanded a right to decide the priorities.

From 1951 the association's position toward federal aid to medical education was gradually relaxed; in 1955 the association endorsed a proposal for one-time construction grants for educational facilities, but nothing came of this proposal.[21] President Eisenhower's message on health of 26, January 1956 endorsed a five-year program of construction grants for medical school teaching facilities as well as for research facilities. But while the latter was translated into the Health Research Facilities Act of 1956 (P.L. 84–835) the former was not heeded. Nor was the president's later request for aid for construction of teaching facilities, when the 1956 act was extended in 1958 (P.L. 85–777). Throughout the 1950s, therefore, at a time of rapidly expanding medical school research budgets, there were no major federal grants for construction or for operation of the schools as teaching institutions.

THE MEDICAL SCHOOL AS A RESEARCH CENTER

The expansion of research by members of the faculty of medical schools, like the AMA attitude toward medical education, was a reflection of the

20. Editorial, "Enrollments in Medical Schools," *J. Amer. med. Ass., 142* (1950), 420. See also editorial, "The Alleged Shortage of Physicians," ibid., pp. 111–13, and editorial, "Conference of Academic Deans," ibid., p. 183.

21. Proposals for construction grants and student loans were presented to Congress each year between 1951 and 1962, but did not clear both houses. The 1955 bill (S.1323, H.R. 4743) would have authorized 50 percent construction grants for existing schools and grants of up to 66.67 percent for new schools. Another bill, S.434, would have added operating expenses. Similar requests continued until their ultimate passage of the Health Professions Educational Assistance Act of 1963 (P.L. 88–129). For analysis of the AMA's role in debates over federal aid to medical education, see Rayack, pp. 81–100, from which this discussion draws. Rayack argues that the source of AMA hostility to federal aid was primarily one of economic restrictionism, a reaction against increased physician supply. It is argued here that, whereas restrictionism was clearly a vital factor in the AMA's views during the 1950s, this was not an end in itself. Rather, it was one symptom in a network of attitudes toward professionalism which had been crystallized during the pre- and post-Flexner decades—in short, that the AMA was reacting with a preconditioned set of attitudinal responses, rather than with a reasoned Machiavellianism.

definitive scientific function of a medical school as stated in the Flexner report. By 1930 the faculties in the best schools had become scientific investigators, as indeed they have remained. Occasionally, medical schools received earmarked foundation grants for support of specified research projects. But in large part medical schools made no distinction in their departmental budgets between teaching and research up to World War II. Then, however, an accelerated, focused program of medical research, sponsored both by private organizations and by various governmental departments for wartime needs, led to separate accounting for research in the schools, and thus to a separation of the research function from the regularly expected role of teaching. By 1948 almost all the schools had separate research budgets.[22] Drawing income from major charitable and tax sources, the medical schools were actively building up their research programs. The stage was set for the extraordinary subsequent growth of research programs, sponsored by the governmental National Institutes of Health.

The Institutes trace their history back to 1887, when a laboratory for bacteriological studies was created as part of the U.S. Public Health Service; this became, with enlarged functions, the National Institute of Health in 1930. The creation of the National Cancer Institute under an act of 1937 set up an additional organization. It had, moreover, the additional functions, which were to become central to the function of the present Institutes, not only of operating direct on-site research and training programs but also of making extramural research grants to individuals and institutions. The Cancer Institute also set the precedent for the development of further *specialist* research programs focused on specific conditions or diseases which developed after World War II. From these modest beginnings the National Institutes of Health developed into fourteen research institutes and major research divisions, together with the National Library of Medicine and five divisions designed to stimulate the research and training of health manpower. By 1968, the NIH employed over 13,000 full-time persons, and was responsible for a budget of $1.6 billion, of which $254 million was spent on its own direct operations.[23]

22. Federal Security Agency, Public Health Service, *Report by the Surgeon General's Committee on Medical School Grants and Finances* (Washington, D.C., 1951); Deitrick and Berson, pp. 33–45 and passim.
23. The National Institute of Mental Health was authorized by the Mental Health Act of 1946. (This institute, because of its expanding role in the 1960s of administering grants for mental health centers and other services, as well as research, is no longer considered part of the NIH and is now administratively organized within the Health Services and Mental Health Administration, a branch of the U.S. Public

At the same time, the program of NIH subsidies to universities for medical research transformed the research functions—and altered the balance of faculty interests—in the nominally independent medical schools. By 1955, one-third of the income of medical schools was coming from outside research grants, chiefly from the federal government. Not only had the contributions by NIH become essential to the continued existence of the schools; the activities of the faculty had substantially changed. In 1949–50 the average medical school had a full-time faculty of approximately 70, a substantial increase from nine or ten years earlier. In 1959–60, the average full-time faculty was over 120 per school; of the total of 10,468 faculty thus represented, 1 in 7 received more than half of his salary from federal sources, with federal money concentrated in the lower academic ranks. By 1968–69, the total number of full-time faculty had reached 23,014, or over 250 per school. There was more than one full-time faculty member for every pair of medical students, but many, if not most, of the faculty were not regularly involved in teaching medical students at all. A substantial bloc of faculty were solely or primarily engaged in research, and these research interests were reflected in the patterns of funding. In 1968–69, just under half of the faculty of medical schools received some of their salary from federal support, predominantly for sponsored research. Nearly a third of the full-time faculty received the majority of their salaries in this way, and there was a substantial minority (3,466 faculty out of the total of 23,014) who were totally dependent on federal support.[24] While the AMA had been opposing federal aid for medical education, using as one argument distrust of increased governmental control over a traditionally professional responsibility, the medical schools had de facto become extensively dependent on the government through the back door of research subsidy.

The accumulation of knowledge, the stimulation of excellence, and the focus on scientific achievement in the medical schools were aims

Health Service which is parallel to the NIH.) The National Heart Institute and the Dental Research Institute were authorized in 1948; the Institute of Neurological Diseases and Blindness and the Institute of Arthritis and Metabolic Diseases in 1950; the Institute of Allergy and Infectious Diseases in 1955; the Institute of General Medical Sciences and the Institute of Child Health and Human Development in 1962; the National Eye Institute in 1968, the Institute of Environmental Health Sciences in 1969. See *Congress and the Nation, 1945–1964*, pp. 1123–25; James Shannon, "The Advancement of Medical Research: A Twenty Year View of the Role of the National Institutes of Health," *J. med. Educ., 42* (1967), 97–108; National Institutes of Health, *1968 Annual Report* (Washington, D.C., 1969), pp. 58–60.

24. Deitrick and Berson, p. 195; "Medical Education in the United States and Canada," *J. Amer. med. Ass., 159* (1955), 574–75; ibid., *174* (1960), 1433, 1438; ibid., *210* (1969), 1478–79, 1561.

which were consistent with the AMA's position toward a higher quality of medical education. But it was not the AMA but other lobbying efforts which dominated the development of biomedical research in the two decades following World War II. The so-called Lasker Lobby—a powerful combination of Dr. James Shannon, director of NIH in its crucial developing period, Representative John E. Fogarty of Rhode Island, Senator Lister Hill of Alabama, and Mrs. Mary Lasker, a wealthy New Yorker dedicated to expanding health programs, together with a close group of her influential physician and nonphysician friends—provided a pressure group for large-scale expansion of focused research into particular areas, from mental illness through cancer to blindness, which proved to be of overwhelming success.[25] Biomedical research attained for a short period almost the sacrosanct status of American motherhood, as one large appropriation was succeeded by one of even larger proportions. From the 1940s to the 1960s, as the NIH budget shot up from $2.5 million (1945) to $285 million (1960), on its way to its current $1.6 or $1.7 billion, there was little effective criticism of NIH. But at the same time, this extraordinary program had a substantial impact on the operation and function of the medical schools. By 1960 the medical schools had become in large part arms or branches of NIH. Their faculties and their interests responded to the availability of an apparently never-ending stream of federal wealth, channeled through a complicated, byzantine system of national peer-review groups and advisory committees.

The successful accumulation of federal grants by principal investigators on the faculties of medical schools created a system in the schools of powerful baronies built around specific research projects and interests. At the very time that medical schools were demanding effective full-time administration, with decisions as to their long-term educational and service functions, the power of making decisions was decentralized—even scattered—among virtually autonomous senior faculty members whose interests lay in relatively esoteric realms of research. Project grants had grown without a sufficient administrative structure to weld the research activities into a part of the medical school activities; indeed, at the beginning of the 1950s, there were many schools which still had part-time deans, whose vision, administrative ability, and financial acumen were not always commensurate with the task before them.[26]

25. The full story is yet to be written, but see Elizabeth Brenner Drew, "The Health Syndicate, Washington's Noble Conspirators," *Atlantic Monthly* (Dec. 1967), pp. 75–82.
26. See Deitrick and Berson, pp. 126–28.

The general appearance of the full-time administrator-dean was a phenomenon of the extraordinary development of medical schools from the 1950s; and he was soon joined by university provosts or vice-presidents for health affairs, and by full-time associate deans with specially assigned responsibilities. But while this strengthened structure might seem to have heralded a new age of effective planning for medical schools and medical education, the budgetary situation of medical schools left the deans with relatively little influence. The balance of income became a continuing headache to the deans, not least of which was the relationship between special federal project grants and the university contributions. There was concern that while universities received large amounts for research projects, these did not cover the total costs of the projects; thus the medical schools were forced to subsidize research from their proportionally dwindling general income.[27] The more this happened, the less chance there was of creating new leadership and educational policies within the individual medical schools. Attempts by university administrations to "regain control" over medical schools were inevitably doomed to failure. The federal government was proving as rigid an influence on the schools—although for different reasons and through different means—as earlier professional dicta on the nature and shape of the medical curriculum.

The deficiencies in federal research grant financing of medical schools led to two types of recommendations for change in the 1950s. The first was that the system of project grants for medical research should gradually be replaced by institutional block grants; the second, the incorporation of more realistic indirect cost allowances in research grants, to pay for general university overhead.[28] Both raised substantive issues of the nature and function of research in medical schools. The introduction of a block

27. See e.g. AMA Council on Medical Education and Hospitals, *Money and Medical Schools* (Chicago, 1961).
28. Five-year institutional grants to be made on the basis of an approved general research proposal submitted by each institution were recommended by the Second Hoover Commission on Organization of the Executive Branch of the Government in 1955. The commission also suggested that there should be a federal council of health within the Executive Office of the President with responsibility for facilitating federal health research programs. Neither recommendation has, at least yet, been put into effect. Commission on Organization of the Executive Branch of the Government, *Task Force Report on Federal Medical Services* (Washington, D.C., 1955), pp. 10–11, 17–23. Payment by the federal government of the full costs of research was one of the recommendations made by the Secretary's Consultants on Medical Research and Education in 1957, on the grounds that such research was done by the universities as a general public service and that universities should be treated similarly to industrial concerns which also accepted federal money for scientific and medical research. Bayne-Jones Report (reference below), p. 71.

grant system to medical schools would recognize, and legitimate, the existence of a general government subsidy for medical research and education, instead of the existing series of focused projects radiating from NIH, each with specified starting and termination dates. To replace the project grant system with a general subsidy would be to recognize relative institutional excellence rather than the potential contributions of individuals. It would decentralize the formally centralized system of supervising and stimulating medical research. It would hand fiscal power to the deans. At least in theory, it would allow each school to take a new look at its overall purpose of teaching, research, and service. Block grants could thus be seen as having an integrative impact on medical schools. On the other hand, suggestions for complete coverage of the overheads of project grants would emphasize the existing isolation of research from teaching and service in the schools. By asking for fiscal independence of sponsored research, the medical schools accepted such research under their umbrella as small research institutes rather than as an integral part of faculty activities.

In both recommendations, there was the crucial question of the purpose of federal proprietorship. Were federal grants for biomedical research primarily a means of aiding the schools in building up their own research, as part of a well-rounded educational process, or were they part of a federally directed research program? If the former, federal assistance to the schools for research should be tied into plans for both research and education, and the relationship of the two functions in each school closely reexamined. If the latter—that is, if research grants were not to be viewed primarily as subsidy to medical schools but as part of a national research effort—the medical school would be well advised to recognize the existence of separate, affiliated research institutes whose purposes were quite distinct from the school's primary responsibility of teaching. Neither posture was set in the 1960s; nor indeed has it been to the present. There was, however, a growing movement to reexamine the missions—and funding—of medical research and medical education.

FEDERAL AID TO MEDICAL EDUCATION

The implications of building up federal research support to medical schools, while there was at the same time only a slow expansion of medical education, received serious scrutiny with the publication of two major governmental reports between 1958 and 1960: the Bayne-Jones report in 1958 and the Bane report in 1959.[29] Neither of these groups

29. *The Advancement of Medical Research and Education through the Department*

attempted to formulate a blueprint for balanced development of medical schools; indeed, the Bayne-Jones committee expressed itself appalled at such a prospect, given the complexity of the subject and the time available. Nevertheless, by coming to similar conclusions, the reports had a major impact on prevailing attitudes toward medical education and research in the schools, in the AMA, and—by no means least—in the Congress. They set the tone of debate for the 1960s.

On biomedical research support the reports were cautiously optimistic. There were calls for developing a diversity of grant support by attempting to attract new money for research from private sources; recommendations for increased use of outside advisers in the disbursement of federal grant support; and suggestions that, while research grants to individuals should continue, a greater amount of general research support be given to universities, thus enabling deans and departments to develop their own programs without the detailed direction from outside through project grant support. There was, however, no indication from the committees that the expanding federal effort should be slowed down or discontinued. It was noted that total national expenditures on medical research had risen no faster in the 1950s than had the total amount of money being spent on all national research and development programs.[30] Biomedical research was thus tacitly grouped with other major scientific expansions of the cold war period. In a decade of relative conservatism, the Congress had recognized a commitment to biomedical research as a national political asset. While concern was expressed over the evolving relationship between the government and the university, federal sponsorship of biomedical research appeared in these reports as justified became of its *national* or *federal* purposes, rather than in terms of a need for university subsidy.

Endorsement of federal grants for research was, however, only one of the two major national themes stressed in the reports. The second theme was concern over the production of physicians—a concern which

of Health, Education, and Welfare, Final Report of the Secretary's Consultants on Medical Research and Education, U.S. Department of Health, Education, and Welfare, June 1958, p. 71 (hereafter cited as Bayne-Jones report). *Physicians for a Growing America* (Bane report) Report of the Surgeon General's Consultant Group on Medical Education, U.S. Department of Health, Education, and Welfare, 1959. See also U.S. Congress, Senate, Committee on Appropriations, *Federal Support of Medical Research,* Report of the Committee of Consultants on Medical Research, 86th Cong., 2d sess., 1960.

30. Total national medical research in 1947 (i.e. from all sources) was estimated at $0.088 billion and rose to $0.330 billion in 1957. In the first year this represented 3.8 percent of all research and development programs; in the latter, 3.3 percent. Bayne-Jones report, p. 21.

was logical in terms of building up national biomedical resources. In other scientific fields receiving major governmental research support, education was also heavily subsidized. The National Science Foundation, set up under legislation of 1950 (P.L. 81–507), included manpower development programs in mathematics, physics, medicine, biology, engineering, and other fields; during the 1950s, moreover, the educational scope of the foundation was steadily broadened. The successful launch of the first Russian sputnik in 1957 sparked considerable concern in the Congress that America was falling behind in scientific education. One result was the National Defense Education Act of 1958 (P.L. 85–864), with policies for federal educational grants and scholarships, passed by Congress and endorsed by President Eisenhower in the interests of national security. There was an assumption of national responsibility for producing strategic manpower, even though these were produced and would work in private industries or institutions rather than in a streamlined public service. At the same time, the universities were becoming accustomed to building up their scientific departments, hiring teaching faculty, and granting scholarships, through the availability of federal funding. Both of these movements had potential parallels in the medical sciences, where there was also an assumption of research development as a national priority. The acceptance of federal responsibility for scientific manpower and the dependence of universities on availability of federal teaching as well as research funds were two important factors in the ultimate introduction of federally sponsored medical manpower programs.

At the same time, there continued to be a partially related movement for increasing the supply of physicians, which was growing around the buildup of concern over the adequacy—rather, the inadequacies—of the nation's health *services*. While the AMA continued to insist in the 1950s that there was not a doctor shortage, a strong body of opinion contended otherwise. Estimates by Mountin, Pennell, and Berger of the U.S. Public Health Service in 1949, on the basis of bringing understaffed areas up to an acceptable physician-population ratio, estimated a shortage of between 17;500 and 45,000 physicians. The President's Commission on the Health Needs of the Nation (1953) indicated a shortage of physicians as high as 59,000 by 1960.[31] Hospitals sensed a doctor shortage in their increasing and unmet demands for house staff. In the rather crude terms of physician-population ratios, moreover, the supply of doctors *fell* between 1950 and 1960, from 149 to 148 physicians per 100,000 popula-

31. See Herbert Klarman, "Requirements for Physicians," *American Economic Review: Papers and Proceedings* (1951), p. 635 and passim; Fein, p. 9 and passim.

tion.[32] Far from being a physician excess, there was evidence of a physician deficit, and it was this evidence which was seized on in the Bayne-Jones and Bane reports.

The assumption was made that the existing ratio of physicians to population was a minimal social requirement, which must at least be maintained to assure a reasonable future supply. While it could just as well be argued that there had been too *many* physicians in 1950, or that physician productivity had increased sufficiently to make increasing the number of physicians less important, the findings were politically persuasive. In a context of anxiety that American youth were less scientifically proficient than their Russian counterparts, and in mounting interest in the social provision of health services, there were few who were likely to cavil over the need for more rather than less physicians. The hearings of the Senate Subcommittee on Aging in 1958 and concurrent discussions of the Forand-Kennedy-Anderson bills for health insurance for the aged publicized the deficiency in health services, at least to the elderly population; and it seemed reasonable to suppose that one remedy would be to improve the number of physicians. The Bayne-Jones and Bane reports made a strong case for national responsibility for the number of physicians—and thus, by implication, for medical education. The reports concluded that between fourteen and twenty new medical schools were needed immediately if the relative supply of physicians was not to drop further. At the same time, there should be a rapid expansion of students in the eighty-five existing two-year and four-year M.D. schools which, together with the six schools of osteopathic medicine, represented the national resources for physicians. Altogether, it was considered that there should be an increase in the number of graduates from 7,400 a year in 1959 to about 11,000 in 1975—a 50 percent increase in a short sixteen years.[33]

To effect what was virtually a national crash program in medical education would require substantial federal subsidy, both in building and maintaining the new schools and in student grant support. Here, then, was a strong, virtually incontrovertible case for pushing the passage of federal aid to medical education. Here, too, was an assumption of national responsibility for assuring to the public an adequate production of physicians. Physician supply, following biomedical research, was moving from the private domain to the public sector.

32. Physician-population ratios are confusing in that AMA figures tend to include only MDs, excluding the osteopathic physicians. The figures given here include both MDs and DOs. The rate of MDs to population fell from 134 per 100,000 in 1950 to 133 in 1959. *Health Resources Statistics* (1968), p. 123; Rayack, p. 71.
33. Bayne-Jones report, p. 2; Bane report, p. 13 and passim.

At the same time, professional attitudes were changing. The shadow of the Depression was finally passing. Physician incomes were large and stable. Debates in Congress over an expanded federal role in health care documented unmet needs for personnel. Perhaps the sheer reiteration of there being a manpower and a health care crisis during the 1960s was a potent factor in attitudinal change. Whatever the reason, the official view of the American Medical Association was modified in the late 1950s from its earlier hostility to any suggestion that more doctors were required to recognition that there was in fact a physician shortage. The Council on Medical Education greeted the Bayne-Jones report in 1958 with a judicious statement on the need to consider the possible expansion of schools and development of new facilities; by the following year, the council was stressing the need for expanded educational facilities.[34] The AMA's position was, however, still one of action through private initiative rather than through the public sector, and of endorsement of construction funds but not of student scholarships and loans. Making its position clear in congressional hearings in 1960 and 1962, the association remarked again—with justification—on the danger of control over medical education which would result from federal funding, and stated its opposition to the use of monetary incentives on the grounds that expanded enrollment implied reduced quality.[35]

The medical school deans, on the other hand, strongly supported the legislation through the Association of American Medical Colleges. Their authority had been eroded by the fragmentation of their budgets into sponsored research projects and other tied funds. At the same time, their teaching funds had slowly evaporated—indeed their endorsement of the

34. Interestingly, the same process was happening in England, under a very different health service system. The professional viewpoint in the early 1950s was, as in the United States, that too many doctors were being produced; indeed, this view was reinforced in a government-sponsored committee (the Willink committee) in 1957. It was followed, however, by immediate concern that there was in fact a serious physician shortage; at the same time, the government was being forced to assume greater manpower responsibilities. The timing and the scenario were thus very similar in the two countries, a product most probably of lingering professional attitudes of the 1930s rather than of any similarities in the two health systems. See Stevens, pp. 242–56. On changing AMA attitudes, see Rayack, pp. 94–95.

35. U.S., Congress, House, Subcommittee of the Committee on Interstate and Foreign Commerce, *Medical and Dental Schools: Hearings on H.R. 6906, H.R. 10255, H.R. 10341, H.R. 11651,* 86th Cong., 2d sess., 1960, pp. 111–13; *Training of Physicians, Dentists and Professional Public Health Personnel: Hearings on H.R. 4999, H.R. 8774, H.R. 8833,* 87th Cong., 2d sess., 1962, pp. 340–41 and passim. In line with the wish to maintain the independence of the medical schools from federal control, the AMA also supported the development of unrestricted research development grants to medical schools (*H.R. 10341*).

Bane report was an empty gesture without such funds. Hence the deans, far from seeing the possibility that federal funding of teaching would lead to federal interference, felt it might redress the imbalance in the educational process caused by the extensive federal funding of medical research. The practitioners were finally losing ground. It was becoming evident that federal aid to medical education had not been defeated but merely delayed, and the proposals were successful in the Health Professions Educational Assistance Act of 1963 (P.L. 88–129); the long cycle was complete. The legislation authorized a three-year program of matching federal grants for construction and improvement of medical schools, together with a six-year program of loans to students in medicine, osteopathy, and dentistry. The aim of the new program was twofold: to increase the number of students in the stated health professions and to increase the quality of their education.[36]

DECLINE IN RESEARCH SUPPORT

But even while the star of educational support was rising, that of research support was beginning to wane. From the early 1960s, congressional concern and criticism of research grant administration began effectively to be expressed. The catalyst of criticism was the House Intergovernmental Relations Subcommittee, chaired by Rep. L. H. Fountain of

36. President Kennedy had included a program of grants for construction and expansion of medical schools, together with scholarships and educational subsidies, in his special message on health in 1961, and again in 1962; although the proposed scholarship program was amended to a student loans program during the 1962 hearings, the administration bill died at the end of the 87th Congress in 1962. The 1963 bill (H.R. 12) followed the format of previous legislative recommendations, including both construction grants and student loans provisions. A Republican-led effort to debate the student loan provision—encouraged by letters from the AMA to each representative on the day before the bill was voted—was defeated in the House; the bill cleared the Senate; it was signed into law in September 1963. After the years of gestation and debate, the program, once launched, was soon expanded. Student optometrists were added in 1964 (P.L. 88–654). Amendments to the act in 1965 (P.L. 89–290) finally set up a program of scholarships. At the same time, two new grants programs were created, again on grounds of improving both quality and quantity in medical education. Basic improvement grants were now made available to schools (a specified sum for each full-time student), on the basis of assurances from schools that they would increase their student enrollment by 2.5 percent a year over the grant period. Special improvement grants were also made available to improve the quality of teaching. Finally, the amendments included a "forgiveness" principle for student loans where students practice in areas defined as needy. Amendments of 1966 (P.L. 89–751) allowed a cancellation of 15 percent a year, up to 100 percent of the loan and interest, so long as the physician practices in a rural area of low family income as designated by the secretary of Health, Education, and Welfare. Two years later, the various provisions of the 1963 legislation were incorporated into the Health Manpower Act of 1968 (P.L. 90–490).

North Carolina. It was not immediately evident; but the halcyon days of federal funding of medical research were beginning to draw to a close.

The first Fountain report, of 1961,[37] was a cold shock to researchers in the medical schools who had become used to receiving federal largesse as an expected by-product of a faculty appointment. The report criticized the administration of grant programs, insufficient technical review of the financial side of grant applications, lack of contact between NIH and grantees in relation to continuation proposals, and an uneven application of indirect or overhead costs. While there was little criticism of the research effort itself, the conclusions and recommendations focused on methods of reducing inefficiency and increasing public accountability. The Fountain report's comments and criticisms were accepted by NIH and the Public Health Service at hearings in 1961, but little was done to tighten up research grant administration. Quite apart from the lack of experience in financial review within NIH, in the medical schools, and on the review committees, there was an inbuilt resistance among the researchers—who were simultaneously reviewers, administrators, and recipients of research funds—to any greatly improved system of grants management.

But the Fountain committee was not to be deterred, and the relative inactivity was exposed at a second, more detailed round of hearings in March 1962. This time the committee, armed with the findings of a detailed audit which revealed misuse of grants, excessive payments, purchase of unnecessary equipment, and inadequate administrative review by NIH, took a stronger line and sounded for the first time a warning which penetrated NIH complacency and was in the late 1960s to become a reality. Congress, it was intimated, had been "overzealous" in appropriating money for health research.[38] The days of unexamined increase in research support were slowly coming to a halt

There was a continuing difficulty in reconciling the aims of an efficient national biomedical research program with the general financial underpinning of research in universities and other independent institutions. Over the years the NIH had developed its role as one of stimulating research potential rather than buying a particular product or service; re-

37. U.S., Congress, House, Committee on Government Operations, 2d rept., *Health Research and Training: The Administration of Grants and Awards by the National Institutes of Health,* 87th Cong., 1st sess., 28 Apr. 1961, H. Rept. 321. For a review of the role of federal aid in the context of all the sciences, see Harold Orlans, *The Effects of Federal Programs on Higher Education* (Washington, D.C., 1962).

38. U.S., Congress, House, *Administration of Grants by the National Institutes of Health (Reexamination of Management Deficiencies),* 87th Cong., 2d sess., H. Rept. 1958, p. 26 and passim.

search grants had become a form of educational investment or grants-in-aid. This direction had been encouraged in 1960 by legislation (P.L. 86–798) which authorized institutional grants for general research and training in universities and other institutions; the move followed similar action by the National Science Foundation. The relative importance of such funds was small (6 percent of NIH research support funds in 1962); nevertheless, here was a promise of greater general subsidy of medical schools in the future, with (presumably) reduced direct project support. The Fountain committee, more interested in the benefits derived to society from so much federal aid, continued to insist on tighter federal research controls.[39] The committee's views were supported by other reports on the administration of NIH, including hearings in 1965 by the Intergovernmental Relations Subcommittee of the House, and in 1967, a second, more critical Fountain report was released.[40]

This report focused on excessive payments made by NIH to grantees in the form of indirect costs as a symptom of "weak central management." Grants to the Sloan-Kettering Institute, a private institute for cancer research in New York City, were used as an example of the impact of government prodigality on outside institutions. Sloan-Kettering had been receiving NIH money in 1965 from forty-one grants and three contracts, each for earmarked research and training projects, and each therefore subject to separate and independent NIH review; fourteen other grants had been applied for and turned down in the span of two fiscal years. For this fragmented pattern, NIH substituted in January 1966 a single large grant for an initial five-year period, with annual amounts ranging from $4.3 to $4.7 million—almost half of the Institute's total operating budget—with provisions for further cost increases and expectations of additional grant requests. In short, grants to individuals had been replaced by an institutional subsidy. The case was important, for it established a major precedent which could be followed in the university medical schools, with their multiplicity of applications, projects, and proposals.

The Fountain committee condemned this process as reducing public accountability for individual research efforts. All research projects funded should, it was emphasized, be in the range "excellent to good"; this statement implied the continuation of a centralized rather than institutional evaluation of what was "good." In terms also of costs and

39. U.S., Congress, House, Special Subcommittee on Investigation of the Department of Health, Education, and Welfare, *Investigation of HEW*, 89th Cong., 2d sess., H. Rept. 2266, p. 130 and passim.
40. U.S., Congress, House, Committee on Government Operations, 9th rept., *The Administration of Research Grants in the Public Health Service*, 90th Cong., 2d sess., 20 Oct. 1967, H. Rept. 800, p. 2.

benefits, it was recommended that training grant programs to institutions would be examined in relation to the actual training output of those institutions. The second Fountain report recommended that besides this process there should be a separate effort by federal agencies to give technical assistance to help institutions plan to improve their scientific education and research, and particularly to improve the academic quality of weaker schools. This sensible recommendation remains, however, still largely unexplored. Block or institutional grants for various purposes continue to be discussed; but they continue to be of only minor importance in the total funding of medical schools.

The pattern of NIH grants from the cold war period had favored certain projects and individuals over others, on the basis of peer-group definitions of excellence. Since the best researchers tend to gravitate to the major centers, one effect of the grants policy of the last twenty years has been to favor certain institutions over others; the most highly regarded medical schools are also de factor those doing the most research. In fiscal year 1968, Harvard Medical School received $11.9 million from the Department of Health, Education, and Welfare for support of research. At the other end of the scale, established schools such as Creighton University School of Medicine, Loma Linda, Meharry Medical College, and Howard Medical School (the last two primarily serving black students) each received less than $400,000.[41] A second result is evident in the present structure of medical school faculties and departments as clusters of people whose focus is a research project rather than the institution by which they are technically employed. A third has been the development of a growing cadre of biomedical research scientists. An estimated 71,000 professional workers at the M.D. or Ph.D. level were engaged in biomedical research in 1970, at an expenditure of $41,000 per worker; these figures are expected to rise by 1985 to 150,000 and $104,500, respectively.[42] Such figures not only give rise to speculation as to whether, and on what grounds in relation to other social priorities, this huge amount of effort is justified—How much knowledge is enough?—they also emphasize a fourth factor in the federal grants policy of the last decades, which is the commitment to basic rather than applied medical research. As the current state of health services in the United States graphically illustrates, the advancement of knowledge itself does not imply better services for the average citizen. In one direct way, indeed, the focus on biomedical research has cut

41. *DHEW Obligations to Medical Schools FY 1968*, p. 59.
42. USDHEW, NIH, Office of Resource Analysis, *Resources for Medical Research, Report No. 11, Biomedical Research Manpower—for the Eighties*, 1968, p. 37.

into the supply of available physicians. A recent NIH manpower model expects almost one of seven of the freshman medical students of the 1960s to spend at least part of their careers in biomedical research.[43]

By far the most important factor of research grants policy has, however, been the increasing dependence of all medical schools on federal support. The balloon began to deflate in the mid-1960s, under the combined impact of a variety of factors, including the general budget retrenchments in the face of the Vietnam War, the recognition of more urgent domestic social priorities, the concerns of the Fountain report of the efficiency and rationale of biomedical support, and the lessening in power of the Lasker Lobby. The expansion of NIH appropriations for research began to level off in 1966, and then actually to decline. Support of medical schools for research and development from the Department of Health, Education, and Welfare dropped by $9 million between fiscal years 1967 and 1968, with fifty-three medical schools receiving less for research in 1968 than they had the previous year, in some cases with losses of over 50 percent.[44] Since then the cutbacks have continued, becoming acute in the delayed and trimmed Nixon budget for the Department of Health, Education, and Welfare for fiscal year 1970, which was not signed until the year was almost at an end. They continue to remain in a state of crisis.

The impact on the medical schools is critical, not only in terms of the breaking up of established research projects and teams, but at the very core of the institutions. The full implications cannot yet be measured, partly because of the patterns of funding themselves. Because of the complexity of the project grant system, funds are being reduced not across-the-board but in small, persistent bites; one faculty member may for example have funds coming from separate sources, only one of which is withdrawn. The medical school may then try to subsidize him from other sources. Because of the intertwining of research with teaching, the latter function is threatened with the former. The federal government has not recognized a responsibility for medical school funding; the medical schools have thrust themselves into the present crisis. Yet there is a de facto government responsibility, if only in negative terms. If action is not taken quickly to shore up medical schools, some institutions may be forced to close.

Thus the peculiar situation developed where it is on the one hand federal policy to reduce support to medical schools, and on the other to increase the supply of physicians, the latter possibly having gained

43. Ibid., pp. 85–87.
44. *DHEW Obligations to Medical Schools FY 1968.*

momentum after the passage of federal aid to health professions education in 1963. In an important health message of 7 January 1965, President Johnson called for at least a 50 percent increase in the number of graduates from medical schools and a 100 percent increase of dental graduates by 1975. The number of professionals was coming increasingly to be seen as an aspect of overall health services development— a factor emphasized in the appointment of the presidential National Advisory Commission on Health Manpower in 1966, and strongly evident in the subsequent recommendations of this commission in November 1967. The commission estimated that physician supply would increase by about 18 percent in the period 1965–75, but that this would be more than offset by increasing population and increasing consumer demands for service. Even with a parallel increase in physician productivity, more doctors would be necessary.[45] Thus the movement to increase supply continued. The Health Manpower Act of 1968 (P.L. 90–490) expanded the Health Professions Educational Assistance Act by including new conditions to encourage medical and nursing schools to increase their student enrollments and enlarged the scholarship and loans programs.[46] In fiscal year 1968, however, federal funds for teaching in medical schools represented on average only about 12 percent of the schools' budgets.[47] Moreover, much of the increased money is being directed to the establishment of new medical schools, rather than to any major realignment between research and teaching funds in established schools.

Since 1968, medical schools, legislatures, and private groups have responded with alacrity to the sense of urgency over increasing the number of physicians; the number of medical schools is beginning to swing back to pre-Flexner levels. By 1970, there were 100 four-year medical schools in the United States, in full or partial operation or in development. Of these, 69 were founded before 1910; another 14 appeared over the next fifty years, that is between the Flexner report and 1960. In the

45. *Report of the National Advisory Commission on Health Manpower I* (Washington, D.C., 1967), pp. 13–15.
46. The Health Manpower Act amended and consolidated the provisions of five existing health laws. Besides the Health Professions Educational Assistance Act of 1963, amendments were made to the Public Health Service Act of 1956, the Nurse Training Act of 1964, and the Allied Health Professions Personnel Training Act of 1966. The new legislation increased the proportion of the federal share from one-half to two-thirds of construction costs in cases when schools are experiencing financial difficulties, set up a competitive scheme among schools so that schools which increase their enrollment the most receive the greatest share of federal funds, and allowed special project grants for innovative teaching programs which promise to expand and to improve manpower supply.
47. *DHEW Obligations to Medical Schools FY 1968,* pp. 2, 61, 63.

last decade, as many as 16 new four-year schools have been founded, together with 4 two-year schools of basic medical sciences, and at least 12 more two- or four-year schools are being considered at various institutions around the country. Since 1960, therefore, the call for 20 new medical schools has been met, although most of these schools are as yet far from their full capacity. At the same time, the older schools have made some efforts to expand their enrollment; the number of medical students increased from under 30,000 in 1958 to nearly 38,000 in 1969.[48] Given an average length of medical education of eight years—four years of medical school, a one-year internship, and a three-year residency—it will not be until the late 1970s and early 1980s that the expanded supply of physicians will begin to make an impact on full-time medical practice. Nevertheless the buildup is evident. Medical schools have taken on a major commitment to increase the number of physicians, even though present resources cast doubt on their ability to sustain this commitment, unless educational funds are rapidly increased.

THE MEDICAL SCHOOL

The traditional roles of medical schools are teaching, service, and research, presumably in that order of priority. The great era of research funding, 1950–66, put particular emphasis on the last. In the past decade, there has also been increasing emphasis on the medical school as a service center, not merely as an adjunct of undergraduate teaching but as an essential cog and catalyst of the developing health care system. Indeed, in the Eighty-ninth Congress, university-based hospital regions surfaced effectively as a possible framework for restructuring the American hospital system. Legislation of 1965 (P.L. 89–239) enabled cooperative arrangements to be made among medical schools, research institutions and hospitals for research, education and demonstrations of patient care (but not general patient care) in heart disease, cancer, stroke, and related diseases. This was accomplished through federal grants on the basis of applications for new regional medical programs. At present forty such programs are in operation; another fifteen are in the process of becoming operational. In the same period university medical centers have become involved in the development of neighborhood health centers and comprehensive child health services for poverty populations, funded by the Office of Economic Opportunity and the Children's Bureau; in establishing community mental health centers sponsored in part by

48. "Medical Education in the United States," *J. Amer. med. Ass., 214* (1970), 1512.

the National Institute of Mental Health; in developing prepaid group practices; and in other innovative service schemes.[49] These programs, most of which are still in the process of development, have given a new role to medical schools, new federal responsibilities, and a new impetus for the revision of undergraduate medical teaching. On the one hand is the research component, pushing toward knowledge and further specialization; on the other hand are the new applied service programs that require generalists in family practice, pediatrics, and psychiatry. The undergraduate medical curriculum is poised uneasily between.

Seen in terms of the natural history of professionalism, recent developments in medical education represent a striking success. The average doctor has been transformed in sixty years from an incompetent physician, whose strength lay in the "bedside manner" of his mystique, to a specialist internist, surgeon, or endocrinologist whose own competence is buttressed by an array of diagnostic and treatment aids and techniques. American doctors are among the best trained, perhaps *the* best-trained technological physicians in the world. Together, however, they are not providing optimal medical care; and it is this factor which has become the educational paradox—the manpower crisis—of the 1970s. Traditional goals of professionalism are no longer enough. If the medical schools are to meet their role as public service corporations, the inbuilt conflict between the goals of professionalism and the improvement of health services has to be resolved.

This process began seriously in the 1960s with the passage of federal aid to medical education, appreciation of the role of government vis-à-vis the schools, and the growing awareness of the organizational problems and social inequities of American medical care. The medical schools themselves have begun to exert effective leadership with the strengthening of the Association of American Medical Colleges. The Association produced a landmark report in 1965, which called for a broader and enlarged responsibility in that group and for a wider social and educational role by individual medical schools, extending from undergraduate to graduate and continuing medical education.[50] The AMA meanwhile was becoming concerned about the undersupply of physicians, a concern emphasized by the passage of Medicare in 1965 and the promise of increased social demands on medical services in the future.

Meetings between the AMA Board of Trustees and Council on Medi-

49. The background legislation and development of programs are described and developed in chapter 20.
50. Lowell T. Coggeshall, *Planning for Medical Programs Through Education* (Coggeshall Report), Association of American Medical Colleges (1965).

cal Education with AAMC representatives resulted in an epochal joint statement on health manpower released in the spring of 1968. For the first time, it was noted, "both associations endorsed the position that all medical schools should now accept as a goal the expansion of their collective enrollments to a level that permits all qualified applicants to be admitted," [51] a condition which has not been met since before the Flexner reforms. The associations stressed that to do this would require adequate financing from both private sources and the federal government, for construction, operation, and experimentation in the medical schools. Education, it was emphasized, should be given increasing emphasis in the medical schools, to the end that their mission of medical manpower production be given the highest possible priority. Once again the situation which prevailed during the Flexner reforms has been attained. The leading medical schools, the AMA, and leading public organizations (in this case the federal government) are in agreement on a single professional goal—this time, a rapidly increased production of physicians.

The medical schools are now thus once again in a state of rapid functional transition. Efforts are being made in the older schools to reform the curriculum toward a greater emphasis on community or general medicine and toward more flexibility and earlier specialization. The student's first patient used to be a corpse in an anatomy class; the trend now is to introduce students very early to the patient, and not only on the wards but in clinics and physician offices. The new schools are freer to develop new curricula; the new University of Arizona College of Medicine, the Milton S. Hershey Medical Center at Hershey, Pennsylvania, and the School of Medicine of the State University of New York at Stony Brook are three notable examples. These schools are seizing the opportunity for teaching first year students by contact with patients; for emphasizing patient care with research as an adjunct (rather than vice versa); for developing medicine as a humanity as well as a science; and for building medical education as one of a series of educational programs for all health professionals. In a sense the wheel has come full circle from the 1870s to the 1970s—away from the homogenization of students and advancement of science which were the hallmark of the Flexner reforms, and back (or forward) to differential curricula, a widening in the type, background, and interests of students, and a return to the primary apprenticeship aspects of medical education.

The curriculum itself is not, however, by any means the most striking implication of the long and curious history of medical schools and medi-

51. Joint AMA–AAMC statements were released on 5 Mar. 1968 and 16 Apr. 1968. *J. Amer. med. Ass., 206* (1968), 1970.

cal education. Nor is it the only future answer to realignments between professional structures and attitudes and the emerging physician manpower structure. The federal government has become tacitly responsible for the number of medical students, and for the basic financing of medical schools. The production of physicians is thus firmly in the public as well as the professional arena—in financial fact, as well as by philosophical implication. There is a national manpower policy, strongly endorsed by the major professional associations, to increase the supply of physicians. Strong governmental and professional action is now urgently required to translate the accepted policies into effective action, preferably before one or more medical schools fold under the present fiscal restraints. A stated explicit and effective national funding policy is essential, through a responsible national council for medical education. Federal block grants to medical schools should be reexamined. The fragmented funding pattern for research, even if continued, should be constantly evaluated, and regulated, in terms of its institutional implications. In short, the implicit aspects of federal intervention in medical education, as de facto proprietor of the medical schools and as delineator of manpower policy, should be rapidly made explicit. Clearly in this process the professional associations themselves would need to play a major role.

The institutional issues are manifold—whether there should be separate research faculty and institutes in medical schools; whether community practitioners and medical scientists are best trained in the same or different schools; how (and by whom) funding is to be controlled. The professional issues both connect and follow. The question of who is to decide on the number of physicians, and by what means, depends on the future structures of federal health policy as a whole, and on the emerging health care system as much as on professional prerogatives. (A centralized national health insurance scheme might, for example, have its own manpower and educational funding divisions with representatives of governmental, professional, and consumer groups.) But—as always—the number and basic education of physicians is only one of the evolving issues of professionalism. Professional regulation, in the form of licensing, accreditation, and certification, continues to be as important as the structure of undergraduate medical education. The medical schools may produce more, and differently educated physicians with the M.D. degree. Yet the new graduates still have four or more years of graduate education before them, and ultimately specialist certification; their experiences in this period as well as in medical school will determine their ultimate medical careers, and thus the success or failure of the professional system in meeting society's demand for physicians. The crucial area is now graduate medical education.

The evolution of the medical schools, the role of federal support in medical education, service, and research, the future of the specialty boards, are thus all tied together. The debates over whether there are too few or too many physicians (proved by experience to be more a question of opinion and expedience than of any objective measurement), whether abdominal surgeons should have a specialty board, whether there should be general practice residencies, whether health insurance is needed, are fragmented but interconnecting reactions from within the medical profession to the changed milieu of medical care, each a direct product of medical specialization, in its turn the product and stimulator of scientific excellence. The problems of medical schools as of other professional institutions are the products not of a failure in medicine, but of releasing the potentials of the technological successes of the previous 30 years in a medical system which has been developing for over 300 years, and which could not easily bend to change. At issue now is how the pieces are to be linked together.

CHAPTER 17

Graduate Medical Education

Developments in scientific specialization, in public demands for a subsidized and organized health service, and in the transformation of medicine into a series of specialties created a volatile situation within the medical profession of the 1950s and 1960s which was not unlike the situation existing before World War I. The scattered, unevenly educated, and largely uncontrolled medical profession of the earlier period had been integrated and standardized by the AMA and the Flexner reforms, through a partnership of professional associations, leading medical schools, and private foundations. But with the development of specialties, accelerating after World War II, a new system of professional demarcations and stratifications was built. The fragmentation was now inside the confines of one profession. But once again the profession was scattered and apart. Once more there was a need for reintegration of the purposes and functions of medical education in terms of the numbers, standards, and kinds of physicians appropriate to medicine's scientific and social contexts.

In the 1960s, however, the questions of redefining the medical profession and of "standardizing" medical education were far more complex than at the time of earlier professional reforms. At the crux were still the desired shapes and purposes of the physician's vocational education, and definition of responsibility for physician numbers, distribution, standards, and trends. But these decisions could no longer rest at the undergraduate level of medical education. The future of graduate medical education was now as important as had been the future of M.D. education at the time of the Flexner reforms. Questions of medical manpower, likewise, could not be limited to the number of students entering medical schools, for no longer could the assumption be made that one graduate would be similar as a physician to another. The days of producing a standardized "safe general practitioner" were long gone; instead, the medical schools were educating for a multitude of possible careers. As a result, improving the supply of physician services did not merely rest on increasing the number of medical students—the assumption made in the passage of the Health Professions Educational Assistance Act of 1963—it depended also on the physician's ultimate career choice, in terms of specialty as well as practice location. Manpower decisions of the 1970s have to be extended to the appropriate balance and mix of specialists, including the specialty of primary care. And this in turn depends on the emerging development of medical care financing and organization.

All these elements are combined in discussion of the role and future of graduate medical education. The old definitions of the internship as the learning period for general practitioners and of the residency as preparation for consulting practice for a minority of physicians became obsolete; yet the old structures remained. But beyond this, there have been growing pressures to consider the function of graduate medical education—as undergraduate medical education was considered long ago —in terms of the production of adequate physician manpower with appropriate skills for the practice of modern medicine. And in this last consideration are issues not only of education but also of providing the hospitals with house staffs and of developing professional organizations which can in turn produce a specialist manpower structure tailored to meet health service needs.

THE INTERNSHIP

Through years of university neglect of the education of interns, residents, and practicing physicians, graduate medical education was preempted by organized professional groups. The internship was claimed halfheartedly from time to time as the fifth year of medical school, although by the 1950s most medical schools (though not licensing boards) had dropped a requirement for the internship as part of the M.D. degree. The specialty boards put their stamp on residency programs, which now represented the sixth to eighth, ninth, or tenth years of medical education, depending on the specialty. In 1960, only 38.1 percent of internships and 53.9 percent of residencies were in hospitals affiliated with university medical schools.[1] Moreover, even in affiliated hospitals, the continuation of graduate medical education as a journeyman apprenticeship sharply distinguished the interns and residents from their juniors who were full-time university students working toward the M.D. degree. Interns and

1. See below table 7.

residents were technically students; they had been so designated in the GI bill and were regarded as incompletely trained by the specialty certifying boards. Yet the great majority were not enrolled in an institution of higher learning, nor were they preparing for a university certificate or degree.

With the lengthening of the educational span into specialty training for virtually all physicians came increased focus on house staff appointments as the true vocational training period. Between 1940 and 1960, at a time when entry into medical schools was being tightly controlled, the number of physicians in internship and residency training programs trebled, from less than 12,000 to nearly 38,000, four times the number of undergraduate medical students (see table 4). By the latter year, one

Table 4. *Physicians in Approved Training Programs, U.S.,
Selected Years, 1931–1969*

	1931	1940	1949	1960	1969
All physicians	158,406	178,643	206,277	249,989	305,047
Physicians in training programs	7,200	11,800	23,448	37,843	51,816
Physicians in training programs as percent of all physicians	4.5	6.6	11.4	15.1	17.0

Source: U.S. Department of Health, Education, and Welfare, *Health Manpower Source Book*, sec. 14, Medical Specialists, table 5; American Medical Association, *Distribution of Physicians in the U.S. 1969*, vol. 1, table 1.

of every seven physicians was an intern or resident. These "graduate students" had become an essential part of hospital staffing patterns, providing the necessary twenty-four-hour on-call service in the modern community hospital and performing the increasing battery of preliminary diagnostic tests. By 1960, internships and residencies were offered in 1,400 hospitals which contained among them almost half of the hospital beds in the country. These hospitals, together with their attending medical staffs, had a vested interest in retaining the scattered system of graduate apprenticeship which had become the basis for half of the physician's professional education. Thus the medical profession itself—or at least that substantial part of it which relied on house staffs to give invaluable professional service to their own hospitalized patients—had little incentive to suggest radical change.

The average doctor of 1910 had been threatened by an educational system which produced, in his eyes, too many doctors. He had thus been amenable to draconic measures for educational reform which, inter alia, rapidly reduced his competition. The average doctor of 1960 (or for that matter of 1971) was, in contrast, aided by a decentralized, local system of graduate medical education which provides house staff in local hospitals. As a result, the AMA Council on Medical Education has been unable to employ for graduate education the sanctions it so forcefully used to stamp out proprietary medical schools half a century ago. In the crucial period of expansion of internships and residencies to accommodate the expanded number of wartime students and of veterans returning after World War II, the AMA Council on Medical Education imposed no controls over the total number of house staff positions offered; nor over the number of approved teaching hospitals. The council viewed its own role as one of accreditation of all programs which met rather minimal educational criteria; there was no educational rationing process, as had for long existed in undergraduate medical schools. In sharp contrast to the competitive entry to medical school, there were more approved internship and residency positions than there were physicians ready to fill them. From the hospitals' point of view, there was particular concern over a shortage of interns, the backbone of the ward staffing structure. In 1940, more than 90 percent of internship positions were filled; in 1950 the proportion was less than 70 percent.[2] As competition became more intense, with hospitals inventing ingenious methods of recruitment and inducement, some degree of control over entry into graduate medical education became essential. The question was of how much control, for what purposes, and by whom control should be exerted.

One resolution, referred to the Council on Medical Education in 1948, would have set up a rationing system for house staff on the basis of a hospital's annual patient admissions. In theory, this scheme would have given small hospitals a better chance of attracting interns and residents, against the competition of large, more prestigious institutions. But this suggestion could hardly appeal to those interested in developing the internship as an integral and excellent part of the system of medical education, irrespective of the service needs of hospitals. Instead, as a measure to regulate competition among hospitals and to introduce some order into the selection process for prospective interns, the National Intern Matching Program was set up in 1951. This developed, under the guidance of the Council on Medical Education, the Association of American Medical Colleges and hospital organizations, a procedure and

2. In 1968–69, 74 percent of available internship positions were filled. "Graduate Medical Education," *J. Amer. med. Ass., 210* (1969), 1494, 1510.

a set of rules for hospitals and prospective interns to make their selections, respectively, of house staff and posts, including an agreed time for hospitals to offer their appointments.[3] The matching plan brought a welcome degree of organization out of chaos, protecting both hospitals and interns. Medical students could now become interns through a process of orderly change. The process did not, however, affect the nature of the internship itself, poised uneasily between undergraduate education and specialist residencies, and between an educational experience and a job.

The difference in goals between the hospitals and the educators dominated discussions of the internship throughout the 1950s, the one looking for the service of house staff and the prestige of educational accreditation, the other viewing interns more in the light of graduate students, who might more properly be educated in a relatively small number of institutions. The dichotomy of views was reflected in the differing pronouncements emanating from the AMA House of Delegates and from its Council on Medical Education. While the internship was losing its educational justification, its continuance was guarded carefully by the practitioners in the house of delegates; there was an organizational stalemate within the profession. If the council had been able to gain control over the number of interns, it could have taken a strong position over the future nature of the internship as an educational program. It could, for example, have developed a ranking system for internships according to their assessed quality, as had been done earlier for medical schools, gradually eliminating the weaker teaching hospitals. As it was, the wide range in educational standards for internships was well known, but there was little leverage for improvement.

The Council on Medical Education suggested in 1951 that there should be an overall reduction in the number of available places for interns in approved hospitals; more than 2,000 approved places for interns were then lying vacant. In hospitals approved for intern training only, it was suggested that the number of internships to be offered in 1952–53 would

3. Internships and residencies begin on 1 July of each year. In choosing an internship the medical student registers with the matching plan and makes applications to the hospitals of his choice. The student then sends to the matching plan a list of the hospitals to which he has applied, ranked in order of his preference. The hospital in turn ranks its applicants and files these with the matching plan. On a specified date in March hospitals and students receive the results of the matching of these two lists. From February 1968, the matching plan has also been available for residents, and is currently being so used for the specialists of radiology and orthopedic surgery. Details are given in the AMA's annual *Directory of Approved Internships and Residencies*.

be cut back to 80 percent of the number offered in 1950; and in hospitals approved for both internships and residencies the number was to be reduced to 70 percent.[4] But this plan, not surprisingly, held little appeal to medical staffs in approved hospitals, whose staffing might be threatened; and no action was taken. The number of available internships continued to exceed the number of applicants.

Instead of the number of places being consolidated and reduced, there was an inbuilt incentive for hospitals to seek applicants for vacant house staff positions from other sources. Since the supply of new M.D.s from American schools was strictly limited, one obvious solution was to attract medical graduates from foreign schools into approved graduate educational positions. The educational structure of medicine was becoming topsy-turvy. At the very time that there was supposedly an excess of doctors in practice, and efforts to reduce the supply of medical students, there was a "shortage" of house staffs. This shortage, however, had little to do with the future production of private physicians; for it was a shortage of house staff *per se,* not necessarily a shortage of trainees in different specialties. In 1968–69, over 14,000 internships were offered by American hospitals; 10,500 were filled, but of these, only 7,200 were filled by American graduates.[5] The internship thus continued to have features which were totally different from student recruitment and deployment in undergraduate medical education.

Meanwhile, there was continuing reluctance from professional groups in the 1950s, as there had been in the 1940s, to abolish the internship altogether, in favor of one system of graduate medical education leading to specialism. An advisory committee of medical school teachers, appointed by the Council on Medical Education to review the internship in 1951, suggested that it be regarded as the first year of a two-year graduate program for all physicians, whether or not they subsequently specialized. This committee also recommended that the Council on Medical Education continue to limit its surveillance of the internship by merely approving or disapproving each post; that it should not introduce any kind of qualitative ranking of positions (it being considered that guidance to good-quality internships was a responsibility of the medical schools); and that, in approving internships, the council should place no weight on whether a hospital was attached to a university, but

4. For hospitals approved after 1950, a formula was to be developed. "Establishment of a Quota Basis for the Appointment of Interns," *J. Amer. med. Ass., 146* (1951) 865–66. And see AMA, *Digest,* p. 421.
5. AMA, Directory of Approved Internships and Residencies (1969–70), Table 4, p. 4.

merely on the educational facilities and opportunities offered in the hospital.[6] In short, there was approval of the status quo. The committee did, however, recommend successfully that internship programs should be dropped from approval if they failed to fill the stated number of openings by a factor of two-thirds for two successive years; and this new rule was incorporated into the council's "essentials" for internship approval. But, under pressure from the AMA House of Delegates, the two-thirds rule was quickly dropped, in the interest of correcting apparent inequalities and injustices to the attending staff of community hospitals which were not affiliated with medical schools, and which had the most difficulty filling their internships. The committee had begun to look like a medical school plot. There was a continuing division of objectives between teachers and practitioners.

To obtain a more acceptable view of the internship, the AMA House of Delegates set up a new group to represent private practitioners who were not connected with medical schools or their affiliated hospitals. The new Ad Hoc Committee on Internships reported to the house of delegates in December 1954 and June 1955. This group also upheld the value of the internship as a separate educational period, unaffiliated with either the undergraduate or specialist training years, but acting as the fifth year of medical education. The committee came out firmly against any quota system for interns, or any "arbitrary scheme designed to allocate interns to hospitals." [7] It did, however, endorse the principle that any hospital not filling one-fourth of its complement of interns in two successive years be dropped from the approved list, and this was incorporated into the "essentials" in 1955. The committee also suggested that university-affiliated hospitals be studied with a view toward a "voluntary reduction" in the number of internships they offered, or even a possible elimination of internships from these hospitals; and that the possibility of discontinuing approval of intern programs in veterans hospitals be considered. Taken as a whole, the recommendations were a strong plea for strengthening the position of interns in voluntary hospitals outside the major university teaching centers.

If the internship were regarded as a working apprenticeship, there was much to be said for this view. Medical schools and their affiliated

6. The Advisory Committee on Internships was chaired by Dr. Victor Johnson, who had been secretary of the Council on Medical Education (1943–47) and a member of the executive committee of the Advisory Board of Medical Specialties. "Report of the Advisory Committee on Internships to the Council on Medical Education and Hospitals of the American Medical Association," *J. Amer. med. Ass.*, *151* (1953), 499–510; and see AMA, *Digest,* p. 423.

7. AMA, *Digest,* pp. 424–26.

hospitals were already a labyrinth for students of many different kinds, and in some specialties there was keen competition among students for providing patient care. The obstetrics department, for example, was the learning laboratory not only for interns and residents in obstetrics but sometimes also for medical students, nurses, and sometimes nurse midwives, all competing for available deliveries. The patient in a university-affiliated hospital might be seen by an intern, by medical students, by assistant and senior residents, and by university professors in the department, often eliciting similar basic facts. During the 1950s and 1960s, moreover, as health insurance reduced the availability of the old "charity" or ward patients, it also became customary for university-related hospitals to teach students at the bedside of private and semi-private patients. The private patient was thus subject to the whole spectrum of students and teaching physicians, plus the attendance of his private physician. The intern stood in the middle, servant both of the attending physician and of the university department to which he was attached. An influential study by Saunders in 1960 documented the financial and professional exploitation of interns in university hospitals. Surgical interns were allowed to perform procedures as if this were a favor on the part of the surgical staff. Obstetrics and gynecology was a particularly poorly planned field, with interns only rarely getting more than preparation for doing uncomplicated procedures. There was a lack of connection between the various parts of medical education. (Nor was this confined to university-based internships.) Saunders concluded his observations with cogent arguments for recognizing the internship as the first year of residency, thereby developing an integrated program of graduate education.[8] Logically, as education, this would be based on universities. But it could equally well be held that at least the initial stages of graduate medical education should be removed from the hard-pressed medical schools altogether, into well-organized graduate medical centers.

Again, the organizational structure of medical practice militated against objective and innovative discussion of such issues. Graduate medical education was located in hospitals because it had developed in hospitals. As a result future physicians, who would spend most of their time in office practice rather than in hospitals and dealing chiefly with patients who would not require hospitalization, were still being trained on the hospitalized sick. Except in the emergency room, these patients were usually classified into a broad category of sickness through their

8. Richard Saunders, "The University Hospital Internship in 1960: A Study of the Programs of 27 Major Teaching Hospitals," *J. med. Educ., 36* (1961), 642–43.

assignment to a particular specialist department of the hospital. Even in a rotating internship, the young graduate was experiencing a situation which was quite different from the average patient mix in private office practice. He might be receiving an excellent education to become a resident or a permanent member of the hospital staff, but the training was not necessarily appropriate to his future professional practice. If graduate medical education was to be regarded as an apprenticeship (parallel, say, to the first post taken by a new law student who aimed to enter private practice), a more appropriate assignment would probably be as a junior associate in a group practice of specialists who also formed the staff of a community hospital—the form, for example, of the Kaiser Permanente group practice model. But this alternative was not, at least as yet, organizationally available. Nor was it in line with the traditional mold of teaching physicians which was of the "baptism by fire" variety; there seemed to be an assumption that the good physician was one tough enough to make judgments in the face of life-and-death crises on the wards, and to survive these judgments, while himself suffering from long hours and little sleep. This was, after all, what existing private physicians had themselves experienced, the entry ritual into the society of physicians.

Quite apart from the appropriateness of training, however, was the question of which professional organization or group had the responsibility of speaking for graduate medical education. The question remained open, for up to 1965 only a minority of the internships offered were in hospitals affiliated with medical schools. If the internship were an associateship, the appropriate group was probably the practicing physicians; if the intern were a graduate student, the educators (including those on specialty boards) were the more logical determiners of curriculum and quality. Both views were current through the 1960s. Partly as a reflection of this there were continuing attempts from within the AMA House of Delegates to change the structure of the Council on Medical Education from its predominance of university teachers by requiring half of its membership to be private practitioners who were not connected with university-affiliated hospitals. But these moves were unsuccessful. In its turn, the council meanwhile tried, unsuccessfully, to cut itself free from the practitioners in the House to relative independence as a council of the board of trustees.[9] This atmosphere of mutual dis-

9. Under AMA bylaws of 1948, the council consisted of seven members or service fellows, at least one of whom had to be a private practitioner who was neither a faculty member of a medical school nor a staff member of a university-affiliated hospital. Membership was increased to ten members in 1952, but with no further stipulations about private practitioners. In 1953, the reference committee on medi-

trust between the council and the delegates was scarcely conducive to authoritative consideration of graduate medical education, and it was only after 1959, when the council began a deliberate program to improve relations between medical education and practice, and as the structure and functioning of graduate medical education increasingly demanded review and reform, that the situation began to improve.

The official AMA view toward the internship in the 1950s was the encouragement and retention of the rotating internship, which could be regarded, though increasingly unrealistically, as preparation for general practice. This view complemented other suggestions in the house (described in chap. 14) which were likewise designed to stem the decline of general practitioners. A 1956 resolution of the house of delegates, apparently reflecting distrust of the Council on Medical Education's position toward the internship, asked the council to increase its efforts to encourage rotating internships and to publish the results of these efforts each year.[10] These efforts kept the types of internship fairly constant up to 1960, with rotating programs accounting for about 75 percent of all internships (see table 5). The council approved straight (i.e. specialist) internships only in medicine, surgery, pediatrics, and pathology, and these were chiefly in university-affiliated hospitals. The questions of university or nonuniversity responsibility for the internship and of retention or rejection of a general internship thus overlapped. They were part of an older division of university specialist interests versus the generalists in the community; and there was a presumption (not unfounded) that university-based graduate medical education would automatically favor specialties. It was only with the recognition of general practice itself as a specialist field, with its own residency program, that this stance became modified, and that the tensions surrounding the future of the internship lessened.

---

cal education felt it necessary to issue a long statement about the council's functions. One tart remark in the statement was that those not familiar with the council's history in education "frequently assume that the Council's chief function is to protect the interests of the medical profession against any movements in medical education that physicians may feel are inimical to their personal interests."

The struggle between practitioners and educators continued into the 1960s. A resolution to the house in 1961 that the council include five private practitioners was not acted on. The question of the ratio of private practitioners in unaffiliated hospitals to "salaried personnel of a medical school or university" on the council was raised again the following year, and similarly in 1963, both times without any action being taken. The council continues as a standing committee of the house of delegates, whose members are nominated by the AMA Board of Trustees. It has ten members, on five-year terms. AMA, *Digest,* pp. 464–66; and AMA, *Supplement Digest,* pp. 192–94.

10. AMA, *Digest,* p. 427, and see pp. 429–30.

Table 5. Types of Internship Programs Offered, 1959–1969

| | Types of Programs | | | | | | | | |
| | Rotating; no major emphasis | | Rotating; emphasis on a specialty[1] | | Straight | | General practice | | |
	No.	%	No.	%	No.	%	No.	%	Totals
1959–60	816	75	33	3	246	22	0	0	1,097
1960–61	817	70	69	6	276	24	5	*	1,167
1961–62	737	61	107	9	359	30	9	*	1,212
1962–63	697	56	133	11	391	32	14	1	1,235
1963–64	661	52	153	12	432	34	17	1	1,263
1964–65	658	50	189	14	467	35	14	1	1,328
1965–66	641	45	251	17	531	37	17	1	1,440
1966–67	568	24	1,211	51	582	24	17	*	2,378
1967–68	563	20	1,502	54	687	25	16	*	2,768
1968–69	581	21	1,504	54	703	25	0	0	2,788

1. Listed in tables previous to 1966–67 as "mixed" internships.
* Less than 1%.

Source: American Medical Association, *Directory of Approved Internships and Residencies*, 1969–70, table 3.

There was still, however, no guiding organization to make policy decisions about the internship, in terms of its own development or in relation to other aspects of medical education. The Internship Review Committee, set up in 1954, brought together various professional groups concerned with intern training—the Council on Medical Education, the Federation of State Medical Boards, the American Hospital Association, the American Academy of General Practice, and the Association of American Medical Colleges—but this was a judicial rather than a policy committee. Like the residency review committees which were developing at the same time, it received the reports of inspectors from the Council on Medical Education on each program, together with supporting data from the hospital, and approved, provisionally approved, deferred action on, or put on probation each program individually, according to the rules set out in the "Essentials of an Approved Internship." [11] The great majority were approved. There was no attempt to cluster internships in particular teaching centers or specific areas.

11. The Essentials set out guiding principles, as well as concrete requirements, for an approved internship program. Stress is placed on: (1) the primacy of the educational function of the internship; (2) the unique educational character of the internship—neither a fifth year of medical school nor a first year of specialty training; and (3) organization of the internship in such a way as to provide the intern with a progressive increase in responsibility for the care of the sick. An

THE RESIDENCY

The purpose of the residency, dependent as it was on the specifications for training set out by the specialty certifying boards, was much more clearly definable. The residency was the training period in which physicians reached reasonable competence in a specialty, and thus to practice as a physician. Residency training was the modern equivalent of the undergraduate medical education envisaged in the Flexner report. The organizational structure for residency approval was, however, little better prepared for taking leadership toward the development of a well-planned program for graduate medical education than was that for the internship. Residencies were scattered over 1,400 hospitals. But besides geographical diffusion, there continued also to be a lack of coordination in training in related specialties—the result of diffusion of responsibility for the specification of standards for training, and of the accreditation of particular training programs among the independent certifying boards. One hospital might, for example, have four specialist residency programs. While broad general standards for training were set out in the "Essentials of Approved Residencies" of the AMA Council on Medical Education,[12] each specialist group had its own criteria; thus

approved internship must be at least 12 months in length and may be either "rotating" or "straight." A rotating internship is one which provides supervised training in internal medicine and at least one of the following: surgery, pediatrics, obstetrics and gynecology, psychiatry, pathology, radiology, and anesthesiology. In rotating internships lasting 12 months, at least 2 months in duration must be spent on the emphasized specialty areas. A straight internship is one which concentrates on a single service, with the possible inclusion of one or more related subspecialties. These are given in: internal medicine, surgery, pediatrics, obstetrics-gynecology, and pathology. Hospitals offering straight internships must be approved for residency training in the specialties involved.

To be eligible for approval, hospitals seeking to offer internships must have a capacity of 150 beds and a minimum of 5,000 annual admissions, excluding the newborn. In addition three of the four major clinical divisions must be represented, and an organized outpatient service on a continuous basis must be available, either within the hospital or through affiliation with another hospital. The hospital must also maintain an autopsy rate of at least 25 percent of its deaths. Each clinical department should have a chairman who serves for a minimum of a year and is responsible for the general conduct of the clinical work in his department and assists in formulating and carrying out the internship program. All hospitals offering approved internships must be accredited by the Joint Commission on Accreditation of Hospitals. "Essentials of an Approved Internship," in AMA, *Directory of Approved Internships and Residencies* (1969–70).

12. According to the "Essentials of Approved Residencies," graduate medical training in the various specialties should be of sufficient duration and educational content to enable the resident to begin the practice of his specialty upon completion of his training. With the exception of a few specialties, such as pediatrics, a well-organized, comprehensive program should include three or more years of formal

the hospital had to comply with four separate sets of requirements. For the large hospitals, of course, with as many as eighteen specialist training programs and additional subspecialty components, the process of reviews and regulations was compounded.

By 1950, all but two of the specialty boards had joint arrangements for residency approval with the AMA, but these arrangements appeared more cohesive on paper than they did in practice.[13] Hospitals were still subjected to the visits of inspection teams from the Council on Medical Education and from the various specialty boards. And there were other organizations (notably the American College of Surgeons) which were also interested in improved training standards. But some reforms were in sight. In 1950, after two years of discussion, the Joint Conference Committee on Graduate Training in Surgery was named, with equal representation from the American Board of Surgery, the American College of Surgeons, and the Council on Medical Education. This development of a unified committee for residency review, albeit in one specialty, was a breakthrough in cooperative arrangements, obviating the need for multiple hospital inspections. In its first year, the committee approved 224 four-year residency programs in general surgery and 258

residency work. Daily contact with both patients and the attending staff, participation in an organized educational program, and the assumption of responsibility are the most important aspects of a residency. Therefore, as the resident demonstrates his ability, an increasing degree of reliance should be given to his judgment in diagnosis and treatment, as well as in the teaching of interns, nurses, and medical students. The training of residents should emphasize personal instruction at the bedside, in the operating room and in the delivery room, together with related laboratory studies, teaching rounds, departmental conferences or seminars, clinical-pathological conferences, demonstrations, and lectures. In addition, the resident staff should have definite assignments in the scheduled clinics and an active role in the emergency service.

One of the most important requisites for a hospital engaged in providing residency training is a well-organized and well-qualified staff. There should be an educational committee of the staff which has the responsibility for organizing, supervising, and directing the residency program, and for correlating the activities of the resident staff in the various departments of the hospital. All hospitals applying for approved residency programs must be accredited by the Joint Commission on Accreditation of Hospitals. "Essentials of Approved Residencies," in AMA, *Directory of Approved Internships and Residencies* (1969–70).

13. The two were ophthalmology and preventive medicine. Joint arrangements in fact meant approval in concurrence with the boards, rather than unified action. The council procedure was to process applications from hospitals, send a brief form to be filled in, and, if this looked satisfactory, arrange for an inspection. Prior to the inspection, hospitals were asked to fill out a long form. Edward H. Leveroos et al, "Approved Internships and Residencies," *J. Amer. med. Ass., 142* (1950), 1145. For a general review of cooperative arrangements, see E. L. Turner, "Background and Development of Residency Review and Conference Committees," *J. Amer. med. Ass., 165* (1957), 60–64.

three-year programs; it attempted to stimulate four-year graded (i.e. progressive) residency programs and developed a guidebook on residency training.[14] The conference committee took on the educational or training functions, while the specialty board was freed, at least in theory, to concentrate on basic standards and on examination techniques.

The tripartite conference committee began to take hold. By the middle of 1958, the American College of Surgeons and the Council on Medical Education had established similar joint relations with the American Board of Otolaryngology, the American Board of Plastic Surgery, and the American Board of Obstetrics and Gynecology. On the prompting of the American College of Physicians, moreover, a joint educational committee in internal medicine was reactivated in 1949 whose membership consisted of the College, the council, and the American Board of Internal Medicine. In 1953 the name was changed to the Residency Review Committee in Internal Medicine.[15] As an outcome of these residency review committees, other specialty boards grew interested in similar arrangements. The Council on Medical Education endorsed the proposal of such joint arrangements in 1952 and suggested to the other boards that they form bilateral residency review committees with two or three members from the board and from the council. By October 1958, eleven specialty boards had established such committees, and there was also a committee to review the small number of GP residencies; the latter included representatives of the council and the American Academy of General Practice. A residency review committee in thoracic surgery was announced in November 1966, leaving only pathology—at the request of the American Board of Pathology—with the old collaborative arrangements of residency review.

The residency review committees, empowered to act in approving residency programs on behalf of their constituent organizations, formed a new pattern of specialist regulation and a new link between the individual boards and the Council on Medical Education. The committees were also free to make recommendations as to requirements and training programs in the specialties (although the specification of such requirements remained the responsibility of the boards), and several of the

14. Editorial, Warren H. Cole, "The Conference Committee on Graduate Training in Surgery," *J. Amer. med. Ass., 171* (1959), 843–44.
15. Plans for a joint committee of the Council on Medical Education, the American College of Physicians, and the American Board of Internal Medicine were made in 1939, and the first organizational meeting was held in February 1940. This committee evaluated residency programs in internal medicine until the outbreak of war, when its function was disrupted. During the war the council continued to approve residencies in cooperation with the board. Weiskotten and Johnson, *History,* p. 33.

committees issued training guides for the use of program directors in hospitals. At least in part, the residency training function was recognized as a joint professional responsibility, a move that was hailed by medical educators as a major accomplishment in graduate medical education. The system also put the Council on Medical Education squarely back into the field of graduate training and hospital review, for not only was it the common denominator of the residency review committees, it was also a crucial participant in the Advisory Committee on Internships. In terms of accreditation there was the long-term possibility of linking review of graduate training within the confines of one specialty, and, indeed, arrangements were completed for review of straight internships by residency review committees in the relevant specialties in 1969. But the council's difficulties within the AMA, and the continuing chauvinism of specialty boards in reaction to urging that they cooperate more fully in the Advisory Board for Medical Specialties, militated against the establishment within existing organizations of one dominant organization for all aspects of graduate medical education. It was unlikely that the council alone would be allowed to provide any effective coordination of graduate education as a whole. Indeed, the same questions and constraints which inhibited the council's control over the number and distribution of internships applied equally to residencies. Residency review was, moreover, a limited function: a matter of accrediting positions in given specialist areas rather than developing broad educational policies. Field staff of the Council on Medical Education, on behalf of the residency review committees, looked at a total of between 1,700 and 2,200 residency programs each year during the 1960s.[16] The review committees were not, and are not, linked together; each works separately and independently. If anything, the residency review committees, instead of unifying graduate medical education, further fragmented it by making the existing fragmentation more efficient.

The implications of fragmentation on future manpower development became more urgent as residency positions became the de facto gateway to medical practice. About 80 percent were filled. In recognition of the fact that residency training lasted an average of three years, there were by the 1960s three times as many residents as interns (see table 6). The number of residencies rose from under 20,000 in 1950 to more than 40,000 in 1970. Half of the residencies offered in 1960 were in university-affiliated hospitals, with the proportion rising to more than three-quarters by 1970 (see table 7); but the residency, like the internship, relied chiefly on training by apprenticeship and associateship rather

16. "Graduate Medical Education," *J. Amer. med. Ass., 210* (1969), 1498.

Table 6. Number of Approved Internships and Residencies in the United States and Its Territories and Possessions, Selected Years, 1942–1968[1]

Year	Internships		Residencies	
	No. offered	% filled	No. offered	% filled
1942	8,180	64	5,796	60
1950	10,004	68	19,464	75
1954	11,648	78	25,486	80
1957	12,325	83	30,595	82
1960	12,547	73	32,786	87
1963	12,229	79	37,357	79
1966	13,569	76	39,384	81
1968	14,112	75	42,644	83

1. Figures from 1960 include residents in other than hospitals.

Source: U.S.D.H.E.W., Health Manpower Source Book, sec. 9, Physicians, Dentists, and Professional Nurses; American Medical Association, Directory of Approved Internships and Residencies, selected years.

than on an academic graduate program. The focus was on the hospital, rather than on the university. There was no master plan as to the desired distribution of physicians among the specialties.

The specialty distribution of residencies has arisen out of decisions made to give residency approval to specific specialty departments of different hospitals, and this in turn reflects, at least in part, the hospitals' perceptions of their staffing needs and training facilities. The breakdown

Table 7. Internships and Residencies in Hospitals Affiliated with Medical Schools, U.S., Selected Years, 1960–1971[1]

Year	Internships			Residencies		
	Total no.	No. in university-affiliated hospitals	Percent in university-affiliated hospitals	Total no.	No. in university-affiliated hospitals	Percent in university-affiliated hospitals
1960–61	12,547	4,779	38.1	32,620	17,588	53.9
1962–63	12,024	5,907	49.1	36,162	22,373	61.9
1964–65	12,728	4,964	39.0	38,373	18,622	48.5
1966–67	13,569	7,615	56.1	38,895	24,854	63.9
1968–69	14,509	8,329	57.4	42,889	27,208	63.4
1970–71	14,683	9,457	64.4	46,250	35,803	77.4

1. Number of positions offered.

Source: American Medical Association, Directory of Approved Internships and Residencies, selected years.

into specialties between those in training and those in practice is given
in table 8. The resulting patterns have no necessary relationship to what
either a professional group or a public group might indicate as appropriate patterns for the development of medical manpower in the future.
Nor was their any reason why the residency review committees, as
accrediting rather than planning agencies, should shoulder a wider responsibility.

Nevertheless, there were increasing pressures for some body or group
to review the implications of the emerging residency system in terms of
its vocational implications and social needs, for with his choice of residency the physician made his choice of a specialist career. The types
and numbers of residencies offered were thus of great importance in reviewing the emerging character of the whole profession. In 1970–71, for
example, there were more residency openings for urologists than for
general practitioners. There were more residencies offered in radiology

Table 8. Physicians in the United States and Possessions, Dec. 31, 1969

	All Physicians				
Specialty	Total no.[1]	%	No. in training	%	Of total MD's in each field %
All	302,966	100	51,816	100	17
General practice	58,919	19	1,397	3	2
Internal medicine	38,258	13	7,992	15	21
General surgery	28,603	9	7,106	14	25
Psychiatry	20,328	7	3,506	7	17
Obstetrics; gynecology	18,084	6	2,639	5	15
Pediatrics[2]	17,926	6	3,398	7	19
Radiology[3]	12,367	4	2,611	5	21
Anesthesiology	10,434	3	1,497	3	14
Pathology	9,826	3	2,327	4	24
Ophthalmology	9,578	3	1,343	3	14
Orthopedic surgery	9,227	3	1,893	4	21
Others	69,416	23	16,107	31	23

1. Excludes those inactive (19,895), unknown (2,081).
2. Includes pediatric allergy, pediatric cardiology.
3. Includes diagnostic radiology, therapeutic radiology.

Source: American Medical Association, *Distribution of Physicians in the U.S. 1969*,
table 1.

than in pediatrics; more residencies in pathology than in obstetrics and gynecology; there were more places for dermatologists than for specialists in physical medicine. Almost one-fourth of all residencies offered were in general surgery, or in neurological, orthopedic, plastic or thoracic surgery (see table 9). These proportions were unlikely to

Table 9. Number of Approved Residencies Offered in the United States and Its Territories and Possessions, by Specialty, Selected Years, 1940–1970

Specialty	Number of Residencies Offered			
	1940	1950	1960	1970
Total	5,118	18,669	31,733	46,785
Allergy		12	28	99[1]
Anesthesiology	109	731	1,413	2,099
Aviation medicine			21	115
Cardiovasc. disease	6	37	135	
Contagious diseases	49	60		
Dermatology	62	238	330	577
Gastroenterology		9	71	
General practice		94	717	980
Internal medicine	728	3,751	5,525	7,970
Malignant diseases	71	116		
Neurological surgery	31	181	384	564
Neurology	68	200	420	914
Obstetrics; gynecology	419	1,522	2,572	3,070
Occupational medicine		2	16	86
Ophthalmology	150	493	784	1,354
Orthopedic surgery	194	779	1,261	2,102
Otolaryngology	274	422	506	1,008
Pathology	302	1,001	2,638	3,727[2]
Pediatrics	373	1,092	1,862	2,920[3]
Physical medicine	2	55	240	508
Plastic surgery	5	39	121	245
Proctology		18	36	32
Psychiatry	416	1,754	3,658	5,964[4]
Public health			78	305[5]
Pulmonary disease	267	372	306	
Radiology	232	970	1,781	3,136
Surgery	808	4,150	5,872	7,654
Thoracic surgery	26	86	207	355
Urology	123	485	751	1,001

1. Includes pediatric allergy.
2. Includes forensic pathology.
3. Includes pediatric cardiology.
4. Includes child psychiatry.
5. Includes general preventive medicine and public health.

Source: U.S.D.H.E.W., Health Manpower Source Book, sec. 13, Hospital House Staffs, table 8; and American Medical Association, Directory of Approved Internships and Residencies 1969-70, table 10.

be reasonable reflections of society's demand for physicians. They were, rather, reflections of hospital staffing and teaching interests.

FOREIGN MEDICAL GRADUATES

Nowhere was the cumbersome structure and lack of centralized responsibility for graduate medical education more evident than in consideration of the increasing flow of foreign medical graduates into internship and residency positions. In 1951 there were over 2,000 foreign graduates in internship or residency positions; by 1956 there were over 6,000; and in 1969 there were over 14,000, out of a total of 45,000 interns and residents on duty. In this last year, foreign house staff represented 31 percent of all filled internships and 32 percent of all residencies (see table 10). The existence of such a large and increasing number of visitors,

Table 10. House Staff Positions Filled by Graduates of Foreign Medical Schools in Relation to All Filled Positions, 1951–1969

| Year | Foreign house staff[1] | | Foreign interns | | Foreign residents | |
	Number	Filled positions %	Number	Filled positions %	Number	Filled positions %
1951	2,072	10	722	10	1,350	9
1952	3,349	14	1,116	14	2,233	14
1953	4,388	18	1,353	18	3,035	18
1954	5,589	21	1,787	22	3,802	20
1955	5,036	17	1,761	19	3,275	16
1956	6,033	19	1,859	19	4,174	19
1957	6,741	20	1,988	20	4,753	21
1958	7,622	22	2,079	20	5,543	22
1959	8,357	23	2,315	22	6,042	23
1960	9,457	25	2,545	25	6,912	25
1961	9,935	26	1,753	19	8,182	29
1962	8,996	24	1,273	16	7,723	26
1963	8,731	23	1,669	19	7,062	24
1964	9,168	25	2,566	27	7,052	24
1965	10,974	27	2,821	28	8,153	26
1966	11,494	28	2,361	24	9,133	29
1967	12,295	29	2,793	27	9,502	30
1968	13,540	31	2,913	28	10,627	31
1969	14,501	32	3,270	31	11,231	32

1. Includes graduates of Canadian medical schools; excludes American graduates of foreign schools.

Source: U.S.D.H.E.W., Health Manpower Source Book, sec. 13, Hospital House Staffs, table 10; American Medical Association, Directory of Approved Internships and Residencies, selected years.

and yet the continued gap between the number of positions offered and the number actually filled, underlined the "shortage" of interns and residents—the gap between house staff supply and what the hospitals felt they could use.

By 1950 the supply of returning veterans from World War II, on whose behalf the number of residencies had been greatly increased, was coming to an end. The supply of American physicians for house staffs was further affected by the beginning of the Korean War. Meanwhile, as part of the rhetoric of the cold war, the United States government was promoting international exchange, on the assumption that bringing foreign visitors to the United States would give the world an introduction to freedom and democracy. The programs encouraging exchange visitors which followed the Smith-Mundt Act of 1948 made it easier for foreign medical graduates to enter the United States at the very time, coincidentally, that hospitals were searching for replacements for the dwindling supply of American physicians.[17] Foreign physicians, ostensibly as students, were actively wooed by many hospitals, at least in part to meet their staffing needs. Indeed, without substantial aid from abroad many hospitals would have had to function without house staffs, thus developing a very different staffing system. With the deliberate recruitment of

17. According to provisions in the Smith-Mundt Act, any sponsor of an educational exchange program might apply to the secretary of state to have it officially designated an Exchange-Visitor Program. Shortly after the first government programs were established, many such requests were received, and in the late 1940s the department began to grant this designation to programs sponsored by both individuals and private firms which met the primary objectives of the act; namely, promoting the better understanding of the United States abroad and increasing mutual understanding between the people of the United States and other countries. In making these designations it was emphasized that the intent of the Exchange-Visitor Program was that the participant should come to the United States for training and then return to his homeland to utilize that training. It was not intended to help meet staffing needs, and program designations would be denied or revoked if it became apparent that this was the sponsor's real aim in seeking such a designation. While the State Department would ensure the proper operation of the private programs, selection of the participants would remain the responsibility of the sponsor. By 1961 there were over 2,600 private programs so designated to about 135 government ones. Of this number, approximately 1,300 were sponsored by hospitals. That such a high proportion of these private programs were run by hospitals was in large part due to an Immigration and Naturalization Service ruling restricting foreign interns and residents to a J visa, which could only be obtained through participation in the Exchange-Visitor Program. In light of this ruling alone, the State Department agreed to designate Exchange-Visitor Programs for hospitals, as otherwise aliens chargeable to oversubscribed quotas would be denied access to American medical training. For a full discussion of the immigration problems raised by the influx of foreign medical graduates, see U.S., Congress, House, Committee of the Judiciary, Subcommittee No. 1, *Immigration Aspects of the International Educational Exchange Program: Report Pursuant to H. Res. 56,* 87th Cong., 1st sess., 17 July 1961, H. Rept. 721.

foreign physicians for accredited educational programs, there was a real danger of the residency changing from its old educational function to a form of cheap hospital labor; nor could this be controlled under the existing professional accrediting procedures.

There was some qualititative as well as quantitative evidence that the foreign graduate was acting as a backstop to his American counterpart in staffing the hospitals. Was it really the educational preference of the visitor to gravitate toward residencies in the specialties in which there were the most vacancies (see table 11)? The evidence would suggest that a more likely reason for a higher concentration of foreign medical graduates in specialties such as anesthesiology (50 percent of whose positions were filled by foreign graduates in 1968), general practice (55 percent), pathology (48 percent), and pediatrics (42 percent), was the hospital's defined service needs. Did foreign graduate students wishing to

Table 11. Hospital Residencies, by Specialty, U.S., 1968[1]

Specialty	Total filled Sept. 1, 1968	Positions filled %	Foreign graduates in filled positions %
Anesthesiology	1,502	78	50
Colon & rectal surg.	29	85	55
Dermatology	512	95	9
General practice	402	45	55
Internal medicine	6,163	86	35
Neurological surg.	504	92	22
Neurology	684	82	26
Obstetrics; gynecology	2,503	87	37
Ophthalmology	1,238	96	7
Orthopedic surgery	1,758	94	12
Otolaryngology	873	95	12
Pathology	2,230	62	48
Pediatrics	2,185	86	42
Pediatric allergy	65	75	22
Pediatric cardiology	125	80	53
Physical medicine	277	58	40
Plastic surgery	201	92	22
Psychiatry	3,620	75	29
Psychiatry, child	473	71	19
Radiology	2,240	85	20
Surgery	6,064	90	37
Thoracic surgery	279	91	25
Urology	867	91	25
Totals	34,794	83	32

1. Total residency appointments, all years. Table includes hospital residencies only; another 253 residencies were filled outside hospitals in 1968.

Source: Directory of Approved Internships and Residencies 1969–70, table 10.

further their education deliberately seek out hospitals which were not affiliated with medical schools? A reasonable man would suppose the answer would be no. Yet of the 3,270 foreign-educated interns in the United States in 1968, two-thirds (2,039) held positions in nonaffiliated hospitals. Residents were differently divided, with 3,984 in nonaffiliated, and 7,217 in affiliated hospitals;[18] but even so the proportion was much more uneven than that for American graduates. There were nearly three times as many American graduates as foreign graduates acting as residents in affiliated hospitals in 1968; in the nonaffiliated hospitals, in contrast, there were more foreign-trained than American-trained residents (see table 12). Again, the answer was one of hospital recruitment

Table 12. Residencies in Affiliated and Nonaffiliated Hospitals by Size of Hospital, September 1, 1963, and September 1, 1968

	Total filled		Positions Filled %		Foreign medical graduates in filled positions %	
	1963	1968	1963	1968	1963	1968
Affiliated						
Combined Hospitals		10,741		89		21
Less than 200 beds	1,130	609	84	80	10	17
200–299	989	785	82	80	20	39
300–499	3,927	4,132	79	79	19	34
500 and over	10,970	11,367	85	86	17	27
Total	17,016	27,634	84	85	17	26
Nonaffiliated						
Combined Hospitals		1,043		77		37
Less than 200 beds	917	388	70	64	41	59
200–299	1,654	765	69	73	50	66
300–499	3,400	2,072	68	70	40	66
500 and over	6,308	2,892	79	76	25	52
Total	12,279	7,160	74	73	34	56
Grand Total	29,295	34,794	79	83	24	32

Source: American Medical Association, Directory of Approved Internships and Residencies 1964–65, table 35; ibid., 1969–70, table 13.

and job availability, rather than of the action of a teaching network. It was doubtful whether the foreign medical graduate himself was receiving adequate education to meet his needs of direct relevance to his country of origin, to which it was assumed he would eventually return.

The wide variation in the basic skills of visitors, in terms of language and of education in schools all over the world, which ranged from ex-

18. AMA, Directory of Approved Internships and Residencies (1969–70), tables 2, 11.

cellent to poor in terms of American education, made a process of initial evaluation essential. Not only were the hospitals and licensing agencies interested in this question; it was also of immediate importance to the policies of specialty boards in accepting or rejecting foreign candidates for their certification examinations. The influx of a large number of house staffs from abroad thus raised new questions. At first the AMA Council on Medical Education and the Association of American Medical Colleges attempted to meet the problem by publishing a list of recognized medical schools overseas (1950–53). But it was impossible to keep this list complete and current, and in any event the list was only advisory. This fact was made clear when the Brydges Act was passed in New York State in 1952, allowing hospitals to appoint foreign house staffs irrespective of their educational qualifications by exempting them from licensing requirements. There was some doubt in this situation as to where responsibility lay for the guarantee of professional competence. It appeared that the medical profession was losing its prerogative to define standards, in favor of job responsibility as defined by the employing hospitals. At the same time there was still no effective effort to link the question of foreign medical graduates with graduate medical education as a whole, nor this with an assessment of the interlocking educational and service aspects of the residency in terms of medical manpower.

Instead, the professional response was to set up a new, quasi-licensing scheme, designed to test foreign medical graduates. After much debate, the Educational Council for Foreign Medical Graduates (ECFMG) was created in 1957, sponsored by the Council on Medical Education, the Association of American Colleges, the Federation of State Medical Boards, the American Hospital Association, and government agencies. The National Board of Medical Examiners, after some reluctance, agreed to supervise the screening examination; and the first examination was given in 1958.[19] The Council on Medical Education set 1 July 1961 as

19. The examination, which was given only in the United States, consisted of 400 multiple-choice, objective questions, given on one day in morning and afternoon sessions. The questions were chosen from a pool of those previously used on the National Board Examinations. Thirty-five percent of the examination was concerned with clinical medicine, 20 percent with surgery, 15 percent with pediatrics, 15 percent with obstetrics and gynecology, and the final 15 percent with the six basic medical sciences. A score of 75 was needed to pass. In addition, the ECFMG attempted to test English proficiency.

Fifty-one percent of those taking the first examination passed. A breakdown of the figures for the second exam, which was given overseas as well as in the United States, showed that those who took the exam abroad had less favorable results than those taking it in the United States. In light of this, the ECFMG Board of Trustees voted to issue a temporary certificate to those candidates passing the English test and scoring 70–74. This certificate would be good for admission to an internship

the deadline for the completion of the ECFMG temporary or standard certificate by interns and residents from foreign medical schools, in order for both hospitals and hospital educational programs to remain accredited.

The council, in consultation with other educational groups, has since stated that ECFMG certification is to be considered as indicating medical knowledge at least comparable to the minimum expected of graduates of American or Canadian medical schools.[20] How far this is so in fact remains debatable. But what was most notable in the new program was its deliberate approximation to the basic medical license. There was no attempt in the ECFMG mechanism to do more than this, for example to provide a forum for discussion and planning of the distribution of foreign medical graduates, to sponsor orientation programs for the graduates on their arrival, or to develop policy statements on this substantial section of graduate medical education on the behalf of the profession. Graduate medical education was becoming littered with accrediting and testing processes which did not work together.

Whether, and how far, foreign medical graduates were eligible for certification by the specialty boards was a case in point. Here were physicians accepted into avowed training posts, which in turn were approved by the internship review committee and the appropriate residency review committee as education toward specialty certification. Yet in most cases foreign graduates were automatically excluded from board eligibility because of the boards' requirements of U.S. citizenship, graduation from an approved medical school, and a U.S. license to practice. The various specialty boards had long discussions in the 1950s on whether they should make any concessions for foreign graduates; in at least one board there was a strong feeling that the boards did not, and should not develop international functions. The Advisory Board for Medical Specialties discussed arrangements for foreign graduates in 1955 and on other occasions, but characteristically nothing definite was done. Each board was left to make its own arrangements.

---

or assistant residency program for a period of two years. If within this period the candidate did not retake and pass the exam with a score of 75 or better, he would be expected to return home. For more information on the development of the ECFMG see D. F. Smiley, "The Educational Council for Foreign Medical Graduates: A Report on Its First Four Years," *J. med. Educ., 37* (1962). See also Harold Margulies and Lucille S. Bloch, *Foreign Medical Graduates in the United States* (Cambridge, 1969).

20. "Foreign Medical Graduates: Significance of ECFMG Certification," *J. Amer. med. Ass., 198* (1966), 203. On related problems of licensing foreign graduates in the United States, see Robert C. Derbyshire, *Medical Licensure and Discipline in the United States* (Baltimore, 1969), pp. 134–50.

402 PROFESSIONAL STRUCTURES REEXAMINED

The nature of these arrangements became of particular importance with a State Department ruling of 1959 limiting the stay of foreign medical graduates who were in training as interns and residents to a maximum of five years. Added to previous (1956) requirements that foreign exchange students entering the United States on the common J visa would not be allowed to become permanent residents unless they left the United States for two years, there was a tight limitation on the availability of training time.[21] Five years was not long enough for a physician to take even the internship and residency training for some specialties (most notably general surgery), but in addition the boards commonly required one or two subsequent years of practice experience prior to final examination and certification. Even if other eligibility requirements were dropped by the boards, the foreign medical graduate could not possibly meet the time requirements.

Simultaneously, however, the new visa status helped to clarify in one important respect the views of the specialty boards toward foreign graduates. With limitation on their length of stay in the United States, foreign medical graduates ceased to be potential future competition to American physicians in private practice. This latter was a matter of some importance in the professional ambience of physician oversupply in the late 1950s. The foreign graduates ceased to be a threat; they could be welcomed into needed intern and residency positions but then they would conveniently take themselves away. There had been some fear that foreign medical graduates who achieved board certification would pressure the licensing boards to give them an American license to practice, on the basis of specialty proficiency and their foreign license; indeed, such a course would not be unreasonable. Restrictionist measures by specialty boards, on grounds of quality education, were thus tied in with wider questions of restricting and upgrading manpower supply; this was particularly true of board requirements for the holding of a U.S. practice license (and not just the ECFMG), since this almost invariably required U.S. citizenship. During the 1960s, the boards relaxed the licensing requirements for foreign nationals in favor of the ECFMG, the holding of a license to practice in the candidate's country of citizenship, National Board examinations, or other equivalents. Some curiosities remain however; one specialty board, for example, developed a compromise of allowing a foreign candidate to sit for the oral examination but not telling him whether he passed or failed until he was either back in his own country or had achieved a U.S. license.

21. Amendment to the U.S. Information and Educational Exchange Act of 1948, 84th Cong., 4 June, 1956, P.L. 84–555.

On the advice of the Advisory Board for Medical Specialties, prompted by the State Department, several specialty boards developed special certificates for foreign medical graduates; such certificates were granted by eight of the nineteen specialty boards in 1961, and five in 1970. By the latter year, however, several of the specialty boards had or were developing new examination structures which make it possible for both American and foreign medical graduates to take the examinations earlier in their career, within a total five-year span which includes both internship and residency. It is perhaps relevant that meanwhile the dominant professional attitude toward physician supply have changed firmly to acceptance that there is an acute physician shortage. The foreign medical graduate is finally being brought into the certification system on equal terms. Difficulties remain, however, in defining the competence as well as the educational structure for foreign graduates.

In theory, the ECFMG examination, followed by a carefully supervised period of specialist training in an approved residency and success in the written and oral examinations of a specialty certifying board, would seem to indicate a level of recognized skill and competence. Two flaws remained, however, in this reasoning. One question was whether the board examinations were sufficiently comprehensive to measure quality, a claim not made by any of the boards, nor by the hospitals which accepted on their staffs physicians who were "board eligible" even if they had failed the board examinations. The second, more serious, flaw lay in the period of specialist training. Lacking constant supervision and teaching, and sometimes with serious difficulties in communicating in English, foreign medical graduates could not automatically be assumed at the completion of their residency to be the technological equal of their American counterparts. In many instances, of course, foreign medical graduates were better than Americans. Nevertheless, because of the deficiencies in the residency, resting as it did largely on self-learning, the assumption could not be made that one product of a residency (for example, a residency in a small community hospital all of whose residents were foreign graduates drawn from several countries) was of the same standard as another (say an American physician in a large university hospital). There was as yet no standardization of the residency as had long ago been achieved for undergraduate medical education.

One measure of evening up the quality would be to provide education of foreign medical graduates by American-trained peers, and vice versa. Following the report of another ad hoc advisory committee on internships and hospital services set up by the AMA to close the gap between supply and demand, and also State Department concern that foreign graduates were not mixing sufficiently with Americans, the Council on Medical Education tried in 1962 to impose a quota-mix system on hospitals, dependent on the citizenship of its interns and residents. The committee report included a requirement that a hospital's total house staff of interns and residents should include at least 25 percent American or Canadian graduates; and that failure to fill this proportion for two successive years would endanger subsequent program approval. The Council on Medical Education, in endorsing the report, stated its belief "that all hospitals with approved programs share equally in the moral responsibility to participate in the educational exchange program." [22] But, once again, as in previous suggestions for quotas, the AMA House of Delegates did not agree; the council was instructed the same year to drop any such requirement. Instead, in June 1963 the house of delegates merely adopted a general statement which urged hospitals to appoint a reasonable number of foreign medical graduates into their training programs. "Reasonable" was not defined.

REASSESSMENTS

By the mid-1960s there was clearly a crisis in graduate medical education, a crisis not only of function of the internship and residency but also of responsibility for making any necessary change. Both the Advisory Board for Medical Specialties and the AMA's Council on Medical Education had reached a stalemate in their relations with other important professional groups. Yet the questions of graduate medical education were too important to be delayed. Nor were these the only organizations interested in change. The medical schools' official spokesman, the Association of American Medical Colleges, was gaining momentum as an alternative focus for educational change. The National Board of Medical Examiners was another professional group which was being drawn toward increased consideration of graduate medical education, through its own examinations as well as through its connections with the ECFMG and specialty board examinations. The impetus for organizational reform was thus not only to clarify the issues but also to assign intraprofessional responsibilities and to bring all the various strands together—the future of the internship, the structure and location of the residency, the problems of foreign medical graduates, and the lack of a specialist manpower policy. The various organizations were already working together in a number of capacities, including a liaison committee

22. Reported in AMA, *Supplement Digest*, pp. 184–85.

to accredit medical schools of the AMA and AAMC, the internship and residency review committees, the ECFMG, and the liaison committee to examine applications for new specialty boards between the Council on Medical Education and the Advisory Board for Medical Specialties. But the time was ripe for a larger change. And in the background there was the long-term possibility of a governmental interest in graduate medicine.

In 1963, the year in which (coincidentally) federal aid to undergraduate medical education was to be achieved, the opportunity for such change was finally provided by the AMA Board of Trustees. On the recommendation of the Council on Medical Education, the AMA Board of Trustees announced the establishment of the independent, but AMA-financed, Citizens' (Millis) Commission on Graduate Medical Education. The terms of reference of this committee were very wide, including estimation of the quantitative distribution of physicians among different types of practice, the definition of graduate educational programs in medicine, and proposals for attaining the "ideal." The gestation of the commission was shrouded in secrecy. Initially it had been thought that the committee should include all interested professional groups, but this would clearly have been unwieldy. Thus a decision was taken by the board of trustees to approach the problem from a completely different point of view, using the Flexner report—an outside, independent survey—as a prototype. Indeed, it was hoped that the impact of its report would be similar to that which the Flexner report had had on undergraduate education in 1910.[23] An approach was made by AMA staff to the Carnegie Foundation for the Advancement of Teaching, of which Dr. John S. Millis, president of Western Reserve University, was chairman of the board, but this time the foundation did not have funds to support such an enterprise. It was Dr. Millis who suggested instead the creation of a committee similar to an English Royal Commission—that is, a group of carefully selected citizens given a particular problem, holding hearings and producing recommendations. The idea went back to the Council on Medical Education, thence to the AMA Board of Trustees, who agreed to finance such a commission on the condition that Dr. Millis himself would be responsible for the membership. Dr. Millis agreed, and gradually collected a group of eleven, including himself, selected from the fields of medicine, education, science, and representatives of the public interest. The commission held its first meeting in October 1963.

The problems confronting the commission in its deliberations over

23. "Report of the Council on Medical Education and Hospitals, 1963," *J. Amer. med. Ass.*, *186* (1963), 168–69.

the next two and a half years were different from those confronting Flexner, who had before him actual models of teaching situations as then existed in Germany and in the Johns Hopkins Medical School. The Millis commission had no obvious model; nor did anyone else. It had to develop its own models through the process of round-the-table discussion on the basis of presented reports. The commission was based at Western Reserve University, and one member, Dr. Edgar Bowerfind, acted as secretary, but there was no staff to initiate and undertake research. One result of this was an early decision by the commission to concentrate its aims on qualitative rather than quantitative aspects of graduate education. It decided not to pursue manpower and distribution problems in favor of a conceptual analysis of graduate medical education. The commission received position papers and heard evidence during 1963 and 1964 from representatives of specialty boards, the Colleges, the specialist societies, from hospital administrators, and by representatives from medical schools. The commission was guided in its questioning and discussions by Dr. Walter Wiggins, secretary of the AMA Council on Medical Education, who (in his role as consultant to the commission) attempted to keep the interest focused on questions the council had been unable to solve. Gradually the focus of the meetings began to crystallize around the need for a new type of generalist practitioner and on how he should be trained; on the organization of an authority to challenge accepted traditions in graduate medical education (the specialty boards); and on the purpose of the internship. These issues were to become the main points for recommendation in the commission's report published in 1966.[24]

The publication of this report, on the heels of the Coggeshall report (on the role of the Association of American Medical Colleges, and that of the medical schools) of 1965 [25] and in the midst of concurrent moves by the general practitioners to press for a certification board, marked the beginning of a new stage in graduate medical education. The Millis report, adopted by the AMA House of Delegates, reached conclusions which were compatible with, and extensions of, the Coggeshall report. Both reports stressed early educational specialization, in medical

24. Citizens' Commission on Graduate Medical Education, *The Graduate Education of Physicians*. For background materials on the Millis commission I am indebted to Dr. John S. Millis, Dr. Edgar S. Bowerfind, and Dr. Walter S. Wiggins. 25. The Coggeshall report is referred to in chapter 16. A third influential report was that of the Council on Medical Education's Ad Hoc Committee on Education for Family Practice (Willard committee) which produced recommendations consistent with the Millis commission, a liaison facilitated by Dr. Wiggins's connection with both groups. *Meeting the Challenge of Family Practice* (1966).

school and in the first year of graduate medical education. Both put emphasis on the development of teaching for primary medical care; both pinpointed the need for a stronger national responsibility for the directions and impacts of medical education. The Millis commission put the final touch to the decline of the rotating internship by recommending not only its abolition but the end of the internship itself as a distinct portion of medical education. Instead, it was suggested, graduate medical education should be regarded as one integrated and graded program (i.e. with a program of education appropriate for the first year, the second year, the third year, and so on) designated as a residency. Graduate medical education would thus be regarded as entirely specialized. One such specialty would be for "primary physicians," the new or emerging medical generalists, on a similar level of training to other specialties. It was with this endorsement that the American Board of Family Practice moved to official approval.

The report, while not envisaging total university control of graduate medical education (the implication of the Coggeshall report), espoused the university medical school as the hub of new educational programs, with responsibilities for developing a committee on graduate medical education for each hospital or appropriate group of hospitals, and for stimulating curricular innovations and teaching techniques. Nationally, it was suggested, there should be a commission on graduate medical education, with membership drawn from a variety of sources but appointed by the AMA Council on Medical Education. To this commission would be transferred major responsibility for developing policies in graduate medical education. The establishment of such a commission would have a major impact on the specialty certifying boards, the Advisory Board for Medical Specialties, the residency review committees, and the AMA Council on Medical Education.

Taken together with the report of the Ad Hoc Committee on Education for Family Practice, the Coggeshall and Millis reports legitimized and publicized prevailing views from within the dominant medical organizations which were quite different from those of fifteen years earlier. In the area of graduate medical education, as in physician supply, the views of the AMA and AAMC now coincided. Family practice became recognized as a specialty. The rotating internship, with no major emphasis on a specialty, rapidly declined; other internships for general practitioners were dropped. By 1968–69 eight of ten internship programs were classified as "straight," i.e. in one specialty, or as rotating but with emphasis on a specialty. The straight internship, while remaining in name, was becoming de facto the first year of the residency.

In 1970 it was so recognized by six of the twenty specialty certifying boards. Both internships and residencies are coming increasingly under the umbrella of universities. At present, seven of every eight of the first year residents who are graduates of American or Canadian medical schools are in hospitals affiliated with universities. The majority of foreign medical graduates, too, are now in university-affiliated hospitals.[26] The AMA has also established the Commission on Foreign Medical Graduates to examine their situation. Medical residents are not enrolled for university degrees, nor necessarily under close medical school supervision. Nevertheless, graduate medical education appears finally to be taken under the wing of the medical schools, although as yet the movement is still far from complete.

The characteristics of this movement were emphasized at an AAMC conference on graduate medical education in 1968.[27] In many respects the progress of graduate medical education was proving similar to the reform of education and testing at the M.D. level which began one hundred years ago. The development of new testing techniques by the American Boards of Orthopaedic and Neurological Surgery, and more flexible educational requirements by the American Boards of Pediatrics and Internal Medicine, heralds a less rigid control over educational curricula by the specialty boards (just as the state licensing boards long ago relinquished formal control over the undergraduate curriculum). The logic of university-based graduate medical education echoes similar concerns over undergraduate education at the beginning of the century. And the need for centralized responsibility and coordination for the specialties in the 1970s is as great as was the call for a unified profession in 1910. Here, though, the similarities end; for the regulation of a profession which is in effect a federation of fifty or sixty specialties is far more complex than the establishment of a coordinating base for a profession of generalists.

In the last three years the reform movement in graduate medical education has gathered strength. In 1969 the major organizations concerned with graduate medical education—the AMA, AAMC, and the specialty boards—began to discuss appropriate forms of organization, through some form of permanent association or commission which would review future developments in graduate medical education. These discussions are still in progress. One promising action was the change of name of the Advisory Board for Medical Specialties to the American Board of Medi-

26. "Graduate Medical Education," *J. Amer. med. Ass., 210* (1969), 1500.
27. *The Role of the University in Graduate Medical Education,* ed. Cheves Smythe, Thomas D. Kinney, Mary H. Littlemeyer (Evanston, 1969).

cal Specialties in 1970—though whether this actually means greater coordination among the boards remains, as yet, to be seen. Over and above this, the staff of both the AMA Council on Medical Education and the AAMC have developed position papers on possible structures for a joint commission on graduate medical education, which would also include related organizations, such as the National Board of Medical Examiners and the American Hospital Association. The scenario is reminiscent of that of much earlier days when the question of specialty regulation was first aired. As before, there will undoubtedly be protracted discussions over how many representatives from each organization should be on the joint board, how it will be financed, where it should be located, and what its authority will be in relation to existing groups, particularly the Council on Medical Education. This time, however, so great is the need for coordination and so real the possibility of future governmental intervention in the field of specialist education that joint action finally promises to be realized.

Until such action is taken, control of medical education will continue to be fragmented and largely undirected. The medical schools and the federal government share in the development of undergraduate education. Hospitals continue to offer internships and residencies. Specialty boards provide examinations for certification and specify the duration (and in part the content) of training. Residency review committees, answerable to the specialty associations and the Council on Medical Education, accredit graduate training programs. Medical schools are nominally connected with most graduate training positions, but have as yet exerted little authority. Physicians are licensed halfway through their professional education. Board certification acts as a secondary stage of regulation, used in some ways (especially by hospitals in making staff appointments) as a license, but without official recognition. This professional system is the result in large part of actions taken in the 1920s and 1930s, designed to produce specialists whose concern was to focus on the sick rather than—as now—the vocational base for all physicians.

TRENDS IN MEDICAL SPECIALIZATION

The tangled past has produced an oddly structured medical profession in America. The decline of general practice is one phenomenon. A second notable characteristic is the predominance of surgeons in American medicine, the result in part of relatively open access of physicians to hospitals, in part of open access by individuals to surgical training, in part perhaps to prevailing interests developed by students in medical schools. In 1931 only 10 percent of physicians practiced in fields characterized as surgical specialties—general surgery and related specialties, orthopedic surgery, ophthalmology, otolaryngology, obstetrics/gynecology, urology, anesthesiology; the proportion had risen to 26 percent in 1960, to over 30 percent in 1968.[28] In short, nearly one out of every three physicians in the United States is in a field that involves surgery; a number of general practitioners are doing some surgery as well. This increase promises, moreover, to continue. Of all the American graduates in first year resident and fellowship programs in 1968, over 40 percent were in surgical specialties,[29] even though there has been no indication of shortages in surgical fields that would make their current expansion a priority over other specialties. Not only are there twice as many surgeons but twice as much surgery is done in an average American city as in an English city, with no immediately apparent benefits.[30] Even within the United States, self-contained health service systems—the large prepaid groups—include only half as many surgeons proportionally as are generally available.[31] Indeed, if the specialty distributions of the prepaid group practices were extended to the population at large there would be a glut of surgeons, which would get worse as more poured out of their existing training posts. At the same time there would be acute shortages of generalists and of physicians in various other fields, most notably otolaryngology and physical medicine. There are other interesting features of recent specialty trends. For example, the number of psychiatrists has doubled since 1960; the number of physicians in the medical spe-

28. There were 91,932 physicians active in the surgical specialties (including anesthesiology) in 1968, out of a total pool of physicians in active practice of 298,401. AMA, *Distribution of Physicians, Hospitals and Hospital Beds in the U.S., 1968*, p. 39.
29. Of 8,573 graduates of U.S. and Canadian medical schools who were in approved first year residencies in American hospitals in 1968—that is, virtually one complete cohort of American physicians—3,684 were being trained in surgical specialties. See John C. Nunemaker, Willard V. Thompson, George Mixter, Ike Mayeda, Rose Tracy, "Annual Report on Graduate Medical Education in the United States," *J. Amer. med. Ass. 210* (1969), 1–30, Table 11A.
30. See John P. Bunker, "Surgical Manpower, A Comparison of Operations and Surgeons in the United States and England and Wales," *New Engl. J. Med. 282* (1970) 135.
31. A survey of six prepaid medical groups in 1967 indicated that for general surgery and its subspecialties alone, six or seven physicians were sufficient for 100,000 enrolled population; in the same year for the country at large (excluding interns and residents) there were over thirteen physicians in general surgery and its subspecialties (neurological, plastic and thoracic surgery) per 100,000 population. See *Health Manpower, Perspective: 1967*, U.S. Department of Health, Education and Welfare, Public Health Service Publication Number 1667, 1967, Appendix Table 6, page 75; and J. N. Haug, G. A. Roback, *Distribution of Physicians, Hospitals, and Hospital Beds in the U.S., 1967*, AMA 1968, Table 1.

cialties has been steadily increasing. Nevertheless the outstanding features of current trends in the United States are the ones remarked: the decline of general practice and the substantial and continuing focus on surgery.

The question must arise: Is this balance appropriate? But the next question must be: Appropriate to what? And the next still: Who is to make the estimations? And here is the nub of the issue of professional development versus service expectations. From the service point of view no adequate, detailed manpower projections by specialty yet exist, nationally, regionally, or by area. A number of specialist and service groups have made projections for staffing needs in their own fields, but as yet there is no specialist manpower policy in the form of a master plan.[32] Some such policy is becoming increasingly necessary as a basis for modification of specialist trends, for—in at least the instances of general practice and surgical specialties—there is evidence that the pressures of specialization are running counter to the expressed statements of need for services from both the public and the medical profession. Stratification into specialties is no longer primarily a question of education.

Such comments may seem self-evident; they need emphasis because the development of new forms of medical education, while deriving increasingly in the future from articulated policies and from governmental intervention, will be more or less effective insofar as they build on the strengths of existing educational and regulatory systems of medicine. It is essential to understand the predominant characteristics of the American medical profession, as they have developed over many years, in order that they may be used constructively in effecting change. That change is on the way is obvious. While the developing strains and stresses of technological development have been pushing the traditionally professional aspects of medicine—education, licensing and certification—into the public sector, the increasing costs of specialized medicine have brought public interest firmly to bear on how medical services should be financed, and (more recently) on how they should be provided. Both the educational and the organizational spheres of medicine are thus concurrently in rapid transition; indeed, now as earlier in history, the two movements are closely connected.

In terms of the professional structures themselves there are three basic approaches to regulating graduate medical education. One is through a coordinated system of program accreditation, used as a stringent

32. For a pioneer attempt to pull together the various activities, see J. H. Knowles, "The Quantity and Quality of Medical Manpower: A Review of Medicine's Current Efforts," *J. med. Educ.* 44 (1969) 81–118.

gauge of teaching quality, on the familiar lines of the earlier Flexner reforms: all programs failing to meet high standards would promptly be dropped. The implications of this are a recasting of the functions (and possibly the membership) of the existing residency review committees and of the regulation of those committees by a strong commission on graduate medical education, which would set policy on the number and types of training centers to be approved, and the criteria for approval. The accreditation machinery could be used to build up teaching centers of excellence in particular specialties or related areas. It could also be used, if necessary, to restrict (and thus to redistribute) the supply of physicians in certain specialties and geographical areas, much as accreditation was used to reduce physician numbers and eliminate proprietary schools in the period 1905–20.

The second approach relies on a correcting factor being applied to the residency through the operation of specialty board examinations. This argument assumes that the specialty boards are able, in their tests, to evaluate competence, but recent developments by the boards point to an increasing ability to do so. If and when adequate tests are generally available, it will be possible to reconsider board certification as a form of specialist licensing. To do this, however, demands either a shift in the nature of the boards from "professional" to "public" agencies, including a release from their dependence on specialist associations, or the development of the boards as operating agents of a national association (such as a commission on graduate medical education) which would make major decisions on the types and kinds of examinations. Specialty certification again could be used to limit or encourage the supply of specialists. The major drawback of this course is that physicians fully trained in a specialty might be denied certification and would have to take a second type of training.

The third, and in some ways the most promising, approach toward the residency is to reorganize it as an educational rather than as an apprenticeship process, just as in the late nineteenth century the undergraduate apprenticeship was replaced by teaching in the medical schools. In this model, the university accepts real, as well as nominal, responsibility for educating the specialist by developing and overseeing regional graduate educational curricula. One great advantage of increased university responsibility for graduate education is the prospect of flexibility, and thus of the development of different kinds of educational plans. A major issue for discussion and resolution is, however, whether the universities, or their affiliated hospitals, would be left to decide what kinds of specialist training to develop. The universities may continue to prefer to teach pediatric cardiologists rather than general practitioners.[33] Again, there may be a case for the development of some quota-mix system—from the accrediting bodies, from exhortations from a commission on graduate medical education, or from the development of incentives which will encourage the development of some specialties over others, in terms of the apparent demands of the health care system. The demands could be expressed directly by the system; for example, the development of family practice centers might encourage the expansion of family practice education. Another, not unrealistic, possibility is the extension of federal responsibility for medical education to the graduate level, in the form of subsidy or financing, either by direct grants to medical schools or for individual graduate fellowships. In this case, a structure can be envisaged of a publicly organized or delegated council for medical education (as envisaged in chap. 16) with responsibility for funding virtually the whole of medical education.

These various approaches, taken together, are no more stringent than the accepted controls over medical education at the undergraduate level—accreditation of medical schools by professional groups (in that case the AMA and AAMC), the existence of the medical license, the independence of medical schools with respect to curriculum requirements, and the dependence on government funding in relation to overall operation and broad directions. All or most of these functions could be assumed by a strong joint professional committee, acting on behalf of the public as well as of the profession, and with strong two-way ties to emerging governmental policy.

The structures and their purposes are still fluid, but the message is clear: the medical profession is at the beginning of its second major educational revolution in this century. In the whole process of reassessment of medical education—really of the medical profession itself—from the 1950s to the 1970s, the fruit of enormous technological successes, has come the recognition of medicine as an interdependent, not independent, profession and as one consisting of a complex of specialties rather than one general discipline. If the medical profession does not rapidly develop its own policies for medical specialization, these functions will be subsumed by government. Indeed, it is not unreasonable

33. There is also the question of different attitudes toward practice which may be engendered in the hierarchical university teaching setting and the much more independent, competitive milieu of the community hospital. See e.g. Emily Mumford, *Interns: From Students to Physicians* (Cambridge, 1970), pp. 69–93 and passim.

to suppose that public monies, channeled so substantially into medical schools, should be extended to produce a socially desirable manpower mix at the graduate level. Here lies a major challenge to the professional organizations of medicine as the nation moves toward national health insurance.

PART V: THE MEDICAL PROFESSION AND MEDICAL CARE

CHAPTER 18

Medicine and the Public Voice

The Financing of Medical Care

The movement for national health insurance lost momentum in the 1950s, gathered speed with the passage of Medicare in 1965, and appears in the 1970s as a political imperative. Thus even while the various associations and groups within the medical profession were struggling to redefine general practice, medical education, and the stratification of the profession into specialties, major readjustments in attitudes were being demanded toward the framework in which medicine should be delivered. The ordinary physician was caught up in change on all sides. The political attitudes of organized medicine, in particular, demanded redirection; for these, like prevailing attitudes toward specialist certification, were the product of an earlier era. We are now in the middle of these redirections.

The lingering of earlier attitudes affected the responses of organized medicine to articulated public interest in medical care financing and organization from the 1940s to the 1960s, and only now are changes evident. Within the profession was a seeming paradox. On the one hand, the dominant professional reaction to education for the specialties was relatively progressive. No sooner did a new specialty appear than efforts began to establish new forms of education; the problem was of containing such developments, not of stimulation. In contrast, the prevailing mood toward adapting health services to accommodate the specialties was conservative; the specialists, once trained, gravitated to a form of practice which was more suited to their general practitioner predecessors. In the 1950s, through the 1960s and even into the 1970s, when the increase in specialist function was demanding greater organizational cooperation in and among health services, the dominant pattern of professional behavior continued to be that of 1910. The pattern is one of fee-for-service, independent private practice, hedged with professional (but few public) restraints, the archetype an independent entrepreneur who espouses the rhetoric of a free enterprise market system, but refutes its economic implications; indeed, like their colleagues in other professions, physicians have gone to some trouble to deny themselves the normal elements of free-market competition, most notably mergers and advertising. One result of the continuance of noncomprehensive, independent solo practice (a not unreasonable form of practice when most physicians were general practitioners) was that physicians long excluded themselves from much-needed experiments in both large-scale and small-scale practice organization.

A second, equally important result was the increasing rift between the "public interest" as defined by organized medicine, and as it appeared in the growing challenge of organized consumers. In the long debates over health care financing from the 1940s to the present the profession continued to be strongly wedded to earlier ideas of private practice in its official views toward proposals for government-sponsored health insurance. The voice of representatives of the public was raised meanwhile in response to one inescapable result of modern specialized techniques—the skyrocketing costs of medical care. In the now historical debates the word "private" as used by officers of the AMA assumed two definitive meanings, neither of which, incidentally, implied a return of medicine to a private market system. On the one hand, following the precedent set in and before the Wagner-Murray-Dingell bills, private practice continued to be taken as the opposite of governmental control or socialized medicine; this meant a continuing endorsement of voluntary health insurance, which supported the independent fee-for-service system, and opposition to legislative intervention which might threaten it. On the other hand, and perhaps of deeper psychological importance to physicians most closely involved in the long debates which preceded Medicare, private practice was taken to mean professional *privacy*—the privilege of a responsible profession to regulate its members and to dictate its destiny, as indeed it did in the educational area. The debate was in large part an exploration of the appropriate limits of professionalism, in terms of describing the relative roles of public intervention in health services and of delegation to the doctors of responsibilities which had been so expanded through technological innovation that they bore little relationship to professional responsibilities in the Age of Flexner.

THE GROWTH OF INDEPENDENT GROUPS

The public voice rose on the issue of health service costs and financing. Year by year, in large part a reflection of technological advances in medicine, the costs of medical care inexorably advanced, while at the same time the health system itself became more complex; at the same time, the other side of the coin, medical care became more valuable as a social resource. In 1940, the total expenditure on health services and related research and construction in the United States was about $4 billion. National health expenditures reached $18 billion in 1955, were over $40 billion in 1965, had reached $64 billion in 1969, and continue to climb rapidly.[1] The provision of health services has become a vast, yet uncoordinated industry, employing almost 3 million people, or about 4 percent of the entire civilian labor force, and accounting for 6.9 percent of the gross national product.

By the mid-1960s, physicians represented a small minority of the persons providing medical services; for every physician, there were four other health professionals (see table 13). This pattern could have reflected the transformation and strengthening of the physician into the skilled manager of a carefully picked team. The old general practice might have been replaced by groups of pediatricians and internists, with a full complement of nurses, social workers, technicians, consultants, and aides, as the standard modern rendering of what used to be encompassable in solo practice. But this had not happened by the early 1960s. The average general practitioner, internist, or pediatrician continued to work in solo practice or in a small partnership, dispensing a highly personalized, one-to-one service and directly using the services only of a nurse or a receptionist. Only 11 percent of physicians engaged in patient care were practicing in single or multi-specialty groups in 1965.[2]

Instead, then, of physicians dominating and leading the development of imaginative large-scale health systems, where clusters of professionals and other health workers could operate new types of health care institutions, up until the mid-1960s physicians as a group continued to take the stand of isolationism, surveying with jaundiced eyes and outraged complacency the social facts of medicine in the second half of the twentieth century. But while the private medical practitioner remained an isolationist, other cooperative medical care organizations did develop. The increasing number of allied health personnel reflected an expansion and concentration of medical services in hospitals and the development out-

1. Dorothy P. Rice and Barbara S. Cooper, "National Health Expenditures, 1929–70," *Social Security Bull. 34* (Jan. 1971), 5.
2. AMA, *Survey of Medical Groups in the U.S., 1965,* table 33. The best analysis of the dynamics of medical organization at the local level is still the study by Oswald Hall, "The Informal Organization of the Medical Profession," *Canad. J. Economics political Sci., 12* (1946), 30–44.

Table 13. Persons Active in Selected Health Professions, U.S., 1900–1969

Year	All health professionals	Physicians (MD & DO)	Other professional personnel			
			Total	Dentists	Professional nurses	Pharmacists and others[1]
			Number active			
1900	197,140	123,500	73,640	29,700	640	43,300
1910	307,500	152,400	155,100	40,000	50,500	64,600
1920	408,700	151,300	257,400	56,200	103,900	97,300
1930	600,800	162,700	438,100	71,100	214,300	152,700
1940	692,400	174,500	517,900	71,000	284,200	162,700
1950	895,600	220,000	673,900	77,900	375,000	221,000
1960	1,156,500	260,500	899,200	89,200	504,000	306,000
1966	1,504,400	297,000	1,207,400	95,400	640,000	472,000
1969	1,663,600	314,700	1,348,900	101,900	700,000	547,000

Year	Physicians per 100 in all health professions	Number per 100 physicians			
1900	63	60	24	1	35
1910	50	102	26	33	43
1920	37	170	37	69	64
1930	27	269	43	132	94
1940	25	297	41	163	93
1950	25	306	35	170	100
1960	23	345	34	193	117
1966	20	407	32	215	159
1969	19	429	32	222	174

1. Includes pharmacists and other persons who are college educated or in professions which may have baccalaureate or post-baccalaureate preparation: employed as biological scientists, biostatisticians, chiropractors, clinical psychologists, dental hygienists, dietitians, health educators, medical laboratory technologists, medical record librarians, optometrists, podiatrists, rehabilitation counselors, sanitary engineers, social workers (medical and psychiatric), veterinarians, and therapists (occupational, physical, speech, and hearing).

Note: The table does not contain a strictly comparable set of figures. These for 1900-60 (except for the physician figures for 1950 and 1960) are census figures as of the census date (April 1st in recent years) while the 1950 and 1960 figures for physicians and all 1966 and 1969 figures are as of December 31st.

Source: U.S.D.H.E.W., Division of Manpower Intelligence, Bureau of Health Manpower Education, National Institutes of Health.

side hospitals of independent services (such as visiting nurse associations), on which a physician could draw, but for which he was not administratively responsible. More persons were working in hospitals in 1960 than had been working in the whole of the health service industry twenty years before.[3] The hospital, not the physician, gained power as the central focus for health services; patients were recognizing an institutional focus for medicine even if physicians were not. The number of hospital outpatient visits swelled rapidly in the 1950s and 1960s,[4] creating a new form of the much earlier phenomenon of "hospital abuse." This time, however, the initiative lay with the patients themselves rather than with competing medical personnel inside and outside hospitals; indeed, the typical general hospital has no desire to expand its costly and complex ambulatory services. While only about 10 percent of all patient visits were in hospitals in the late 1960s, compared with 70 percent in private physician offices (the remainder representing telephone contacts, home visits and other sources), hospital outpatient care was becoming an institutional focus for an important minority of patients in the urban ghettos.[5] In the process, the physician has rapidly become not the core of medical care but only a cog in a complex system. This fractional role for physicians is emphasized in the physicians' own proclivity to uncoordinated specialization. Of the 271,000 MDs who were giving patient care in the United States at the end of 1969, all but 58,000 were limiting their practice to a specialty. Most were engaged in independent private

3. The number of persons in health service occupations, as classified by the Bureau of the Census, was 1.1 million in 1940. In 1960, the total was 2.6 million, of whom 1.7 million were in hospitals. The great rise in the number of hospital personnel was, incidentally, a major factor in concurrent increases in hospital costs. Hospital personnel numbered 2.4 million in 1968, compared with only 830,000 in 1946. This represented a proportional change from 73 to 180 persons employed for every 100 hospital beds. See *Health Manpower Source Book, sec. 20, Manpower Supply and Educational Statistics for Selected Health Occupations* (1969), p. 3; *Hospitals, J.A.H.A. Guide Issue 44* (1970) Part 2, p. 472.
4. Comparable figures on hospital outpatient visits are not available for the period 1945–1970. One study of a sample of short-term nonfederal general hospitals between 1945 and 1958 found a rise of 160 percent in the number of visits to emergency rooms in this period, and of 128 percent to outpatient departments. P. A. Skudder, J. R. McCarroll, P. A. Wade, "Hospital Emergency Facilities and Services: A Survey," *Bull. Am. Coll. Surg. 46* (1961) 49. Data collected by the American Hospital Association from 1962 show total outpatient visits at all kinds of hospitals to have increased from 99,382,000 in 1962 to 163,248,000 in 1969, a 64 percent increase in a seven-year period. *Hospitals J.A.H.A. Guide Issue 44* (1970) Part 2, p. 472.
5. This was particularly true of persons living in the urban ghettos surrounding major general hospitals. National household survey data for 1966–67 showed an inverse relationship between income and utilization of hospital outpatient care, and a marked difference in relation utilization between whites and nonwhites; under 8 percent of physician visits by whites were in hospital facilities, compared with over 25 percent of those by nonwhites. U.S. Dept. of Health, Education, and Welfare, National Center for Health Statistics, *Volume of Physician Visits United States, July 1966–June 1967*, Vital and Health Statistics, Series 10, Number 49, pp. 9, 30.

practice; and, despite a steady rise in the number of group practices, only about 24,000 physicians were attempting to coordinate their skills in partnerships or group practices which included more than one specialty.[6]

The continuation of a medical profession which is largely made up of independent entrepreneurs had an inevitable effect not only on the profession's attitudes toward health insurance, but also on the types of health insurance proposals which were generated, up to and including Medicare. Had the medical profession not been a "profession," that is, if its members had been free to set up combinations of skills and types of personnel, without the formal restraints of licensing laws and medical ethics and the informal restraints of guild fraternalism, the most congenial American pattern for organizing health services would almost certainly have been independent, voluntary associations of specialists and other health personnel, organized on efficient business lines and offering a clearly specified range of services. As an inducement, such organizations could have offered prepayment, extended payment and credit plans. In this event, health insurance plans (at least for the middle class working population) would be organized on a local basis, as illustrated in the handful of significant prepaid group practices which did develop in the United States. Given such a decentralized system of health insurance, the governmental role might be focused on such matters as standards of care and ensuring that members of the population who were poor in income or as health risks would not be excluded from such organizations.[7] At it was, the diffuse system of practice organization stimulated demands for a centralized governmental role in paying for medical care. Put another way, the adherence by the medical profession to the old ethic of solo private practice was itself a factor in encouraging so-called socialized medicine.

The few earlier group practice prepayment schemes were joined by a few others during and immediately after World War II, but interest lagged in the 1950s, and only picked up again in the mid-1960s. Out of the exigencies of the ship-building industry in World War II, the Kaiser Foundation Health Plan in California, Oregon, and Hawaii (and now Cleveland) was developed and proved to be the most successful experiment in this country of the feasibility of a prepayment scheme with relatively comprehensive benefits provided through a group medical practice based on a hospital. Other interesting forms of organizational develop-

6. AMA, *Distribution of Physicians, Hospitals, and Hospital Beds in the U.S., 1969*, p. 25; Mary E. McNamara and Clifford Todd, "A Survey of Group Practice in the United States, 1969" *J. Amer. med. Ass., 60* (1970), 1308.
7. For a development of this viewpoint see Milton Friedman, *Capitalism and Freedom* (Chicago, 1962), chap. 9.

ment are also chiefly the products of the years immediately following World War II. The Health Insurance Plan of Greater New York (HIP), also a group practice prepayment scheme, was started by Mayor La-Guardia and a group of distinguished physicians and laymen in 1947. Group Health Cooperative of Puget Sound in Seattle, a prepaid group practice based on a consumer cooperative, was established out of pre-existing organizations in 1947; the rather similar Community Health Center in Two Harbors, Minnesota, in 1944; and the Labor Health Institute in St. Louis, a union-sponsored group practice scheme, organized in 1945.[8] John L. Lewis began to develop a medical program for the United Mine Workers in 1946; subsequently the UMWA Welfare and Retirement Fund stimulated the development of group practices and hospital construction in the mining areas of Pennsylvania, Ohio, and West Virginia. But in the 1950s there were few new major efforts. Prepaid group practice continued to be an interesting and apparently successful organizational response to medical specialization, but one of limited application. By 1968 it was estimated that prepaid group practice plans were offering ambulatory services to only 4.6 million people—2 percent of the population.[9]

In part, the reluctance by physicians to develop prepaid group practices was a reflection of continuing antagonism by the AMA to what was a potent form of competition to traditional fee-for-service practice. The "closed-panel" characteristics of such groups were supposed to deny the patient a free choice of physician. There was thus an argument on the one hand for encouraging a free market for consumers, and on the other for discouraging competition among the providers of care. As noted above, this logically untenable position was successfully challenged in the courts in the 1940s, over plans in Washington, D.C., Seattle, and New York. But considerable professional resistance (and some prohibitory state legislation) remained, continuing in some areas and cases to the present day,[10] even though AMA policy toward prepaid group practice

8. For a useful review of the development of prepaid group practice, see William A. MacColl, *Group Practice and Prepayment of Medical Care,* pp. 17–56.
9. Louis S. Reed and Willine Carr, "Independent Health Insurance Plans in 1968, Preliminary Estimates" *Research and Statistics Note,* Oct. 6, 1969, table 3.
10. A study of state legislation in 1969 found that in less than half the states was the situation sufficiently defined to enable prepaid consumer-sponsored group practices to be developed without concern about possible legal restraints. In some states, the law requires a majority of the board of directors of such plans to consist of physicians, and in some there are requirements that all physicians in an area have the privilege of joining the plan should they so desire. Other restrictions hinged on organizational and fiscal requirements of the plans, including questions of limited liability, tax and insurance. See Health Law Center, Aspen Systems Corporation,

was officially changed in 1959. The new policy—developed from recommendations of a committee headed by Dr. Leonard W. Larson (himself a member of a practice group)—allowed the patient "free choice of policy or plan," thus redefining the earlier "free choice of doctor." [11] This important modification finally removed prepaid group practice from the shady realms of medical ethics, and also finally allowed for the development of all types of group practice arrangements. The AMA, while warning that the physician practicing in a group might be subject to closer ethical scrutiny by his fellow colleagues than his fellow practitioners in solo practice, cooperated with the Association of American Medical Clinics (an organization for group practices) in producing in 1962 guidelines for physicians interested in forming or joining a medical group. Moreover, since then the AMA view has been generally supportive of group practice.

AMA endorsement encouraged the new development of group practice during the 1960s, whether or not these practices were linked with prepayment insurance schemes. The number of groups, including single specialty and multi-specialty groups and those with and without prepayment schemes, rose from at least 1,546 in 1959, to at least 4,289 in 1965; the number of physicians in groups more than doubled in the same period, from 13,009 to 28,381, and has since continued to rise (see table 14). In terms of *prepaid* group practices, however, there appears to have been relatively little change, although a flurry of interest is evident. In 1969, only 85 groups could be identified in which over 50 percent of activities was organized on a prepaid basis. Nor were the groups evenly distributed. Almost three of every four physicians in prepaid groups were in the Middle Atlantic South Atlantic and Pacific Census Divisions.[12] Both the number and geographical distributions of prepaid groups promise to change during the 1970s as a number of new practice groups now being developed into full operation. But even so there is no indication that—without deliberate efforts by the federal government to fund such developments directly or through national health insurance—prepaid groups will form the major locus of practice by 1980.

Looking back to the critical period of debate which preceded Medicare it is evident that professional endorsement of group practice came

Group Practice and the Law, A Digest of State Laws Affects the Group Practice of Medicine (1969).

11. AMA, "Report of Commission on Medical Care Plans" *J. Amer. med. Ass.* Special edition, Jan. 17, 1959.

12. McNamara and Todd, pp. 1309–12.

Table 14. *Physicians in Group Practice, Selected Years, 1946–1969*

	1946	1959	1965	1969
No. of groups	404	1,546	4,289	6,371
Single specialty[1]	36	392	2,161	3,953
Multi-specialty	368	1,154	2,128	2,418
No. of physicians in groups	NA	13,009	28,381	40,093
Single specialty	NA	1,562	8,956	15,744
Multi-specialty	3,493	11,447	19,425	24,349

1. Includes general practice groups, of which there were 784 in 1969, including 2,691 physicians. The 1959 figures, however, combine general practice and multi-specialty groups.

These figures, derived from four special surveys, should be interpreted cautiously, with underreporting possible for each of the four years; they are however the only figures which exist on the development of groups in the United States. Definitions also vary. The 1946 and 1965 surveys required three or more full-time physicians in order to be classified as a group. The 1959 survey required only that there be three physicians; two part-time physicians were counted as one full-time. The 1969 survey required three or more physicians, formally organized, with joint use of equipment and personnel, and with their group income distributed according to predetermined criteria.

Source: American Medical Association, *Survey of Medical Groups in the U.S. 1965*, pp. 78, 81; Mary E. McNamara and Clifford Todd, "A Survey of Group Practice in the United States, 1969," *J. Amer. med. Assn. 60* (1970), 1303–13. See also G. Halsey Hunt and Marcus S. Goldstein, "Medical Group Practice in the United States," ibid., *135* (1947) 904–09; U.S.D.H.E.W. *Medical Groups in the United States 1959*, Public Health Service Publication no. 1063, July 1963.

too late. Instead of the 1950s being a time of radical change in the health service system (as in many European countries which developed new financial payment schemes), they were a time of acrimony, of a polarization of views between the professional associations and public interest groups. Instead of joint professional and lay cooperation in towns and cities across the country to establish tailored health service schemes, there was a continuing confrontation at the national level between would-be reformers of health services through Congress and the embattled AMA.

At issue was the authority to determine the future nature of health services, an authority which in actual practice physicians had largely lost. In the 1950s, as in the 1940s, the AMA found itself in a position not of offering innovative plans for responding to the health service system's increasing industrialism (in terms of its economics, its staffing, its importance, and its size) but of exerting the considerable power of the AMA to block the efforts of those who wished to innovate from outside its charmed circle. The AMA thus had a negative effect. Implicit in its efforts was the wishful and erroneous assumption that medicine was "above politics." On the contrary, it was certain that politics and medicine could no longer be divorced.

PROPOSALS FOR STRENGTHENING PRIVATE HEALTH INSURANCE

Inevitably, political debate over health care has hinged on methods of paying the accelerating medical bills of modern medicine. The AMA's lavish national educational campaign from 1949 to 1952 lobbied successfully against plans for a federal health insurance system for all age groups; in three and a half years, the AMA campaign cost $4,678,000, providing a landmark in the annals of public relations, if not in health development.[13] Thereafter, less draconic measures were required to stop the introduction of national health insurance. The demand for governmental health insurance for workers, still favored by the labor unions, became less urgent with the growth of private health insurance through collective bargaining. Enrollment in private insurance for hospital bills (by far the most expensive item of medical care) rose rapidly. About 32 million people had hospital insurance in 1945; the total reached 105 million in 1955, and rose to over 175 million people in 1969, representing over 88 percent of the civilian population. In 1957, private health insurance premiums were valued at almost $6 billion; by 1967 they were about $17 billion, of which more than $10 billion flowed through the commercial insurance companies.[14] This expansion of health insurance, through commercial insurance companies and through the nonprofit Blue Cross (hospital bills) and Blue Shield (medical bills) plans, was a strikingly successful feat of salesmanship. The provision of health insurance under government sponsorship had been a leading and controversial issue in the 1949 Congress; after this the movement lost momentum.

As in the earlier proposals for compulsory health insurance, the AMA, while the leader of the opposition, was not alone in its reluctance to jump into massive governmental financing of health services. It was joined not only by other powerful interested parties, including the American Dental Association, the American Pharmaceutical Association, and organizations representing profit and nonprofit health insurance, but also by other groups (such as the Chamber of Commerce) and individuals who, all things considered, preferred solutions outside the governmental

13. For the flavor as well as analysis of the AMA's political position on national health insurance, see Stanley Kelley, *Professional Public Relations and Political Power*, pp. 67–106; and R. Harris, *A Sacred Trust*, pp. 31–63.
14. Health Insurance Institute, *1970 Source Book of Health Insurance Data* (New York, 1971), pp. 15–16, 37.

framework or through the exercise of only minimal governmental regulation. The prevailing mood of the country was toward conservatism. Compulsory health insurance was an election issue in 1952, stigmatized in the Republican party campaign for its "crushing cost, wasteful inefficiency, bureaucratic dead weight, and debased standards of medical care." [15]

Instead of direct governmental intervention in health services, there were efforts during the Eisenhower administration (1953–61) to build on the success of private health insurance. The health financing proposals of the new administration's proposals were designed to recognize a public-private mix of funds, with the public funds reserved as far as possible for the poor. Private health insurance would be the third-party payer of medical bills for the middle class. At the same time, there would be efforts to expand the existing system of federal grants to the states to provide medical care for those on public assistance. Ideally, most of the population would thus have at least some of their health expenses covered. Federal grants to states for payments to hospitals, doctors, and other providers of medical care for health services given to public assistance recipients were $51.3 million in fiscal year 1949–50. With the added increment of federal grants for "vendor payments" under the 1950 Social Security Administration, the federal share rose to $311.9 million in 1954–55, and to $492.7 million in 1959–60.[16] If this system were extended and improved to ensure that the health needs of all the poor were met, and if the private sector could cover or be encouraged to cover the mass of the income-producing population through adequate and suitable health insurance policies, governmental national health insurance would prove to be unnecessary. The debate centered on whether, and how far, those conditions could be met.

Extending federal grants for public assistance recipients was a more straightforward process than encouraging the private health insurance plans—nonprofit and profit—to offer reasonably comprehensive health insurance policies. Inadequate individual insurance contracts were the major flaw of the private system—one, moreover, which was camouflaged by the impressive rise in enrollment figures. The mysterious deficiencies in insurance coverage of medical bills, even for those who had health insurance, had become a stock joke by the 1950s.[17] According to one study, half of the families who spent $500 or more on health services

15. Quoted by Sundquist, *Politics and Policy*, p. 290.
16. Cooper, "National Health Expenditures," table 3.
17. A good example is the joke by Phil Leeds: "I have health insurance. If a giraffe bites me on the shoulder, I get $18, provided I am pregnant at the time." Quoted by Richard Carter, *The Doctor Business* (New York, 1958), p. 96. There were—and remain—many variations of this theme.

in 1953 had insurance coverage for less than 20 percent of their expenses. Taking expenditures as a whole, only 3 of every 100 insured families with health expenses could count on being reimbursed as much as 80 percent of their bills.[18] There was thus a significant insurance gap. Indeed, in no year yet have private health insurance plans managed to cover more than a third of the total medical bill of private patients.

Moreover, as health costs rose—from an average expenditure of $84 per capita in 1950, to $149 in 1960, to $250 in 1967 [19]—the amount of out-of-pocket expenditure on medical bills, particularly for those with low incomes, assumed greater significance. Generally speaking, the richer the family, the larger the amount of money spent on health; but at the same time, health expenses represent a much larger proportion of the poorer person's income. One study of family expenditures on health in 1957–58 showed an average annual expenditure of $165 for families with incomes of under $2,000. This was half the amount spent by those with incomes in the $5,000–$7,500 range, but it represented no less than 13 percent of the poorer families' total income.[20] Medical bills were, moreover, not evenly spread even within different income categories. It was estimated in 1963 that 8 percent of all families accounted for 36 percent of health expenditures; the larger the bill, moreover, even with health insurance coverage, the more chance there was of the individual family going into debt.[21] Private health insurance alone was not doing an adequate job of protecting the population against high medical costs. To be effective, any proposed social policy which would equalize or neutralize the effective demand for and receipt of medical services through health insurance—whether it was tagged "public" or "private"—would take account of such financial inequities.

There was no reason why the health insurance industry should on its

18. The percent of the bill covered in the high-expense range rose steadily in the 1950s under the impact of major medical insurance. But, even in 1963, only 12 percent of families with expenses of $500 or more were covered for 80 percent or more of their bills. Broken down by category of expenses, it was found that in fact two-thirds of those receiving hospital benefits—by far the most expensive item of medical care—had 80 percent of these charges covered. Nevertheless, the loopholes in coverage remained considerable. Nor was the patient with a crippling, largely uninsured hospital and surgical bill likely to be heartened by apparent improvement in the overall benefit average. See Ronald Andersen and Odin W. Anderson, *A Decade of Health Services,* pp. 95–97.
19. Dorothy P. Rice and Barbara S. Cooper, "National Health Expenditures 1950–67," *Social Security Bull., 32* (Jan. 1969), table 6.
20. Anderson, Collette, and Feldman, *Changes in Medical Care Expenditures and Voluntary Health Insurance* HIF-NORC (1963), Tables 4, 6.
21. Andersen and Anderson, pp. 52–59; 115–17.

own initiative shoulder responsibility for what was becoming a major social service. Insurance as a business depends on a realistic balance between premium income and benefit expenditures, estimated on the basis of actuarial risk. On this basis, the healthier person is a better "risk" for health insurance, as he is for life insurance, or as the man with no accident record is for automobile insurance. A social service, on the other hand, is designed by its very nature to provide services for those who need them most—in this context, the highest, or worst, insurance risks. Individual risks may be pooled by designing insurance contracts to cover large population groups, for example through industry-wide union-negotiated contracts; by 1969, 68 percent of the health insurance business of insurance companies was in group as opposed to individual or family policies.[22] But these, too, excluded many people who needed health services the most: the unemployed, those working independently or in non-unionized employment, those with partial health insurance but with low incomes, and—of increasing political as well as social importance—the aged. The nonprofit Blue Cross and Blue Shield plans, which covered under half of all those insured, had similar problems, although they paid out a higher proportion of their premium income in benefits and on the whole had wider health benefits than the commercial insurance plans.[23] Neither type of plan could claim success as an alternative to governmental intervention if the ultimate goals was comprehensive insurance coverage —comprehensive, that is, in terms both of services and of the enrolled population.

The Eisenhower proposals were designed to help insurance plans through public reinsurance, regulation, and initial subsidy: in short, to give a boost to the private sector through a public-private partnership which would harness the social responsibilities of the federal government to the supposed efficiency and ingenuity of private enterprise. So doing, moreover, the insurance system would remain free of obligations to

22. Health Insurance Institute, *1970 Source Book of Health Insurance Data*, p. 41.
23. In 1955, Blue Cross–Blue Shield plans covered 43 percent of those with hospital insurance, 39 percent with surgical insurance, and 49 percent with insurance for physician in-hospital visits. The nonprofit plans were however gradually losing ground to the insurance companies. Through large, collective bargaining, group insurance contracts, the insurance companies were able to sell policies to the relatively healthy working population and their dependents, leaving the nonprofit plans with a greater than average proportion of those who were likely to be sick. In 1969, Blue Cross–Blue Shield plans covered 36 percent of hospital insurance, 36 percent of surgical services, and 41 percent of physician in-hospital visits. Louis S. Reed and Willine Carr, "Private Health Insurance in the United States, 1967," *Social Security Bull.*, *32* (Feb. 1969), 11; Marjorie Smith Mueller, "Private Health Insurance in 1969: A Review," ibid., *34* (Feb. 1971), 6.

modernize the way in which health services are provided. The proposals emerged in concrete form in 1954, in turn building on suggestions made four years earlier by Harold Stassen. Under the Stassen proposals, 2 percent of private insurance premiums, together with a donation from federal general revenues, would be channeled to a new federal health reinsurance corporation. In turn, the corporation would reinsure nonprofit health insurance agencies on the basis of agreed service and population criteria. The corporation would then become liable for two-thirds of each insurance claim of over $1,000 for the hospital or medical care benefits of any individual in any twelve-month period. As a result, insurance companies would be protected against unusual financial losses. The Eisenhower proposals were a variation on this theme. They would have reimbursed both profit and nonprofit companies, and on the basis not of individual bills but of a carrier's average losses on reinsured contracts.[24] Through this mechanism it was hoped that health insurance companies could be encouraged to extend their coverage from the rich pool of unionized workers to high-risk and hard-to-reach members of the population, particularly those with low incomes and those living in rural areas. At the same time, the companies might be encouraged to experiment with the development of broader and larger health benefits.

The federal reinsurance principal, a legacy of the Depression, had been accepted for the protection of banks and for home mortgages granted by savings and loan associations. Direct use of public money as a subsidy to make good the social deficiencies of private enterprise was also widely accepted by the 1950s, for example, in Hill-Burton construction grants to hospitals, in housing, and in aid to independent schools and colleges. But while the principle of public support of the private sector was endorsed for health in the Eisenhower proposals, the proposals themselves appealed to none of the major interest groups. The bill was opposed by the AMA as being the first step toward socialized medicine, for the association could see little difference between a direct national health insurance program and a program which in effect made the private insurance industry an agent of the federal government. In both cases efforts could be made to exert control over private practice. Others, dedicated to the principle of national health insurance, saw the Eisenhower bill as the

24. The Stassen proposals were incorporated in a 1950 bill sponsored by Rep. Charles K. Wolverton (R., N.J.), H.R. 8746 of the 81st Cong., 2d sess. The Eisenhower proposals were presented as H.R. 8356—S. 3114 of the 83d Cong., 2d sess. The proposal suggested that the government lend the reinsurance fund an initial $25 million, but the system was designed to be self-sufficient. For further analysis, see Brewster, pp. 2–5 and passim.

development of an undesirable approach to the financing of medical care. Even spokesmen for health insurance companies opposed the bill, on the basis of its vagueness and uncertain long-term implications.[25] As a result, the bill died in the House. Nor were later reincarnations any more successful. The administration proposals reappeared in 1955 (H.R. 3458, H.R. 3720, S. 886), the most notable difference being the establishment of four separate funds instead of one—one fund for plans for low- and average-income families, one for major medical insurance contracts, one for plans dealing with rural areas, and one for other plans. Similar bills appeared in 1957 (S. 1750, H.R. 6506, H.R. 6507); but no action was taken.

Nevertheless, the encouragement of health insurance coverage through subsidy of, or guarantees to, the private insurance sector remained appealing to those who saw this as a more logical approach to income protection than any major swing to a completely governmental payment system. In 1956 a bill was sent to Congress by the secretary of Health, Education and Welfare, Marion B. Folsom, with a modified proposal. This suggested that small insurance companies and voluntary health insurance groups be allowed to pool their resources and thereby expand their coverage. But while this too was unsuccessful, there were continuing calls for governmental strengthening of private health insurance.[26] In terms of the number of people who had some type of health insurance coverage, private health insurance continued to expand rapidly during the 1950s. But without public subsidies or public regulation, it was evident that neither the nonprofit "Blue" plans nor insurance companies, or both together, were able to provide a complete answer to paying for the popu-

25. U.S., Congress, House, Interstate and Foreign Commerce Committee, *Hearings,* 83d Cong., 2d sess., 31 Mar. 1954.
26. President Eisenhower requested the Folsom bill (S. 4172) again in 1957, but no action was taken. Other proposals in the early 1950s included the Flanders-Ives bills (1949–55) for a voluntary national prepayment program with federal subsidy, using existing nonprofit prepayment plans such as Blue Cross (for hospital bills) and Blue Shield (doctor's bills). The Hill-Aiken bills (1949–53) suggested that the government pay voluntary health insurance contributions for those unable to afford them. Suggestions arose from the American Hospital Association and Blue Cross Association in the mid-1950s that there be federal grants for experiments and demonstrations by private insurance carriers and for government subsidy of insurance for low-income families and for the aged. The Republican (Flemming) proposals of 1960 suggested a federal-state program, which included as one option the purchase of health insurance for the elderly needy. And the AMA endorsed federal and state purchase of private health insurance for the aged in its Eldercare proposals of 1965. Meanwhile, from 1949 (81st Cong., 1st sess., S. 1969) there was a series of proposals, continuing to the present, which would allow individual exceptions or credits on federal income tax for money spent for private health insurance premiums.

lation's medical care. Meanwhile, rising costs of medical care continually ate into apparent gains in insurance coverage.

PROPOSALS FOR A NATIONAL INSURANCE SYSTEM

The difference between those who favored subsidized private insurance and those who endorsed a governmental insurance scheme was in part a matter of political philosophy. Private insurance, backed by federal aid to the poor, was the official Republican position of the 1950s. This could be regarded as part of a wider stand of favoring wherever possible the provision of goods and services through private sources rather than the public economic sector. Proposals for governmental national health insurance, on the other hand, were largely identified with liberal Democrats, men such as Sen. Wagner and Murray and Representative Dingell in the 1940s, and Sen. Forand, Anderson and John F. Kennedy in the 1950s and early 1960s. But there was more to the question of private versus public responsibility for health care financing than a difference in political commitment; also at issue were the basic purpose and implications of collective health care financing.

The issues were similar to those raised in the health insurance debates before 1920 and reflected in the debates of the 1930s and 1940s. If health insurance is seen merely as a form of income maintenance, designed to protect individuals against potentially heavy financial loss in time of sickness, the mechanics of insurance are more or less immaterial. Private health insurance or public health insurance would be judged solely on the basis of which, or which combination, is more likely to do the job efficiently and economically. If, on the other hand, the method of financing is seen as a means of creating widespread changes in the way health services are distributed, a national health insurance scheme is clearly a more powerful and concentrated instrument than the dissemination of responsibility for financing through numerous nonprofit plans and insurance companies. The debates in the 1940s had been in terms not merely of central third-party financing of medical bills but of establishing in America a government-sponsored health service system. It was this aspect of financing which the AMA and others saw as creeping socialism, the thin end of a wedge of government-controlled medicine.

The change of tack in the Democratic party from the early 1950s, away from comprehensive national health insurance for the whole population toward the more limited goals of hospital insurance for the aged,[27] confused what had been a clear-cut issue of favoring or not favoring

27. See chapter 13.

health service reform. Both Democrats and Republicans were arguing in the late 1950s on the basis of maintaining the incomes of the aged, rather than in terms of restructuring the health system. The argument was whether private or governmental schemes could serve the aged the best. This was translated in the Congress in terms of whether the needs of the elderly could be met through existing insurance mechanisms, with or without expanded public assistance programs for the indigent; or whether a more sweeping public program was necessary.

There were cogent reasons for concentrating on the special needs of those sixty-five years of age and over. Those over sixty-five were twice as likely to have chronic health conditions as the younger age groups, and had two and a half times the number of days of restricted activity; they also suffered a substantial amount of acute illnesses, predominantly from respiratory conditions and accidents. Yet less than half of the elderly were covered by any type of health insurance and, as with the general population, the coverage was partial and inadequate, especially for those with the lowest incomes.[28] These facts had implications not only for the financial survival and individual dignity of those who were retired, but also for the issue of whether they received health services. A national survey of old people between 1957 and 1959, excluding those in institutions, found that half of those with chronic bronchitis and visual impairments were not under medical attention; 43 percent of cases of paralysis were unattended; over 40 percent of the hearing impairments were not under medical supervision; and there were substantial inadequacies in medical attention with respect to other major disease groups.[29] These gaps alone would have pointed to increased social provision of health services to the elderly. But the facts did not have to stand alone. For the first time in American history the elderly themselves were becoming an important political force. Increasing longevity had raised the proportion of elderly people from 4 percent of the population in 1900 to 8 percent in the early 1950s; in terms of the proportion of the voting population the latter percentage was much higher. Moreover, the elderly were becoming politically articulate. Their voices raised through senior citizens clubs and other organizations, the elderly became the "deserving poor"

28. See U.S. National Health Survey, *Duration of Limitation of Activity Due to Chronic Conditions United States, July 1959–June 1960*, USPHS, Publication no. 584–B31 (Washington, D.C., 1962); *Disability Days, United States, July 1959– June 1960*, Publication no. 584–B29 (Washington, D.C., 1961); *Interim Report on Health Insurance, United States, July–December 1959*, Publication no. 584–B26 (Washington, D.C., 1960).

29. U.S. National Health Survey, *Older Persons, Selected Health Characteristics, United States, July 1957–July 1959*, USPHS, Publication no. 584–C4 (Washington, D.C., 1960).

of the newer generations. Their pleas could not be ignored. Both Democrats and Republicans rallied—each in their own way—to improve the health and economic situation of the aged.

The program of federal grants to states for medical vendor payments for public assistance recipients was extended in 1956, thus increasing the amount of money available for medical care for the elderly who were eligible for Old-Age Assistance. But it was not those on welfare, but those who were living precariously on small pensions and savings who were hardest hit by serious illness—and who were the most vocal representatives of those over sixty-five. They developed into an effective pressure group for the introduction of national health insurance, financed through the Social Security system and available as an entitlement which would accompany the long-accepted old-age retirement benefit.

The movement for government-organized hospital insurance for the aged gained momentum with the Forand bill of 1957.[30] The bill proposed that Social Security contributions should be raised to provide up to 120 days of hospital and nursing-home care and necessary surgery for those receiving Social Security retirement pensions. It was strongly backed by organized labor, in a climate of increasing sympathy for the plight of the aged as a group. The proposal was much narrower than the earlier proposals for health insurance for the whole population. Nevertheless it could be seen as a beginning of a national health insurance scheme, and the AMA and other critics were realistic in their claims that the Forand bill could be the thin end of the ever-present wedge. Hearings on the Forand proposals were held in 1958 as part of general hearings on the Social Security Act. No action was taken, but they provided an opportunity for publicity and discussion of the proposals, and groundwork for hearings by the House Ways and Means Committee on a new Forand bill in 1959.[31] In the same year, moreover, the Senate Committee on Labor and Public Welfare held hearings in different parts of the country to elicit the community's point of view on the problems of the elderly. The elderly were achieving massive and continuing visibility.

The various points of view slowly crystallized. As might be expected, the Eisenhower administration opposed the Forand bill, continuing to

30. 85th Cong., 1st sess., H.R. 9467; introduced by Rep. Aime J. Forand (D., R.I.). For analysis of the congressional and extrapolitical congressional background and actions from the Forand bill to Medicare, see especially R. Harris, *A Sacred Trust*, pp. 71 ff.; Sundquist, pp. 296–321; Theodore R. Marmor, "The Congress: Medicare Politics and Policy," in *American Political Institutions and Public Policy*, ed. Allan P. Sindler (Boston, 1969). This account draws from all of these. Useful documentation of the various viewpoints is also to be found in Eugene Feingold, *Medicare: Policy and Politics, a Case Study and Policy Analysis* (San Francisco, 1966).
31. 86th Cong., 1st sess., H.R. 4700.

support instead the viability of private health insurance. The AMA claimed that the needs of the elderly were being exaggerated, and that under the existing system of private practice and charity care, no one need be deprived of adequate services. Dr. Leonard Larson, speaking for the AMA in 1958, condemned health insurance benefits through Social Security as "unwise" and "unnecessary," and "not in the public interest." [32] Meanwhile, groups of senior citizens were presenting a different viewpoint, encapsulated by one senior citizen in Detroit: "It is not an American heritage to suffer in pain and be stripped of life savings by any organization and then tossed back into society still sick and a complete social problem." [33] By 1960, compulsory national hospital insurance for the aged had become a major political controversy.

Against the growing pressures of the Forand bill, the Eisenhower administration developed an alternative proposal to expand medical aid to the elderly. A proposal developed by Health, Education, and Welfare Secretary Arthur Flemming and supported by presidential candidate Richard Nixon was outlined to the president in March 1960, and subsequently developed in detail. This proposal set out a plan for federal matching grants to the states for state-administered programs of medical care which would cover catastrophic medical expenses, after a substantial deductible, for all those sixty-five and over whose income was under $2,500 ($3,800 for a couple).[34] The scheme thus had a double purpose. On the one hand it would maintain the place of private health insurance for those who could afford it. On the other hand, it recognized the limitation of private insurance for large bills and for protecting those in lower-income brackets; the federal government, through the states, would provide major back-up protection. This plan was termed voluntary as opposed to compulsory, because it included an individual option of receiving cash toward the purchase of voluntary (i.e. private) health insurance. But in its use of federal and state authority to protect the incomes of the elderly, the bill was more paternalistic than the Forand proposals—which, at least formally, relied on a self-balancing fund with specified contributions for recognized benefits. Sen. Barry Goldwater of Arizona remarked that hiding behind the word voluntary was a "dressed up" version of "socialized medicine." [35]

32. U.S., Congress, House, Committee on Ways and Means, Social Security Legislation, *Hearings,* 85th Cong., 2d sess., June 1958, p. 890.
33. U.S., Congress, Senate, Committee on Labor and Public Welfare, Subcommittee on Problems of the Aged and Aging, Mr. Bill Russell, *Hearings,* 86th Cong., 1st sess., 10–11 Dec. 1959, pt. 8, p. 2087.
34. *Congressional Quarterly Almanac, 1960,* p. 155.
35. Quoted by Sundquist, p. 305.

In any event, both the Forand and the administration proposals were rejected by the powerful House Ways and Means Committee. Instead, the committee returned to an earlier concept, which had appeared in the Taft bills of 1946 to 1949, of providing medical care to selected members of the population through an enlarged public assistance program. It now suggested that the system of federal grants to states for health services for the poor would be expanded up the income scale to cover elderly persons who were not actually indigent (i.e. on public assistance) but who could be considered medically indigent, in that they could pass a means test showing inability to pay their medical bills.[36] In other words, there would be a special category of poverty, contingent on the risk of expensive illness. Such a category would, it was thought, meet the needs of the elderly who were faced with large medical bills which, through no fault of their own, they could not pay. It would also, at least in theory, serve to keep this group of people financially solvent, and thus off the general roles of public assistance. If the income limits for medical indigence were defined sufficiently broadly by the individual states, the federal proposal could lead to a generous provision of publicly financed medical care for the elderly. Unlike the previous administration proposal, however, no federal guidelines were set as to what the income limits should be.

The new proposal, strongly supported by Rep. Wilbur Mills, chairman of the House Ways and Means Committee, was an effective political compromise. It passed the House in June 1960. In the Senate, Sen. Clinton P. Anderson of New Mexico, supported by Sen. John F. Kennedy of Massachusetts, offered as an amendment a revised version of the Forand proposals. But this failed, as did an amendment from Sen. Jacob Javits, based on the principles of the administration bill. Sponsored by Sen. Robert S. Kerr of Oklahoma, the Mills proposals passed the Senate and were signed into law in September 1960.[37]

The Kerr-Mills Act—forerunner of Medicaid—provided for additional federal matching grants to the states for vendor medical payments under their Old-Age Assistance programs, together with a new matching program, Medical Assistance for the Aged, for vendor payments for those over sixty-five who were judged as medically indigent, according to means-test standards to be set by each state. This solution, an extension of long-accepted welfare medical programs, was supported by the AMA.

36. The Taft bills were: 79th Cong., 2d sess., S. 2143; 80th Cong., 1st sess., S. 545; 81st Cong., 1st sess., S. 1581. The 1960 proposal was added to an omnibus Social Security bill, H.R. 12580.
37. P.L. 86–778.

In theory it could have provided extensive medical services to a substantial proportion of the elderly population. Indeed, the provision of open-ended grants to states for health programs for as large a proportion of the elderly as each state decided to include opened the door to substantial public (socialized) medical programs. But in practice it became clear that the new program was ineffective, even for those it supposedly served. After three years of operation, only twenty-eight of the fifty states had the program in operation; only four of these were judged to have a comprehensive program.[38] Tied to the existing administration of state welfare programs, with limited provisions for care, with cumbersome, sometimes humilitating means-test requirements, and with unequal application state by state, the Kerr-Mills program proved to be at best only a partial success, and at worst an unhappy failure.

No-one seriously pretended that Kerr-Mills was the final answer to meeting the health needs of the elderly. Nevertheless the program was disappointing to conservatives and liberals alike. It neither vindicated the view of those who saw the long-term answer to health care financing as a mix of private health insurance backed by public assistance, rather than as of comprehensive national health insurance; nor did it begin to meet the concern of those who looked for a full range of preventive as well as curative services for the elderly as a means of forestalling possible indigence. Under the program, the elderly were forced to spend down to the relatively low and repressive income eligibility limits of the program before receiving any benefits. As Secretary Celebrezze pointed out in the 1963 hearings on hospital insurance for the aged, Kerr-Mills did not prevent dependency but only dealt with it after it had happened.[39]

The Kerr-Mills Act thus proved only a temporary holding operation against renewed attempts to include medical care for the elderly under the old-age insurance provisions of Social Security. Instead of following the concept of private health insurance backed by government assistance to the indigent, the current Medicare program of hospital insurance for

38. The four states were Hawaii, Massachusetts, New York, and North Dakota. Adding to the problems of the scheme, a number of states had used the injection of new federal money as a device to transfer people already on welfare programs into the new category, to take advantage of higher federal matching provisions. There was thus increased expense without a corresponding increase in service. U.S., Congress, Senate, Special Committee on Aging, Subcommittee on Health of the Elderly, *Medical Assistance for the Aged: The Kerr-Mills Program, 1960–1963,* Oct. 1963, pp. 1–2 and passim.
39. U.S., Congress, House, Committee on Ways and Means, 88th Cong., 1st and 2d sess., *Hearings on H.R. 3920,* p. 31. For a review of Kerr-Mills in the context of public assistance medical programs, see Rosemary Stevens and Robert Stevens, "Medicaid: Anatomy of a Dilemma," *Law and Contemp. Problems, 35* (Spring 1970), 348–425.

the aged, passed in 1965, was a direct descendant of the Forand proposals. While limited both in population coverage and in benefits, Medicare established a system of compulsory national health insurance. But at the same time, adding to the confusion of American medical care, federal-state programs for the indigent were to continue on an enlarged basis through the present program of Medicaid.

MEDICARE: TRIUMPH OF THE PUBLIC VOICE

President John F. Kennedy had strongly endorsed hospital insurance for the aged through Social Security in his health message to Congress in 1961. This was followed by an Administration bill introduced in the Senate by Senator Clinton Anderson and in the House by Rep. Cecil King.[40] Opposed on the outside by the AMA and by the Health Insurance Institute and with little chance of support from Representative Mills' powerful Ways and Means Committee, the King-Anderson bill was initially unsuccessful; and a similar proposal offered by Senator Anderson as an amendment to the Public Welfare amendments in 1962 suffered a resounding defeat.[41] Nevertheless, a supporting record was slowly being built up. Hearings by the Ways and Means Committee in 1961 documented the continuing failure of the existing system (including the Kerr-Mills legislation) to meet the medical bills of the elderly. Hospital expenses had risen from $9.39 a day in 1946 to $32.23 in 1960, and were rising increasingly rapidly.[42] Born of the continuing increase in medical costs, and encouraged by the lack of effectiveness of the Kerr-Mills programs, the changed composition of the Senate after the 1962 elections, and perhaps even the sheer familiarity of the continuing phrases and the lessening credibility of the AMA position, support of health insurance for the aged was rising. President Kennedy outlined his proposals for hospital insurance in a special message in February 1963; the King-Anderson bill was introduced again, and the House Ways and Means Committee again held hearings.[43] The following year, after bipartisan efforts to break the

40. 87th Cong., 1st sess., S. 909, H.R. 4222.
41. The Anderson amendment was offered as a revised version of S. 909, as a Senate Floor amendment to the Public Welfare amendments (H.R. 10606) which had already been passed by the House.
42. U.S., Congress, House, Committee on Ways and Means, Hearings on *H.R. 4222*, 87th Cong., 1st sess., vol. 1, p. 40.
43. President Kennedy's proposals were submitted to Congress on 21 February as part of the message "Aiding Our Senior Citizens." He called for Social Security payment of inpatient hospital costs for the elderly of up to 90 days (with some contributions from the patient), of up to 180 days (with the patient making a

deadlock and reach agreement on some constructive health proposal, the Senate for the first time passed a proposal for hospital insurance for the aged as an amendment to the Social Security bill of 1964; but it died in a House-Senate conference committee.

With the Democratic landslide elections of November 1964, the composition of the House of Representatives (and the Ways and Means Committee) was changed in favor of compulsory hospital insurance. President Johnson at once called for action on the King-Anderson proposals— Medicare—as a first priority of business. Hospital insurance for the aged through Social Security appeared as the first bill of both the Senate and the Congress for 1965: bills S.1 and H.R. 1 of the Eighty-ninth Congress. The proposals were incorporated into the overall aims of the new administration's program for a "Great Society." Hearings were held by the House Ways and Means Committee in January and February 1965. While the AMA continued to claim that "We physicians care for the elderly and know their health needs better than anyone else," and that health insurance controlled by Washington was incompatible with "good medicine," [44] the tide was turning in favor of including compulsory hospital insurance as a benefit of Social Security.

Other proposals for financing health care were, however, by no means dead. Indeed, it was the eventual inclusions of several major proposals which was to give the Medicare legislation its peculiar and distinctive character. The AMA, in a last-ditch stand against hospital insurance through Social Security, developed its own "Eldercare" proposal, sponsored in the Congress by Representatives Curtis and Herlong, and by Sen. John G. Tower. This called for a federal-state program which would subsidize private insurance policies for the elderly, for hospital, doctor, and drug bills. A rather similar bill was sponsored by Rep. John W. Byrnes and endorsed by the House Republican leadership. The Byrnes bill, "Bettercare," suggested a federal (rather than a state) program whereby the elderly would be encouraged to contribute part of the premiums of a voluntary health insurance program with public subsidy of the remainder. There were also continuing proposals for tax credits and

---

greater contribution), or all costs for 45 days. The proposals also included up to 180 days of nursing-home care and 240 home health-care visits. The administration bill was introduced by Representative King (H.R. 3920) and Senator Anderson (S. 880) in February 1963; and initial hearings were held in November. *Congress and the Nation, 1945–1964,* p. 1155.

44. U.S., Congress, House, Committee on Ways and Means, Testimony of Dr. Donovan Ward, President of the American Medical Association, *Executive Hearings on H.R. 1,* 89th Cong., 1st sess., Jan.–Feb. 1965, pp. 741–47.

deductions for health insurance premiums, and arguments for expanding the struggling Kerr-Mills program.[45]

Representatives Mills, King, Herlong, Byrnes, and Curtis were all members of the House Ways and Means Committee. The full range of points of view was present in Congress's vital committee, and the outcome of the debate over Medicare was thus by no means predictable. In the event, the bill reported out of the committee was not one bill but a compendium of three originally separate and in some respects competing proposals. The administration's proposals for hospital insurance for the aged, financed through the Social Security system, would provide basic inpatient and nursing-home coverage for all those eligible for Social Security retirement benefits. As a second layer, there would be a system of federal subsidies to enable old people to buy into a voluntary program of insurance for their doctor bills (the Byrnes proposal), with the federal government setting premiums and benefits but with the administration of the scheme being funneled through insurance companies and nonprofit agencies. These two proposals were to become, respectively, part A and part B of title XVIII of the Social Security amendments of 1965. They provided the two interlocking parts of Medicare. At the same time, a third proposal was made, to liberalize and extend the Kerr-Mills program of federal grants to states for the medically indigent not only with respect to those over sixty-five but to others groups of the community as well. This last proposal became title XIX of the Social Security amendments, popularly known as Medicaid. The different points of view over medical care financing were thereby brought together. In one fell swoop the elderly were offered compulsory hospital insurance through Social Security, subsidized voluntary health insurance for their medical bills, and the expanded program of benefits under the rubric of medical indigence. States could take medical indigence much further if they chose. In terms of passage, this strange mixture, brewed by adept political alchemists, proved to be successful. The revised proposals passed the House, survived hearings by the Senate Finance Committee, were voted with some modifications in the Senate, were further modified in conference committee, and were finally signed into law in July 1965.[46] Thus came Medicare and Medicaid.

On 1 July 1966, when parts A and B of Medicare came into effect, the elderly population overnight became eligible, subject to specified deductibles and contributions, for 90 days of inpatient care for each spell of

45. For a full report of congressional history of the different bills, see *Congressional Quarterly Almanac, 1965,* pp. 248–69.
46. P.L. 89–97.

illness, for another 100 days of care in a skilled nursing home following hospitalization, for hospital outpatient services, and for home health services, physicians' services, and other diagnostic services and supportive care. The Social Security Administration was made responsible for both the automatic hospital insurance benefits under Social Security (part A, title XVIII) and the supplementary medical benefits (part B), available to the elderly on a voluntary, contributory basis. Under part A, contributions are made through the usual Social Security contributions paid by the working population. Part B of Medicare is also based on the insurance principle, although it is outside the compulsory Social Security contributory scheme. This part is a federally subsidized insurance scheme (rather like Blue Shield) to which those over sixty-five may contribute on a monthly basis. The federal government matches the voluntary contribution of the subscriber from general revenues. The basic provisions of part B include physician bills (inside and outside hospitals), other medical services such as injections and dressings, and a specified number of home visits.

In the period before Medicare came into effect, the Social Security Administration recruited staff; formulated policies and regulations; negotiated contracts with state health agencies and with the nonprofit agencies and insurance companies which were to act as intermediaries and agents of the government in administering the plan; surveyed thousands of hospitals and other health institutions for the purposes of certifying them as participators in the Medicare program; and launched a massive public information campaign designed to reach virtually all of the 19 million people who were sixty-five years of age or over. These measures reaped dividends. In its first full year of operation, Medicare paid for 34 percent of old people's medical bills; in its second year (fiscal year 1967–68) the proportion was 45 percent. The major impact was on expensive hospital services; in 1967–68 Medicare paid 63 percent of hospital bills for the elderly.[47]

Meanwhile, as the Medicare program was becoming established, Medicaid, the third layer of the Mills' cake, was moving into operation. This program offered to states a federal matching grant of from 50 to 83 percent, based on the variable grant system used in welfare grants-in-aid (in turn based on the per capita income of the states involved) to pro-

47. Dorothy Rice and Barbara Cooper, "Outlays for Medical Care of Aged and Nonaged Persons, Fiscal Years 1966–68," *Research and Statistics Note,* 1969, no. 12. For a review of the setting up of Medicare, see *1st Annual Report on Medicare,* Letter from the Secretary of Health, Education, and Welfare transmitting the first annual report of the Medicare program, 90th Cong., 2d sess., House Document no. 331 (Washington, D.C., 1968).

vide medical care to specified needy persons, including those deemed medically indigent. Medicaid was not limited to the older members of the population although it was expected to have a special impact in this group. As the expanded successor to the Kerr-Mills Act of 1960, Medicaid is based on public assistance to the indigent and medically indigent, whereas Medicare covers all beneficiaries, rich and poor. Medicaid is a state rather than a federal program, and therefore subject to wide variations. Its chief provisions are the integration of previously fragmented public assistance medical provisions under one program, the standardization and expansion of medical assistance, and the abandonment of relatives' financial responsibility for the elderly as well as of state residence requirements.

With Medicare offering benefits for expensive health services, and with Medicaid as a backstop for those most in need, the elderly achieved substantial protection against economic loss due to medical bills. The 1965 amendments offered an important program for income maintenance. In including hospital benefits under Social Security, moreover, the long cycle of the compulsory health insurance movement was at least partially complete. The door was open for possible extensions of health insurance to other segments of the population. But at the same time, Medicare did not attempt to effect major changes in the health service system. As set up, it provided a financing mechanism for individuals, a credit card for the purchase of care, rather than any means for large-scale development in the organization of health services. The time for basic changes among providers was still to come.

In the long process of debate, however, had come a clear and loud enunciation that it was the general public and not the professional voice which was to determine how health services would be financed, and thus in the long run how they would be provided. The success of the AMA's political position from the 1940s to the mid 1960s delayed effective reappraisal of the old set of professional attitudes. Seduced by the elusive image of small-scale, fee-for-service, private practice, the American medical profession of 1965 was running in its political thinking at least three decades behind the social implications of specialized medicine. Medicare provided the opportunity for a period of reappraisal in which the attitudinal emphases of the professional associations might be realigned in terms of current social and political necessities. At the least this meant a redrawing of professional functions in terms which were consistent with consumer definitions of the public interest. Before 1965, report after report from governmental and other sources exposed the plight of the elderly, but the AMA had continued to take the position the aged (and other dependent groups) were by no means as sick, as in need of medical attention, or as financially needy as other groups were claiming. This attitude was more than a rationalization of pecuniary narrow-mindedness or vested interest; it was a statement that organized medicine was the proper interpreter of the nation's health. Finally, however, with Medicare, the public emerged as the dominant decision maker. There was both a crisis in medical care and—part and parcel of the same scientific, technical, and social movements—a watershed in the long history of medical professionalism. The passage of Medicare marked the beginning of a new era.

CHAPTER 19

Shoring up the System

Medicare

The passage of Medicare proved that the development of payment schemes for health care is politically as well as socially important. Since 1965, the argument has been one of the shape health insurance will take in the future rather than of its necessity. There are now opportunities for shared-risk prepayment schemes through private insurance plans (including prepaid group practice), through compulsory insurance for the elderly, and through federal-state medical assistance schemes administered through a means test for those who are poor; and each of these methods of financing is capable of extension, through federal organization, regulation, and subsidy, so that eventually the entire population could be covered through a shared-risk scheme for the payment of much or most of their medical bills. More important, the potential recipient of medical care, the patient, has become increasingly aware of the costs of health services and of the deprivation of not receiving services when in need.

The Medicare program has been an important ingredient in this awareness. But in the process both Medicare and Medicaid appear increasingly as health care programs in transition. Marked by charges of extravagance, fraud, and waste, the programs point toward a future health insurance system in which more stringent controls will be exerted by government over the private medical sector, or in which the private sector—most notably, organized groups of physicians—will act as recognized public agents. As this book goes to press, the future form of health services in the United States is in doubt. On the one hand are sweeping proposals for national health insurance which would foster organized health systems through prepaid group practice, through medical society foundations and other recognized service groups. Under these, national health *insurance* would be interpreted, as it has in many western European countries as being a form of national health *service,* even though hospitals, physicians, and other facilities and personnel need not be directly employed by the government. At the other end of a spectrum of potential governmental intervention are suggestions for expanding individual protection against crippling medical bills (in the form of tax credits or offsets for the purchase of health insurance premiums), but without concomitant intervention into the way in which medical practice is organized.

There are many other suggestions in between these proposals. But the argument is the old one. If physicians and hospitals can and will respond to demands for adequate and efficient health services without government controls or incentives, then only health insurance is necessary. Every member of the population could be required to hold a specified package of health insurance benefits, with or without government subsidy, just as every child is required to have an education. If, on the other hand, the health care providers seem unable to respond with more effective services, even to the increased demand generated through more generous insurance benefits, then more direct government action may prove socially desirable and politically necessary. As in all the previous debates over health insurance in the United States the initiative lies in the private rather than in the public sector. It is here—in the responses of a largely private health service system to massive infusion of public funds—that the experiences of Medicare and Medicaid were to prove so important.

THE FISCAL STRUCTURE

The federal government took over no hospitals or other facilities, nor does it directly employ any doctors under Medicare. The same is true with respect to the state governments under Medicaid. The new scheme was thus not socialized medicine in the sense of creating a nationalized, governmental service; quite the reverse, for as third-party reimbursement schemes, both Medicare and Medicaid mimicked the private insurance system. Doctors continued to practice as they had before. With the exception of nursing homes, whose development blossomed under the impact of additional funding, no separate clinics or centers were set up for the elderly (as was happening for the poor with the establishment of federally-financed neighborhood health centers). Physicians accept Medicare patients into their private offices or in hospitals, where they may also be private patients, and the billing mechanisms set up are similar to those for other, nongovernment, types of health insurance. Those doctors who choose to see Medicare patients (the great majority, if not all, of those who previously saw patients over 65) merely fill in a different form from that usually requested for patients covered by private health insurance, and continue to be paid on a fee-for-service basis.

The real difference wrought by Medicare lay not in the doctor's office, nor even in the hospital, but in the administrative structure set up between the federal government and the health providers. The legislation as written broke down medical services into two separately-administered sectors, those connected with hospital care and those primarily concerned with physician services. Under Medicare part A (hospital insurance) groups of hospitals, extended care facilities,[1] and home health agencies which offer services under the plan are able either to deal directly with the Social Security Administration for their payments or to nominate an organization (subject to government approval) to act as a "fiscal intermediary." The functions of the fiscal intermediary as defined in the original law include reimbursing providers for their services; providing consultative services to hospitals and other participating agencies to help them set up the appropriate records systems and qualify for the program; establishing a channel of communication and information for providers of care, and between them and the secretary of Health, Education, and

1. New health programs seem destined to coin new phrases. An "extended care facility" is a nursing home or rehabilitative institution recognized as eligible under Medicare for up to 100 days of skilled nursing care for patients discharged from hospitals after at least three days' hospitalization. Information presented at the 1965 hearings by the chief actuary of the Social Security Administration and a representative of the private health insurance industry indicated that such care was envisaged as an alternative to more expensive hospitalization; indeed, it was hoped that the provision of extended care would reduce hospital utilization. U.S., Congress, House, Committee on Ways and Means, *Medical Care for the Aged: Executive Hearings,* 89th Cong., 1st sess., Jan.–Feb. 1965, H.R. 1 and other proposals for medical care for the aged, pp. 436–41. By January 1967, when this part of the program came into effect, 2,607 institutions had qualified to participate as extended care facilities; of these, 1,968 were nursing homes, with a required level of skilled nursing care as defined by the Social Security Administration, and most of *these* were proprietary (profit-making) institutions. *Medicare Newsletter,* USDHEW, Social Security Administration, 13 Jan. 1967. By July 1969, 4,776 extended care facilities were participating. The detailed development of Medicare is outside the scope of this study. It should be noted, however, that one effect of the inclusion of "extended care"—which tended to be defined in the early medical period as skilled nursing-home care per se rather than as strictly an alternative to hospitalization—was a rapid development in the construction of nursing homes, and thus in the utilization and costs of nursing-home care. For a review, see U.S., Congress, Senate, Committee on Finance, *Medicare and Medicaid, Problems, Issues and Alternatives,* Report of the Staff, 91st Cong., 1st sess., Feb. 1970, pp. 91–96 and passim (hereafter cited as *Medicare and Medicaid Report,* Feb. 1970).

Welfare; and auditing providers' records.[2] The fiscal intermediary accepted functions which would otherwise have had to be established through vastly expanding the Social Security Administration's district offices, which handle direct Social Security cash payments to beneficiaries. The intermediary deals primarily with the paperwork of Medicare part A, receiving and paying claims for hospital care on behalf of Medicare patients and in turn being reimbursed for these payments (together with administrative costs) by the federal government.

The use of private fiscal agents rather than government regional or district offices was logical in that the latter had no experience in handling hospital and medical claims. But the result of the legislation was to entrench Medicare firmly into the structures of private health insurance. The great majority of hospitals (6,876 of 7,906) nominated the Blue Cross Association as their intermediary through their membership in the American Hospital Association. Over half of the extended care facilities and home health agencies also selected the Blue Cross Association, the remainder choosing commercial insurance companies; only a sprinkling of facilities chose to deal directly with the federal government. As a result, the seventy-five local Blue Cross plans, which are the components of the Blue Cross Association, together with twelve other principle private intermediaries, became agents of a major government program. While national responsibility and regulatory power remain with the government, it is the private organizations which are the organizational pivots of a program of hospital insurance for the aged whose estimated annual cost reached $5.8 billion in 1970.[3]

A similar pattern was followed for Medicare part B (medical insurance), although the private insurance agents were termed "carriers" rather than intermediaries, and the choice made in this instance not by the providers of care but by the secretary of Health, Education, and Welfare. The majority (33 of 49) of the part B carriers so designated are Blue Shield plans. Each carrier covers a particular geographical area, usually a state. Part B carriers are responsible for making payments for physician and other services from the national supplementary medical insurance trust fund which, in turn, draws its income in equal parts from monthly contributions from those sixty-five years and over and from the federal government. The sum of $1.25 billion dollars flowed through this system in fiscal year 1967; as much as $2.49 billion

2. P.L. 89–97, sec. 1816. The part A intermediaries are paid administrative costs for these services by the government, a sum of $76 million in fiscal year 1969. For the initial selection and establishment of the intermediaries, see Somers and Somers, *Medicare and the Hospitals,* pp. 25–42.

3. *Medicare and Medicaid Report,* Feb. 1970, pp. 30, 113, 261.

is estimated for fiscal year 1971.[4] The major intermediaries and carriers appointed full-time directors of their Medicare operations and developed sizable payment units. This channeling of government funds through the private sector was one of the major features of the new two-headed Medicare program. But it was to become one of its major headaches in terms of oversight and regulation.

In terms of provider acceptance, however, the program was an immediate success. Medicare itself, once passed, was rapidly absorbed into the physician's accepted environmental structure of office and hospital, based as it was on preexisting insurance patterns and on the payment of physicians according to their fees in private practice. Under the 1965 legislation, physicians might bill their patients as usual, and the patient would then pay the doctor and claim a refund from the Medicare carrier of 80 percent of the reasonable medical charge, over and above the standard $50 deductible for part B. This method left the physician free to establish his own individual charges. Alternatively, the physician might choose to claim his fees directly from the carrier, in which case he would accept as his full fee the reasonable charge as determined by the carrier. In terms of time as well as cost, this latter method, known as "assignment," benefits the patient, for the initiative for making Medicare claims rests with the physician. But the former is financially advantageous to the physician, providing he can collect his fees; and during the first eighteen months of Medicare, only 38 percent of part B bills were paid by assignment.[5] The direct billing method was modified in the Social Security Amendments of 1967 (P.L. 90–248) to enable patients to present an itemized bill to the carrier for reimbursement, instead of having to pay the doctor's bill first and wait for payment. But the two methods still remain. Under both methods of reimbursement the fiscal intermediaries and carriers act as an important buffer-zone between hospitals or physicians and the government.

PAYMENT OF PHYSICIANS

The "how" and the "how much" of paying for physician services is a crucial question in the establishment and effective operation of any

4. Part B carriers were paid administrative costs of $117.4 million in fiscal year 1969. Thus the total additional revenue into the private insurance sector (nonprofit and profit) in 1969 was $193.4 million. Ibid., pp. 4, 37–39.
5. Forty-one percent were paid to the Medicare beneficiary, and the remainder to the hospital (for outpatient services and physician billing through hospitals) and other sources. During 1967, assignment became more popular. Figures for the spring of 1968 indicate marked differences by carrier (and thus by area), ranging

governmentally operated system of health financing. By adopting the system of private intermediaries and carriers, Medicare avoided in one fell swoop the prospect of long discussions and potentially acrimonious confrontations with physician organizations on standard methods and amounts of reimbursement for services. Instead of a national professional group or local groups negotiating over fee scales, part-time salaries, capitation fees, or contracts in advance with the Social Security Administration, open-ended responsibility was delegated to the participating private insurance organizations, not the government, to pay fees which seemed reasonable. Instead of a public organization decreeing the relative value of an office visit to a psychiatrist, an ophthalmologist, or a neurological surgeon, prevailing fee customs remained. The structure capitalized on the interests of both organized medicine and the private health insurance system, by making Medicare as structurally "private" as was possible. Fee setting itself rested on the integrity of the medical profession. Indeed, in about 96 percent of cases, Medicare has paid the fees charged by physicians.[6]

The intermediaries and carriers also welcomed the arrangements. The board chairman of the National Association of Blue Shield Plans, a practicing physician, commended the framers of the bill in 1965 for their "keen understanding" of the role of voluntary health insurance organizations in the implementation of the Medicare program, for recognition of Medicare part B as the antithesis of socialized medicine, and for allowing the aged population to continue in accustomed patterns of prepayment.[7] Medicare was thus seen as an extension of existing mechanisms rather than a strange or alien system, or even at times as being a governmental system at all. Blue Shield plans, it was noted, were already collecting information from local physicians as to prevailing medical charges in different places, and were accustomed to working with mediation and other evaluating groups organized by local medical societies to resolve fee problems and to control utilization of medical services. Thus, by implication, the private-public mix would build not only on established insurance procedures but also on the existing patterns and controls of organized medicine. Since Blue Shield—the so-called Doctors' Plan— was a system set up and approved by medical associations, Medicare part B imposed a major responsibility upon, and extended the concept of,

from Massachusetts Blue Shield with 83 percent claims paid by assignment, to Cleveland Blue Shield with 23 percent. Russell J. Myers, *Medicare,* p. 243; *Medicare and Medicaid Report,* Feb. 1970, pp. 322–23.

6. Myers, p. 244.

7. U.S. Congress, Senate, Committee on Finance, Statement of Dr. Russell B. Carson, *Hearings* on H.R. 6675, 89th Cong., 1st sess., 1965, pp. 391–98.

professional self-regulation at least for services to the elderly. It provided a challenge to the effectiveness of the private insurance sector as a future vehicle for national medical insurance and to physicians as controllers of medical services in their own areas.

The carriers were instructed to pay physicians for a covered service under part B an amount that represented a "reasonable charge." The establishment of this charge was to be made in the context of customary and prevailing charges for similar services in the area and was supposed not to exceed comparable charges paid for similar services under the carrier's existing insurance programs.[8] The carriers were also made de facto responsible for seeing that the charges paid were for appropriate and proper services. But this responsibility was not spelled out, in terms either of setting up necessary information systems or of possible fines and other disciplinary action for inappropriate or wasteful care and billing. In consequence, the individual physician was given extraordinary freedom to prescribe, treat, and charge for services under Medicare. Except for routine physical examinations (which were not initially covered, this being a sickness insurance plan rather than one designed to reassure the well) and psychiatric care (which has fiscal limitations), no limits were built into the legislation with respect to the types of services physicians might perform under the program.[9] There are no conditions for physician participation by dint of special experience or graduate training. All licensed physicians became eligible to participate, for all services. The general practitioner could be reimbursed for undertaking major surgery; the specialist in internal medicine, dermatology, etc., for giving perfunctory or inappropriate care. As with other forms of insurance, and, indeed, with uninsured medical practice, judgments of the propriety and costs of care were left to individual physicians, with correcting factors being applied if necessary after the event: through controls and audits by the payment plans, through new utilization review committees in participating hospitals, through medical society procedures for complaints by patients over fees and over competence, and in the last resort through legal actions. Except for hospital utilization review (a requirement set up by the Medicare legislation), these patterns followed those long accepted in Blue Shield and other private insurance plans.

The primary impact of Medicare on individual physicians was not,

8. P.L. 89–97, sec. 1842.
9. Psychiatric care outside the hospital was limited in any calendar year to the smaller of $250 or 50 percent of the expense. Other physician services were allowed without a numerical limit. The major limitation on part B was the patient's pocketbook, with the patient paying the first $50 of covered expenses and 20 percent of the remaining charges.

therefore, one of federal control but of increased professional flexibility. Physicians were now free to see elderly patients without concern that the patients would be impoverished by submitting to treatment, or that their own services would go unremunerated. More than 15 million elderly people used part B services in 1968, chiefly in physicians' offices; during fiscal 1969, Medicare paid 72 percent of the physician bills of those aged 65 and over, and about half of all their health care expenditures.[10] The value of such services to the patients is inestimable in terms of the effect of the services themselves, the release of the income of the elderly for other purposes, and the reduction in anxiety of people faced with the threatening possibilities of expensive sickness. But there were two related impacts of the system on the responsibilities and behavior patterns of physicians. One sprang out of the phenomenon that under Medicare a group of persons who had been poor in their ability to purchase medical services suddenly became comparatively rich. The other lay in the responsibility of organized groups of physicians to review the appropriateness of fees on behalf of fiscal intermediaries.

Medicare had been introduced to protect the incomes of the elderly. But since physicians were encouraged through the new system to charge for care of the elderly on the same basis as they charged other, more prosperous members of the population, Medicare, supported by developing Medicaid programs for the poor, evened up the financial status of the population. One byproduct of Medicare was to support and increase the incomes of physicians. By 1970, part B of Medicare, 90 percent of which is for physician services to the elderly, was paying out amounts which averaged $7,000 per physician. A second byproduct of income protection was to reduce the traditional Robin Hood argument whereby professionals have the privilege of setting differential fees according to the ability to pay by different members of the population. Put baldly, Medicare abolished a large segment of charity medicine.

The logic of this argument, certainly if applied to the whole population, would be for physicians to be reimbursed on standard fee schedules according to standard and accepted procedures. Such fees could be weighted according to additional factors which took into account an

10. "Current Medicare Survey Report, Medical Insurance Sample," Social Security Administration, *Health Insurance Statistics,* 27 Jan. 1970, p. 2; Barbara S. Cooper, "Medical Care Outlays for Aged and Non-Aged Persons, 1966–69" Ibid., *Research and Statistics Note,* 18 June, 1970. The highest per capita reimbursement in 1969 was in California, where an average of $136 per enrolled was paid out through Medicare Part B; the lowest, Iowa and South Dakota with $54. Louis B. Russell, "Health Insurance for the Aged: Amounts Reimbursed by State, Fiscal Years 1967–69," Ibid., 15 April, 1970.

evaluation of competence of the physician, or even his popularity. But Medicare did not openly face the possibility of equal pay for equivalent work. Indeed, the complex method of setting up ranges of reasonable and customary fees for each physician under Medicare was an attempt to continue differential fee charging within the confines of a public system. The doctor may still charge the rich senior citizen more than the poor, even under the assignment method. This outcome is an odd reflection of the compromises wrought between equality of service for patients in a social insurance system and the safeguarding of professional "freedom." The ultimate test is, however, not one of political philosophy but of how well the system works in providing patient care and in assuring physician participation. In both these instances the Medicare system of payment to physicians provided initial satisfaction. For both patient and physician the Medicare recipient was a full-fledged private patient.

The concept of usual and customary fees for physicians as the basis of a large-scale public medical program was further strengthened in the early development of the federal-state programs for Medicaid. Of twenty-seven Medicaid programs approved by the Department of Health, Education, and Welfare in 1966, fifteen proposed a physician fee structure of usual and customary charges rather than agreed fee schedules (a trend since reversed).[11] These actions could be interpreted, from the recipient's point of view, in terms of social dignity and equality. The poor, like the elderly, were to receive their care in the "mainstream" of medicine (private practice), rather than in inferior or segregated conditions. But on the other hand, the implicit abandonment of physician charity arrangements, and the needed development of individual and local statistical profiles of physicians' charging practices for both Medicare and Medicaid, emphasized the responsibility for fee regulation by individual physicians, by local medical associations, or by their representatives on Blue Shield and insurance company advisory committees. Not only did Medicare (and to a lesser extent Medicaid) enlarge the physician's ability to prescribe the best treatment for the patient without fiscal restraints; it imposed an enlarged responsibility for medical costs on physician organizations. There was a potential rebirth of local physician responsibility for establishing what used to be called "fee bills" in the nineteenth century—the creation of accepted levels of payment for specified procedures and services, even if these rates varied from physician to physician, and policing to ensure that these were carried out. Nor, in contrast to the time honored discretion and secrecy of charging

11. USDHEW Social and Rehabilitation Service 1966, personal communication.

practices in the days when physicians used to charge patients what the market would bear, was there any reason why such rates should be secret.[12]

Fee review itself was largely left to the carriers, just as hospital reimbursement, which was on the rather similar basis of "reasonable costs," was left to the part A intermediaries. Herein, indeed, lay much of the initial advantage of Medicare's administrative mechanism. In the first four years of Medicare, the Social Security Administration showed reluctance to put pressure on the carriers to standardize the concept of usual and customary fees; the crucial decisions remained in the private sector, with the government acting primarily as a reimbursement agency. The assumption was, however, that the private agents would carry out their duties efficiently. But there was increasing evidence that the carriers and intermediaries did not see themselves as government inspection agencies. While some carriers surveyed local physicians with inquiries as to what were their customary fees, many others did not, on the grounds that any survey would produce "anticipatory bias" on the part of physicians, leading automatically to fee inflation.[13] The Utah Blue Shield plan was unusual in its use of its experience with non-Medicare patients as the source of information for payments for Medicare. Most Blue Shield carirers did not use for Medicare the fee schedules already established for Blue Shield's own operations, instead relying on individual physician judgments as to their own billing practices. The idea of customary charges was thus translated (subject to review by carriers for obvious overcharging practices) into the charges made by individual physicians who had little basis for assessing how far their own fees fitted prevailing patterns in the community. In the absence of other controls (including effective controls through organized professional regulation) the individual actions of 300,000 physicians became a key to the developing costs of Medicare. This was true, moreover, not only in the case of physician fees

12. The medical ethics of publicizing (or rather not publicizing) charges has also been closely tied to the anathema of unrestricted professional competition through underbidding. The elements of competition have now, however, largely disappeared —a factor of a recognized physician shortage, as well as of the provision of additional sources of funding. The present confusion is illustrated in the answer to a question posed by a physician to the AMA in 1967, whether he might ethically post a list of his charges in his waiting room. He was warned that the "very nature of medical practice prevents the rigid establishment of inflexible fees for the many services which may be rendered to any individual," that posting a schedule might tend to degrade the profession, and that it would not be in the profession's best interest. Reasons for these statements were not given. "Questions and Answers," *AMA News,* 18 Dec. 1967.

13. *Medicare and Medicaid Report,* Feb. 1970, pp. 65–66.

but also in the determination of hospital and nursing home utilization and in the prescription of diagnostic tests, drugs, and other services. Instead, then, of the development of relatively independent and effective local agencies for the administration of Medicare, with strong physician participation and leadership, Medicare evolved swiftly into an amorphous network of handouts to medical providers, and then in turn to congressional publicity, anxiety, and confrontation about the apparent lack of administrative responsibility for an increasingly expensive medical program. The idea of decentralized administration and control of health insurance payments through carriers and intermediaries which was built into both parts of Medicare was overtaken, particularly since 1968, by one of increasing federal supervision and regulation.

It is true that some federal regulations were developed at the beginning of the Medicare program, for the purpose of setting basic standards and guidelines for hospitals and other facilities to participate for reimbursement.[14] But the early regulations only peripherally affected physicians. In January 1967, regulations were developed specifying that payments could only be made for institutional care under Medicare when there was a physician's certification that such care was necessary (it was pointed out by the Social Security Administration that this action was "consistent with information issued at the start of the program to the medical profession," and that no standard form for doing this was required).[15] The following month, efforts were made to clarify the meaning of customary and prevailing charges; the former being the charges usually made by a particular physician, the latter those used by all physicians in an area. The acceptable top level for prevailing charges was defined as being no more than one standard deviation above the mean of the customary charges in a locality. But no major efforts were made to impose federal control over the part B carriers; indeed, it was

14. These were issued as "Conditions of Participation" for hospitals, extended care facilities, home health agencies, and laboratories by the Social Security Administration. The extended care facility regulations, for example, required at least one registered professional nurse or licensed practical nurse on duty at all times. Responsibility for certifying facilities for participation was vested in the state health departments. Regulations have also been developed for reimbursement procedures, to clarify, particularly for hospitals, what elements of hospital costs might be included for reimbursement. All regulations are published in the *Federal Register*. See e.g. *Federal Register*, 22 Nov. 1966; 16 Dec. 1967.
15. *Medicare Newsletter*, 31 Jan. 1967. The proposed regulations appeared in the *Federal Register*, 20 Jan. 1967. Physician certification of the medical necessity for hospital outpatient services and admissions to general hospitals was removed, as being unnecessary, under the Social Security amendments of 1967 (P.L. 90–248), except for recertification provisions after a specified length of stay, for patients in institutions.

noted that carriers "do not negotiate or set up special fee schedules for Medicare." [16]

The rising costs of medical services soon began, however, to puncture this relative freedom. Physician fees increased from an annual average of 3 percent between 1956 and 1965 to an apparent rise of 6.5 percent between June 1965 and June 1967;[17] it appeared that the average physician had taken advantage of the establishment of the new program to raise his charges. In part to meet the rising expenditures the monthly premium paid by the elderly for services under part B of Medicare was increased from the original $3 in 1966, to $4 as of April 1968, and again to $5.30 in July 1970, these sums in each case being matched from general federal revenues. Including the first $50 which a patient pays for care under part B, the person sixty-five years and over now has to pay $113.60 a year before receiving any services, compared with $86 of four years ago.

The overall amount of Medicare money going to physician services is relatively small and less pressing than the concurrent rise in hospital costs; moreover, the development of the Medicare program as a whole is in better financial condition than concurrent concerns and collapses in Medicaid. Nevertheless, because part B is a specific insurance program contributed to by those sixty-five and over, the impact of rising costs on the beneficiaries has been more evident than for part A, whose costs are spread among Social Security contributions from the total working population. The question of doctors' fees is also simple and visible. In at least some cases, moreover, the amounts received by physicians have been staggering.

Senator Anderson of New Mexico, a member of the Senate Finance Committee, asked the Social Security Administration in 1969 to publish the names of doctors in his state who participated in Medicare in 1968, with the amounts received under the program. The Social Security Administration was reluctant to do this on the grounds that the appearance of a large amount against a physician's name might be interpreted as evidence of wrongdoing.[18] A list of all payments made to physicians of $25,000 or more under Medicare was, however, made available to the Senate Finance Committee, with the amounts attributed to account numbers, not physicians' names, and was published in 1970. There were

16. *Medicare Newsletter,* 28 Feb. 1967; 6 Oct. 1967.
17. U.S. Congress, Senate, Committee on Finance, *Staff Data Relating to Medicaid-Medicare Study,* 1969, pp. 26–27.
18. U.S., Congress, Senate, Committee on Finance, *Medicare and Medicaid Hearings,* 91st Cong., 1st sess., July 1969, pp. 190–91 (hereafter cited as *Medicare and Medicaid Hearings,* July 1969).

4,284 such physicians in 1968, excluding physicians known to be in group practice. Of these, a select 18 received at least $150,000 from Medicare, in one instance for treating fewer than 350 beneficiaries.[19] Such figures were produced together with other testimony indicating abuse of Medicare, so-called gang visits when a doctor would sweep through a nursing home and charge Medicare for a visit to each patient, and the development of higher fees under Medicare than under similar Blue Shield schemes.[20] A small but significant minority of physicians was clearly abusing Medicare, making what in other occupations would be considered a fortune, and (the last indignity) getting away with it. Moreover the private carriers, which were officially the government's agents, appeared to be doing little to correct abuses, and in many respects were themselves inefficient and wasteful; some carriers spent $6 or more merely to process a bill for payment. The tone of the Finance Committee hearings and staff report was of shock and of the need for administrative stringency. The desirability of more detailed centralized information on individual physician fee practices was stressed, and the establishment of fee schedules was recommended. These moves suggested a much more forceful role by the federal government in administering Medicare.

Along the same lines during 1969 the Health Insurance Benefits Council (the statutory advisory committee to the Social Security Administration) recommended tightening up the Medicare program by cutting off practitioners who abused charges and by setting professional qualification standards for certain kinds of services.[21] The message was loud and clear. Without effective regulatory action from within the private sector—either by carriers and intermediaries or by groups of physicians—there will be a continuing polarization between a Congress concerned about rising costs and a profession which, except for its political machinery in the AMA, is inadequately organized and diffuse. And there will be increasing governmental regulation.

MEDICARE AND PRIVATE REGULATION

Medicare, with its parts A and B, its limitation to the elderly, and its uneasy approximation of a governmental program to a private system,

19. *Medicare and Medicaid Report,* Feb. 1970, pp. 153–54. The names of those who received $25,000 and more under federal health programs also began to be reported to the Internal Revenue Service in 1969.
20. These were developed during congressional hearings, and in the public press, in 1969 and 1970. See *Medicare and Medicaid Hearings,* July 1969; *Medicare and Medicaid Report,* Feb. 1970.
21. Reported in *Washington Report on Medicine and Health,* 30 June 1969.

is a health payment program geared to the debates of the early 1960s
rather than the health needs of the 1970s. Its structure, born in congressional compromise, was sufficient to launch the program but not in the
long run to sustain it. But Medicare can claim substantial victories. Between 1966 and 1970, government-sponsored health insurance, at least
for the elderly, was fully accepted. The official AMA position continues
to be of opposition to the form of the Medicare program as a prototype
for universal health insurance, but by no means to its substance. Instead, the association's position from 1965 to the present has been one
of enabling and subsidizing individuals to purchase private health insurance policies on their own initiative; that is, of government subsidy
of private health insurance rather than use of the latter as governmental
agents. It is unfortunate that experience with Medicare part B throws
doubt on the ability of the private sector of carriers and organized
groups of professionals to organize a medical payment system any better
than any other private or public mechanism.

In defense of the carriers, it must be remarked that there has been a
fallacy in the assumption that, through Medicare part B, government
money has indeed replicated private health insurance; such has not
strictly been the case. The Medicare structure, with its open ended
budgeting and lack of fee scales at the local level is significantly different
from self-sufficient insurance scheme which have to match outflow to
income. With the few exceptions of prepaid group practice plans, which
act both as insurer and provider of services, the government does not
contract with the part B carriers (or for that matter the part A intermediaries) for a specified package of services for a specified sum; it
makes the carrier a mere conduit or administrative agent.[22] Budget bal-
ancing is done only at the level of the Social Security Administration,
and on a post facto basis. As a result, the carrier is responsible neither
for raising its income nor for keeping within a preassigned budget; the
normal checks of a private system do not operate; and the structure has
inbuilt pressures toward inflation. This is true for both profit and
nonprofit carriers. Blue Shield, for example, in selling and operating
its own insurance packages, has customarily expected physicians to

22. Carriers submit their administrative costs to the Social Security Administration
at quarterly intervals. Surveys of administrative costs of part B carriers by the Department of Health, Education, and Welfare for 1967–68 found costs ranging from
an average of $2.33 per payment record processed (Pennsylvania Blue Shield) to
$6.14 (Delaware Blue Shield). The latter's administrative costs represented almost
16 percent of benefit payments. Administrative costs in the large plans were huge;
the largest, California Blue Shield, with benefit payments of $109 million in 1967,
was reimbursed administrative costs of $7.7 million. *Medicare and Medicaid Re-
port,* Feb. 1970, pp. 294–95, 314–16.

accept reduced fees as full payment for medical bills if the outflow of payments exceeds the income of the Blue Shield plan. Local physicians have thus through Blue Shield accepted a tacit system of cost controls. This is reinforced through requirements for official approval of rate increases through insurance departments of the states. Such expectations and local arrangements were not generally transferred to Medicare. Nominally, Medicare made full use of an experienced private system. It did so, however, with the benefit neither of tight requirements for public accountability nor of adequate private restraints.

Some formal professional regulation of fees and services was envisaged in the Medicare legislation. But, in the expectation that the intermediaries and carriers would assert effective controls, and in the initial downplaying of governmental intervention into medical practice, they were abandoned or ineffectively used. The 1965 legislation authorized the establishment of a national medical review committee (with appropriate staff) for the specific purpose of studying the utilization of health services inside and outside hospitals under both parts of Medicare, with a view to recommending changes in the patterns of utilization and in administration of the programs. It was intended that a majority of the nine members of this committee would be physicians, and that the committee would include outstanding professional leaders and representatives of professional organizations.[23] This group might have developed into a powerful professional organization, working closely with national data and with local utilization groups, medical societies, carriers, and intermediaries. The committee was, however, not set up by the secretary of Health, Education, and Welfare, reportedly because no judgments about utilization of services could be made until the program was well established, and information available as a basis for study.[24] But at least of equal importance was the sensitivity of the whole area of governmental "policing" of professional services, in the face of the needed cooperation of physicians in the implementation of the Medicare program.

The law itself declared that there would be no supervision or control by any federal office or employee over the practice of medicine or the manner in which medical services are provided. The AMA cooperated fully in the establishment of Medicare, with representatives serving on technical committees of the Department of Health, Education, and Welfare to develop appropriate regulations, and on the association's own

23. P.L. 89–97, sect. 1868.
24. U.S. Congress, Senate, Committee on Finance, *Social Security Amendments of 1967: Report to Accompany H.R. 12080,* 90th Cong., 1st sess., Nov. 1967, pp. 101–02.

Advisory Committee, but its leaders were naturally wary of government encroachments. Opposition continued to be expressed to the very concept of a governmentally operated payment program, because of its very real dangers of centralization, inflexibility, and controls. Effective review of services was thus politically unfeasible—at least for Medicare's first three years, even by a professionally dominated review committee. There was particular distrust of the establishment of statistical data systems, which were vital for appraisal of performance and service.[25] It was in a climate of dissatisfaction expressed by AMA leaders that the requirement for a national medical review committee was repealed in 1967. Instead, the functions of medical review were transferred to the Health Insurance Benefits Advisory Council, which was established following the 1965 legislation to advise the secretary on general administrative policy and regulations for Medicare (and on which the AMA has a representative).[26] This council is now pressing for more centralized direction and management of Medicare. In the interim, however, major responsibilities and activities for review of services remained in the relatively permissive ambience of the carriers and intermediaries.[27]

The focus on cost controls by the Congress was an inevitable reaction to a large governmental program which constantly overran its budget estimates. For example, the estimate made in 1965 for part A costs in 1970 was $3.1 billion; this was steadily revised upward to $5.8 billion in 1970; part B costs, meanwhile, doubled between 1967 and 1971.[28] Costs themselves were, however, only one element (and of relatively small importance in a well-run social system) in the total complex of the provision of health *services*. A national medical review committee (as local medical review committees) would presumably have been ex-

25. See e.g. U.S. Congress, House, Committee on Ways and Means, Statement of Charles L. Hudson, M.D., *President's Proposals for Revision in the Social Security System: Hearings on H.R. 5710*, 90th Cong., 1st sess., Apr. 1967, pp. 1652–67.

26. The AMA initially supported an expansion in membership of the National Medical Review Committee, but changed its position during the 1967 hearings. The Health Insurance Benefits Advisory Council was enlarged from 16 to 19 members. P.L. 90–248.

27. The Social Security Administration demanded little management information from the carriers until July 1968, when data on payments to physicians was requested by the staff of the Senate Finance Committee. A number of Blue Shield plans initially refused to identify by name physicians who had been paid $25,000 or more from Medicare in 1968, on the grounds that they did not have the physicians' authorization to do so. It was pointed out that the government rather than the physician was the trustee of Medicare funds, and the materials were made available. *Medicare and Medicaid Report*, Feb. 1970, p. 120.

28. The federal share of part B costs were $623 million in fiscal 1967. They were expected to rise to $1,245 million in fiscal 1971. In each case the amounts are matched by contributions made directly by the elderly. Ibid., p. 4.

pected to evaluate the kinds of services available to beneficiaries, the reasons for demanding them, their quality, effectiveness, and apparent areas for improvement or service deficiency. In short, how far is the Medicare program meeting the apparent needs of the elderly?

For hospitals and extended care facilities (under part A), the Medicare legislation required "utilization review" procedures as a condition of participation—that is, a review of the use of the hospital (or nursing home) and hospital services by individual medical patients. Each institution had to establish a utilization review committee which was supposed to consider both the medical necessity of services and the use of health facilities. Medicare thus set up a new organizational structure for hospital medical staffs. The committee may be either a group, including at least two physicians, organized from within the institution (the pattern usually followed by hospitals), or organized on a visiting basis by a local medical society or another group approved by the secretary of Health, Education, and Welfare (a method followed by small nursing homes). Community hospitals, with their organized medical staffs, were already engaged in various review mechanisms—tissue committees, "death" committees, medical records committees, and others.[29] Such activities were stimulated by the development in the early 1960s of computerized analysis of patient care and physician treatment profiles, drawn from abstracts of patient records. The utilization review committee (into which in some cases elements of these other committees have been drawn) extended the concept of review from a process of technical self-evaluation and education among physicians to one concerned with wider elements of patient care, including service costs and administrative mechanisms.

The predominating function of such committees under Medicare (at least as seen from the Congressional viewpoint) was not quality but cost. Effective action by a utilization review committee supposedly enables swift referral of Medicare patients from expensive to less expensive types of care—from hospital to extended care facility, and from the latter to their homes. A primary activity of the committees as they developed in the early years of Medicare was thus examining how long patients stay in hospitals. The potential of such physician groups in reviewing the work of the institutions, including all elements relating to the quality and planning of medical care, was thus significantly narrowed. In the Congressional debates of 1967, 1969 and 1970 cost controls became in-

29. See P. A. Lembcke, "Evolution of Medical Audit," *J. Amer. med. Ass., 199* (1967), 543–50.

extricably linked to utilization review as an administrative policing mechanism.[30]

The requirement—and springing up of—utilization review committees was not the same, however, as their widespread effective operation. As yet, few efforts have been made to push for their development as crucial evaluating agencies in the operation of Medicare. Instead of welcoming the opportunity to review the effectiveness of services, there has been local physician resistance to controls over the individual's prerogatives to practice medicine. A survey of hospitals by the Social Security Administration in 1968 found that almost half of the hopsitals were not reviewing any admissions, although this is a statutory requirement;[31] mechanisms for extended care facilities were even less developed. Part A intermediaries have been as loath as their part B counterparts to take a hard line when their traditional relationships with providers are concerned. Their dilemma has been somewhat like that of the foreman in industry, caught between sympathy for the rank and file and the exigencies of the management. To continue the metaphor, it may be remarked that any company which does not have effective administrative and quality controls at the shop-level would be advised to step up controls from higher management; otherwise it may find itself bankrupt. This, in a capsule, is the developing dilemma of Medicare.

But besides the large questions of centralized federal control of costs and standards versus renewed attempts to decentralize the administration of Medicare on a more effective basis, there are unresolved questions as to what is the appropriate role for physician organizations in administering publicly-subsidized medical care. The relationship between carriers and physicians is not always clear. In many cases medical associations, or medical committees nominated by the medical associations, have acted as agents of commercial insurance companies or nonprofit plans, both for Medicare and for Medicaid. Los Angeles County Medical Association, for example, reviews for insurance companies selected claims from a pool of 10,000 area physicians. The association's committee acts for the companies chiefly in relation to the appropriate level of fees; but it can also refer to other association committees ethical

30. This interpretation of "utilization review" has been particularly clear in relation to the adoption of Medicare procedures into state Medicaid programs under the 1967 Social Security Amendments (P.L. 90–248). The intention was that this would "safeguard against unnecessary utilization" and ensure that payments would be "not in excess of reasonable charges consistent with efficiency, economy, and quality of care." sec. 1902 (a) (30).
31. *Medicare and Medicaid Report,* Feb. 1970, pp. 106–08.

problems appearing in a review of physician records, utilization abuses and questions of potential incompetence.[32] The Sacramento County Medical Society, through its corporate subsidiary, the Medical Care Foundation of Sacramento, manages and staffs a regional claims office for Medicaid under a sub-contract with the State Department of Health Care Services and California Blue Shield; it has also developed a standard health insurance plan, in consultation with insurance company representatives, and a schedule for certifying appropriate lengths of stay for hospital admissions. Another notable example of medical society administration of physician payment programs in California is the San Joaquin County Foundation for Medical Care, which administers Medicaid payments for the state on a prepaid basis. Indeed in California alone there are more than 30 medical society foundations. Such activity from medical societies is in evidence, with more or less enthusiasm, in counties and states from Florida to Oregon and in respect of both Medicaid and Medicare.[33] Indeed, so great has been medical society responsibility in some instances that there have been complaints that carriers have been abdicating their own responsibilities by dumping claims on the societies.[34]

Yet by no means all medical societies relish the role of claims review or administration. The Louisiana State Medical Society, for example, was recently reported as favoring the limitation of professional review to the settlement of disputes between physician and physician, physician and patient, or physician and third parties; this follows the more traditional view of the disciplinary role of the medical society, with the major sanction against offenders being expulsion from the medical society. A spokesman from the Louisiana Society remarked that fiscal review of claims by insurance carriers and other third parties without the patient's written consent "violates the ethical relationship between patient and physician." [35] Meanwhile other medical societies are proceeding to act as primary advisers to (if not agents of) insurance carriers and thus ultimately, in the case of Medicare and Medicaid, of the federal government.

At the same time other groups of physicians, acting as hospital utilization review committees and as utilization review committees for nursing

32. *Am. Med. News,* 26 Oct., 1970.
33. For a review of current developments see *U.S., Congress, Senate, Committee on Finance, Hearings on Medicare and Medicaid,* 91st Cong., 2d sess., Apr.–June, 1970.
34. See e.g. testimony of Mr. William C. White, Jr., Ibid., pp. 283–85.
35. *Am. Med. News,* 26 Oct., 1970.

homes under Medicare, extend further the professional role, for these too are de facto agents of the intermediaries. While the hospitals would argue that their committees are in fact agents of the hospitals (since professional review of a hospital's activities is an essential part of its administration), and while neither type of committee is yet in generally effective operation, the two parts of Medicare have spawned potentially powerful foci for professional regulation, at least with respect to fee levels and hospital utilization. The existence of hospital utilization review committees emphasizes the potential strengths of hospital medical staffs as a basis for stimulating health services improvement and change; the delegation of physician fee determination to the part B carries creates another potential focus for local medical review. Each of these groups has available to it basic (indeed, invaluable) information on service patterns and utilization by the elderly; the hospital committees through hospital records, the carrier committees through the physician billing process. But the next step, of developing full-fledged data analysis systems—an essential, and surely reasonable, component of medical practice in the current environment of multispecialist medicine—has not yet been taken on the local level.

CHANGES, ACTUAL AND POTENTIAL

As has been remarked, Medicare was dropped into a professional system whose responses to medical specialization were, if not embryonic, at least incomplete. While the program was supposedly not to increase governmental intervention in the health care system, it could not avoid questions of the ultimate direction of organizational change. Indeed, any scheme as large as Medicare—representing by 1970 between 10 and 15 percent of all medical care expenditures in the United States—could not fail to have some impact on the health care system, and thus on the way medical care is provided. But much of its impact has been peripheral or unintended. As a limited program it has been able to avoid the issues which have to be faced in any scheme of national health insurance: of ensuring adequate services, of building mechanisms for quality review and cost control. Nevertheless, there have been changes in the health care system which are directly attributable to Medicare. The growth of utilization review committees and of medical society review committees are but two examples.

These two types of professional organization were, moreover, one reflection of the division of Medicare into part A and part B according to recognized divisions between "hospital insurance" and "medical insurance." This division was epitomized in the separate development of Blue Cross and Blue Shield insurance plans. But, apart from their history, such a division has little logic or continuing justification. One early effect of Medicare was thus to freeze an outmoded form of organization. Outpatient services were a case in point. Hospital outpatient diagnostic services were originally included under part A (hospital insurance), while other diagnostic medical services were included under part B. One result was that the patient who sought diagnostic services in a hospital clinic was responsible for the first $20 of costs, together with 20 percent of costs above this amount, for each series of diagnostic services by a hospital during a 20-day period. In contrast, the patient who received diagnostic services in a physician's office was responsible for the first $50 for all services under part B, and then for 20 percent of the remainder. After a period of confusion (not least of which was in the hospital accounting offices) all hospital outpatient services were transferred to part B in April 1968. But the broader divisions in Medicare remained. In terms of administrative costs alone there is a strong case for merging Blue Cross and Blue Shield, and for commercial insurance companies to be required to offer both parts of Medicare. But as yet few plans are able to offer the whole package of Medicare. In almost all states Blue Cross and Blue Shield plans continue under separate administration, each with its own office to process claims for Medicare and each with its claims review mechanisms.

Administrative convenience was, however, a relatively minor affair compared with the furor over payment of hospital-based physicians under Medicare. Implicit in parts A and B was a division between hospital care and physician services; this fact reawakened bitter professional disputes in the case of physicians whose work was primarily or totally based on hospitals, and who were not therefore engaged in fee-for-service private practice. Before Medicare, anesthesiologists, pathologists, radiologists, and psychiatrists were being paid increasingly by hospitals on salary or contract; and in many cases their services were included for reimbursement by hospital (rather than physician) insurance plans. These arrangements would undoubtedly have been extended had Medicare not been passed. Instead Medicare, in its need to formalize practice arrangements, evoked vehement demands by the hospital-based specialists that they should be reimbursed on the same basis as other physicians; that is, through an identifiable professional fee, paid through Medicare part B. The root of the issue was summarized by Senator Curtis in the 1965 hearings, in a remark that "these four are picked out to be classi-

fied as hospital employees while all other doctors are independent practitioners." [36]

Professional rationale hinged on the long struggles for increased status
compared with the fee-for-service private practice enjoyed by other specialties. It was not that there was anything sacrosanct in a fee, or a contract, or even a salary (the latter mode of payment having long been
accepted by clinicans who are university professors); nor was there any
indication that physicians might enjoy a higher income under part B
than part A of Medicare. Rather, there was a lingering fear of the
hospital as a dominant institution in medical practice, harking back to
the old battles of the corporate practice of medicine, and a disinclination
to distinguish professional independence from fee-for-service practice.
The specialists were included under part B of Medicare from its inception, although the hospital could still collect for the physician's services.
But as a result of this action and of the subsequent moves in 1966 by
professional groups to return all physician services to independent, private
billing, the patterns of physician-hospital relations in these specialties
were changed.[37] In this case, therefore, the existence of the two parts of
Medicare had a deliberate impact on the organization of medical practice.

While, then, Congressional committees were looking with concern at
Medicare's accelerating costs, and while consumer groups were pressing
for expansion of coverage and services, basic professional issues remained. Some expansion of services was made available through the
Social Security amendments of 1967.[38] The Johnson administration also
recommended that the population eligible for Medicare should be expanded from those sixty-five years of age and over to the 1.5 million dis-

36. U.S. Congress, Senate, Hearings on H.R. 6675, Apr.–May 1965, p. 313. For a
description of the debates on this issue, see Somers and Somers, *Medicare and the
Hospitals*, pp. 130–53.
37. The AMA House of Delegates passed a resolution in June 1966 which would
make it unethical for a physician to displace any hospital-based specialist who was
bargaining with a hospital for private billing for his fees, but this resolution was
promptly vetoed by the AMA's legal advisers as endangering the AMA in actions
in restraint of trade. See Wesley W. Hall, "Letter from the Chairman of the Board
to Members of the House of Delegates," *J. Amer. med. Ass., 197* (1966), 791–92.
Meanwhile the professional societies in the specialties continued to press for "independence," and some shifts were observable in physician income arrangements,
particularly for radiologists. See Robin Elliott, Richard Ross, and Frank van
Dyke, "Medicare and the Hospital-Based Specialist: Pathologists' and Radiologists' Arrangements with Hospitals, 1965–1968," *Inquiry 6* (March, 1969), 49–59.
38. Most notably, inpatient hospital benefits under part A were modified to give
patients, over and above their eligibility for 90 days of hospital care for each spell
of illness, a life time reserve of 60 days of care, to be used when the 90 days were
exhausted.

abled persons who were under sixty-five but receiving Social Security benefits. Among other possibilities the question of including outpatient drugs under part B was also raised.[39] Both of these questions have continued as possible extensions of the existing program. Logically, Medicare would be extended to cover all Social Security beneficiaries; this could be joined, as has been suggested by a number of reformers, by coverage of children. Indeed, eventually Medicare could be expanded to the whole population, thus being, as was once feared, the thin end of the wedge of national health insurance. But each or all of these measures would of themselves do little to approach Medicare's underlying inconsistencies, which rest in turn on inconsistencies in the professional organization of medicine. In brief, these are the continuing administrative division of services given by hospitals and by physicians in private practice, and the disorganization of physicians in private practice. The continuation of private practitioners as small-scale entrepreneurs has meant that there is as yet, with few exceptions, no effective organizational focus for the development of cohesive local services. As a result, the insurance plans, not the physicians or health care organizations, have become Medicare's intermediaries in fact as well as for fiscal reasons.

For physicians themselves it is doubtful whether control of their charges (and to a lesser or greater degree their practices) through an insurance agency is any more desirable or acceptable than direct control through a government agency. So far the issue has been largely skirted because the insurance agencies themselves have been permissive rather than efficient. A Senate Finance Committee report of 1970 described a situation of deficiencies, abuses, "lack-luster administration" in paying for physician services, besides the widespread failure to apply utilization review procedures.[40] This was followed by a report similar in tone from the House Ways and Means Committee which supported inter alia the imposition of limits on provider costs, the termination of payments to hospitals and physicians who abuse services, and the stopping of Medicare payments for patients found by utilization review committees to be unnecessarily hospitalized.[41] Indeed, already there has been alarm as to effect of a more efficient role for the carriers and intermediaries, in the refusal in some instances of an insurance company to make Medicare payments for nursing home care which has been deemed unnecessary, but which has been sanctioned by the patient's physician (and which the patient may already have received). As the tide moves toward greater

39. See Myers, pp. 70–71, 316–18.
40. *Medicare and Medicaid Report,* Feb. 1970, pp. 4, 10, 18 and passim.
41. U.S., Congress, House, Committee on Ways and Means, *Report on H.R. 17550.*

or more efficient control over costs, the question is Control by Whom? The continuation of a diffusely-organized medical profession suggests increasing controls exerted by Congress and enforced through Medicare carriers and intermediaries.

It is in this context that two major proposals for changes in Medicare appeared in 1970. Both were designed (though for different purposes) to provide a middle layer of organization between individual physicians and Medicare's existing administrative structures. The first proposal appeared officially in March 1970 in a statement from John Veneman of the Department of Health, Education and Welfare which set out a number of measures to strengthen the operation of Medicaid and Medicare. The statement included a proposal to develop a new and alternative form of payment to providers, originally entitled Medicare part C.[42] Under the proposal, contracts would be developed by the Social Security Administration with "health maintenance organizations," on a negotiated capitation basis instead of through post facto reimbursement of bills which is the hallmark of parts A and B. The health maintenance organization option was incorporated into the Social Security Amendments of 1970 (H.R. 17550), but died with the 91st Congress. The concept has, however, remained as a viable organizational answer to both the costs and the structures of specialized medicine.

The health maintenance organization was not clearly defined in the legislation; the term itself was new. Mr. Veneman cited as possible examples existing prepaid group practices such as the Kaiser plans, medical society foundations such as San Joaquin or Clackamus County, Oregon, and new medical service organizations such as that being developed in the new town of Columbia, Maryland. The name "health maintenance" reflected a concern that Medicare payments should be used to encourage health as well as to pay for sickness. Under the option, therefore, organizations would be expected to emphasize preventive medicine.

Implicit in the proposal were, however, two other dominant ideas. On the one hand there was a growing concern within (and outside) the Department of Health, Education, and Welfare that control of health services in the United States was becoming increasingly centralized. Both Medicare and Medicaid were prime examples of a shift to increasing federal authority over fee-setting and standards of care in the absence of effective action by insurance agents (for Medicare) and by the states (for Medicaid). Deliberate encouragement of local health service systems (health maintenance organizations) could provide a

42. Statement by John G. Veneman, before the House Ways and Means Committee, March 23, 1970.

needed middle layer of agencies which would provide or organize health services independently, and in turn contract for payment, at least for Medicare and Medicaid, directly with the government. Built into the legislation was a stipulation that a health maintenance organization would only be recognized for such contracts when at least half of its enrolled population were under sixty-five years of age. These organizations, assuming they developed rapidly, could therefore become the nucleus of a decentralized health service system which would counter the trend toward control from Washington, and could eventually form the basis for a national health insurance program.[43]

The other dominant idea in the adoption of health maintenance organizations was the concern by major Congressional committees, notably the Senate Finance Committee and the House Ways and Means Committee, over controlling high medical costs. Contracts between independent health service corporations and the government would fix Medicare budgets in advance. There would not be the inflationary slippage which has been a major characteristic of Medicare's operation; cost controls would be shifted to the health maintenance organizations. As an added ingredient the legislation also stipulated that health maintenance organizations would be reimbursed for Medicare enrollees at a level of only 95 percent of the prevailing local payments for Medicare under parts A and B.

At the time this book goes to press the regulations for health maintenance organizations have not been issued, and their development remains a matter for speculation. How far existing prepaid group practices, medical foundations, hospitals and neighborhood health centers will find it advantageous to develop services and to accept the health maintenance option of capitation contracts for Medicare instead of being reimbursed under parts A and B, is a question at the moment of some doubt. It can probably only be resolved by the merging of all parts of Medicare into one integrated reimbursement system. In the meantime the acceptance of the option will undoubtedly be affected by the rigor of controls set up over payments made to providers under parts A and B. What is important, however, is the *idea* of a health maintenance organization as a free-standing, locally-controlled health service. In this respect Medicare has had a direct influence on conceptual approaches to changing the American health care system. One may expect the development of a program of federal grants and contracts for setting up health maintenance organizations which is independent of Medicare.

43. See Paul M. Ellwood, Jr., "The Health Maintenance Strategy," *Medical Care,* May–June, 1971.

A second major proposal for change has stemmed from the medical profession's own concern over the lack of organization in Medicare at the local or intermediate level, a concern stimulated by the consistently bad press concerning the physician's role in increasing Medicare costs and fees. Out of this concern has developed a proposal from the AMA to set up a formal, quasi-public network of professional peer review organizations which would focus the responsibility for policing physician performance (chiefly in relation to fees) on standardized and recognized groups outside the control of the insurance agencies.

The history of this proposal is one of frustration from the AMA leadership over the irresponsible behavior of some physicians. A report of the AMA Board of Trustees, approved by the house of delegates in June 1967, spoke unavailingly but with some urgency of the physician's responsibility for controlling costs, in terms of holding down days of hospitalization, choosing low-priced instead of high-priced drugs, and stabilizing professional fees. It noted, moreover, that "the privilege of a physician to charge usual and customary fees will continue to require prudence." [44] But such warnings fell on deaf ears. Nor was it realistic to expect physicians individually to keep costs and charges low when other physicians were raising their fees. Instead, the AMA debates focussed increasingly on more organized means of policing fees and other forms of health care utilization. These debates were crystallized in a statement approved by the AMA House of Delegates at its annual convention in 1970, in favor of so-called professional review organizations. These organizations would have three primary characteristics. They would ensure review of the performance of physicians by fellow physicians (and not by insurance or governmental agents); primary responsibility for review would rest in the first instance with state medical societies; and the review would not attempt to include utilization of services in hospitals or other institutions.[45] This definition of peer review was built into the national health insurance proposals supported by the AMA and designed to provide health care coverage through allowing tax credits against individual income tax for the purchase of private health insurance, and for subsidizing insurance premiums for those at low income levels.[46] Indeed, the provision of effective peer review was a necessary counterbalance to a voucher plan which would contain fewer formal controls over costs than Medicare.

44. This statement was introduced as part of the AMA evidence to the hearings on the Social Security amendments of 1967, on H.R. 12080, pp. 761–63.
45. *Am. Med. News,* 26 Oct., 1970.
46. These proposals, popularly known as Medicredit, were incorporated in the 91st Congress into three bills: S. 4381, S. 2705, and H.R. 18567.

Under the proposals the Secretary of Health, Education, and Welfare would contract with a state medical society or its designated agent to establish a review organization, which would develop appropriate administrative and advisory machinery at the state and local level. The organization would assume responsibility for assessing questions of the need, quality, and costs of medical care actually given to patients by reviewing their medical records. Such activities would be done in accordance with specified national requirements or by approval of a state plan by the Secretary, and the review organizations would be appropriately reimbursed for their activities. In addition, the organizations would be responsible for hearings over disputes and for discipline of physicians, the latter subject to approval by the Secretary of Health, Education, and Welfare. In short, review of physician activities under major public medical programs would be removed from insurance organizations, and the medical societies would become formal government agents.

This willingness to be socialized emphasizes not only how far the official attitudes of medicine's leading professional organization have traveled since 1965, but also the irrelevance of the old connotations. The issue that was raised in the early debates over compulsory health insurance at the time of World War I is finally having to be faced. Specialized medicine has dual effects: on the one hand of rising and unequal costs (the justification for insurance) and on the other of coordinated services. Peer review itself does not directly organize services. Nevertheless, by setting up organizational networks for medical records review, by designing and enforcing standards of care, and by developing through computerized information services profiles of medical care received in an area, state and local peer review organizations can provide a basis for further coordinated service development; the activities of some existing medical society foundations are a case in point. Taken together with the prospect of physician involvement in health maintenance organizations, the organized involvement of physicians in health care administration appears not to be receding under increasing governmental programs, but to be increasing significantly.

The idea of professional peer review organizations has, moreover, now received public sanction. During hearings of the Social Security Amendments in August, 1970 Senator Wallace F. Bennett introduced his own proposals for peer review, developed with the help of Senate Finance Committee Staff.[47] The Bennett Amendment proposed the establishment of a national, state and local network of professional

47. Amendment No. 851, 91st Cong., 2d. sess., H.R. 17550.

standards review organizations which would be responsible for reviewing both professional activities *and* institutional medical services given under Medicaid, Medicare, federal-sponsored maternal and child programs, and any other designated federal programs. These organizations, it was suggested, would have the responsibility of approving in advance elective hospital admissions and other costly forms of care inside and outside hospitals. Norms for care and treatment would be developed through a national review organization (with technical assistance from the department of Health, Education, and Welfare); and fines or exclusion from the program could be imposed on recalcitrant physicians.

These provisions would have joined together the mechanisms for hospital and out-of-hospital review. But such a juncture was opposed both by the American Hospital Association (who did not want to subject hospitals to administration scrutiny by medical societies) and by the American Medical Association, whose own proposals also excluded review in hospitals. Nor was the AMA in favor of other elements of the amendment, particularly the requirements for prior review of treatment, federal ownership of medical records, and the possibility that through direct contracts with local medical associations state medical associations might be bypassed. Following negotiation between physician and other spokesmen and the Senator, the amendment was modified to conform more nearly with the AMA specifications. Again, as this book goes to press, the shape and importance of professional review organizations is uncertain. What does seem clear, however, is that the provision of such organization for major public payment programs will stimulate the development of medical society foundations and will pull the medical societies themselves more firmly into health care planning and policy. On the impetus of the Bennett amendment, therefore, professionally-organized health maintenance organizations may be generated.

Looking back over the five years since Medicare began, it is evident that enormous strides have been taken in relation to professional organization as well as to consumer concerns and expectations. It is true that much of the impetus for change has come from outside Medicare. Nevertheless, the Medicare experience has been particularly important as the prototype or stimulator of other forms of national health insurance. In its development a number of issues have been sharply delineated. These can be stated as simple maxims. The first is that no major public insurance scheme can fail to affect the way health services are organized. The second, that government spending will always be accompanied by government scrutiny and potential controls. The third, that American health services lack an essential layer of middle-level or community organization, without which there will be increasingly centralized health care administration. The fourth, that the logic of greater government intervention is a more structured and organized medical profession.

CHAPTER 20

Medicaid

Promise and Experience

An important and concurrent aspect of developments in Medicare, and a joint if not major stimulator of the present national health insurance movement, has been the rapid rise and fall in expectations of Medicaid. Medicaid was set up as a program of federal grants to states for the expansion and consolidation of existing scattered programs for vendor payments for medical care on behalf of persons on public assistance and for those who were not on assistance but whose financial situation could not withstand major medical expenses. The latter had been termed medically indigent in the Kerr-Mills program for the aged, established in 1960. Medicaid extended the concept of medical indigency to other groups of the population. It provided more generous federal matching grants to states than previously available, and specified services to be offered by participating states across the board to those persons who are eligible according to state means-test levels.

IMPLEMENTATION

When the 1965 legislation was enacted Medicaid, as an expanded version of the previous Kerr-Mills program, attracted less interest than Medicare. Federal-state health programs for the indigent and medically indigent were well accepted.[1] The major questions raised by the new program pivoted on the level of the means tests to be adopted in the states and the comprehensiveness of services to be offered.[2] In theory

1. By January 1965 Kerr-Mills (medical assistance for the aged) was in effect in 44 of 54 possible jurisdictions, although only 5 provided comprehensive medical services, U.S., Congress, Senate Committee on Finance, *Hearings on H.R. 6675,* 89th Cong., 1st sess., 1965, pp. 163–64.
2. Under the initial Medicaid program, states could include the following groups in order of priority: (1) people on public assistance (old-age assistance, aid to fami-

Medicaid was a powerful rival to Medicare, for it could cover a substantial section of people as medically indigent under tax-supported services. If the means test were placed at a sufficiently high level, the concept of federal-state health programs might eventually lead to a national health service system—i.e. socialized medicine, rather than a national *insurance* system. The option lay with the state legislatures, for the federal matching grants were initially open ended.

One of the first states to take advantage of the new legislation was New York, which already had relatively generous eligibility standards for vendor medical payments on behalf of its public assistance recipients and those not on public assistance but eligible for medical assistance to the aged. From 1963 the New York State Department of Welfare allowed payment for hospitalization expenses to families with annual incomes of up to $5200. In March 1966, in anticipation of Medicaid, income standards of $5700 for a family of four were adopted under the existing programs; it was this figure which was proposed for the new Medicaid program by Governor Rockefeller. The New York bill was finally passed by the primarily Democratic assembly and the primarily Republican senate—after arguments from Assembly Speaker and Democrtaic leader Travia, backed by Sen. Robert Kennedy, that the eligibility limits were too low and that the program should be administered by the health department and not the welfare department (to avoid the stigma of relief) —with eligibility for a family of four set at $6000.[3] This eligibility figure was not greatly out of line with previous experience in New York. It was, however, very high in terms of the existing means tests for public assistance and medical assistance to the aged in other states. Even the rich neighboring state of Connecticut, which also set up a Medicaid program in 1966, adopted a means test for the medically needy family of four of only $3800; and in most states the levels were well below this.[4]

---

lies with dependent children, aid to permanently and totally disabled, aid to the blind); (2) people in the above categories not on assistance, but medically indigent; (3) all medically needy children under 21; (4) "substantially all" of a state's medically needy to be included by 1975. Services to be included were: (1) inpatient hospital services; (2) outpatient hospital services; (3) other laboratory and x-ray serviees; (4) skilled nursing-home services; (5) Physicians' services. State plans were to provide "comprehensive care and services" by 1975. The plan had to operate though an entire state, under a single state agency. P.L. 89–97. For reviews of the early implementation of Medicaid, see Advisory Commission on Intergovernmental Relations, *Intergovernmental Problems in Medicaid* (Washington, D.C., 1968) Tax Foundation, Inc., *Medicaid: State Programs After Two Years* (New York, 1968).

3. *New York Times,* 21 Mar. 1966; 23 May 1966.
4. For a general review of the program in the states from 1966 to 1970, see Rose-

The New York action, which was well publicized in the press, under-lined the problems inherent in viewing the Medicare-Medicaid legislation as one package. One function of Medicaid was to fill in the gaps of serv-ices left by Medicare, for the eligible medically needy person over sixty-five and for those on public assistance. These included the deductions under part A and part B of Medicare; the patient's part payment of serv-ices for other bills; and the provision of services which were not covered by Medicare, such as drugs for outpatients, or care in nursing homes which does not require skilled nursing attention. The states were also encouraged to pay the part B premiums for public assistance recipients and for the medically indigent, although in the latter case the state does not receive federal matching funds under Medicaid for this purpose. As a result, for those sixty-five years and over, virtually all health services may be provided free of cost to the patient, depending on the income levels for eligibility under Medicaid and the services available through the program, and these are in turn dependent on the state in which the person lives.

The high New York eligibility level emphasized that there would be continuing variations by state in the medical services available free of charge or as a right to the elderly, including those with moderate incomes. Medicare is a national program; the combination of Medicare with Medicaid is not—a fact which gathered importance with the growing interest by the Nixon administration in 1969 and 1970 in the establish-ment of a federal welfare program to replace at least in part the federal-supported income assistance programs in the states. Medicaid developed out of public assistance as a supplementary program of income main-tenance, and while welfare programs continued to be organized by the states, it was logical that there should also be state variations in health assistance. By 1966, however, Medicaid had come to be regarded—partly because of its joint passage with Medicare and partly because of its wide-open potential as the basis for large federal-state health plans for the general population—as a health rather than an income mainte-nance program. With the relatively liberal federal matching funds built into the legislation and continuing federal encouragement, Medicaid was capable of expansion into an interlocking network of federal-state health plans in the different states. The New York Medicaid program thus had a second notable impact as a precedent under which pressure might be brought for programs of similar scope in other states.

mary Stevens and Robert Stevens, "Medicaid: Anatomy of a Dilemma," *Law and Contemp. Problems, 35* (Spring 1970), 348–425.

Criticism and alarm at high income eligibility levels thus had national implications. But there was also immediate criticism within New York, where 45 percent of the state's population (8 million people) would reportedly be eligible. This was taken in the ensuing controversy, in Albany as well as by other opponents of state medicine throughout the country, not as evidence of a very high poverty rate in New York, nor even as an indication of the realities of the high cost of medical care, reflected as potential indigence, but as a widespread movement toward free medical care and away from the traditional limitations of medical assistance. The New York Medical Society, however, gave the Medicaid program its general support, subject to guarantees that patients would have freedom of choice of institutions and professionals, and that there would be adequate professional representation on state and local Medicaid advisory committees—both of which the society gained. Initial enrollment by physicians was slow, in part at least because of the vagueness of the program and growing concern about governmental supervision.[5] But the program took hold. In the year ended June 1969, despite a series of cutbacks in the program in the interim, New York's Medicaid budget was $1.29 billion, of which 42 percent was provided from federal funds.[6]

Much of the initial expansion of Medicaid in the "liberal" (and richest) states was facilitated by what was in effect expansion of programs through transfer of a proportion of the costs of existing vendor payments being borne by the states to Medicaid's more advantageous federal matching program. States with large medical assistance programs had an immediate incentive to move into Medicaid, for through budgetary transfers they could expand services without additional income being required initially from the states. But in turn, this put additional financial pressures on the federal government, thus creating continuing attempts by each agency to impose increased fiscal responsibility on the other. The federal situation was exacerbated because, as with Medicare, there were unfortunate discrepancies between initial federal cost estimates and actual experience. In

5. New York Times, 15 May 1966; 5 Dec. 1966; 18 Dec. 1966. This caution was justified. By late 1969, the New York City Medicaid program had an auditing staff of 134 professionals, 60 paraprofessionals, and 143 clerks (for all aspects of the program). Auditing includes on-site visits of private physician offices with a high volume of Medicaid patients, the first and only Medicaid program to do so. Lowell E. Bellin and Florence Kavalar, "Policing Publicly Funded Health Care for Poor Quality, Overutilization and Fraud—the New York City Medicaid Experience," Paper presented to American Public Health Association, Philadelphia, 11 Nov. 1969.
6. "Source of Funds Expended for Public Assistance Payments and for the Cost of Administration, Services, and Training, Fiscal Year Ended June 30, 1969," DHEW, Social and Rehabilitation Service, NCSS Report F-2.

January 1967, the president's budget for fiscal year 1968 predicted total payments in forty-eight states of $2.25 billion; but as of January 1968— only halfway through the fiscal year, and with only thirty-seven Medicaid programs in operation—the cost estimates had risen to $3.41 billion; and the actual expenditures were $3.54 billion.[7] Almost from the beginning, therefore, Medicaid provoked budgetary concern in the Congress. Major concern hinged on coverage of the able-bodied working population. The House Ways and Means Committee and the Senate Finance Committee —unlike the leadership within the Department of Health, Education, and Welfare, of which John Gardner was then secretary—tended to view Medicaid as part of the states' responsibility for public welfare, that is, as a relatively small program for unfortunates, and not as a program to supplant private health insurance being provided through collective bargaining. The prevailing congressional mood was thus one of retrenchment rather than expansion.

Meanwhile the Medicaid program was differently interpreted in different states. The New York program, despite its size, was a relatively modest extension of previous health programs provided through Kerr-Mills and other vendor payment programs to all covered groups and with a somewhat higher income level. California, in contrast, substantially changed its previous programs in the nature and extent of health services offered. Medi-Cal became the second largest Medicaid program ($808 million in fiscal year 1969, of which 50 percent was from federal funds), with wide health coverage, from prevention to rehabilitation.

The California program, more than that in any other state, attempted to use Medicaid as a vehicle not only for expanding services to the poor but also, and importantly, for removing health services administration and delivery as far as possible from the stigma of public relief. The program was designed to take the poor out of second-class citizenship and enable them to use private health services. The philosophical basis of the early Medi-Cal program was thus of an entitlement to regular middle-class medicine (such as it is), rather than of the minimal services provided at least cost which are the usual trappings of services available for welfare recipients. Thus Medicaid was approximated in design to Medicare, although the services offered by Medicaid were wider than those of Medicare. Public assistance recipients were encouraged to use physicians' private offices and to enter private hospitals. The latter policy reversed a long history in California of treatment of the indigent in public hospitals. The program (as were a number of other Medicaid programs) was channeled through fiscal intermediaries, thus paralleling the "usual

7. *Medicare and Medicaid Report,* Feb. 1970, p. 42.

and customary" fees of the Medicare program, and administered by the California Health and Welfare Agency, a step above the department of welfare.[8] In California, unlike New York, relatively limited services were made available to the medically indigent. Nevertheless, the size of the population, the scope of benefits, the emphasis on care with dignity for the poor, and the relative caution or inactivity in developing Medicaid programs in many other states in 1965 and 1966 put national emphasis on Medi-Cal as well as on the New York program.

Medicaid thus began almost immediately to reveal the strains of rising expectations. The optimistic might view the new program as a mandate for establishing a base of comprehensive health services to the poorer members of the population, which could gradually be expanded upward (just as earlier European health insurance schemes were expanded) to cover middle-class members of the population. In this sense, Medicaid could be viewed as the "sleeper" of the 1965 amendments, a term which gained a short-lived popularity. On the other hand, the adherents of the welfare approach—and Medicaid is technically a welfare program—became increasingly concerned about the flagrant lack of fiscal control in programs which were being simultaneously expanded because of rising eligibility levels in the cash payments of public assistance. President Johnson's War on Poverty was geared to the basic and urgent needs of income, jobs, housing, and food for the poor whose plight, whether in the ghettos of the northern cities, in the base levels of subsistence in the rural south, or in the camps for migrant labor in the southwest and west, was dramatically rediscovered in the 1960s, shaking the mood of complacency and prosperity of the previous decade. While adequate health services are also one of the basic needs of reasonable human existence, and a necessary element in breaking the cycle of sickness leading to poverty and poverty to sickness, the difference between minimal and middle-class or "mainstream" medical care is of less immediacy than the provision of an adequate income. Given the choice, an individual might prefer to receive an extra ten dollars in cash rather than to have additional payments made to his physician, for services now regarded as private rather than as charity.

The choice of where welfare money would and should be channeled is not usually made in such simple or direct terms. Nevertheless, the dual

8. See A. C. Barnes, *A Description of the Organization and Administration of the California Medical Assistance Program: Title XIX* (Department of Health Administration, University of North Carolina School of Public Health; mimeograph 1968); Margaret Greenfield, Medi-Cal, *The California Medicaid Program* (*Title XIX*) (U.S. Department of Health, Education and Welfare; 1969).

pressures on state welfare budgets for medical care and for cash payments, and thus in turn on federal matching appropriations, emphasized the peculiar status of Medicaid in an era of rising health care expectations. It was becoming clear that if one standard of health service were to be made available to the whole population even within a state, the financing of health care and the financing of welfare schemes would have to be divorced. But in addition, besides differences in health services within states there were also significant differences in services made available under Medicaid from one state to the next. This argued for eventual federalization of the Medicaid program, into a national program of health care assistance.

By the end of 1966, there were twenty-six Medicaid programs with federally approved plans; another eleven followed in 1967.[9] A number of other states continued with their previous vendor payment programs. But the programs varied widely. A 1967 study indicated per capita costs ranging from $3.39 in West Virginia to $35.46 in California.[10] Almost half of all federal payments flowing to the states for Medicaid went to New York and California.[11] Even in 1970 there were still two states (Arizona and Alaska) without a Medicaid program, and two-thirds of the federal contributions to the Medicaid program was flowing into six or seven states. Medicaid did not therefore develop as a universal or general program for paying for medical bills, even for the poor; the concept of medical indigence did not take hold as the basis for health provision for the whole population. For the poor themselves, other means of health service provision have continued to be discussed and developed, including federally funded neighborhood health centers for low-income populations, even in states with relatively generous Medicaid provisions. There is now a de facto recognition of the inability of Medicaid as a state program to achieve acceptable national goals.

MEDICAID'S RISING COSTS

Of all the factors affecting Medicaid—in its initial rise in the enthusiasm of the early years of the Johnson administration, through a period of retrenchment from 1967 to the present, to the plans of the Nixon administration to introduce a scheme of family health insurance as part of a

9. *Medicaid* (Tax Foundation) p. 19 and passim.
10. Ibid., p. 11.
11. U.S., Congress, Senate, Committee on Finance, *Social Security Amendments of 1967: Hearings on H.R. 12080,* 90th Cong., 1st sess., Aug.–Sept. 1967, pp. 300–01.

national family assistance (welfare) program—the one great factor has been cost. Legislators and their staffs at all levels of government were unprepared for Medicaid's budgetary impact.

Federal payments to the states for medical assistance increased from $555 million in fiscal year 1965 (before the impact of Medicaid) to $2.8 billion in 1970, with parallel increases by state and local governments.[12] In the fall of 1966, when most programs were barely off the ground, the House Ways and Means Committee issued a report calling for a brake to rising costs.[13] The concern was twofold: to put a lid on federal open-ended matching assistance and to stem any broad extension of the program to people with moderate incomes. In an atmosphere of growing congressional concern over the costs of all Great Society programs, the Senate Finance Committee held hearings in 1967. The committee chairman, Sen. Russell Long, reiterated his concern in further hearings in 1969:

> We want the Medicaid program to provide help to people who need it and we want the Medicare program to look after the medical needs of our senior citizens. We want that care to be of high quality. But, we think it should be provided on a basis that is efficient and economical, not on a basis which is wasteful and extravagant.[14]

Questions of the administration of Medicaid, including supervision by the federal and state governments, and of cases of abuse and fraud by service providers, joined similar concerns about the operation of Medicare.

These concerns were translated into legislation in the Social Security amendments of 1967 (P.L. 90-248) which, among other attempts to control costs, and in a political climate moving back toward a more repressive view of welfare than that of 1965, limited federal sharing to the present 133⅓ percent of the state's maximum levels for the payment of aid to families with dependent children. There was thus a federal definition of medical indigence, and it was tied to a level used for public assistance. The short attempt to bring welfare patients into the mainstream of private medicine was ending.

Under the 1967 amendments the Medicaid program was widened in the provision of federal grants for service in "intermediate care facilities." This term invented another classification for nursing homes, to fall somewhere between the skilled nursing home recognized as an extended care

12. *Medicare and Medicaid,* Feb. 1970, pp. 3–4 and passim.
13. *Limitations on Federal Participation under Title XIX of the Social Security Act,* 89th Cong., 2d sess., 11 Oct. 1966.
14. *Medicare and Medicaid Hearings,* July 1969, p. 3.

facility under Medicare and services which were merely room and board or custodial care. But again the argument was of reduction in costs. Just as it was assumed that the inclusion of extended care facilities under Medicare would enable patients to be moved to less expensive skilled nursing homes instead of staying in hospital, it was now assumed that patients would be transferred, when appropriate, from skilled nursing homes to the less expensive designation of intermediate care. The continuing optimism that there would be such disinterested rationalization of services proved in both cases quite unjustified. The total costs of hospital care for the elderly rose from $4.17 billion in fiscal year 1967 to $6.53 billion in 1969; and that of nursing homes from $1.52 billion to $2.17 billion in the same period.[15] Only skilled nursing-home care after hospitalization is available through Medicare, and most of the nursing-home care of the elderly has thus fallen to Medicaid. Nursing-home costs have become a major headache in the developing administrative problems of Medicaid and represent 30 percent of the costs of all federal, state, and local vendor payments.

The Medicaid program was doomed, then, to be seen in terms of expense rather than as a social service. Of twenty-three states providing care to the medically needy, eleven cut back or adjusted their income eligibility levels following the 1967 amendments; these included California and New York.[16] In both states, as elsewhere, the federal cutbacks, combined with state budgetary retrenchments, created an acute financial situation. Governor Reagen reacted by cutting back services in Medi-Cal against the opposition of numerous citizens and groups including the California Medical Association and other professional associations. The cuts were finally restored after an action in the California courts, brought by a client of California Rural Legal Assistance against the state.[17] But the long-term costs issue was not relieved. Medical vendor payments represented less than one-third of state welfare costs in 1965. By 1968 they had risen to almost half of the states' welfare budgets, and it was reported that one of every three states had been forced to raise state taxes, at least in part because of the rising costs of Medicaid.[18] Medicaid quickly threatened a crisis in state budgetary arrangements.

15. On the purposes of intermediate care facilities, see *Social Security Amendments of 1967, Report of the Committee on Finance, U.S. Senate on H.R. 12080,* 90th Cong., 1st sess., Nov. 1967, pp. 188–90. Of the nursing-home costs in 1969, Medicare covered $400 million, and other public programs (chiefly Medicaid) another $1,249 million. Barbara S. Cooper, "Medical Care Outlays for Aged and Non-Aged Persons, 1966–69," *Research and Statistics Note,* 18 June 1970.
16. *Intergovernmental Problems,* p. 34.
17. See Greenfield, pp. 56–59.
18. *Staff Data Relating to Medicaid-Medicare Study,* 1969, p. 8.

Governor Rockefeller's position was particularly embarrassing. On the one hand he himself had sponsored Medicaid; on the other, the New York eligibility levels for Medicaid were well above the level of federal matching funds now available. State budgetary concerns came first. The New York legislature amended its law in 1968 reducing the income limits to about 140 percent of the highest Aid to Dependent Children levels. Further reductions were made in 1969 to an eligibility level of $5,000 for a family of four, and in addition coverage was eliminated for all persons between twenty-one and sixty-four years of age. All told, against a background of rising living costs and accelerating medical charges, the number of people eligible for Medicaid in New York was reduced by about 40 percent. The state also tried to require Medicaid outpatients to pay 20 percent of their bills, but this was blocked in the courts in a suit challenging its constitutionality.

The problems besetting Medicaid were epitomized in New York City, where the costs of welfare and Medicaid payments doubled between 1965 and 1969 and where one million people are on welfare and another 900,-000 deemed medically indigent. The changes in Medicaid forced additional people into the city's already overwhelmed hospital system, developing still further the chronic understaffing and underfinancing facilities. In the Congress, meanwhile, there were continuing and rising claims of administrative inefficiency, abuse, and fraud. In the fall of 1969, federal auditors claimed that New York City had wasted $9.7 million because of procedural violations and laxness.[19] At a less dramatic level, similar actions were taking place in other states. Cost increases in Medicaid between 1968 and 1970 were estimated to be three times as great as the increases in the number of people served.[20]

FROM FEDERAL SUBSIDY TO NATIONAL CONCERN

The initial federal role in Medicaid was one of developing minimal programs of technical advice to the states and of administering federal grants-in-aid. This followed the pattern of federal–state relations under other welfare programs. Against a background of publicity and rising costs from 1967 Medicaid, like Medicare, became more directly federally regulated. Sen. Russell Long called in 1968 for reductions in Medicaid of $500 million on the grounds that the states "with the connivance and cooperation [of HEW] have found ways to make all kinds of people

19. See Myers, *Medicare,* pp. 292–94; *American Medical News,* 21 July 1969, 8 Sept. 1969.
20. *Medicare and Medicaid Hearings,* July 1969, pp. 8–9.

eligible that nobody in Congress ever intended to make eligible." [21] The various exchanges illuminated the range of views toward Medicaid, from a minimal welfare supplement to a reasonable health care program. While no further action was taken to restrict Medicaid in 1968, Senator Long's Senate Finance staff began a probing survey of the administration of both the medicaid and medicare programs.

Attempts to control the costs of Medicaid were stepped up from the beginning of the Ninety-first Congress, in the wider frame of the Nixon administration's attempts to control increases in federal appropriations. In March 1969, it was announced that utilization review procedures for hospitals and nursing homes would be required for state Medicaid programs, as well as for Medicare.[22] At the same time, the Nixon administration's review of the Johnson budget for fiscal year 1970 proposed limitations of federal payments under Medicaid for patients in state and other public mental institutions (thus putting more fiscal responsibility on the states), special reviews of Medicaid patients in nursing homes with a view to cutting costs, and changes in physician fees under Medicaid; the suggestion was that the lowest prevailing Blue Shield payments for nongovernmental service would be adopted.[23]

Physicians as a group had fared well under Medicaid, as under Medicare. The amount paid to physicians for medical assistance increased fivefold between 1965 and 1969, from $122 million to $523 million.[24] The proposal for fee schedules could not be expected to please physicians, who had fought for the establishment of usual and customary fees in Medicare and Medicaid. Fee schedules for physicians under national programs came one step nearer. Already Senator Aiken, who took credit for inspiring the Medicaid fee limitation, had introduced a bill (S. 111) which would impose fee schedules on Medicare. In June 1969, Secretary of Health, Education, and Welfare Robert Finch announced regulations limiting payments to doctors under Medicaid.[25] The link to Blue Shield was dropped; instead, the regulations tied Medicaid fees to 75 percent of

21. *AMA News,* Oct. 7, 1968.
22. For hospital and extended care facilities participating in Medicare, existing utilization review committees would be used. For other nursing homes, state utilization review procedures are being developed. The regulations were published in *Federal Register,* 4 Mar. 1969.
23. Reported in *Washington Report on Medicine and Health,* 21 Apr. 1969.
24. *Medicaid, Fiscal Year 1969,* NCSS Report B-5, Table 1.
25. The regulations also eliminated for both Medicaid and Medicare a 2 percent "cost-plus" payment which had been allowed by government to nonprofit hospitals and nursing homes above identified costs; also eliminated was a similar 1.5 percent cost-plus favor to proprietary institutions. See *Congressional Quarterly Almanac, 1969,* p. 204.

physicians' average charges in January 1969. This mandatory action was different from concurrent suggestions that carriers under part B of Medicare should only change the level of prevailing charges at fixed intervals, thus allowing overall fee increases over a period of timed steps, rather than as a continuous process. The Medicaid regulations actually froze physician fees at a given level, although administratively that level was difficult to define. It thus set up a form of personalized fee schedule applicable to each participating physician. With the new regulations, two levels of service were recognized, with lesser fees for the poor. For the elderly who were entitled to Medicare, part of whose medical bills were picked up under Medicaid,[26] the situation was anomalous. On the one hand they had recognized entitlements to care in the private sector; on the other, they were once more welfare patients.

The meeting of the AMA House of Delegates in New York City in July 1969 attempted to grapple with the interconnected problems of Medicare and Medicaid as they affected the physician. In a letter to Secretary Finch the previous April, the AMA president, Dwight L. Wilbur, had assured the government of the AMA's cooperation in planning for the health needs of the people but had warned of the dangers of "freezing the process and stifling it," especially in relation to wage and cost controls. The emphasis instead, wrote Dr. Wilbur, should be on ways of encouraging needed manpower to flow when it is most needed and can do the most good.[27] The new regulations took the opposing view. The AMA was no longer however in a dominant bargaining position with the government. The association suffered from the unfavorable publicity received on its apparent blocking of the appointment of Dr. John Knowles as assistant secretary for Health and Scientific Affairs in the early months of 1969. Dr. Knowles' appointment was withdrawn in June. It was remarked at the time that AMA lobbyists had reminded leading Republicans of the association's substantial contributions to the party; the AMA "cashed in $2.5 million worth of chips." [28] While the AMA president stated that the association as an entity had never opposed the nomination,[29] there were inevitable repercussions. The new Medicaid regulations slipped through while the Knowles affair was at its height.

The AMA proposals for curtailing Medicaid abuses, as for building

26. In the month of November 1969, for example, nearly 2.2 million persons aged 65 or over were reported as recipients of medical vendor payments "Medical Assistance Financed under the Public Assistance Titles of the Social Security Act, November, 1969," NCSS Report B-1 (11/69) Table 1.

27. *AMA News,* 28 Apr. 1969.

28. *Washington Report on Medicine and Health,* 30 June 1969.

29. Quoted in *Medical Tribune,* 17 July 1969.

better controls into Medicare, were to develop better professional methods for physician peer review. In 1969, however, these proposals were rhetoric rather than fact. And there was increasing evidence that the group to gain most from the health programs of the 1965 legislation was physicians. Unfavorable comments on physician fees under both Medicare and Medicaid in the press cast doubt on the ability of physicians to act as governmental agents in cost controls.[30] The AMA was being buffeted on all sides. The internal management of the association had been subjected to a critical review from outside management consultants and a change in key administrative personnel. The AMA was also once again concerned about the rising importance of specialist associations in relation to its own development. It was in this atmosphere that the association met in 1969 to consider its own policy directions in relation to health care for the poor and, nearer at home, to physician payment mechanisms.

The meeting was disrupted by protesters, including physicians, nurses, and medical students, who assailed the AMA's conservative leadership,[31] but in fact the association's positions on health services were more progressive than ever before. The outgoing president, Dr. Wilbur, spoke of the inseparability of medicine and society, the national commitment to health and the further commitment ahead, the importance of the physician self-appraisal and peer-review committees, the social responsibility of physicians to overcome barriers to health services met by the poor, the need for physicians to work with consumers of care, the importance of community health centers, and the leadership required of the association to protect the right of the patient to health care as well as the right of the physician to professional independence. His speech was received with a standing ovation.[32] Both Dr. Wilbur and the incoming president, Dr. Walter C. Bornemeier, called for the treatment of the poor through one health service system (private practice). This was to be achieved through the endorsement of proposals for a system of federal income tax credits so that the poor might purchase comprehensive medical insurance.

---

30. Physicians received abundant evidence of this bad press through their own publications. The *AMA News,* for example, was filled with reports of apparent kickbacks, overcharging, duplicate billings, and other apparent abuses of Medicaid. E.g. the report of the State Attorney-General of California on unethical abuses of Medi-Cal (2 Dec. 1968); complaints of huge sums to individual providers in Massachusetts (9 December 1968); the investigation of fraud by physicians, dentists and pharmacists by the Attorney-General of Maryland (23 Dec. 1968); quotation from the *Chicago Tribune* of cheating by "unscrupulous doctors and sticky-fingered functionaries" (21 July 1969); etc.
31. *New York Times,* 14 July 1969.
32. *Proc. AMA House of Delegates* (July 1969), pp. 12–19.

This proposal had been officially endorsed by the AMA House of Delegates in December 1968.[33] Both the leadership and the delegates of the AMA were therefore now committed to the principle of national health insurance, at least for the poor.

One result of the administrative problems of Medicare and Medicaid was thus a strong AMA commitment to the rapid development of private prepayment plans, in which physicians could be reimbursed through usual and customary fees. But at the same time, it was recognized that even in private insurance plans, effective utilization and fee review procedures would be essential. The AMA made peer review its major topic of the clinical convention held in Denver in December 1969. Dr. Roger Egeberg, whose nomination as assistant secretary in the Department of Health, Education, and Welfare had followed successfully on the withdrawal of that of Dr. Knowles, set the keynote. If physicians did not evaluate themselves, the agents of the consumer would take over: "Peer review is going to take a lot of sacrifice by the medical profession, but who the hell else is going to evaluate physicians?" [34]

Almost inexorably, therefore, a number of different movements were coming together. The cost problems of Medicare and Medicaid eliminated much of the previous conceptual differences between those who favored medical care by insurance and those by assistance. The large-scale problems of Medicaid tended to invalidate the second method. Sen. Clinton Anderson of New Mexico, a state which for a time actually suspended its Medicaid program for lack of funds, successfully introduced an amendment in 1969 which allowed states flexibility in the number of services to be developed for their Medicaid programs, and put back the planned development toward comprehensive services, from 1975 to 1977.[35] Thus chances were further reduced for resurrecting Medicaid as a basis for comprehensive federal-state coverage for health services. In July 1969, the same month as critical Senate hearings on abuses and costs in both Medicaid and Medicare, a task force on Medicaid was set up by the Department of Health, Education, and Welfare, chaired by Dr. Walter McNerney, the president of the Blue Cross Association. This group produced an interim report in November 1969 which castigated the flabby federal role in administering Medicaid, urged more efficient procedures for cost controls and review and simplified administration, and

33. See *American Medical News,* 16 Dec. 1968; 20 Nov. 1969.
34. Quoted in *J. Amer. med. Ass., 210* (1969), 2335.
35. The amendment was attached to a tax measure, P.L. 91–56. States could not eliminate the basic five Medicaid services, but they were now able to cut back or eliminate payments for services such as drugs and dentistry. See *Congressional Quarterly Almanac, 1969,* pp. 201, 385.

suggested innovations in the delivery of care including primary health care developments, prepayment plans, and earmarked funds for the improvement of service; increased federal matching funds were suggested. The implications of the report were that Medicaid should be a national basic health program, albeit under state administration.[36] The following month, the Advisory Commission on Intergovernmental Relations (a bipartisan body established by Congress in 1959) stated that the federal government should assume full financial responsibility for Medicaid, as well as for other public assistance programs.[37] If both Medicaid and Medicare are, however, to be federal programs it would be logical that administration of the two programs should be combined, or at least coordinated.

TOWARD REFORM

The various arguments and strands for reform of health service payment systems continue in the 1970s. Medicaid, with its continuing discrepancies in coverage and service by state, even for public assistance recipients, creates at best a patchwork health payment program, at worst a major gap in existing income maintenance programs.[38] Medicaid and Medicare are absorbing increasing public funds, with smaller apparent gains in services and coverage. A study by the Social Security Administration estimated that as much as 61 percent of the $2.1 billion increase in hospital expenditures for the elderly between fiscal years 1966 and 1968 was the result of price changes, and another 7 percent was attributed to the population increase in that period; this left only 32 percent

36. USDHEW, Office of the Secretary, *Recommendations of the Task Force on Medicaid and Related Programs,* November 1969.
37. *American Medical News,* 15 Dec. 1969.
38. For those receiving cash under federally supported public assistance, by July 1970 programs had to provide seven basic services: inpatient hospital care, outpatient hospital services, other laboratory or X-ray services, skilled nursing home services for those over 21, screening and treatment for those under 21, physician services, and home health services. But beyond that, States had great latitude. Mississippi provided no services other than the required ones to the groups compulsorily covered while Wyoming offered only transportation by way of additional service. New Mexico offered to welfare recipients home health services, drugs, dental services, eyeglasses, hearing aids, prosthetic devices, physical therapy, private duty nursing, optometrist services, podiatrist services, chiropractic services, clinic services, transportation and other diagnostic devices. California, Connecticut, Minnesota, New York and North Dakota went further, in offering every additional service for which a federal contribution was available. Taking all Medicaid recipients (those on cash assistance and others deemed medical indigent) New York State in 1968 spent $63.95 per inhabitant for medical assistance programs, while 21 States spent less than $10 per inhabitant. See Stevens and Stevens.

of the increased expenditure reflecting a change in the provision of services.[39] Similar inflation appears to be the case in other aspects of health payment programs. The Senate Finance Committee continues to be the major congressional watchdog on service management and service costs. A detailed and thorough report from the committee staff in February 1970 described the deficiencies in the Medicaid as well as the Medicare program. The result of audits in sixteen states (including the largest) revealed weaknesses whose minimal questionable dollar impact (that is, public waste) was in the region of $318 million. Set against these figures was the listing of total Medicare-Medicaid payments to physicians of more than $25,000 in 1968; a substantial number of physicians had received at least $100,000 in that year from the two programs.[40] In many cases these payments were justified in terms of the enormous number of services to the elderly and the poor. Nevertheless, the publication of these figures raised questions of the morality of Medicare and Medicaid as public service programs—services which are in some respects parallel to those of other publicly organized and important social institutions such as elementary education or the police, whose professionals are paid a fraction as much. For the first time in the United States the *incomes* of physicians have thus come under public scrutiny and concern. Nor will this concern necessarily cease with evidence of the stabilization of physician fees, so long as there are large, governmentally subsidized health service payment programs. In this respect, as in others, physicians have crossed the dividing line between the private and the public sector, as they have in other advanced industrial countries. If health care is to be regarded as a social service, physicians must recognize a role as public servants.

Yet if the only problems in American health services were of lax management of public programs and high incomes to physicians, there would be little cause for the sense of massive urgency which has infused the health care situation in the United States in the past five years. The problems themselves go far deeper, to the purpose of medical payment schemes and of medicine itself—the provision of good quality medical care to the whole population. Not only has the package of programs which was passed in the Medicare legislation of 1965 as Medicare part A, Medicare part B, and Medicaid proved unexpectedly expensive; except for the elderly there is little evidence that the new programs, by

39. Dorothy P. Rice and Barbara S. Cooper, "Outlay for Medical Care of Aged and Non-Aged Persons, Fiscal Years 1966–68," *Research and Statistics Note,* 16 July 1969.

40. *Medicare and Medicaid Report,* Feb. 1970, pp. 82, 245, and passim.

infusing vast sums of money into the private medical sector, have served to improve the operation of that system in terms either of service or of income maintenance. Even the elderly have not benefited as much as they might have expected. In fiscal 1966, the year before Medicare came into effect, the elderly spent an average of $293 per capita on medical care out of their own pockets or through other private sources; another $130 was spent from public sources. Despite the vast programs of Medicare, backed by Medicaid, the private contributions of the elderly were still $193 in 1969. The public contribution had, it is true, risen very rapidly, to over $499 a head. Nevertheless, the elderly could by no means claim complete protection from medical costs.[41] Indeed, their private contributions for medical care still average more than those of people under sixty-five.

A Social Security Administration study estimated in 1968 that a hypothetical health insurance scheme which included relatively comprehensive hospital and group practice medical benefits, dental care, and drugs (but not nursing-home care or most medical appliances) would cost the average family an annual premium of $850,[42] and this figure is already out of date. Estimates from the Social Security Administration, on the basis of existing patterns of health services in the United States, forecast that the total costs of medical care in 1975 will be double that of 1968.[43] Meanwhile virtually nobody in the United States has health insurance which will pay for services of the range available, for example, under the National Health Service in Britain. Prepaid group practices come closest to providing comprehensive packages in the United States, but they cover only 3 or 4 percent of the population. For most people in the United States the chance of falling sick and being hospitalized for an extensive length of time or for very expensive procedures is a macabre lottery. High medical costs strike equally the working citizen with limited private health insurance and the throng of the poor and near-poor, who have both inadequate means and inadequate insurance coverage. To all

41. Barbara S. Cooper, "Medical Care Outlays for Aged and Nonaged Persons, 1966–69," *Research and Statistics Note,* 18 June 1970.
42. Louis S. Reed and Willine Carr, *The Benefit Structure of Private Health Insurance Organizations, 1968,* Social Security Administration (1969).
43. The low projection of 1975 costs for 1975 is $111 billion; the high projection $120 billion. Figures for 1980 are, respectively, $156 billion and $189 billion. Taking the high projections, per capita costs could rise from the 1968 figure of $280, to $552 in 1975, and $814 for 1980. Averages have to be interpreted with caution but it may be helpful to translate this last figure into a family unit of four persons, representing average expenses of over $3,000. Dorothy P. Rice and Mary F. McGee "Projections of National Health Expenditures, 1975 and 1980," *Research and Statistics Note,* 30 Oct. 1970.

intents and purposes, the costs of medical care—with hospital service charges alone perhaps reaching $200 a day by 1980—have made almost every American potentially "medically needy." This fact has been a potent force in accelerating the acceptance of a need for national health insurance.

Up to the passage of Medicare, the debates over different forms of health care financing continued almost through their own momentum. There were those who favored health insurance and there were those who did not, and the AMA was numbered among the latter. Since the passage of Medicare, the old antagonisms have changed in the face of the three crucial pressures on health care: costs, the outmoded organization of services, and broader social pressures for civil rights and equal opportunity. Much of the debate has centered on costs, for at root money is the loudest reformer. Both Medicare and Medicaid were passed, however, in a political climate, the mid-1960s, of concern over poverty, racial discrimination, and inequity which has injected its own urgency into medical care deficiencies. Medicare (designed for the high-risk, low-income elderly) and Medicaid (designed to provide medical services to the poor) have exacerbated rather than reduced medical care's cost problems. And neither has tackled the issues of service inequities and maldistributions. Children in poorer families still see the physicians less than those who are richer; people in one area have available to them more health services than those in another. The average white person in the United States sees the physician four or five times a year, the average nonwhite only three times a year; and differences hold at all income levels.[44]

The value of health services as part of income maintenance programs is self-evident. Yet Medicare and Medicaid, by helping to accelerate a preexisting trend to more elaborate procedures and more costly places of care, have actually worsened the state of the low income person without health insurance coverage, a fact noted by the President's Commission on Income Maintenance Programs in its report (the Heinemann report) in November 1969.[45] This commission, in proposing a new federal family assistance program to replace the existing and outmoded categorical public assistance program in the states—a program adopted by President Nixon—did not specifically recommend the inclusion of a fed-

44. See *Differentials in Health Characteristics by Color, United States, July 1965–June 1967,* USDHEW, Vital and Health Statistics, Series 10, no. 56 (1969), pp. 17–18.
45. *Poverty amid Plenty: The American Paradox,* Report of the President's Commission on Income Maintenance Programs (1969), pp. 134–35.

eral medical assistance scheme to match it. But this became an obviously interconnected step; for there can be no national minimum income level while there are major discrepancies in health care provision under Medicaid from state to state. Joe Brown in California could be eligible both for family assistance and free health services; Harry Jones in Mississippi would have to pay his medical bills from his family assistance; thus Joe's potential income would be considerably higher than Harry's. If the principle of a national income level is to be maintained, the extension of family assistance to include federal entitlements to medical care is inevitable. It was following this line of reasoning that President Nixon announced his administration's intention of developing a health insurance plan as an integral part of a national family assistance program for families with young children in his statement on welfare reform in June 1970.[46] As in the administration's income maintenance program, both the nonworking and the working poor would be included; there would thus be in effect a national means test for medical indigence, at least for one section of the population.

Such a scheme would not abolish Medicaid, the majority of whose payments are made on behalf of the old and the disabled who would not be covered under the proposed family health insurance program. Indeed the proposed program would impose an additional public program on a system already bogged down in administrative complexity. What the proposal does do, however, is to emphasize the irrelevance of the old philosophical divisions between proposals for national health "insurance" and proposals for medical "assistance." Inexorably the various viewpoints on health care financing are being fused together.

PROSPECTS FOR NATIONAL HEALTH INSURANCE

The health insurance movement from the 1940s to the mid-1960s was dominated by liberal Democrats and opposed by the American Medical Association. That of the 1970s has a strong Republican as well as Democratic ingredient, and the American Medical Association has its

46. *New York Times,* 11 June 1970. As initially suggested, the family health insurance plan would buy private health insurance through intermediaries, but there would be national administration and national standards. It was suggested that coverage might be free for families with $1600 or less (the basic family assistance level), $70 for a family with $3000 income, and ranging upward to the fee of $500 for a family with an income of $5620. As many as 25–30 million people could be covered. The details of the plan were not developed as this book went to press; legislation is planned for 1971.

own national health insurance proposal, Medicredit, endorsed by the Association at its Clinical Convention of 1968 and designed, it was reported, to reverse the traditional welfare approach to medical care.[47] The widescale cut-backs in Medicaid, the bad publicity being given to members of the profession, and the general failure of effective administration in the states were major factors in the Association's abandonment of the principle of public financing of vendor medical payments. Instead of supporting a separate mechanism to finance medical care for the poor, Medicredit proposes a national insurance scheme for all members of the population under the age of 65. Under the proposal the federal government would provide low income persons with certificates for the purchase of health insurance policies from approved insurance carriers; persons higher up the income scale would receive federal benefits in terms of scaled income tax credits.[48] The Association is vigorously promoting this legislation, together with other means of integrating medical care for the poor with that of other members of the population. In their first joint approach to a Congressional committee, in July 1970 the AMA and the National Medical Association urged the replacement of Medicaid with a national health insurance program subsidized by the federal government.[49] And at its clinical convention later in the year, the AMA President, Dr. Walter C. Bornemeier, called for the establishment of private practice groups in low-income areas, if necessary subsidized by the federal government.[50]

Over the same period other forces have arisen in support of merging Medicaid into a system of health insurance. Following the drastic retrenchments in the New York Medicaid program and fiscal problems with other elements of public assistance, Governor Rockefeller became a dedicated spokesman for federal financing and regulation of welfare programs, and for an alternative to Medicaid which would both provide health care and repair the states' tattered welfare budgets. Governor

47. See *AMA News,* 16 Dec. 1968; 3 Feb. 1969.
48. There are several current proposals for tax credits for the purchase of health insurance. See chap. 19, footnote 47. For an analysis, see Saul Waldman, *Tax Credits for Private Health Insurance: Estimates of Eligibility and Cost under Alternative Proposals* (Social Security Administration, 1969). The AMA version, under the main title "Health Insurance Assistance Act of 1970," appears in its *Proc. H. of Delegates,* 21–25 June 1970, pp. 66–69.
49. Before the Senate Finance Committee. Reported in *Med. Tribune,* 6 July 1970.
50. *N.Y. Times,* 30 Nov. 1970. Acceptance of government grants by medical societies for the development of medical services in their areas, and the administration of government programs through medical society foundations was endorsed by the AMA in 1968 and further strengthened in June 1970. The latest suggestion would merely extend the principle to individual and group practitioners. See *Proc. H of Delegates,* 21–25 June 1970, pp. 139–42.

Rockefeller presented proposals to President Nixon early in 1969 for a national compulsory health insurance system, financed from employer-employee contributions. In September of the same year, largely on Rockefeller's advocacy, a resolution in favor of a national health insurance program was endorsed by the National Governors Conference in Colorado Springs. This was followed in May 1970 by Rockefeller's forming his own Conference on Health and Hospital Services and Costs to develop a detailed plan for health insurance. Meanwhile similar concerns were being pressed by Senator Javits of New York, long an advocate of comprehensive prepaid practice through a private financing system. The Javits proposal, introduced in Congress in April 1970, proposed a health insurance scheme financed by employer-employee contributions up to a maximum of 3.3 percent of annual wages together with a federal government subsidy, and administered by the Social Security Administration. As with Medicare, private health insurance carriers would act as agents of the program.[51] The proposal would absorb both Medicare and Medicaid.

Other groups were also mobilizing into action. In February 1970, Rep. Martha Griffiths introduced a far-reaching health insurance proposal to be financed through the Social Security system and organized without the use of private intermediaries; this bill was supported by the AFL-CIO.[52] Meanwhile an independent group, called together under the leadership of Walter Reuther, was preparing its own rather similar proposals; these were presented to Congress as a "Health Security" proposal in August, 1970 under the sponsorship of Sentaor Edward Kennedy and fourteen other senators.[53] Both bills specified the intention of using government-sponsored health insurance as a means of creating organizational changes to stimulate organized health care systems such as were being proposed in the administration's proposals for health maintenance organizations under Medicare and Medicaid.

In June 1970, too, the Task Force on Medicaid issued its final recommendations to the Department of Health, Education, and Welfare. In tune with the groundswell of movement toward national health insurance, this report stressed that the problems of medical assistance to the poor lie beyond the walls of Medicaid; its analysis thus ranged widely over other aspects of the health care delivery system.[54] The Task Force supported 100 percent federal funding of Medicaid, with the state role

51. S. 3711, 91st Cong., 2d sess.
52. H.R. 15779, 91st Cong., 2d sess.
53. S. 4297, 91st Cong., 2d sess.
54. *Recommendations of the Task Force on Medicaid and Related Programs,* Department of Health, Education and Welfare, Office of the Secretary, June 1970.

being one of providing supplementary benefits; with initial coverage of all persons under welfare extension of Medicare to cover the disabled, and federal coverage of others who are dependent and of low income. Chiefly, however, the report stressed the need for innovations and reorganization within the health care system, including support of health maintenance organizations offering services on a prepaid capitation basis. The need was also emphasized for a uniform system of professional review of services by federal programs, and for appropriate federal reorganization to provide national health services leadership and greater technical assistance. Above all it was stressed that a new national policy for health care financing is essential.

Nor is this by any means the sum of activities toward a more coordinated national payment program. In the Congress in 1970 were more than two hundred proposals for changes of some degree in Medicare and Medicaid, ranging all the way from suggestions that one or another service be included in the programs or that eligibility groups be widened, to the rebirth of comprehensive national health insurance proposals. As this book goes to press, representatives of the insurance industry are discussing the development of federal reinsurance and subsidy of private insurance for low-income groups, proposals for national insurance for catastrophic illness are being discussed, the administration's family health insurance program is being redesigned, and a variety of individuals and groups, including the American Hospital Association and several state medical societies, are developing their own proposals. The journal *Medical Economics* has long since told its readers that national health insurance is a "near-certainty" for the 1970s.[55]

Thus the era of Medicaid as a distinct and limited program is passing; the watershed that was the beginning of Medicare is long past. But while some expanded government subsidy of medical bills seems inevitable, the questions of organizing and distributing medical care more effectively remain. Medicaid was designed as part of a program of income maintenance; so also was Medicare. Together they have proved that to concentrate on income maintenance alone is an inappropriate answer to the problems inherent in a major and essential social service. Any scheme of health care financing in the future, no matter what its historical origins or its philosophical base, its contributory mechanisms, or its apparent emphasis on the public or private sector, will rise or fall on the effect it has on the organization and administration of medical care at the city and neighborhood level. Such systems may be termed health maintenance organizations (under the administration's proposals) comprehensive

55. *Med. Economics* 27 Apr. 1970, p. 10.

health service organizations (under the Health Security proposals), comprehensive health service systems (under the Javits proposals), or health care corporations (the American Hospital Association); the terminology is irrelevant. At issue is how far action taken in Washington can stimulate local initiative.

The experience of Medicaid, then, has thrown the federal role in health into prominence. As local provision of medical services to the poor failed, it was taken over by the states; the states are now looking to Washington for federal intervention. There are thus concurrently movements for centralization of policy and financing with decentralized health care organization. Earlier in this study the organization of health services in the United States was described as being an array of physicians scattered like dots on a map; later these dots were clustered on major urban areas and around hospitals, and joined by the dots of other health care occupations, but there was still little systematic cohesion of services. The great extension of private and public payment schemes for health services in the last two decades has done little to modify this pattern; Medicaid has been no exception. The next step is to achieve effective community health care organization; but to do this effective national policies are essential. It should be noted that this conclusion has already been reached by organized medicine, whose health policies have long been more effectively centralized and articulated than those of governmental agencies; hence much of the AMA's past lobbying successes. Medicredit, a nationally standardized governmental plan, stands or falls on the effectiveness of decentralized professional review mechanisms. Indeed, so persuasive are the arguments for review and for its extension into prepayment plans that the medical society foundation promises to be a necessary component of any future health insurance program. Thus while state welfare departments are trying to hand over their authority to the federal government, the AMA, one step ahead, is strengthening professional authority at the state and local level.

CHAPTER 21

The Federal Government and the Health Care System

In other advanced Western countries in the last two or three decades, the development of governmental schemes of health financing has implied an acceptance of national governmental responsibility for the organization of health services. In England, for example, the National Health Service Act of 1946 put upon the minister of health the duty to establish a comprehensive health service, designed "to secure improvement in the physical and mental health of the people of England and Wales and the prevention, diagnosis and treatment of illness." [1] With this centralization of responsibility came immediate action to coordinate a health service system which was at that time as disorganized as that in the United States today. English hospitals were nationalized, affiliated, and grouped under local hospital management committees, which in turn formed part of larger university-centered hospital regions, covering a service of 2–4 million persons (equivalent to the population of the state of Connecticut). General practitioner services were organized with other professional services through local executive councils and local professional committees; and such practitioners were reimbursed by the government through nationally agreed payment schemes. The GPs themselves, acting as primary or family physicians, contract with the government to provide first-contact and continuing medical care to persons who sign up with them, and are paid for these services through a rather complex system based on capitation fees. Medical specialists are paid by salary through the hospital system and see patients on consultation. Local public health and domiciliary services in England, including home nursing and ambulance services, are provided through local health departments. The system itself, born of preexisting patterns of medical practice and of ideas for organizing medical care which had

1. National Health Service Act 1946, 9 & 10 Geo. Ch. 81 sec. 1.

crystallized in the 1920s and 1930s, was not necessarily transportable anywhere else; it was perhaps not an ideal organizational structure for modern medical care in Britain. Nevertheless, by concentrating responsibility for health services at the national level, the National Health Service began to attack gross discrepancies in available personnel and facilities in different areas, to make services available regardless of income, and to plan its services as a system. By the late 1950s the National Health Service had become an established facet of British life. By the late 1960s, it was time for a reappraisal—a need which continues—of specific organizational forms of the service. Health care had been accepted as one of an array of necessary social services, parallel to Social Security and education.

In the United States, in contrast, there has up till now been little opportunity for wide scale organizational experiment. The financing of medical care has not been centralized or federated to the extent that national or even local planning of health services has been mandated. Federal subsidies for the advancement of medical research are still considered separately from subsidies to medical education. Public subsidy for the building of hospitals comes under different legislation from subsidy for building mental health centers or neighborhood health centers. And apart from the latter there is still no subsidy for group medical practice or primary medical care.[2] Provision for the organized or subsidized payment of bills for individual medical care is scattered across numerous programs, each geared to selected disease or population groups. The federal role has been one not of planning but of prodigality.

This diffusion of energy and efforts is the major feature of American medical care. Even before the burgeoning of health programs of the Kennedy and Johnson administrations, there were federal or state programs for veterans, Indians, servicemen, servicemen's dependents, the merchant marine, public assistance recipients, immigrants, recipients of workmen's compensation benefits, temporary disability insurance, medical rehabilitation services, maternal and child health services, and

2. Proposals for federal loans, grants, or mortgage guarantees to finance construction costs of prepaid groups have appeared regularly in the Congress since 1949, but to the present none has been successful. In 1966, a program of federal insurance for loans was finally passed for financing and equipping nonprofit facilities for group practice of physicians, dentists, or optometrists; but these loans were not restricted to *prepaid* group practice. The legislation (title V of the Demonstration Cities and Metropolitan Development Act of 1966, P.L. 89–754) authorized the new program through an extension of the existing FHA mortgage insurance program. But the plan provides a banking service, not a major subsidy. Subsidy of health maintenance organizations is an obvious target for health legislation in 1971, and after.

school health services. There are state mental hospitals, hospitals for tuberculosis and for other chronic diseases, and programs for venereal diseases and other aspects of public health. A number of counties and municipalities, notably in California and New York, operate public general hospitals. But with few exceptions, no organized health service systems have developed either through public or private initiative, even in relatively small geographical areas.[3] There are exceptions, of which notable examples are the self-contained prepaid hospital-based group practice schemes (primarily for middle-class populations) and more recently neighborhood health centers set up under the Office of Economic Opportunity and other federal agencies (solely for those with low incomes). But even now such organizations have very little impact on the total health care of the country. Instead of logical and innovative networks and systems to help the patient through the maze of specialists, there has been an unimaginative accretion of services (and costs) by independent practitioners and institutions. The health care legislation of the middle and late 1960s, designed to alleviate the needs of yet more elements in society (notably the poor and the elderly), added to the organizational disarray. Some might see in the actions of the Johnson administration an invisible hand weaving a great society, but as far as health services were concerned any such hand was weaving a tangled web of increasing complexity. While the costs of health services continued to mount, and while deficiencies continue to be identified, there remains no national health policy, no national health service for the general population, such as many European countries have enjoyed for several decades.

In a statement on the health of the nation's health care system in July 1969, Secretary of Health, Education, and Welfare, Robert Finch, and Assistant Secretary, Dr. Roger Egeberg, stated baldly, "This Nation is faced with a breakdown in the delivery of health care unless immediate concerted action is taken by government and the private sector." The increasing demand for services accompanied by crippling inflation in medical costs (both in part attributable to Medicare and Medicaid) were, it was noted, not only causing vast increases in governmental health expenditures for little return, but also—and significantly—raising

3. A detailed legislative history of the entire network of publicly financed health programs in the United States has yet to be written. For analyses of aspects of the network, see Ralph Chester Williams, *The United States Public Health Service 1798–1950* (Washington, D.C., 1951); George Rosen, *A History of Public Health* (New York, 1958); Somers and Somers, *Doctors, Patients and Health Insurance;* Odin Anderson, *The Uneasy Equilibrium: Private and Public Financing of Health Services in the United States 1875–1965* (New Haven, 1968).

private health insurance premiums. Without concerted efforts (including the federal cost controls over Medicare and Medicaid which were proposed at the same time) the "pluralistic, independent, voluntary nature of our health care system" would be endangered by pressures for "monolithic government-dominated medical care." [4] This statement puts in a nutshell the characteristics of the strains and stresses on the American health care system—costs, demand, inflation, inflexibility, waste. But it also reflects the tone of the debates over health services in the late 1960s and early 1970s. Health services are now "political," in the sense not of party politics—Republicans and Democrats are equally concerned over the need for health services provision—but of impending and needed legislative reform. Such reform is, moreover, predicated not on one basic assumption for change but on a variety of issues. These include questions of income maintenance (of both the poor and the middle class), of equal rights, of community development, of controlling costs and making existing programs more efficient, of stimulating organizational change to meet the demands of specialized medicine, of centralized versus decentralized regulation of the health care system, and of the appropriate roles of public, private and professional enterprise. The political situation in American medicine in the 1970s is much more complex than that in England (or for that matter in the United States) in the 1940s, when the advancement of a national health service could be justified as one plank in the platform of social reforms which together formed the British Welfare State. In the United States the political mood of the 1970s is, if anything, moving away from governmental regulation of social services toward at least a flirtation with concepts of laissez-faire. Discussion of voucher schemes for the purchase of health insurance (and even education) is a case in point; the concept of independent health maintenance organizations is a further example; proposals to replace student grants-in-aid by a system of loans is a third.

There has, moreover, been no massive disruption of health services in America such as there was in England during World War II, a factor which facilitated the establishment of the National Health Service. Health services in the United States were not sufficiently disturbed by World War II, nor later by Korea or Indochina to the point of needing radical action to sustain them. Hospitals have been propped up by private health insurance, and sustained by Medicare, Medicaid and other public programs, rather than by direct government control. Nor

4. USDHEW, "A Report on the Health of the Nation's Health Care System," mimeographed statement, 10 July 1969.

has there yet been, in the face of the more impelling social issues of income, food, and discrimination, a concentration of public sentiment demanding immediate health service reform. Poor health services in the black urban ghetto were described in the Kerner report and elsewhere as a contributing factor to poor health conditions, which in turn was a contributing factor to the summers of violence in major cities in the middle 1960s.[5] But such indirect assertions, politics and vested interests being what they are, will not alone effect a vast reorganization of health facilities for all income groups. Yet at the same time a slow-burning sense of crisis has been engendered, born not of social revolution but of administrative chaos. The combined effect of one piece of legislation after another, poured into an unconnected health service system, has been to produce increasing dysfunction in the way the system works. Rising costs of medical care have begun to provoke middle-class support of proposals for national health insurance; how widespread this support now is may be tested in the national elections of 1972. Of itself, however, national health insurance, like Medicare and Medicaid, could serve to increase further both the demand for services, and their costs, in an inflationary spiral, rather than necessarily affect the operation of the health care system. It is in the latter that reform is now chiefly needed. Change is demanded not primarily to take a great leap forward in creating a new health system—as in Britain over twenty-five years ago—but by rationalizing, at all governmental and community levels, the unwieldy accretions of programs and services which are already in existence.

THE FEDERAL HEALTH ESTABLISHMENT

The pattern of medical care in the United States twenty years from now may not be one of federal domination of health services, in the sense of a monolithic or centralized governmental health service, as in England. Nevertheless, the key to health services organization is inevitably the present and future actions taken by the federal government. Indeed, the time has long passed in the United States when it could be debated whether or not there should be federal governmental intervention in health services. Federal government involvement in the development of health care facilities, educational institutions, and payment plans for deprived population groups is already important and substantial. Under the impact of Medicare, Medicaid, and other public

5. *Report of the National Advisory Commission on Civil Disorders* (Government Printing Office, 1968), pp. 136–37.

medical programs of the 1960s, federal expenditures on the operation and construction of medical services jumped from $2.9 billion in 1959–60, to $15.1 billion in 1968–69, to $20.6 billion in 1970–71, a sevenfold increase within eleven years. Taking all expenditures together, public spending (federal, state, and local) already represents more than one of every three dollars spent on personal medical care and on the construction of health facilities. Even without sweeping new public health programs, such as national health insurance, the proportion appears to be steadily rising. Much of the public money feeds into private medical institutions, in turn stimulating new construction and thus having a multiplier effect in the private as well as the public sector.[6] Whether one approves of governmentally influenced health services or not, the United States is on the way to having a publicly financed health care system.

Logic might suggest that federal outlays of over $20 billion—10.5 percent of all federal expenditures—would be matched by close and careful planning and control in Washington. That such is not the case is a heritage of two important factors. The first is the perceived role of the federal government in public welfare spending. Sundquist has noted that before 1960 the typical federal assistance program, whether it be for land grant colleges, highways, vocational education, agricultural support, crippled children services, or vendor medical payments under public assistance, did not involve an expressly stated national purpose.[7] Federal programs were designed to support state or local efforts, financed through formula and other grants, and with federal advice but not control. Medicaid proved a prime example of the continuation of this assistance philosophy; it was designed to help the states rather than to establish a federal health or welfare program. But Medicaid also offers

---

6. Total expenditures on health and medical care in 1968–69 were $60.3 billion. Of this, $37.7 billion represented private expenditures, including insurance benefits and expenses, direct payments for services, and other private expenses, including research and construction. Public expenditures accounted for $22.6 billion, including Defense Department medical services ($1.6 billion) and construction ($59 million); veterans services ($1.5 billion) and construction ($55 million); and civilian medical care research, construction through Medicare, Medicaid, and other programs ($19.4 billion). Federal expenditures accounted for $15.1 billion, state and local expenditures for $7.5 billion. Barbara S. Cooper, "National Health Expenditures," *Research and Statistics Note,* Nov. 1969, table 2, 3. See also U.S., Congress, Senate, Committee on Government Operations, Subcommittee on Executive Reorganizational and Government Research, *Health Activities: Federal Expenditures and Public Purpose* (Pursuant to S. Res. 320), Committee Print, 91st Cong., 2d sess., June 1970, pp. 39–40 and passim (hereafter cited at *Health Activities*).
7. James L. Sundquist, with the collaboration of David W. Davis, *Making Federalism Work* (Washington, D.C., 1969), p. 3 and passim.

a case study of the changing role and expectation of federalism which was the result of massive increases of federal spending in the 1960s. Like air pollution control (1963), community action programs (1964), neighborhood youth corps programs (1964), neighborhood facilities programs (1965), demonstration cities (1966), and the many other federal assistance activities developed in the 1960s, effectiveness depends on local coordination, planning, and control; in short, a diffuse federal bureaucracy must be matched by strong state and community initiative. But at the same time, to encourage such initiative, coordination is required among assistance programs at the federal level so that they do in fact provide assistance and support to local groups. In administering many of the programs of the Great Society of the mid-1960s, neither effective local initiative nor effective federal assistance has been forthcoming; again, Medicaid provides a classic example. As a result, what were assistance programs have begun, under the spearing of congressional questioning and concern, to acquire the burden of national programmatic responsibilities. In the last ten years therefore, the concept of governmental decentralization has partly given way to that of centralization, at least in terms of effective federal analysis, monitoring, management, and coordination of domestic welfare policies.

In turn, it has become evident that even the stimulation of decentralized planning of social welfare services, whether it be for city air pollution programs, legal aid services, or community health services, requires a shift from federal passivity to federal action, if only to bring to the community the full resources of federal support. The operation and implications of federal grants and contracts to medical schools are an important but typical example of the attempts to keep federal assistance "pure," in terms of assistance to local programs, but of the chaos which results as uncoordinated assistance programs proliferate without any sense of coordinated federal responsibility. The present situation is thus one of a need for a national policy (for science, for health, for city planning, for welfare) which will provide for sufficient *de*centralization of services, while providing at the same time centralized direction, standards and control.

A direct outcome of a historically weak federal role has been the diffusion of health subsidies over a patchwork of legislation dealing with federal health assistance and service programs. Pockets of federal action are now scattered across 221 different federal agencies and departments. These represent, moreover, a series of distinct approaches as to what the federal role should be. An initial thrust of federal involvement (1935–46) stressed categorical grants-in-aid for maternal and child health programs and state and local health departments. This was followed by a period of investment (1946–63), during which federal aid was provided for hospitals in the Hill-Burton program, for massive support of medical research through NIH, and through increasing funding of health manpower programs. The short but active years of ferment of the early Johnson administration (1963–66), produced Medicare, Medicaid, community mental health centers, maternal and infant care projects, neighborhood health centers, regional medical programs, comprehensive health planning agencies, and the National Center for Health Services Research and Development. The present decade is one of transition, in which the costs and complexities of these and other health-related programs demand consolidation and an approach to local and regional comprehensive health care systems.[8] Altogether this process can be described as the decades of federal intervention in health, accelerating from the middle 1960s, and demanding major realignments in federal and local health care organization. For the structures of federalism, as well as of professionalism or community action, have not kept pace with the constant accretions of programs which are in turn responses both to social activism and to the costs of specialized medicine.

By far the biggest federal department concerned with health is the Department of Health, Education, and Welfare. DHEW has responsibility for over 70 percent of the federal health dollar, including Medicare, Medicaid, and most of the health programs of the 1960s. There are, however, major divisions, compartmentalisms, and even rivalries within this department, which are a direct result of the transposition of old attitudes of passive federal assistance into federal administration, and of the development of health services around a variety of different social welfare programs. A Congressional report of 1970 noted the phenomenon that the assistant secretary for Health and Scientific Affairs, the highest-ranking spokesman on health within the department (and the government), is connected only with the divisions which arose out of the old U.S. Public Health Service. The department's two major programs, Medicare and Medicaid, are not in his domain; as a result he is a spokesman for only 22 percent of the department's health budget.[9] Medicare, as an offspring of Social Security legislation,

8. The terms have been adapted from *National Advisory Commission on Health Facilities: A Report to the President* (Government Printing Office, 1968), p. 6 and passim. And see William L. Kissick, "Health Policy Directions for the 1970's," *New Engl. J. Med., 282* (1970), 1343–54.
9. See U.S., Congress, Senate, Committee on Government Operations, Subcommittee on Executive Reorganization and Government Research, *Federal Role in*

is operated by the Social Security Administration, and Medicaid, off-spring of public assistance programs, by the separate Social and Rehabilitation Service; the latter also administers a number of maternal and child health services. Each program is administered in its own pocket of operations, in the context of its own piece of legislation and its own congressional committees.[10] The disconnections of the federal bureaucracy in health can be readily appreciated by anyone who has attempted to compile a list of all federal involvement in specific health activities (for example, in federal support of medical graduates in training in all fields and specialties, or of current federal interest in physician assistant training programs) or have asked the governmental switchboard for general information. While there are now national centers for health statistics, health services research and development, social statistics, and social security research and information, there is still no central informational service nor ongoing analysis of all federal health programs.

Lack of coordination among federal departments and offices would not matter if there were clear-cut divisions in their span of operations. In that event, the beneficiary would usually deal with only one federal officer or adviser, and programs could be evaluated independently of each other. But the nature and number of programs mean that there are constant problems of overlapping functions and jurisdictions. Despite the coordination of various pieces of legislation in the Health Manpower Act of 1968, as many as 14 separate federal departments and agencies are engaged in programs of health training and education. When asked by a Senate subcommittee for a list, moreover, the Department of Health, Education, and Welfare was only able to identify 12, and even departments with manpower programs did not always identify them correctly.[11]

Health: Report Pursuant to S. Res. 320, 91st Cong., 2d sess., 30 Apr. 1970, S. Rept. 91–809, pp. 8, 11, 29, and passim. This report details the responsibilities of the different agencies and their responses to specific questions. It is notable that such information is not readily available anywhere else.

10. In the 91st Congress, for example, hearings on health services were held in the Senate by the Committee on Labor and Public Welfare, Antitrust and Monopoly Subcommittee, the Finance Committee, and two subcommittees of the Committee on Aging. The major committees in the House are the Ways and Means Committee and the House Commerce Committee.

11. Licensed practical nurses and nurses' aides, for example, are being trained through funds channeled through the Indian Health Service and the National Institute of Mental Health (USDHEW, Public Health Service), Bureau of Vocational Programs (USDHEW, Office of Education), Economic Development Administration (Department of Commerce), Manpower Administration (Department of Labor), Office of Economic Opportunity, Veterans Administration, and elsewhere. Professional nurse training is supported by a much larger number of programs. The number of programs itself is immaterial. Not until 1969, however, did the Department of Health, Education, and Welfare compile its own list of health training

An observer of federal health policies, Dr. James Shannon, former director of the National Institutes of Health, has estimated that in the Johnson administration alone, Congress enacted 51 pieces of health legislation, administered through 400 different authorities.[12] Not surprisingly, federally supported health services are a potpourri of activities. Even the national ("socialized") health care systems for certain members of the population—the hospitals and clinics operated by the Department of Defense for military personnel and their dependents, the Veterans Administration health care system, the Indian Health Services, and Public Health Service Hospitals—are not interconnected. Nor are such disconnections observable merely at the federal level. One of the two physicians serving the fourteen-bed Fort Yuma Indian Hospital near Yuma, Arizona, was asked recently about his relations with the neighboring ten-bed army hospital and five-bed marine dispensary serving populations in the same area. He replied, "I have never even talked to the people at the Army or Marine facility." [13] These characteristics of a lack of coordination of health programs at the federal level matched by a lack of coordination locally, run through all elements of the health service system. They are the result of the development of separate pieces of health legislation over the past thirty years; they provide the impetus for reform.

The problems of overlap are self-evident. The Small Business Administration and the Hill-Burton program (DHEW) have for example in some instances made grants and loans to competing hospitals in the same communities, with a resulting overexpansion and thus waste of their facilities.[14] By 1970 such action was interpreted in congressional committees not so much as evidence of lack of effective local hospital planning, which was clearly the case, but as a breakdown in the purposes and administration of federal assistance. The same charges of lack of effective central management are being made with respect to programs of hospital construction through the Senate Committee on Government Operations as are being made with respect to Medicare and Medicaid by the Senate Finance Committee, and were exposed in the Fountain committee investigation of federal biomedical research

programs, and the list itself contains relatively little information of use either for analyzing the effectiveness of the programs in total, or for the assistance of community or health service groups anxious to receive appropriate support. See *Federal Role in Health,* pp. 11–12, 127–39.

12. Ibid., p. 18.

13. Ibid., p. 27.

14. Notable examples were at Vallejo, Calif., and Belle Glade, Fla., in both of which it was alleged that federal grants to competing hospitals had served to produce more hospital beds than were actually needed. Ibid., pp. 23–25.

grants management during the 1960s.[15] All are part of the combined pressures toward a new definition of federal health responsibility.

From the viewpoint of the city or neighborhood, the federal health establishment offers a maze of almost incredible entanglement. It is difficult, if not impossible, for local citizen groups or groups of physicians or other health service providers to develop a well-integrated health service scheme for an area or neighborhood which would utilize all appropriate governmental resources now available. Suppose, for example, that a far-seeing group of concerned politicians, physicians, community leaders, and others decides to develop a cluster of interrelated neighborhood health services which would include a health center providing all income groups in the population with a wide variety of specialist services, dental care, community health and home health services, special services for maternity and infant care and for children and youths, school health services and health education, out-of-hospital mental health programs, day hospital facilities for the old and sick, and physical, mental, and vocational rehabilitation services. To do this, they would need help in raising the initial capital and some operating subsidy with respect to services for the poor. Elements of all of these services are eligible for governmental grant or subsidy. Such is the number of agencies and programs involved, however, each with differing requirements in terms of the form and routine of applications, the amount of matching funds required, the requirements for participation in the program, the scrutiny of perhaps a score of independent grant-reviewing groups and so on, that any major attempt to link the programs together as one unit is doomed to frustration, at least as yet.

Dr. John Knowles, director of the Massachusetts General Hospital, described in 1968 the difficulties of even that venerable and authoritative institution, in working "through the multiplicity of funding arrangements from the Children's Bureau to the OEO to the other departments of the HEW," in a proposal to develop coordinated health services for 16,000 people in the Charlestown area of Boston.[16] It took nearly six years of planning before even the children's portion of the program could be funded, even though the authorization for federal funding of components of the project was already available and even though special arrangements were made by the assistant secretary for health, Dr. Philip Lee, in developing and coordinating the application. (Indeed

15. See chapter 16.
16. U.S., Congress, Senate, Committee on Government Operations, Subcommittee on Executive Reorganization, *Health Care in America: Hearings,* 90th Cong., 2d sess., Apr. and July 1968, pp. 702–03 (hereafter cited as *Health Care in America*).

Dr. Lee and his associate, Dr. George Silver, suggested assigning a special governmental coordinator to the project who would test the ability of the department to respond to an application for comprehensive health services in a poor area, rather than with categorical services geared toward specified diseases or age groups.) Such an anecdote, involving an initial budget of $2 million in a total HEW health budget which was then 7,000 times that size, illustrates what is meant by the ungovernability of the Department of Health, Education, and Welfare (a feature by no means confined to health). But it also has disturbing implications for local health development. Most people, even those in prominent local positions, do not have the kind of access to the federal establishment as that held by a medical leader of prominence such as Dr. Knowles, or by other members of the department's well over 300 recognized health advisory committees, whose membership of about 3,000 forms an advisory oligarchy or exclusive club, drawn primarily from established health programs, schools, and institutions.[17]

The advisory committees themselves are, however, no better coordinated with each other than the programs they advise. Indeed, they serve to emphasize and legitimize organizational separatism. Individual members who are on more than one committee may be better informed about federal programs than those on the outside, or even those inside government; but presumably the function of the committees is to give advice, not to provide an informal system of communication. In any event, the most evident organizational result of the massive infusion of federal funding in health in the past decade has been the creation not of a monolithic force, dominating and rigidifying the health care system into predetermined molds, but of a many-peopled labyrinth, whose guides know only part of the system and to which only perhaps the initiator has an effective map. Each and every health program has its own stated purpose and is designed to help individuals in need through the process of creative federalism. Taken together, however, federal programs, not least of which are Medicare and Medicaid, are contributing to health care inflation, waste, and inefficiency—the denial of public accountability.

17. During Senate Finance Committee hearings in 1969, a table was produced by Sen. John J. Williams showing a total of 407 advisory groups to DHEW in fiscal year 1970. These had, it was claimed, a gross membership of 5,514 people and a cost in that year of $7.2 million. The U.S. Public Health Service accounted for 334 of the committees (almost two-thirds of which were advisory to the National Institutes of Health) and 3,830 of the gross membership, some advisers being members of more than one group. No studies have been published of who sits on these committees, what are the decisions that are made, and what are their actual functions and purposes. *Medicare and Medicaid Hearings,* July 1969, p. 171.

Meanwhile, studies continue to show that despite the influx of federal (and private) dollars, people are receiving far from adequate medical care.[18] Indeed, studies are not necessary (except perhaps to build up the sense of well-documented crisis in the Congress and the press), for the deficiencies in American health services are everywhere evident: the small-business man having to sell his business to pay for his dying wife's hospital bills; the self-serving expansionism of hospitals in pushing for further capital development without consultation with other institutions and local populations; the lack of home care services, and even of information about where medical care services and aid are locally available; the social discrimination of large city outpatient clinics which now provide a major general medical service for the poorer members of the population; the use by the middle class of a string of independent specialists and facilities without any necessary coordination of treatment; the absence of any medical care in many rural areas; and the wretched conditions and lack of staff in many municipal (and some private) hospitals, chronic disease facilities, and nursing homes. Such conditions are too well known (if only from the battery of congressional and departmental reports in the last decade) to need detailed documentation.

The one-third public investment in health services demands acceptance of public responsibility for such conditions on the grounds of economy, accountability, and consumer protection. Yet the federal government is locked, through historical accident, into a system of federal assistance which is marked by dissemination of funding, diffusion of effort, and disguise of the extent of tax subsidy. A popular form of disguise has been an acceptance that the government can (and should) continue to play the game of grantsmanship; this game assumes that money is available only to those who apply for it, successfully meet the agency's operational and qualitative criteria, and pass the scrutiny of an influential peer group of those to whom money may be presented. An eminent physicist remarked that scientific research is "the only pork barrel for which the pigs determine who gets the pork." [19] While the

18. E.g. a community study group in Monroe County, N.Y., headed by Marion B. Folsom, former secretary of Health, Education, and Welfare, stated in 1968 on the basis of a survey that 41 percent of the elderly in the country who needed health care were either receiving no care or the minimal type of care. In one part of the Bronx in New York there is now only one doctor to every 10,000 people; 20 years ago there were four times the number of doctors and only half the number of residents. Both these examples are given in U.S., Congress, Senate, Special Committee on Aging, Subcommittee on Health of the Elderly, *Costs and Delivery of Health Services to Older Americans, Hearings,* 90th Cong., 2d sess., pt. 3, Oct. 1968, pp. 612, 757.

private foundations themselves have been coming under increasing public scrutiny, major health programs have been built on the similar assumption that governmental money can be disbursed as if health services were a continuing series of charities, emergency relief, or demonstration projects.

Efforts continue to be made to coordinate elements of programs in HEW through departmental reorganizations which attempt to refocus activities around specific problems or issues, such as child development or health manpower training. Regional health directors are being appointed to coordinate local federal programs in each of HEW's ten regional offices. They will report to the HEW regional directors, who in turn report to the secretary's office in Washington. Most of the previous reorganizations of HEW have, however, not altered the functions of particular federal programs; the components have been reshuffled, but continue as before. They have, however, served to emphasize three broad and accepted areas of developing federal responsibility in the health service system: the subsidy of buildings and plant in which to provide medical care, the encouragement of regional and other cooperative health care activities, and the direct provision of services to populations inadequately served by the private sector.

THE FEDERAL ROLE: SUBSIDIZING HEALTH FACILITIES

Building subsidies have long been accepted. But federal involvement has so far been relatively small, designed to supplement rather than to change or dominate the existing system. The Hill-Burton Act of 1946, for example, was a brave but partial attempt to improve the plant and the distribution of hospitals by providing federal grants to hospitals, originally in rural areas. Federal subsidies for construction, limited to one-third of the approved construction cost, are channeled to approved nonprofit hospital corporations through recognized state Hill-Burton agencies, typically the state health department. As a condition of grant approval, each state agency had to develop a statewide hospital plan, based on a ratio of hospital beds to population, and with specified priorities geared toward areas which were apparently in the greatest need. In terms of providing hospitals in rural areas, the Hill-Burton (later Hill-Harris) program has been a great success. Almost half of the

19. Kenneth M. Watson, quoted by Daniel S. Greenberg, *The Politics of American Science* (London, 1969), p. 197.

4,678 projects undertaken in the first twenty years of Hill-Burton were related to communities of under 10,000 population, and less than 10 percent were in communities of 250,000 or more.[20]

Over the years, moreover, the program has been steadily extended. Grants were added for research on hospital utilization in 1949; for construction of nursing homes, diagnostic and treatment centers, rehabilitation and chronic disease facilities (1954); to give hospitals the option of accepting a long-term loan instead of a grant (1958); for constructing out-of-hospital community health facilities (1961); for hospital modernization, and for urban services, developed through regional, metropolitan, or local area plans (1964). Between 1946 and 1968 nearly $3.2 billion in federal funds were channeled to hospitals through the program, representing a total expenditure of over $10 billion, an addition of 425,000 hospital and nursing-home beds, and 2,800 other health facilities; federal obligations under the program in fiscal year 1969 were $272 million.[21] In the absence of a national health program, Hill-Burton provides a major backstop for health service institutional development. In theory, at least, the programs can be regarded as a governmental commitment to the production of necessary and basic health resources. But in practice the commitment to hospital development has been more titular than real. The early proposals (1938–45) for federal grants-in-aid for hospital construction, which predated and led up to the Hill-Burton legislation, were only one part of a proposed national health program; they did not stand alone, but were, rather, an integral component of a program of federal grants to states, or federal health insurance, for general medical care of the population. While the demand for medical services would be stimulated through health insurance, at the same time there would be an improvement in the supply of service through construction and initial operating grants for needed facilities. If a national health program had gone through, there would almost inevitably have been the concomitant of strong local and regional planning

20. Two-thirds of the Hill-Burton funds for general hospital projects went to smaller towns and rural areas, with populations of under 100,000 people. USDHEW, *Hill-Burton Progress Report July 1, 1947–June 30, 1966* (Washington, D.C., 1966), pp. 32–33.
21. The Hill-Burton expenditures included $185.3 million for hospitals and public health clinics, $55.8 million for long-term care facilitities, $16.9 million for diagnostic and treatment centers, $9.7 million for rehabilitation facilities, and $3.9 million for operations and technical services. *Catalog of HEW Assistance Programs Providing Financial Support and Service to States, Communities, Organizations, Individuals,* Department of Health, Education, and Welfare (Washington, D.C., 1969), pp. 6.5.1–5. See also Anne R. Somers, *Hospital Regulation: The Dilemma of Public Policy* (Princeton, 1969), p. 135 and passim.

of health facilities, even though those facilities would have remained under private ownership, because of continuing leverage on the health system through state control of both capital and operating funds. As it was, the construction grants were passed in a vacuum.

Despite the impressive figures, both the funds and the authority of the Hill-Burton program have been limited. Hill-Burton funds, while substantial, have been small compared to the present annual expenditure (public and private) of $2.4 billion on construction of medical facilities. And the program has applied only to assisting in the building, equipping, and (later) modernizing of facilities on the basis of special application by institutions. In large part hospitals choosing to ignore the state plan have been free to develop as they wished. The tide is now beginning to turn, as states such as Rhode Island, New York, and Connecticut are imposing state controls over further hospital expansion, through licensing, bonding authority and other means. But the process has barely begun. For the most part, the states have played a vestigial role in hospital planning and coordination. The impact of Hill-Burton itself has been to improve the distribution of beds and other facilities within the states, without necessarily linking the hospitals together to provide joint services, or affiliating them with other service institutions or medical schools.

The deficiencies and modesties of the Hill-Burton program became increasingly evident as efforts were made from the mid-1960s to relate the various facets of health care—that is, to link health payment schemes with the development of facilities, research, and manpower production. President Johnson expressed alarm in his health and education message of 1 March, 1965 because one-third of the nation's hospital beds were in "obsolete condition," and he rightly predicted that when Medicare came into effect the pressures on many hospitals would "grow even more intense." [22] By 1967, hospital services in the major cities were reaching a point of breakdown. A study by the Department of Health, Education, and Welfare estimated that the cost of modernizing New York City hospitals was $1.25 billion; the city had received only $17.5 million from the Hill-Burton program.[23] Similar concern was being expressed in other major cities. In Chicago, the Hospitals Planning Council estimated that the sum of $255 million was needed for hospital modernization; so far the city had received only $14.1 million in Hill-Burton funds. In Boston, a major reconstruction of the Boston City Hospital was estimated to cost $90 million within ten years; and the Massachusetts

22. Presidential message, *Congressional Quarterly Almanac, 1965,* p. 1256.
23. Ibid., 1967, p. 451.

General Hospital estimated its ten-year capital needs as $70 million, if the money could be obtained.[24] Overall, there was an estimated need for $10 billion for modernization of hospitals, let alone for effective expansion of services to meet the additional demands of Medicare.[25] The sheer size of these figures gives pause for reflection about future responsibility for shoring up a complex of more than 7,000 hospitals, whose annual budget now exceeds $20 billion, and whose charges are the major component of the inflationary costs of medical care.

In terms of its regional aspirations, the Hill-Burton legislation also sadly failed. In character with the ad hoc assistance approach of federal health legislation, other fragmented federal subsidies also developed. The entry of the Small Business Administration into hospital construction has already been noted. There are at least seven federal health construction programs besides Hill-Burton, involving six federal departments or agencies. In all, federal expenditures for construction of hospitals and health facilities rose from $470 million in 1968 to an estimated $712 million in 1971.[26] A report to President Johnson on health facilities published in December 1968, just as that administration was leaving office, recommended that instead of the isolated program of federal construction grants, there should be a deliberate development of systems for the delivery of comprehensive health care.[27] This suggestion has acquired a new importance in current proposals for health maintenance organizations.[28] Hill-Burton itself has also been under fire from the Nixon administration. Secretary of Health, Education, and Welfare, Robert Finch, proposed in March 1969 a "radical redirection" of the grants program to one of guaranteed loans to stimulate private capital to modernize outdated facilities, together with block grants to encourage state expansion and coordination of health facilities.[29] So far efforts by the administration to change Hill-Burton from its emphasis on grants to

24. Testimony of Dr. John Knowles, General Director, Massachusetts General Hospital, *Health Care in America*, p. 700.
25. Robert M. Ball, "Problems of Cost—As Experienced in Medicare," in USDHEW, *Report of the National Conference on Medical Costs* (Washington, D.C., 1967), p. 65.
26. Construction aid is available indirectly through Medicare and Medicaid, and directly through mental health centers, OEO health centers, and programs through the Department of Housing and Urban Development, the Small Business Administration, the Economic Development Administration, the District of Columbia, the Veterans Administration, and the Department of Defense. See *Health Activities*, pp. 8, 28–29, and passim.
27. *National Advisory Commission on Health Facilities, Report*, pp. 68–70.
28. See Chapter 19.
29. For a report on the debates, see *Congressional Quarterly Almanac, 1969*, pp. 868–70.

one on loans has met with considerable congressional (and AMA) resistance. Meanwhile, the questions of both central and local coordination of construction resources—health facilities planning—remain vital to future health care development.

THE FEDERAL ROLE: REGIONALISM

Medicare has encouraged some cooperation between hospitals and nursing homes, in terms of agreement for transferring elderly patients from one to the other. Such agreements have, however, been of minimal success, either in pulling hospital and nursing homes closer together or in establishing coordinated policies for hospital or nursing-home utilization. There are also continuing attempts, through the private initiative of hospitals and through federal regional Medicare programs and comprehensive planning agencies, to begin to pull health care institutions together. Again, so far all these efforts have been only partially successful.

University-based regional medical programs surfaced as a possible framework for restructuring the American hospital system in the Eighty-ninth Congress, around President Johnson's personal interest in heart disease, cancer, and stroke.[30] President Johnson established an ad hoc President's Commission on Heart Disease, Cancer, and Stroke, in March 1964 under the chairmanship of Michael DeBakey, a noted heart surgeon from Houston, Texas. The commission's report, published in December 1964, set out a program of "frontal assault" on problems directly related

30. The Hill-Burton program was posited on filling in the gaps in hospital facilities in relation to the population. The primary conceptual motivation of university-centered hospital regions is the distribution and coordination of scarce specialist services across a substantial service region, coupled with a free exchange of knowledge and specialist personnel. University-based regionalism was as fashionable a concept in this country as in Britain in the years before World War II, but there was no health service framework through which it might be put into effect. Before the war, Tufts Medical College stood alone in effective medical school commitment to the regional concept, through its system of affiliations among hospitals, spreading from Boston deep into rural New England. In the 1940s there were two other notable private experiments. The Commonwealth Fund, long interested in providing hospitals in rural areas, selected Rochester, N.Y. as a demonstration area for a regional hospital plan in 1945, linking medical school and hospitals. The Hunterdon Medical Center originated as an idea in 1946 and was opened in 1953, linking the staff of a rural hospital in New Jersey with the New York University-Bellevue Medical Center. A number of universities also began to develop regional postgraduate educational schemes for practicing physicians. But there was little inducement to do more than this until the 1965 legislation. See Leonard S. Rosenfeld and Henry B. Makover, *The Rochester Regional Hospital Council*; Ray E. Trussell, *Hunterdon Medical Center;* David A. Pearson, *Regional Medical Care: An Inquiry into Conceptual Development and Application with Suggested Characteristics for Future Programs,* unpublished Ph.D. dissertation, Yale University, 1970.

to these diseases, including a national, regionalized network of facilities for patient care, teaching, and research based on university medical centers.[31] In addition, it made wider recommendations for increasing health resources, including the development of manpower programs, the expansion of health research facilities, the development of a medical libraries network, the extension of funds for stimulating health service planning and coordination, and a strengthened and coordinated health policy leadership within the Department of Health, Education, and Welfare. Together these recommendations were designed to provide a framework for disseminating medical knowledge to physicians and patients in order to reduce the impact of heart disease, cancer, and stroke—the nation's three major causes of death. But they might also have provided a federally subsidized regional hospital system, consisting of a network of both private and public hospitals.

The legislation (signed in 1965 as P.L. 89-239) was, however, attenuated during its passage through Congress, and in discussions with administration officers and the AMA. Medicare was in the process of passage, and the Johnson administration was keenly aware of the need for professional cooperation. The amendments resulting from these meetings, together with other amendments arising in the Congress, led to strong statements barring construction of new buildings under the legislation, thus emphasizing the role of the legislation as one of coordinating existing institutions into "regional medical programs" instead of the "regional medical complexes" in the original bill. At the same time, the title of the bill was changed to heart disease, cancer, and stroke "and related diseases" instead of "other major diseases." Under the legislation also regional medical programs (like Medicare) were supposed avowedly not to interfere with existing patterns of medical practice, forms of financing, or hospital administration. Such phrases were scarcely those of major coordination of facilities or reform. The grants for regional medical programs have, however, provided a carrot to encourage voluntary regional planning through cooperative arrangements between medical schools, hospitals, and other appropriate institutions or agencies, with the results dependent on the relative degree of institutional concern from one region to the next.[32] The prospects for university-based

31. President's Commission on Heart Disease, Cancer, and Stroke, *Report to the President: A National Program to Conquer Heart Disease, Cancer, and Stroke,* 2 vols. (Washington, D.C., 1964–65), vol. 1.
32. The activities of regional medical programs include continuing education and training, chiefly for physicians; demonstrations of patient care, such as the development of mobile and in-hospital coronary care units; research and development activities; and planning, coordinative, and evaluative activities, such as the development

regional medical systems are thus ambivalent; the structure is there but it has no teeth.

Meanwhile an alternative, and in some respects competing, federally assisted planning model has been developing in the prospect of areawide and state planning of both hospitals and non-hospital services and facilities. This movement stemmed in part from the widely distributed report, *Health is a Community Affair*, published in 1966 and sponsored by the American Public Health Association and the National Health Council, both private health organizations.[33] The report stressed that communities, a concept defined in terms of a community of solution rather than existing political boundaries, should be responsible for providing comprehensive health services (from detection of disease to rehabilitation, and including environmental control, accident prevention, family planning, and health service information); that each state should have a single official health agency with enough funds to provide a complete range of health

---

of regional data systems, and cooperative arrangements among hospitals. But the prospects for the latter are dim without the possibility of considerably increased authority and funding. The one major success of the program so far is the stimulation of activities for medical education, an area in which medical schools and hospitals can comfortably combine. Indiana University School of Medicine for example used the framework of regional medical planning to design a comprehensive statewide plan to integrate undergraduate, graduate, and continuing medical education. The University of Oklahoma School of Medicine set out to design a multi-institutional health center, in which health service, educational, and research agencies would voluntarily relocate in a functional relationship to the medical center. A number of other programs have been considering setting up programs of itinerant seminars around the state, or stimulating university interest in providing teaching in community hospitals, and are making major efforts to link the aims of the medical societies and the teaching institutions. Over and above this important educational activity, it remains to be seen how far regional medical programs, with the power to educate and stimulate rather than to effect change, will in fact encourage widespread coordination of hospitals and other facilities, and their more effective utilization. For information on programs, see U.S. Department of Health, Education, and Welfare, Division of Regional Medical Programs, "Directory of Regional Medical Programs," *News, Information, Data,* 15 July 1969.

33. The report was written by the National Commission on Community Health Services, set up in 1962 under the chairmanship of Marion Folsom, former secretary of Health, Education, and Welfare. Financed by three foundations and two government agencies, it set up a program of review and study of community health needs, through three advisory committees, six task forces, four regional forum committees, and four community research teams. The study was ambitious, perhaps too ambitious, for it did not produce its final report until April 1966; meanwhile the DeBakey commission had been set up, reported, and had at least some of its recommendations translated into legislation. Once launched, the final report, supported by a number of more detailed publications, quickly absorbed congressional attention. See National Commission on Community Health Services, *Health is a Community Affair, Report of the National Commission on Community Health Services* (Cambridge, Mass., 1966).

services; that there should be effective local planning of community health services; and that one goal of such planning should be to enable every individual to have a personal physician.

The report's key recommendations were ultimately translated into a legislative request. President Johnson called for a program of grants to states to plan for comprehensive health services in his domestic and education message of 1 March, 1966. An administration bill, described as Partnership for Health, was introduced the following day; the bill was signed into law, with few changes during its congressional passage, in November 1966 as the Comprehensive Health Planning and Service Act, P.L. 89-749. This act consolidated preexisting project and formula grants to states through a new system of grants for comprehensive health services, effective in fiscal year 1968. The legislation stipulated a program of federal, state, and local planning for comprehensive health services, including the promotion of local health services. In signing the bill President Johnson underlined the intent of the new legislation as being to "broaden the whole base of our state and local health programs," and to "bring them into line with the achievements of 20th century medicine." [34] The comprehensive health planning agencies offer a needed focus for local coordination of health institutions and personnel into an effective and economic network of service. By July 1969, fifty-two statewide and territorial agencies had been funded under the act, together with ninety-seven areawide health planning agencies. Most, however, are still engaged in developing the appropriate councils and committees, in setting up procedures and protocols for future development, and in developing health planning information. [35]

Like the regional medical programs, the comprehensive health planning agencies (when they exist) have little clout, in the form of available funding of facilities and services, or authority. The legislation provides available federal assistance in the form of grants which will underpin preexisting and necessary local initiative. As with Hill-Burton, NIH grants programs, and other federal categorical programs, the new programs help most those who are most ready to be helped. Comprehensive health planning agencies, with community participation, investment (in the form of matching funds), and control, provide important nuclei for change. But without major changes in health care funding, it is doubtful

34. Quoted in *Congressional Quarterly Almanac, 1966,* p. 325.
35. See Donna Anderson and Nancy N. Anderson, *Comprehensive Health Planning in the States: a Current Status Report,* American Rehabilitation Foundation, Minneapolis 1969; Lana B. Stone, *From Organization to Operation: The Evolving Areawide Comprehensive Health Planning Scene,* Ibid., 1969.

whether they will achieve much more than is being achieved in community agencies which are not federally subsidized, such as community councils or the eighty or more older, private areawide health planning agencies.[36] Like other aspects of federal health policy, health planning has been accepted in theory, but applied only half-heartedly.

THE FEDERAL ROLE: BRINGING MEDICAL CARE TO THE PEOPLE

Federal subsidies for health facility construction and regional or area planning may be grouped with federal grants for medical research and training as a process of developing and sustaining health care resources. On the one hand, the government helps to develop necessary buildings and planning networks, on the other the advancement of basic knowledge and the production of professionals to improve and staff decentralized services. Such programs would continue to be necessary in a scheme of national health insurance. A scheme based on capitation payments to established health maintenance organizations or systems might include a factor for capital financing and modernization as part of the capitation arrangement. But even so there would still need to be machinery for subsidizing construction (and perhaps operation of service) in needy areas, and for stimulating organizational demonstrations and experiments. The major current proposals for national health insurance also assume that manpower development—at least of health professionals—would also remain as a separate national funding program, as would grants for biomedical research. In concrete terms, there might be a national health insurance board, with associated but separate councils for health facilities, manpower, and research. But, as the experience of the 1950s showed,

36. The voluntary hospital council, linking local hospitals for joint discussion of their own interests was a feature of the 1930s. With the expansion of Blue Cross plans in the 1940s and 1950s discussions among hospitals through their state hospital associations also became important vehicles for negotiating hospital reimbursement formulae. But these were functions of trade associations, not planning agencies. Areawide planning of hospitals over large metropolitan areas received widespread publicity in 1961 with the publication of a joint committee report by the American Hospital Association and the U.S. Public Health Service of guidelines for agency organization, followed by a joint report on areawide planning for long-term care facilities two years later. The agencies themselves have been most effective in cities with clear-cut power structures, whose authority can be exerted through the direction of large donations of money into local hospitals and other institutions. See *Areawide Planning for Hospitals and Related Health Facilities,* a Report of the Joint Committee of the American Hospital Association and the Public Health Service, USPHS, Publication no. 885 (Washington, D.C., 1961); *Areawide Planning of Facilities for Long-term Treatment and Care,* USDHEW, USPHS, Publication no. 930-B-1 (Washington, D.C., 1963); Somers, *Hospital Regulation,* pp. 137–38.

the process of investment in health resources alone does not automatically lead to the development of adequate health services; and during the 1960s there were two major thrusts for more direct federal involvement in health care provision. The first was the movement for increased federal programs for the purchase of medical care which led to Medicare and Medicaid. The second was a rather different but interconnected movement to bring medical services directly to the people, or at least to one or another group of specified people whose cause was socially and politically urgent. There developed from 1963 to 1966 a rapid series of federal medical care programs. Few of the new programs were coordinated with any of the others, for they sprang from different sources and were enacted for a variety of reasons, including presidential interest.

It has almost become customary in the United States for the president to espouse a special health cause or disease. President Truman endorsed national health insurance; President Eisenhower lent his weight to public expenditures on biomedical research and education. President Kennedy pressed for services to the elderly and the mentally ill, and ultimately became the "father" of the mental health and mental retardation center. (Later, President Johnson espoused Medicare, heart disease, cancer and stroke, and other health legislation; and President Nixon is pleading the cause of family health insurance as a plank in his welfare reform program.)

Concern over the inadequate and sometimes appalling status of mental health services led to the authorization by Congress in 1955 of a study of mental health facilities, services, and problems. The subsequent report from the Joint Commission on Mental Illness and Health, published in 1961, more than justified this concern. State mental hospitals were custodial rather than treatment institutions, dumping grounds for those whom society had rejected. It was recommended that there should be a national mental health program under which federal funds would be used both to construct facilities and to treat patients. The large impersonal mental hospitals, often more akin to a prison or army barracks than a hospital, would be broken down into, and replaced by, compact and intensive community treatment centers, through which preventive and rehabilitative services would be developed for psychiatric care. President Kennedy's special message on mental health of 5 February 1963 provided the opportunity to develop these themes, and later the same year, with little opposition in either chamber, Congress enacted two major administration proposals which together provided federal matching grants for the development of community mental health centers and mental retardation facilities, and for associated programs for planning, teaching, and research.[37] With this legislation, a new type of health facility was born.

The community mental health center and the community mental retardation center brought organized psychiatric services into the city; they did no less than recognize the reversal of the ancient process of segregation of the mentally ill—preferably in a safe building conveniently out of town. Moreover the centers were intended to serve a defined population, somewhere between 75,000 and 200,000 persons. As part of this process of localizing mental health, a new specialty, social psychiatry, was born, whose laboratory was the classroom and the street, rather than the hospital or private psychiatrist's office. Thus the community mental health center offered an institutional focus for a new movement. There are now almost 400 such centers, spread over the whole country, and offering services to more than 50 million people.[38] But at the same time, the separation of mental health facilities and planning from the development of other health services served to emphasize the ultimate need to develop coordinated policies and plans for health services, at the national, state, and local levels. A further categorical or specialized approach to medical care was provided in the project grants for women in low-income families to receive comprehensive maternity and infant care, as part of the program to prevent mental retardation. Between 1964 and 1970, 55 such projects received support for prenatal and postnatal services.[39] These various projects reflected multiple sources of interest in health services, but the result was a form of congressional dilettantism. Nor was the end by any means in sight.

With increased political awareness of social deprivation in the early 1960s, and with no overall system offering the possibility of good medical

37. The report, *Action for Mental Health,* was published by Basic Books. The Mental Retardation Facilities Construction Act (title I of P.L. 88-164) authorized initial federal grants of up to 75 percent of the costs of constructing research facilities and clinical facilities for treatment of the mentally retarded; this was to be replaced from 1965 with federal formula grants to states for construction costs. The Community Mental Centers Act (title II of P.L. 88-164) authorized federal grants to states for construction of public or private community health centers for the mentally ill in their own communities. The act also contained grants for research and training purposes. The Maternal and Child Health and Mental Retardation Planning Amendments of 1963, P.L. 88-156, authorized a new program of grants to public health agencies for prenatal care for the poor; it also included an appropriation to states for increasing public awareness of mental retardation services and coordinating resources and community activities in the sphere of mental retardation.
38. The average first year grant to a typical center for staffing was $283,000; the average construction assistance, $450,000. *Catalog of HEW Assistance Programs,* (1969).
39. Kissick, "Health Policy Directions," p. 1347.

care to the whole population, came the discovery of other needy population groups, each discovery adding another layer to the separate provision of medical care for different causes, localities, and people. Migrant farm workers and their families in California and other parts of the country had little or no opportunity for obtaining medical care. Their needs were at least partially served under legislation of 1962 (P.L. 87-692) which authorized funds for family health clinics and other health services specifically for migrant workers; hospital care was added in 1965. Cuban refugees were another group given special congressional treatment for medical care, through the Migration and Refugee Assistance Act of 1962 (P.L. 87-510). Grants for the construction and operation of health facilities were authorized for another special poverty group in the Appalachian Regional Development Act of 1965 (P.L. 89-4). Medicare and Medicaid offered improved medical care for the elderly, who were also, inter alia, served by community planning and coordination of programs in the Older Americans Act of 1965 (P.L. 89-73). Grants for neighborhood and community centers, and health stations, in the Housing and Urban Development Act (P.L. 89-117) added to the growing array of special services to low-income groups. They were joined, in the apogee of legislation of the Eighty-ninth Congress, by grants for comprehensive health services or centers for children and youth in the 1965 Social Security amendments (P.L. 89-97) and other programs to develop home health programs and to expand vocational rehabilitation and other special services.

Meanwhile, the neighborhood health center was also developing, offspring of President Johnson's War on Poverty legislation, the Economic Opportunity Act of 1964 (P.L. 88-452). The poverty programs did not initially include medical services as a separate program, but many of the early plans submitted to the Office of Economic Opportunity for Community Action Programs included some elements of health programs, and there was a strong lobby led by Dr. Jack Geiger of Tufts to press for a new program of neighborhood health services. As a result, in 1965, the fragmented approach to health services in OEO was replaced by endorsement of the development of comprehensive neighborhood health centers, specifically designed to tackle the problem of poverty. Such centers were to offer a full range of ambulatory services, work in liaison with other community services, have close working relations with a hospital (preferably one with a medical school affiliation), and, as far as possible, involve the local population in planning, operating, and working in the center. These aims, including the medical school affiliation, were those of the first funded center, under Tufts University College of Medicine in 1965. They were followed by the development of centers in many other parts of the country, including Mound Bayou, Mississippi, the Watts District of Los Angeles, the Bronx in New York, and other locations and cities. Again, selection was by the applicants rather than by the federal agency. In 1970, federal funding was being made to forty-nine OEO neighborhood health centers, serving an estimated 500,000 people a year.[40] These centers thus provide health services to a tiny minority of the poor; they are, moreover, still in an experimental stage, and the prospects of their long-term funding remain in doubt. Nevertheless these, too, like the community mental health centers, represent a new focus for medical practice—and could provide a new long-term source of federal funding for the complex of health resources.

The federal government is now funding a total of 517 health centers, through $289 million in project grants, and serving nearly 2 million persons (1 percent of the population).[41] The great majority of centers do not however offer either comprehensive medical care or care to all age groups in the population. Besides the 49 OEO centers, there are 298 mental health centers, 115 maternal and child health centers, and another 35 general health care centers under Partnership for Health. Responsibility for OEO health centers is shifted from OEO to DHEW when they are fully operational. The objectives of these centers vary. The OEO neighborhood health center, in particular, is only partly concerned with medical care, but is also involved in job training and other aspects of community development. In some respects the rubric of health has been used as a convenient and acceptable device to shelter non-health-related objectives. At the same time the concept of the health center (the old concept of a dispensary or clinic, not a particularly new development) has added a further dimension to the development of American health care resources. The number of persons served in health centers is the equivalent of more than a third of the number of people who are members of prepaid group practice. They are, however, largely different populations, for the idea of bringing medical care to deprived groups has had as a corollary the establishment of separate types of medical organization—the opposite of Medicaid's early assertion to bring everyone into the mainstream of medicine.

The new programs added categories to a system which was already

40. For a useful account of the personalities and issues involved in the development of the OEO neighborhood health center, see Sar Levitan, *The Great Society's Poor Law: A New Approach to Poverty* (Baltimore, 1969), pp. 191–205.
41. *Health Activities*, p. 31.

split into numerous components. Most of the services are contingent on the potential recipient falling into an appropriate category, as a veteran, a crippled child, an Indian, a merchant seaman, a migrant, a Cuban, an Appalachian, a pre-school or school-age child, a person sixty-five years old or over, a resident of an approved low-income area. Thus, while the governmental role has been expanding it has been doing so through setting up a series of programs which rarely take account of other programs. Each new program, while extending the range of available services, has added to the system new requirements, qualifications, and barriers, or (like Medicare) has had inflationary characteristics. Programs for resource development and coordination, particularly regional medical programs and comprehensive health planning, have not yet had the funding to influence existing patterns. The mentally sick go to one building, the poor to another, veterans to a third—all set up under the influence of federal funding; yet avoidance of fragmentation has been very low on the priority list of the federal medical establishment. Diffuse responsibility at the federal level has if anything led to ever increased diffusion of services locally.

BOUNDARIES OF FEDERAL RESPONSIBILITY

Organizational diffusion is of course not necessarily undesirable; it may denote a richness of experiment with new forms of service, allow individual patients to have a wide choice of different facilities, and offer the opportunity for constructive competition among various health care schemes, organizations, and agencies. National planning is not necessarily a valid criterion for efficiency. Well-organized neighborhood, citywide, or multicity health systems, whether under public or private auspices, may offer services which are far superior to any nationally organized service system. The experience of independent health insurance plans built around group medical practices, offering a wide range of health services to a defined population, has demonstrated the feasibility in the United States of the development of health services of good quality and reasonable cost through private initiative and effort. The Kaiser Foundation Health Plans were by 1970 covering 927,000 people in northern California, 835,000 in southern California, 126,000 in Oregon, 76,000 in Hawaii, 40,000 in Ohio and 3,000 in Colorado; the Health Insurance Plan of Greater New York had an enrollment of 757,000; Group Health Cooperation of Seattle, 122,000; Community Health Association in Detroit, 74,000; Group Health Association of Washington,

D.C., 72,000 people.[42] Such plans offer a medical care "package" on a local basis which is similar to (if less extensive than) the national health schemes available through the government in western Europe. In both cases members of the population covered by the plan are entitled, for a standard annual payment (whether collected through direct contribution, through employer-employee benefit contracts, or through tax), to a specified range of services, including physician services and hospitalization. For most people in the United States, however, the assumptions on which medical care is provided have not changed since World War I, when there were similar discussions of the need to coordinate the health care system as well as to finance individual medical care. There is still a disorganized system of private practitioners for the comparatively affluent, a disorganized clinic system for the poor, and a mixture for those who fall between.

There is no blueprint of how a health service system should be constructed. Given the pluralistic nature of American health care institutions, the continually shifting body of technological knowledge, the existence of regional and local differences in health care resources (and perhaps also in the relative financial and social value put on health services by members of the population), one ideal system may never be attainable, and is probably undesirable. General or multispecialist medical firms, health maintenance organizations, hospital-based group practices, and regional health networks are terms which encompass a wide variety of practical implications. In one place, a hospital may expand its outpatient department into a well-organized health service unit. In another, several hospitals will join together to sponsor a system of community medical care through affiliated centers or multispecialist clinics. In a third, effective coordination of services may be provided through comprehensive health insurance in private practice, buttressed by well-organized computerized information and records systems and quality control of available services. In a fourth, physicians in partnership will set up new practice networks and programs, employing appropriate staffs and subcontracting for services that they themselves cannot provide. In one area, leadership for change may be generated by state or local health departments, in another by a medical society, boards of hospitals, community action groups, or industrial leadership, or by a combination of one or more of these.

At the same time, however, the specific organizational forms of any

42. Marjorie Smith Mueller and Maureen Dwyer, "Private Health Insurance Plans Other than Blue Cross, Blue Shield and Insurance Company Plans, 1969," *Research and Statistics Note,* 24 Dec. 1970.

health system are in large part dictated, or at least molded, by preexisting organizational structures, professional traditions, and political realities. The appropriate role of the federal government is a crucial issue in current debates, for the government could act in a variety of capacities, ranging from that of administrator of a comprehensive national health insurance scheme (as under the current Health Security proposals) to that of a financial collection and standard-setting agency (as under Medicredit). Decisions have yet to be made whether financing or subsidy should be through general taxation, Social Security taxation, private insurance plans, or a combination of two or more of these; whether the whole population should be covered, or merely those most in financial need; whether a new plan should absorb or complement Medicare; whether other federal programs designed to stimulate health care resources, such as Hill-Burton or grants to medical schools or neighborhood health centers, would remain separate from the health insurance program; what, if any, central controls, policies, standards and public guarantees of service should be set up for the program; and how far a national health insurance scheme, no matter how the money is collected for its financing, should attempt to be more than a bill-paying mechanism and attempt to guide and restructure the health care system.

These questions are implicit in all the current proposals for national health insurance. Under the tax credit proposals there would be a federally organized program of national health insurance, fairly heavily subsidized from general taxation but administered (as is Medicare) through private insurance plans and companies. A national health insurance advisory board would set guidelines for states to follow in approving plans which would qualify under the system. This board, backed up by the states, could establish services to be covered, and even contribution rates, and thus affect the form of medical practice. At the same time there could be substantial federal control of services and standards through a national network of professional review organizations run by the medical societies. How far such controls would be exerted from the federal level is a matter for speculation. Less directly, the availability to the whole population of a broad health insurance policy, thus giving each person (at least in theory) equivalent buying power and potential demand for services, would also be expected to affect the supply structure of medical care. But there would be no direct attempt to use the financing mechanism to modify the health care system.

Under all of the proposals, however modifications of the system are inevitable, for the hodge-podge of services, programs and facilities which now form American health services cannot readily adjust to the increased demand which would be released through any extended health payment program. The current proposals for national health insurance being supported by Rep. Martha Griffiths and Sen. Edward Kennedy would rationalize the federal roles in health payment and in health care provision by joining them together. Thus the Griffiths proposal would set up national and regional health insurance boards; the latter would contract for services with providers, assisted by professional and consumer advisory groups. The regional offices would also be involved in keeping records of patients, disseminating information about the rights of beneficiaries and providers, maintaining effective relationships with providers, planning and allocating funds for construction of facilities and for manpower development, and for generally overseeing health services in the region.[43] The regional framework would also form a natural channel for the disbursement of federal funds for health services which remain outside the insurance proposals; the emphasis for health care might thus shift from federal intervention on the one hand and local programs on the other to strong regional organizations. Proposals which do not set up such an administrative framework for channeling funds, such as Medicredit, would leave existing federal programs in their present state of chaos. While Medicredit would absorb much if not all of Medicaid, it would retain Medicare and presumably a host of other existing, uncoordinated, construction and assistance programs. The need for coordinating these programs would thus remain. Indeed, the passage of Medicredit would probably have to be matched by a strengthening of federal authority in relation to other government programs. Thus the proposal which appears to have the least immediate impact on the health care system may in the long run lead to the greatest degree of administrative centralization.

This observation points up a problem inherent in present discussions of alternative programs; the debates on the proper role and authority of the federal government (more concretely, of the Department of Health, Education, and Welfare or of a new health agency) continue to be dogged by uncertain rhetoric. The phrases "laissez faire" and "regulation" applied to health services tend to appear as if they are alternatives, somewhat along the lines of capitalism versus socialism. Yet the distinction is dangerously simplistic. Laissez faire in many other industries has led not to small-scale, decentralized local industries (of which the parallel in present medical care technology is the health maintenance organization) but to highly regulated chains, mergers, and national corporations. The issue here is not one of regulation per se, but of whether regulation is best exerted by the private or the public sector, for example by

43. H.R. 15779, 91st Cong., 2d sess., Title VI.

the insurance companies or by a government agency. Laissez faire is also often used to imply elements of free-market competition; in turn, competition presupposes well-informed consumers, making an enlightened choice of purchases from competing suppliers. As has been remarked, these conditions do not hold in the health care industry. In particular, consumer information about health insurance entitlements, accessible health services, relative costs and quality, is generally less available in America than in countries that have "socialized" medical systems.

Finally, the federal role itself has been oddly interpreted. There seems to have been a feeling that the proper role of government in health is one not of efficiency but weakness, not of planning but of grantsmanship, not of statesmanship but of irresponsibility. The curious result has been that the federal role in health has been distinguished by minimal consumer protection and public accountability.

Yet it is evident that to promote the supposed advantages of private enterprise—including decentralized control of health services, competition among health systems, adequate public information, and other measures of consumer protection—a strong governmental role is essential. As it is, the clichés surrounding health care provision still stand in the way of free, constructive debate. It is to be hoped that one of the major achievements of the present political prominence of national health insurance will be to air the practical issues.

What are these issues? The first is the degree of commitment by the public, as represented in the Congress, to the provision of adequate health services at various levels of expected cost. This may seem obvious, but the fact that the United States does not yet have national health insurance reflects a degree of indifference on the subject which is obscured in committee presentations. At the time this book goes to press national health insurance is a "political issue," and a hot one in current debates. But even health insurance does not guarantee the availability of appropriate and effective services, and some commitments tend to be only partial and to diminish with time. Medicaid provides a stark example of public interest in "mainstream medical care" for the poor which sank in the quicksands of budgetary difficulties.

A second question which is still unanswered concerns the role of federal funding and/or direction in the development of local service systems, such as health maintenance organizations (or the current proposals for a larger area-wide coordination through grants to stimulate experimental health care delivery systems) which will assume collective responsibility for providing health services to a population or area. Third, there is the related regulation and development of manpower resources.

And finally there is the willingness to create strategic organizations responsible for developing federal policies in defined priority areas. In all of these instances there is already substantial de jure federal governmental responsibility through the present operation of the funding system. But there has been, at least as yet, relatively little de facto acceptance of a coordinated federal role in developing a nationally organized health care system.

The maze of existing health care legislation and the diffusion of responsibility for programs over so many agencies make coordination of efforts at the administrative level difficult, if not impossible, to achieve. A health service system, in the European sense, will be generated only through the Congress. But the signs of increasing congressional and political concern over health care problems reveal at least the beginnings of a movement for the more effective placing of federal tax dollars in the health care industry. Major reform may not be achieved for many years. Indeed, the confusion of federal programs and services may have to grow much worse before any serious overhauls are made. Nevertheless, eventually, the increased demand for health services, their rising costs, the lack of coordination of programs, will make a more directive notion of the federal role imperative.

CHAPTER 22

American Medicine and the Public Interest

The current situation in medical care in the United States is often referred to as one of crisis. The sense of crisis should be interpreted, however, not as one of imminent collapse of health services—the United States is well-stocked with personnel and facilities and can afford to spend even more on providing them—but as at a critical stage of health care development. Perhaps a more appropriate word is maelstrom. Ideas and proposals are whirling around in profusion, based on a variety of premises, and uncertain as to their ultimate importance and effect; in the confusion the hapless observer may fear to sink. It is precisely here that the historical perspective is important. There is a tendency in American social planning to assume that the past does not exist, or is irrelevant. In health services there is a fashionable pursuit of newness. Enormous efforts are being made to come up with innovative ideas and new solutions. But history is, after all, a review of past politics which influence, if they do not predetermine, present events. Out of the long evolution of professionalism in medicine in the United States, and out of the concurrent definition of the public interest have emerged certain dominant attitudes and patterns which will continue to influence health care development.

In most, if not all countries, whether they have national health insurance or not, the organization of the health system lies as a direct outgrowth of the history and culture of the medical profession. The United States is no exception. Basic patterns of medical care organization, including the relationships between physicians and hospitals and between generalists and specialists, long antedate the growth of what we like to call modern medicine. Professional evolution, interrelationships, attitudes and power structures have had, and continue to have a potent influence on the particular forms of health services, even today. Yet at the same time, political and social pressures on the health system are equally a reflection of the society within which the system operates. The whole current movement toward national health insurance and the dominant shapes which this takes are part of a separate stream of development inside (and outside) the Congress. This stream is influenced not so much by any aspect of the professional history of medicine as by the equally gradual emergence of political attitudes toward welfare and other social services, by the process of legislation and legislative reform in a field of enormous governmental complexity, and above all by the apparent inability of the market to provide health services at a reasonable price through the hallowed machinery of laissez-faire.

In the bad old days when medicine was barely or rarely efficacious, it was possible to consider questions of purely professional development in a context dissociated from social welfare politics. But the Flexner report was perhaps the last true example of this phenomenon. With the remarkable changes in the content and potential of medicine, from the mercantilist faith-healing of the nineteenth century, through the mystique and excitement of specialized medicine in the first half of the twentieth century, to the present age of chemotherapy and precision in techniques, the professional and political aspects of medicine have become inextricably intertwined. It is not the medical profession but Ralph Nader who is calling for tightening in the licensing of medical specialists.[1] The latest report from the Carnegie Commission on Higher Education calls for new types of medical schools and a shortening of the length of medical education; but it also puts particular emphasis on questions which are not within the scope of strictly "professional" responsibilities in the traditional sense of the term: questions such as cutting educational costs, improving the geographical distribution of physicians, and developing health manpower planning.[2] On the other hand the Senate Finance Committee, which has become Congress's chief watchdog of medical costs, has reported out a proposal for national health insurance to cover catastrophic medical bills which is much more conservative than proposals being made by the AMA.[3] The underlying pressures and influences are the same; old sterotypes exist no more.

1. An as yet unpublished preliminary draft by Dr. Robert S. McCleery, *One Life, One Physician* puts forth the recommendations of the Nader task force.
2. *Higher Education and the Nation's Health: Policies for Medical and Dental Education.* A Special Report and Recommendations by the Carnegie Commission on Higher Education (New York, 1970).
3. The proposal, introduced by Sen. Russell B. Long, would provide catastrophe coverage of 80% of all medical bills for any working family if its medical expenses exceeded $2000 a year. *The New York Times,* Dec. 8, 1970.

PATTERNS OF MEDICAL PROFESSIONALISM

The crisis in the professional structures of medicine should not be under-rated. As has been shown, the traditional functions of professionalism are in a period of cumulative stress; the medical profession is still evolving from its nineteenth century structure of a profession of generalists and adjusting to the technological demands of the twentieth century for stratification of the profession into specialties. The specialty certifying boards provide a partial but still tentative approach to the identification of specialists; the AMA coordinates regulation of training posts with the specialty associations; the medical schools are still at the stage of discussing their role in specialist education. The licensing structure for physicians meanwhile assumes that all physicians are omnicompetent. All of these aspects of professional development may change radically in the next two decades, in response to present activities within the professional organizations and pressures for change through external agents, including national health insurance.

Of more immediate importance are the organizational implications of the deep-seated and early development in the United States of a medical profession whose internal social relations are egalitarian. Elitism within the ranks of physicians has been rejected time and again in America: from the early efforts of John Morgan, through the battles over the establishment of the American College of Surgeons and other exclusive groups, to the present recognition of the family practitioner not as a different type of physician but as equal among an array of specialists. The resulting homogenization of medical practice has had effects which will affect politics, power structures and patterns of medical care in the future, as in the past, whatever the form of health care financing.

The first, and perhaps the most important aspect of professional egalitarianism is the future role of the generalist. It has been noted that the general practitioner has been imprisoned in a climate of professional development which has stressed, on the one hand, educational intellectuality and, on the other, an extraordinary freedom for individual physicians to practice a chosen specialty. One current observation is that one or both of these factors must change if the generalist is to be restored to a central place in American medicine. The present situation is one of uncertainty and experimental flirtation. The established scientifically oriented medical schools that set up family practice programs will find it difficult not to try to justify the field in terms of its scientific content— terms in which family medicine may find itself ranked behind the other specialties. In the hierarchy of professional prestige, family medicine may also find itself with curricula which are at least as long as those of other fields; this trend is evident in present specialist certification mechanisms. At the same time, paradoxically, new primary care roles are being developed outside the medical profession through the appearance in many parts of the country of physician assistant and nurse practitioner training programs, whose expertise in primary care may have been acquired in but a few months' formal education. While many of the graduates of these programs will work under the supervision of physicians rather than independently, the issue remains of the ethic as well as the role of the generalist in medicine.

Changing the milieu of practice to encompass the generalist is largely a matter of the form of health insurance and other legislative proposals which will be passed in the 1970s. Evaluating the intellectuality of medical education, length of curriculum, selection of students, encouragement of multiple-track teaching systems, and forms of graduate medical education is still largely the preserve of the professional institutions of medicine. At root these are questions of what, indeed, is a physician. And this question is as yet unanswered. The historical evidence suggests, however, a cyclical adjustment to the long-term effects of the Flexner report; a return in some respects to the educational and social variations in medicine (though not the standards) which were apparent in medical schools of a hundred years ago. In practical terms, this means real acceptance within the medical profession of a role for primary care per se, irrespective of its level of education; continuing and major realignments of curricula and attitudes in the medical schools; and coordinated professional policies for graduate medical education. In the process the long emphasis on standards (and "standardization") will be deemphasized. Quality of medical care will be assessed through services rendered (as through the existing peer review organizations) rather than through the level of the physician's education. It is to be emphasized, however, that to achieve this degree of flexibility, authoritative organizations are necessary. As noted in the various chapters of this book, there is a need for a coordinating policy council for medical schools, an effective specialist manpower council with influence over patterns of graduate education, and (not least) a network of peer review mechanisms. The question of general practice thus ties in to the whole spectrum of professional (and public) regulation.

The uncertain future role of the generalist in American medicine is one result of the heritage of professional egalitariansm in medicine. The relation between physicians and health care institutions is another. The early open-staff arrangements for physicians in America has meant that hospitals form a much more natural focus for medicine in this country than, for example, in England. While closed-staff health care systems are predicted in this country as elsewhere as the pattern of the future, the hospital will play an important role in how these systems develop. On the one hand is the continuing potential of hospital-based service systems; on the other, the existence of hospital medical staffs as a powerful form of professional government, even where other forms of health care organization (such as existing third-party mechanisms, or medical society foundations) are prevalent.

A third continuing aspect of professional egalitarianism is the central role of the American Medical Association. In the absence of rival elitist professional associations, the AMA developed its power base out of both medical education and medical politics, functions which in many other countries are organizationally distinct. It has attempted to be both professional leader and professional representative. Despite the growth of specialties the AMA's centrality has been largely maintained; although from the late nineteenth century to the present, the AMA has been struggling to defend its position as the spokesman for organized medicine against the alternative foci of specialist organizations. But in the last few years, notably from 1966, this position has changed from one of rivalry and concern to one of joint working relationships.[4]

Present signs are that the AMA will become less of a spokesman for medical education and manpower development (the functions on which it rose to eminence); less of a protective trade association (its major public image from the 1920s through the early 1960s); and more of a negotiating body with government, and a governmental agent. In so doing its power will be strengthened, as will that of other groups of physicians.[5]

It is an obvious fact, but one that needs to be stressed, that no national health insurance scheme or local health service system can work effectively without the effective organization of the medical profession. Increasing organization of governmental programs means increasing organization of the medical profession. Even under the most sweeping form of

4. *Proc. H. of Del.* 21–25 June, 1970, p. 49. For example, the adoption in 1969 of a resolution which called on the AMA to coordinate all segments of the medical profession in its relation to the federal government, and the establishment in 1970 of a new department of specialty society services, with a full-time staff, with the office of the AMA Executive Vice-President. Representatives of national specialty groups now meet annually with the AMA Council on Legislation to discuss legislative policy development.

5. Those who would take issue with this statement are referred to Grant McConnell, *Private Power and American Democracy* (New York, 1967), especially chap. 5; and Corinne Lathrop Gilb, *Hidden Hierarchies, the Professions and Government* (New York, 1966), especially chap. 4.

national health insurance, organized physician groups acting as governmental agents would become more powerful rather than less. The professional structure of organized medicine in the United States suggests a potentially critical role for the AMA in administering a national and local health care program. Current patterns suggest AMA representation on national policy groups for medical education, manpower development, standards for health insurance payments, and professional discipline and sanctions in public medical programs. At the state and local level, the peer review movement may be expected to continue. Medical society foundations will continue to be developed for fee payments and control, as agents of public programs, and as a focus for the development of independent health insurance organizations under contract with the government.

The AMA rose as the spokesman of an undifferentiated, egalitarian profession. The structure of the specialties (and specialist regulation) is a fourth important result of early patterns of professionalism. Technological specialization was grafted onto a profession of generalists who were jealous of supposed rankings and insignia, whose mode of professional behavior was solo, private office practice, and who expected open access to hospitals. The specialty certifying boards still tend to regard themselves more as specialist associations than as quasi-licensing or manpower planning organizations. Thus, ironically, the strong professional authority over education and entry which was exerted over undergraduate education at the beginning of the century has not been transferred to control over specialization—at least as yet.

The existing imbalance of medical specialists in the United States has been frequently noted, among others by the President of the AMA.[6] It will become of crucial importance as public funds are used on the one hand for the extension of health insurance, and on the other for extended governmental subsidy of both graduate and undergraduate medical education. Past and present activities in the medical profession point to the necessary merger (or at least effective federation) of the specialty certifying boards into the existing American Board of Medical Specialties, and the strengthening of technical relationships between the certifying agencies and the National Board of Medical Examiners. Indeed, logically the two boards would eventually be affiliated. At the same time, an effective joint professional commission on medical education must finally be created. The most workable proposal now evident for the development of such a commission is an expansion of the existing liaison committee on medical education of the AMA and the AAMC into a strong organization dedicated to reviewing all aspects of medical education from undergradu-

6. Dr. Walter Bornemeier, *Proc. H. of Del.*, 21–25, June 1970, p. 32.

ate education to the education of practicing physicians. This committee's section on graduate medical education (successor to the idea of such a group as delineated in the Millis commission) would work closely with the specialty boards and medical schools; it would take responsibility for the existing residency review committees. Education itself will be the responsibility of the universities.

Manpower development per se is the function of government rather than the profession. Specific types of manpower will be developed through government grants and loans programs. These will probably include funds for medical schools to establish departments or programs of family practice or to focus their entire curriculum on community medicine; grants or loans for residency training in particular specialties; and control of the number of residency training posts in the specialties through certification of hospitals or health care systems for payment under public programs. All of these activities will be undertaken with or through the private organizations of medicine. Thus the existing machinery of professional accreditation has to be tightened to conform more nearly with specified service and manpower policies, which will in turn be developed through a national or regional public-private manpower committee. Specialty certification will also become more important if, as seems probable, it is incorporated as a basic standard of participation in health insurance organizations.

The days of endorsing licensing of specialists are long over; the problems of doing so today would be even more complex than when licensing was seriously considered in the 1920s. Relicensing of physicians in the specialties is, however, likely. It has the advantage of retaining the basic egalitarian license for all physicians, but also of recognizing the specialties, and (by no means last) of providing periodic re-evaluations. The most notable recent suggestion came in 1967 from the National Advisory Commission on Health Manpower. This suggested a system of relicensing physicians and other health professionals on the basis of acceptable performance in programs of continuing education or, for those who so elected, on the basis of challenge examinations in the practitioner's specialty.[7] As in earlier discussions of specialist qualifications, relicensing is logical only on a national basis; it assumes that physician licensing is federalized. But this move is also evident, both through the development of the profession's own FLEX examination as a standard test for state licensing boards,[8] and through the incorporation of federal medical licen-

7. *Report of the National Advisory Commission on Health Manpower,* vol. I, p. 41.
8. FLEX is a new medical licensure examination developed by the Federation of State Medical Boards which was first offered in June, 1968 by seven state medical

sure into legislative proposals for national health insurance. Again, under these changes professional organizations will gain in strength. Relicensing examinations will presumably be conducted by the specialty boards, and certification of participation in continuing medical education programs will be facilitated through the AMA's system of accrediting continuing education programs.

In all of these processes the expected change builds on established professional patterns. Indeed such changes might take place without concurrent social pressures for cost controls in medicine and for national health insurance. Without external pressures, however, the wheels of professional change grind slow. The specialty certifying boards might not decide to pool their resources and authority until (say) twenty years from now. The medical schools, through their affiliated hospitals, might become solely responsible for the residency training of physicians within ten years, but it might take them twenty-five years to develop their own coordinated undergraduate and graduate educational policies. By the end of the century, the profession's joint commission on medical education might be formulating specialist manpower goals and policies and carrying these out through the profession's related education and certification systems. But the present concern over the costs and availability of services cannot afford to wait that long. The social and political pressures on the structures of medical care are accelerating the professional process, and in doing so are urging on it new necessities.

SOCIAL AND POLITICAL IMPERATIVES

It is notable that, despite the political visibility of health issues in the 1970s, the actual ways in which health care might be provided are much more clearly defined by the medical profession than by any body of opinion in the Congress. This is in part because organized medicine has a centralized political structure in the AMA, while responsibility for health matters in the Congress is diffused among competing Congressional

---

boards in lieu of their own examination. The motivation behind FLEX was to provide a uniform and valid examination to evaluate clinical competence and qualification for licensure which could be adopted by all the state medical examining boards. As of April, 1970, 25 state boards had agreed to offer the FLEX examination instead of their own. An additional 10 state boards are favorably disposed to entering the FLEX program but most wait until state legislation is amended in order to participate. Although a special committee of the Federation has established a standard for reporting the FLEX scores so that all candidates' grades will be comparable from one state to another, each state may decide on its own passing level based on these standard scores, thus allowing for state autonomy while providing a uniform standard for measuring achievement.

committees. It is in large part, however, a reflection of the focus of the health insurance movement of the 1970s. The old generalisms about health care are less evident. Health care as a "right" has ceased to have a useful meaning. Does it imply a constitutional right, a moral right, a right for specified benefits under an insurance contract? In today's political context the answers are for practical purposes immaterial. Ray Lyman Wilbur, presenting the final report of the Committee on the Costs of Medical Care nearly forty years ago, could remark that "The quality of medical care is an index of civilization." [9] Such comments have an unreal ring in an age when we hesitate to put our socially-riven society in the context of an ideal "civilization," in which the mainspring of political action is necessity, and the watchword pragmatism.

The dominant political pressures for health insurance are not questions of service but of finance. Cost containment represents perhaps the greatest urgency. Linked with this are parallel discussions, particularly through discussions of welfare reform, of the role of health costs in income redistribution. Further down the line are measures designed to prevent particular groups from going under, such as emergency aid to medical schools, or measures for providing physicians in deprived urban and rural areas. Design of a health *service* per se, through the more effective use of resources, and with a goal of equal health care opportunity, are the primary goals of a minority. American political attitudes of the past as well as the present make it unlikely that health services will ever be viewed in this country as they are, for example, in England as a natural function of a welfare state.

As a result, public controls over the American health care system in the future will tend to be indirect. All of the present proposals for health insurance espouse the principle of decentralization and a minimum of federal intervention. These range from the tax credit and insurance company proposals which would subsidize private health insurance companies, to the proposals for health insurance through the Social Security system which presuppose the development of independent health care organizations at the local or city level. But the proposals, if enacted, may have curious results. It seems self-evident that the passage of a national health insurance scheme which relies on the purchase of individual policies through private insurance companies and minimal controls over the way services are provided will lead in progression to increasing chaos and costs in the health care system, to increasing federal control of the health insurance industry, and thence to increasing centralization. In contrast, proposals which now appear more radical (those sponsored by Senator

9. *Medical Care for the American People,* p. ix.

Kennedy and others, Rep. Martha Griffiths, and to a lesser degree by Senator Javits), could achieve a much greater degree of decentralized regulation by using the health insurance contract to stimulate local health care systems. In short a more courageous leap now into health insurance may lead eventually to a more "moderate" solution. The passage of Medicredit, all else being equal, might lead to socialized medicine within a decade.

For the low-income worker with inadequate health insurance, or for the woman on welfare whose only source of medical care is the busy and impersonal outpatient clinic of a general hospital, such arguments may seem unimportant. They are not; for the type of health insurance proposal which is passed will have one or another effect on the provision of services at the local level. Medicaid, for example, in theory provides equal medical care for the poor as is provided for other members of the population. In fact, welfare patients still largely receive medical care in places different from those used by the more affluent members of the population. National health insurance of itself will not necessarily stimulate more effective forms of health service organization; or it may do so in some areas but not in others.

The political imperatives, then, point toward the imminent extension of national health insurance in the United States. Its major impact will be on those of low and middle income. The social imperatives are less clearly defined. There is a long-term commitment to provide medical services to the poor; there is a recognition of the value of contributory health insurance as a means of risk-sharing; there is concern over the administrative complexity of existing health care programs; but there is little more than this. The general middle-class public has not mounted a lobby for the return of the family practitioner or for prepaid group practice systems. The present flurry of activity in designing local health care systems (a flurry which is by no means universal) derives chiefly from medical school sponsorship and from the foresight of professional and industrial leaders who see the development of health maintenance or comprehensive health care organizations as a logical, perhaps profitable, corollary of standardized health insurance packages. Such a movement will be more or less stimulated depending on the incentives and requirements built into a national health insurance system.

PROSPECT

On the basis of developing patterns of professionalism and of apparent political objectives, what may be the shape of health services in the year

2000 or even in 1980? Government-sponsored health insurance will be in operation. Depending on its success, control of health services will rest at the federal, regional or local level; but there will still be efforts to emphasize health insurance as insurance (that is, as a method for purchasing rather than reorganizing services), and to build effective decentralized systems of medical care. It would be unrealistic to assume a total sweep of traditions and institutions. A new health care system will not spring up overnight; it will, rather, arise out of, or in opposition to, existing institutions. The patterns peculiar to American medicine, developed over three centuries, are thus important in considering particular forms of development.

There are five prototypes for the development of local medical care systems in the United States. The first, and oldest, is the multispecialist group. Up to now the groups with the most visibility have been the large prepaid group practices, drawing their incomes from capitation and other payments at the local level. However, all groups could be "prepaid," in that they might contract to provide specified benefits through population enrollment in national health insurance. This is in essence the structure suggested for Medicare in the health maintenance option. Historically, the multispecialist group is a natural substitute for the old omnicompetent general practitioner.

A second prototype, again deriving from specific patterns of professional development in the United States, is the expansion of hospitals into comprehensive health service systems. In a sense this is the same process as specialist group practice based on hospitals, but this time in reverse. The hospital governing board and medical staff (the latter representing most if not all practicing physicians in the area) would reform and extend hospital ambulatory services, including substations of clinics or private office complexes in the community. To do this the hospital would develop its own insurance corporation which would contract for services with fiscal intermediaries or the government. This system is more complex than specialist group practice, for two reasons. One is that the specialized departmental structure obtaining in most large hospitals is an inappropriate professional structure for the organization of a medical care system whose focus would be primarily outside the hospital. The second is that community hospitals at present tend to serve a distinctive inpatient and outpatient clientele; inpatients are drawn from the community at large, while outpatients tend to be weighted with the poor. Nevertheless the hospital, as the most powerful and most organized institution in medical care does offer a focus of some magnitude. One possibility that could develop under national health insurance would be for the hospital to act as a general contracting organization, with indirect rather than direct control over non-hospital ambulatory care.

The neighborhood health center offers a third possible focus for contractual services under national health insurance, but one of much lesser magnitude. As developed, these centers have become foci only for deprived population groups. Their general development under governmental financing would emphasize a division between health services for the affluent and those for the poor. Such a division should not, however, be rejected out of hand, for the encouragement of such centers may be the only realistic way of bringing services to certain areas.

Primary care units form a fourth potential prototype for comprehensive care, but also one which at the present appears unlikely of general acceptance or development. A health system based on primary care units is being designed in Boston under the direction of Leonard Cronkhite. So far, however, this has only developed care of the relatively poor. How far primary medical care for the middle class will develop depends on professional enthusiasm for setting up such units (an enthusiasm which in the past has been notably lacking), and how far primary care is mandated into a scheme for national health insurance. Any bill which required patients to register with one primary physician would presumably generate interest in institutionalizing this form of care. Thus primary care might be organizationally distinguished from consultative specialist care, as is the case in most of Europe. Without such a mandate, there is little indication that physician primary care will develop outside multispecialist systems.

Finally, and of emerging interest, there is the development of health care networks tied together by a medical information system. This is a potentially important role for medical society foundations. The foundation could, for example, be a contract agency for national health insurance; through its central computer system it could develop as a potent educational force, as a peer review organization, and as a coordinator of care through the development of an areawide patient records system. The foundation could, indeed, also become a manpower planning agency through accepting or rejecting new physicians into the system and through stimulating new forms of practice and organization.

These five systems are possibilities rather than blueprints. Each could be stimulated under existing practice and payment organization, and could be accelerated under national health insurance. The present Kennedy insurance bill specifies as a model prepaid group practice. Other bills are, however, vague as to the exact shape of a desirable health care system. The desirability of pluralism in American society is often stressed, and it is probable that in 1980 elements of all of these models will be in operation.

Other facets of the health care system can also be indicated. Regional hospital planning will be strengthened, at least for superspecialist services such as heart transplant or burns units; cost alone makes this necessary. Special efforts will be made through government financing to establish services in rural areas. Medical schools will become more clearly differentiated from each other; some will remain research institutions, the majority will expand their service activities.[10] The number of physician assistants and other paraprofessional personnel will increase over the next ten years, particularly in the areas of diagnostic care. Greater efforts will be made to attract black physicians and women physicians into the profession. Physician manpower planning will change the balance of the specialties; there will be fewer general surgeons and more internists and pediatricians. Most, if not all, these measures will be accomplished through federal financing. The list could continue; most of these developments are however already evident.

In all of these developments traditional professional patterns and sociopolitical attitudes intermingle. The catalyst for further change will be through the political system; indeed the governmental role cannot avoid becoming more rational if not more extensive. The actual leadership for change will, however, continue to rest largely on the medical profession. Consumer participation and control is a philosophy often expressed, but one which in the health field has as yet had little influence. (Contrast the relative effectiveness of health planning through comprehensive health planning agencies, compared with the potential impact on a community of a reform movement directed by the medical society.) This does not mean a denial of consumer leadership; far from it. It means recognition

10. The 1970 Carnegie Commission report classified medical schools into three models: the Flexner or research model, now generally apparent but outmoded; the health care delivery model in which the medical school is part of a local or regional research, teaching and service system; and the integrated science model, with most of the basic science teaching organized in the main university campus, and with the medical school concentrate on clinical instruction. While many medical schools are a mixture of these models, the classifications are useful in pointing out different functions whose mix may vary in the future among different institutions. Individual medical schools must decide which functions they wish to undertake, and how far their wishes jibe with the availability of federal funding. A further important recommendation of the Carnegie report was the separate development of 126 area health education centers based on hospitals in areas not served by a medical school; these centers would however come under associated medical schools for educational purposes. *Higher Education and the Nation's Health,* pp. 4–5

by the medical profession, locally as well as nationally, of the responsibility thrust upon it to work with public representatives for reform and improvement of the health delivery system.

The strengths and abilities of the American medical profession have been remarked on throughout this history. From its scattered beginnings, to its current concerns over health care financing, staffing and operation, the American medical profession has modified its structures and policies significantly over the years, if still too slowly for the gigantic changes in the technology and the technological implications of medicine. It is in the groping for adequate change mechanisms that professional education, certification, and regulation—the old functions of professionalism—interlock with the concurrent social movement for more effective financing and for more efficient health care organization. The past is history. The present is a time of decision—in the Congress, in the professional organizations of medicine, and elsewhere in the nation. The purpose of this book has been to record, predict, and analyze the rationale and forms of the decision.

STATISTICAL APPENDIX

Table A1. Approved Medical Specialty Boards

	Year of incorporation	Certificates awarded; total to 6 June 1969
1. American Board of Ophthalmology	1917	7,117
2. American Board of Otolaryngology	1924	6,564
3. American Board of Obstetrics and Gynecology	1930	10,901
4. American Board of Dermatology	1932	2,895
5. American Board of Pediatrics	1933	13,045
6. American Board of Radiology	1934	10,606
7. American Board of Psychiatry and Neurology	1934	10,103
8. American Board of Orthopaedic Surgery	1934	6,093
9. American Board of Colon and Rectal Surgery	1934	397
10. American Board of Urology	1935	3,907
11. American Board of Pathology	1936	9,241
12. American Board of Internal Medicine	1936	20,212
13. American Board of Anesthesiology	1937	4,735
14. American Board of Plastic Surgery	1937	907
15. American Board of Surgery	1937	17,496
16. American Board of Neurological Surgery	1940	1,472
17. American Board of Physical Medicine and Rehabilitation	1947	771
18. American Board of Thoracic Surgery	1948	2,258
19. American Board of Preventive Medicine	1948	2,797
20. American Board of Family Practice	1969	
Total		131,517

Table A2. Distribution of Specialty Board Certificates and Number
of Full-Time Specialists, United States, 1940

	Number of full-time specialists	Number of active diplomates	Diplomates as percent of specialists
Total	36,880	15,597	42.3
Anesthesiology	285	86	30.2
Dermatology	974	492	50.5
Internal med. & subspecialties[1]	7,069	2,158	30.5
Obstetrics; gynecology	2,551	1,051	41.2
Ophthalmology; otolaryngology	7,608	4,683	61.6
Orthopedic surgery	1,078	652	60.5
Pathology	987	706	71.5
Pediatrics	2,416	1,470	60.8
Psychiatry; neurology	2,400	832	34.7
Public health	1,555		
Radiology	1,589	1,404	88.4
Surg. & subspecialties[2]	6,645	1,386	20.9
Urology	1,723	677	39.3

1. Includes allergy, cardiovascular disease, gastroenterology, internal medicine, pulmonary disease.
2. Includes colon and rectal surgery, neurological surgery, plastic surgery, occupational medicine.

Sources: *Health Manpower Source Book*, sec. 14, table 6; JAMA *114* (1940), 1663.

Table A3. Number of Full Specialists and Diplomates, and
Percent Relationship, 1949

	Number of full-time specialists	Number of active diplomates	Diplomates as percent of specialists
Total	62,688	32,714	52.1
Anesthesiology	1,231	472	38.3
Dermatology; syphilology	1,609	938	58.3
Internal medicine	12,490	5,396	43.2
Obstetrics; gynecology	5,074	2,595	51.1
Ophthalmology; otolaryngology	9,224	5,362	58.1
Orthopedic surgery	2,035	1,202	59.1
Pathology; bacteriology	1,730	1,444	83.5
Pediatrics	4,315	2,923	65.4
Psychiatry; neurology	4,720	2,932	62.1
Radiology; roentgenology	2,866	2,657	92.7
Surgery	11,127	3,898	35.0
Urology	2,193	1,194	54.4
Other	4,074[1]	1,801[2]	44.9

1. Includes physical medicine, public health, hospital administration, industrial practice, pulmonary disease.
2. Includes physical medicine and public health only.

Source: Building America's Health III (1952), table 214.

Table A4. *Distribution of Specialty Board Certificates and Number of Full-Time Specialists, United States, 1961*

	Number of full-time specialists	Number of active diplomates	Diplomates as percent of specialists
Total	122,573	65,047	53.1
Anesthesiology	5,044	2,132	42.3
Colon & rectal surg.	662	284	42.9
Dermatology	2,571	1,628	63.3
Internal medicine[1]	27,178	11,155	41.0
Neurological surgery	1,150	770	67.0
Obstetrics; gynecology	11,111	5,349	48.1
Ophthalmology; otolaryngology	10,651	7,139	67.0
Orthopedic surgery	4,607	2,905	63.1
Pathology	4,126	3,091	74.9
Pediatrics	9,836	6,188	62.9
Physical medicine	559	337	60.3
Plastic surgery	663	388	58.5
Preventive medicine[2]	4,067	1,172	28.8
Psychiatry; neurology	11,360	5,832	51.3
Radiology	6,071	4,986	82.1
Surgery	17,963	8,686	48.4
Thoracic surgery	879	718	81.7
Urology	3,559	2,180	61.3
Administrative med.	516	107	20.7

1. Includes allergy, cardiovascular disease, gastroenterology, internal medicine, pulmonary disease.
2. Includes aviation medicine, occupational medicine, public health.
Note:
The number of diplomates includes only those who are full-time specialists. In 1961 there were another 1,005 diplomates who described themselves as part-time specialists: the largest group (166) practiced psychiatry, the second largest (161) pediatrics, and the third largest (123) general surgery. The number of specialists excludes those in training programs.

Source: *Health Manpower Source Book*, Section 14, tables 6, 9.

Table A5. Specialty Board Requirements 1941, 1969

A. 1941

Boards	Fees, dollars	A.M.A.	Full citizenship	License to practice	Percent of work in specialty	Case reports	Internship of 1 year	Graduate training	In basic sciences	In clinical work	Additional practice	Certificates offered
Ophthalmology	50.00	+	+	?	?	10	+	3	?	?	0	1
Otolaryngology	50.00	+	+	?	90	0	+	3	?	1–2	2½–3½	1
Obstetrics; gynecology	100.00	+	0	+	100	50	+	3	?	?	2	1
Dermatology; syphilology	50.00	+	+	+	?	0	+	3	?	1½	2	1
Pediatrics	30.00	0	+	?	?	0	+	2	0	2	2	1
Psychiatry and neurology	50.00	+	0	+	0	0	+	3	?	?	2–3	3
Radiology	35.00	+	0	+	70	0	+	3	½	2½	2	4
Orthopedic surgery	50.00	+	+	+	100	0	+	3	?	1⅓	2	1
Urology	50.00	+	0	+	0	50	+	3	?	?	2	1
Internal medicine	50.00	+	0	?	?	0	+	3	?	?		1++
Pathology	35.00	+	0	+	70	0	+	3	0	3	1	3
Surgery	75.00	+	0	?	100	0	+	5	?	4	0	1
Anesthesiology	75.00	+	0	?	100	0	+	2	?	2	2	1
Plastic surgery	75.00	+	+	?	?	0	+	5	?	2	0	1
Neurosurgery	75.00	+	0	?	100	0	+	3	?	2	2	1
	56.66	14	6	8	3	3	15	12	1	8	11	

Years: In basic sciences, In clinical work, Additional practice.

B. 1969

Specialty board	Citizenship	Graduation from approved medical school	License to practice	Approved internship	Years of residency or other formal training	Years of practice or other special activities	Periods of credit in related fields	Credit for military services	Alternative plans for training	Accepted under certain conditions	Board accepts screening by Nat. Bd. Med. Exam., ECFMG, or other method	Special certificate or statement granted	Standard certificate granted	Application or registration fee	Total fee	Stated limitations (years) on applicant's eligibility[g]
Anesthesiology	x	x	x	x	2–3	4–1			x	x	x		x	75	175	7
Colon & rectal surgery	x	x	x	x	4–5	1	x		x	x	x		x	50	200	3
Dermatology		x	x		3		x		x	x	x	x		25	150	3
Family practice (approved Feb. 1969)																
Internal medicine[i]		x			3		x		x	x	x		x	70	225	5

Graduates of U.S., Canadian or Puerto Rican medical schools — *Foreign medical graduates special or additional requirements* — *All graduates*

Neurological surgery	x			x	4	2	x	x x x x	x	25 200	3
Obstetrics; gynecology	x x	x			3	2		x x x x	x	25 225	2
Ophthalmology	x x	x			3	1		x x x x		150 250	3
Orthopedic surgery	x x		x x		4		x	x x x x		25 225	3
Otolaryngology[2]	x		x x		4		x	x	x x	125 255	3
Pathology	x x	x x			4	1	x x	x x x x		200 200	3
Pediatrics[3]	x x	x x			2	2	x x	x x x x	x x	175 175	
Phys. med.; rehab.	x x	x			3	2	x	x x x x		50 200	7
Plastic surgery	x	x	x x		5	2	x	x	x x	75 225	3
Preventive medicine	x				3	1	x	x		50 200	3
Psychiatry; neurology[4]	x	x	x	x	3–5	2–1	x	x x	x	175 325	3
Radiology	x	x	x		3	1	x x	x x	x	200 200	
Surgery	x x	x x			3–4	2–0	x x	x x x	x	50 225	3
Thoracic surgery[5]	x	x	x		2		x	x	x	25 175	3
Urology	x	x	x		4	2	x	x	x	100 200	

1. Also certifies in the subspecialties of allergy, cardiovascular disease, gastroenterology, and pulmonary disease.
2. Limited certification granted at the discretion of the Board.
3. Also certifies in subspecialties of allergy and cardiology.
4. Also certifies in subspecialty of child psychiatry.
5. Certification by American Board of Surgery prerequisite.
6. Applicant may be considered "Board eligible" only for number of years indicated; thereafter, new application must be submitted.

Note:
In this table, those items are marked "X" on which the Board makes specific statement. In most instances, there are additional qualifying statements not indicated in this table. In all instances, refer for details to the board requirements which follow. While all boards may accept the foreign medical graduate under certain circumstances, they do not all specify that ECFMG certification is required. *All foreign graduates who contemplate specialty board certification should correspond with the appropriate board at the earliest possible moment.*

Source: JAMA 116:23 (June 7, 1941), p. 2617; *Directory of Approved Internships and Residences 1969–70,* table 1, p. 339.

BIBLIOGRAPHY

The most valuable sources of material for this research were individuals, unpublished materials made available by relevant medical organizations, and a profusion of articles, editorials, and notes scattered over the years in the many medical and social science journals. This bibliography, including as it does only the more important books referred to in the text, is thus necessarily selective. Specific references are to be found in the detailed footnotes accompanying the text.

Advisory Board for Medical Specialties (renamed American Board of Medical Specialties in 1970). *Directory of Medical Specialists*. Chicago: Marquis, published biennially.

Alexander, F. G., and Selesnick, Sheldon L. *The History of Psychiatry: An Evaluation of Psychiatric Thought and Practice from Prehistoric Times*. 1st ed. New York: Harper and Row, 1966.

Allen, R. B. *Medical Education and the Changing Order*. Cambridge, Mass.: Harvard University Press, 1946.

Altmeyer, Arthur J. *The Formative Years of Social Security*. Madison: University of Wisconsin Press, 1966.

American Academy of Political and Social Science. *The Medical Profession and the Public: Currents and Counter-Currents*. Philadelphia: American Academy of Political and Social Science, 1934.

American Association of Nurse Anesthetists. *Notes on the History and Organization of the American Association of Nurse Anesthetists*. Chicago, 1966.

American Medical Association. *Directory of Approved Internships and Residencies*. Chicago, published annually by the American Medical Association.

American Medical Association. *Digest of Official Actions, 1858–1958*. Chicago: American Medical Association, 1959.

American Medical Association. *Supplement to the Digest of Official Actions, 1959–1963*. Chicago: American Medical Association, 1966.

American Medical Association. Ad Hoc Committee on Education for Family Practice. *Meeting the Challenge of Family Practice*. Chicago: American Medical Association, 1966.

American Medical Association. *Distribution of Physicians, Hospitals, and Hospital Beds in the United States*. Chicago, published annually by the American Medical Association.

American Medical Association. *Survey of Medical Groups in the United States, 1965*. Chicago: American Medical Association, 1968; *1969*, ibid., 1970.

Andersen, Ronald, and Anderson, Odin W. *A Decade of Health Services: Social*

Survey Trends in Use and Expenditure. Chicago: University of Chicago Press, 1967.

Arrington, George E. *A History of Ophthalmology*. New York: M. D. Publications, 1959.

Ashford, Mahlon, ed. *Trends in Medical Education*. The New York Academy of Medicine Institute on Medical Education. New York: Commonwealth Fund, 1949.

Bane, Frank. *Physicians for a Growing America*. Report of the Surgeon General's Consultant Group on Medical Education. U.S. Department of Health, Education, and Welfare, Public Health Service. Washington, D.C.: U.S. Government Printing Office, 1959.

Becker, Howard S., Geer, Blanche, Hughes, Everett C., and Strauss, Anselm. *Boys in White: Student Culture in Medical School*. Chicago: University of Chicago Press, 1961.

Bigelow, Henry J. *Medical Education in America*. Cambridge, Mass.: Welch, Bigelow and Co., University Press, 1871.

Blake, John B. "Origins of Maternal and Child Health Programs." Yale Department of Public Health, mimeographed, 1953.

Blanton, Wyndham B. *Medicine in Virginia in the Seventeenth Century*. Richmond, Va.: William Byrd Press, 1930.

Blanton, Wyndham B. *Medicine in Virginia in the Eighteenth Century*. Richmond, Va.: Garrett and Massie, 1931.

Blanton, Wyndham B. *Medicine in Virginia in the Nineteenth Century*. Richmond, Va.: Garrett and Massie, 1933.

Blumer, George. *The Modern Medical School: Its Relation to the Hospital and to the Medical Profession*. Albany, N.Y., 1916.

Bonner, Thomas Neville. *The Kansas Doctor: A Century of Pioneering*. Lawrence: University of Kansas Press, 1959.

Bonner, Thomas Neville. *American Doctors and German Universities: A Chapter in International Intellectual Relations, 1870–1914*. Lincoln: University of Nebraska Press, 1963.

Boorstin, Daniel J. *The Americans: The Colonial Experience*. New York: Vintage Books, 1958.

Brewster, Agnes W. *Health Insurance and Related Proposals for Financing Personal Health Services: A Digest of Major Legislation and Proposals for Federal Action 1935–1957*. U.S. Department of Health, Education, and Welfare, Social Security Administration, 1958.

Brown, Esther Lucile. *Physicians and Medical Care*. New York: Russell Sage Foundation, 1937.

Brown, Francis H., ed. or comp. *The Medical Register for New England, 1877*. Cambridge, Mass.: Riverside Press, 1877.

Burrow, James Gordon. *The American Medical Association: Voice of American Medicine*. Baltimore: Johns Hopkins University Press, 1963.

Calhoun, Daniel H. *Professional Lives in America: Structure and Aspiration 1750–1850*. Cambridge, Mass.: Harvard University Press, 1965.

Carr-Saunders, A. M., and Wilson, P. A. *The Professions*. Oxford: Oxford University Press, 1933.

Chapin, William A. R., ed. *History, University of Vermont College of Medicine*. Hanover, N.H., Dartmouth Printing Co., 1951.

Citizens' Commission on Graduate Medical Education. *The Graduate Education of Physicians*. Chicago: American Medical Association, 1966.

Clapesattle, Helen B. *The Mayo Brothers*. Boston: Houghton Mifflin, 1962.

Clarke, Edward H., Bigelow, Henry J., Gross, Samuel D., Thomas, T. Gaillard, and Billings, J. S. *A Century of American Medicine, 1776–1876*. Philadelphia: Lea Publishers, 1876.

Clute, Kenneth F. *The General Practitioner: A Study of Medical Education and Practice in Ontario and Nova Scotia*. Toronto: University of Toronto Press, 1963.

Coggeshall, Lowell T. *Planning for Medical Progress through Education*. A Report Submitted to the Executive Council of the Association of American Medical Colleges. Evanston, Ill.: Association of American Medical Colleges, 1965.

Commission on Graduate Medical Education. *Graduate Medical Education*. Chicago: University of Chicago Press, 1940.

Commission on Hospital Care. *Hospital Care in the United States*. New York: Commonwealth Fund, 1947.

Commission on Medical Education. *Preliminary Report*. New Haven, Conn.: Office of the Director of the Study, Jan. 1927.

Commission on Medical Education. *Second Report*. New Haven, Conn.: Office of the Director of the Study, Jan. 1928.

Commission on Medical Education. *Third Report*. New Haven, Conn.: Office of the Director of the Study, Oct. 1928.

Commission on Medical Education. *Supplement to the Third Report*. New Haven, Conn.: Office of the Director of the Study, May 1929.

Commission on Medical Education. *Medical Education and Related Problems in Europe*. New Haven, Conn.: Office of the Director of the Study, Apr. 1930.

Commission on Medical Education. *Final Report of the Commission on Medical Education*. New York: Office of the Director of the Study, 1932.

Committee on the Costs of Medical Care. *Medical Care for the American People: The Final Report of the Committee on the Costs of Medical Care*. Publication no. 28. Chicago: University of Chicago Press, 1932.

Committee on Medical Care Teaching of the Association of Teachers of Preventive Medicine. *Readings in Medical Care*. Chapel Hill: University of North Carolina Press, 1958.

Congress and the Nation, 1945–1964: A Review of Government and Politics in the Postwar Years. Washington, D.C.: Congressional Quarterly Service, 1965.

Corwin, E. H. L. *The American Hospital*. New York: Commonwealth Fund, 1946.

Cushing, Harvey. *Consecratio Medici and Other Papers*. Boston: Little, Brown, and Co., 1940.

Davis, Fred, ed. *The Nursing Profession: Five Sociological Essays*. New York: John Wiley and Sons, 1966.

Davis, Loyal. *J. B. Murphy: Stormy Petrel of Surgery*. New York: G. P. Putnam's Sons, 1938.

Davis, Loyal. *Fellowship of Surgeons: A History of the American College of Surgeons*. Springfield, Ill.: Thomas Publishers, 1960.

Davis, Michael M. *Clinics, Hospitals and Health Centers*. New York: Harper, 1927.

Davis, Michael M. *America Organizes Medicine*. New York: Harper, 1941.

Davis, Nathan S. *History of the American Medical Association from Its Organi-*

zation up to January, 1855. Ed. S. W. Butler. Philadelphia: Lippincott, Grambo, and Co., 1855.

Deitrick, John E., and Berson, Robert C. *Medical Schools in the United States at Mid-Century*. New York: McGraw-Hill, 1953.

Derbyshire, Robert C. *Medical Licensure and Discipline in the United States*. Baltimore: Johns Hopkins Press, 1969.

Deutsch, Albert. *The Mentally Ill in America: A History of Their Care and Treatment from Colonial Times*. New York: Columbia University Press, 1949.

Education for the Allied Health Professions and Services. U.S. Department of Health, Education, and Welfare, Public Health Service Publication no. 1600, 1967.

Ehrlich, J., Morehead, M. A., and Trussell, R. E. *The Quantity, Quality and Costs of Medical and Hospital Care Secured by a Sample of Teamster Families in the New York Area*. New York: Columbia University School of Public Health and Administrative Medicine, 1962.

Evans, Lester J. *The Crisis in Medical Education*. Ann Arbor: University of Michigan Press, 1964.

Faber, Harold Kniest, and McIntosh, Rustin. *History of the American Pediatric Society, 1887–1965*. New York: McGraw-Hill, 1966.

Falk, I. S., Klem, Margaret C., and Sinai, Nathan. *The Incidence of Illness and the Receipt and Costs of the Medical Care among Representative Families*. Chicago: Committee on the Costs of Medical Care, 1933.

Falk, I. S., Rorem, C. Rufus, and Ring, Martha D. *The Costs of Medical Care: A Summary*. Committee on the Costs of Medical Care Publication no. 27. Chicago: University of Chicago Press, 1933.

Fein, Rashi. *The Doctor Shortage: An Economic Diagnosis*. Washington, D.C.: Brookings Institution, 1967.

Fishbein, Morris. *A History of the American Medical Association, 1847–1947*. Philadelphia: Saunders, 1947.

Flexner, Abraham. *Medical Education in the United States and Canada*. A Report to the Carnegie Foundation for the Advancement of Teaching. Carnegie Foundation Bulletin no. 4. New York, 1910.

Flexner, Abraham. *Medical Education: A Comparative Study*. New York: Macmillan, 1925.

Flexner, Abraham. *I Remember*. New York: Simon and Schuster, 1940.

Flexner, Simon and James Thomas, *William Henry Welch and the Heroic Age of American Medicine*. New York: Viking, 1941.

Follmann, J. F. *Medical Care and Health Insurance*. Homewood, Ill.: Richard D. Irwin, 1963.

Fossier, A. E. *History of the Orleans Parish Medical Society 1878–1928*. Privately printed, 1930.

Friedman, Milton, *Capitalism and Freedom*. Chicago: University of Chicago Press, 1963.

Friedman, Reuben. *A History of Dermatology in Philadelphia*. Fort Pierce Beach, Fla.: Froben Press, 1955.

Fulton, John F. *Harvey Cushing: A Biography*. Springfield, Ill.: C. C. Thomas, 1946.

Garceau, Oliver. *The Political Life of the American Medical Association*. Cambridge, Mass.: Harvard University Press, 1941.

Garrison, Fielding H. *Introduction to History of Medicine.* Philadelphia: Saunders, 1960.

Garrison, Fielding H. *History of Pediatrics.* Philadelphia: Saunders, 1965.

Greenberg, Selig. *The Troubled Calling: Crisis in the Medical Establishment.* New York: Macmillan, 1965.

Greenfield, Margaret. *Medi-Cal: The California Medicaid Program (Title XIX).* U.S. Department of Health, Education and Welfare, Washington, D.C., 1969.

Hall, J. K., Bunker, Henry A., and Zilboorg, Gregory, eds., *One Hundred Years of American Psychiatry,* New York: Columbia University Press, 1944.

Hansen, Horace R. *Medical Licensure and Consumer Protection: An Analysis and Evaluation of State Medical Licensure.* Washington, D.C.: Group Health Association, mimeographed, 1962.

Harris, Richard. *A Sacred Trust.* New York: New American Library, 1966.

Harris, Seymour E. *The Economics of American Medicine.* New York: Macmillan, 1964.

Hayt, Emmanuel and Lillian R. *Law of Hospital, Physician and Patient.* New York: Hospital Textbook Co., 1947.

Health Manpower: Perspective, 1967. U.S. Department of Health, Education, and Welfare, Public Health Service Publication no. 1667, 1967.

Health Manpower Source Book. U.S. Department of Health, Education, and Welfare, Public Health Service Publication no. 263. Washington, D.C.

Hirsch, Joseph, and Doherty, Beka. *The First Hundred Years of the Mount Sinai Hospital of New York, 1852–1952.* New York: Random House, 1952.

Hirsch, Monroe J., and Wick, Ralph E. *The Optometric Profession.* Philadelphia: Chilton Book Co., 1968.

Hospital Council of Greater New York. *Hospital Staff Appointments of Physicians in New York City.* New York: Macmillan, 1951.

Hubbell, Alvin A. *The Development of Ophthalmology in America, 1880–1907.* Chicago: Keener, 1908.

Ingelfinger, Franz J. Relman, Arnold S., and Finland, Maxwell, eds. *Controversy in Internal Medicine.* Philadelphia: W. B. Saunders Co., 1966.

Johns Hopkins Half-Century Committee. *The Spirit of Inquiry in Medical Education.* Baltimore, 1925.

Kelley, Stanley. *Professional Public Relations and Political Power.* Baltimore: Johns Hopkins Press, 1956.

Kett, Joseph. *The Formation of the American Medical Profession: The Role of Institutions, 1780–1860.* New Haven: Yale University Press, 1968.

Klarman, Herbert E. *Hospital Care in New York City.* New York: Columbia University Press, 1963.

Klarman, Herbert E. *The Economics of Health.* New York: Columbia University Press, 1965.

Konold, Donald E. *A History of American Medical Ethics, 1847–1912.* Madison: University of Wisconsin Press, 1962.

Larsell, O. *The Doctor in Oregon: A Medical History.* Portland: Binfords and Mort for the Oregon Historical Society, 1947.

Leven, Maurice. *The Incomes of Physicians: An Economic and Statistical Analysis.* Committee on the Costs of Medical Care Publication no. 24. Chicago: University of Chicago Press, 1932.

Lewis, D. Sclater. *The Royal College of Physicians and Surgeons of Canada, 1920–1960*. Montreal: McGill University Press, 1962.

Long, Esmond R. *A History of Pathology*. Baltimore: The Williams and Wilkins Co., 1928.

Long, Esmond R. *A History of American Pathology*. Springfield, Ill.: Charles C. Thomas, 1962.

Lyden, Fremont J., Geiger, H. Jack, and Petersen, Osler L. *The Training of Good Physicians*. Cambridge: Harvard University Press, 1968.

MacColl, William A. *Group Practice and Prepayment of Medical Care*. Washington, D.C.: Public Affairs Press, 1966.

Margulies, Harold, and Bloch, Lucille Stephenson. *Foreign Medical Graduates in the United States*. Cambridge: Harvard University Press, 1969.

Martin, Franklin H. *The Joy of Living: An Autobiography*. Vols. 1 and 2. New York: Doubleday, Doran, and Co., 1933.

Martin, Franklin H. *Fifty Years of Medicine and Surgery: An Autobiographical Sketch*. Chicago: Surgical Publishing Co., 1934.

Mayers, Lewis, and Harrison, Leonard V. *The Distribution of Physicians in the United States*. New York: General Education Board, 1924.

McCleary, G. F. *The Early History of the Infant Welfare Movement*. London: H. K. Lewis, 1933.

McNerney, Walter J., and Riedel, Donald C. *Regionalization and Rural Health Care*. Ann Arbor: University of Michigan Press, 1962.

Means, James Howard, ed. *The Association of American Physicians: Its First Seventy-Five Years*. New York: McGraw-Hill, 1961.

Merton, Robert K., Reader, George G., and Kendall, Patricia L., eds. *The Student-Physician*. Cambridge, Mass.: Harvard University Press, 1957.

Michigan State Medical Society. *Medical History of Michigan*. Vols. 1 and 2. Compiled and edited by a committee: C. B. Burr, chairman. Minneapolis: The Bruce Publishing Co., 1930.

Morais, Herbert M. *The History of the Negro in Medicine*. New York: Publishers Company, Inc., 1967.

Morgan, John. *A Discourse on the Institution of Medical Schools in America, 1765*. reprint ed., Baltimore: Johns Hopkins Press, 1937.

Morgan, William Gerry. *The American College of Physicians: Its First Quarter Century*. Philadelphia: American College of Physicians, 1940.

Morris, Robert T. *Fifty Years a Surgeon*. New York: Dutton, 1935.

Mumford, Emily. *Interns: From Studentst to Physicians*. Cambridge: Harvard University Press, 1970.

Muntz, Earl E. *Social Security: An Analysis of the Wagner-Murray Bill*. New York: American Enterprise Association, 1944.

Mustard, Harry S. *Government in Public Health*. New York: Commonwealth Fund, 1945.

Myers, Russell J. *Medicare*. Bryn Mawr: McCahan Foundation, 1970.

National Advisory Commission on Health Manpower. *Report of the National Advisory Commission on Health Manpower*. Vol. 1. Washington, D.C.: U.S. Government Printing Office, Nov. 1967.

National Commission on Community Health Services. *Health Is a Community Affair*. Cambridge, Mass.: Harvard University Press, 1966.

Norwood, William F. *Medical Education in the United States before the Civil War*. Philadelphia: University of Pennsylvania Press, 1944.

Oberman, C. Esco. *A History of Vocational Rehabilitation in America*. Minneapolis: Denison, 1965.

Noyes, Henry D. *Specialties in Medicine*. Pamphlet. Read before the American Ophthalmological Society, New York, June 1865.

Packard, Francis R. *History of Medicine in the United States*. Vol. 1. New York: Hafner Publishing Co., 1931.

Pease, Marshall C. *The American Academy of Pediatrics, 1930–1951*. New York: American Academy of Pediatrics, 1951.

Peebles, Allon. *A Survey of Statistical Data on Medical Facilities in the United States: A Compilation of Existing Material*. Committee on the Costs of Medical Care Publication no. 3. Chicago: University of Chicago Press, 1929.

Ponton, T. R. *The Medical Staff in the Hospital*. 2d ed. Chicago: Physicians' Record Co., 1953.

Prentice, Charles F. *Legalized Optometry and the Memoirs of Its Founder*. Seattle: Casperin Fletcher Press, 1926.

Puschman, Theodore. *History of Medical Education*. Trans. Evan H. Hare. London: H. K. Lewis, 1891.

Pusey, William Allen. *A Doctor of the 1870s and 1880s*. Springfield, Ill.: Thomas, 1932.

Rayack, Elton. *Professional Power and American Medicine: The Economics of the American Medical Association*. Cleveland: World Publishing Co., 1967.

Reed, Alfred Z. *Training for the Public Profession of the Law*. New York 1921.

Reed, Louis S. *Midwives, Chiropodists, and Optometrists: Their Place in Medical Care*. Committee on the Costs of Medical Care Publication no. 15. Chicago: The University of Chicago Press, 1932.

Riese, Walther. *History of Neurology*. New York: M. D. Publications, 1959.

Riesman, David. *Medicine in Modern Society*. Princeton: Princeton University Press, 1939.

Rodman, John Stewart. *History of the American Board of Surgery, 1937–1952*. Philadelphia: Lippincott, 1956.

Rosen, George. *The Specialization of Medicine, with Particular Reference to Ophthalmology*. New York: Froben Press, 1944.

Rosen, George. *A History of Public Health*. New York: Schumann, 1958.

Rosenfeld, Leonard S., and Makover, Henry B. *The Rochester Regional Hospital Council*. Cambridge: Published for the Commonwealth Fund by Harvard University Press, 1956.

Shafer, Henry B. *The American Medical Profession, 1783–1850*. New York. Columbia University Press, 1936.

Shryock, Richard Harrison. *American Medical Research: Past and Present*. New York Academy of Medicine Committee on Medicine and the Changing Order. New York: Commonwealth Fund, 1947.

Shyrock, Richard Harrison. *The Development of Modern Medicine*. New York: Knopf, 1947.

Shryock, Richard Harrison. *The Unique Influence of the Johns Hopkins University on American Medicine*. Copenhagen: Munksgaard, 1953.

Shryock, Richard Harrison. *The History of Nursing: An Interpretation of the Social and Medical Factors Involved*. Philadelphia: W. B. Saunders Co., 1959.

Shryock, Richard Harrison. *Medicine and Society in America, 1660–1860.* New York: New York University Press, 1962.

Shryock, Richard Harrison. *Medicine in America: Historical Essays.* Baltimore: Johns Hopkins University Press, 1966.

Shryock, Richard Harrison. *Medical Licensing in America, 1650–1965.* Baltimore: Johns Hopkins University Press, 1967.

Sigerist, Henry E. *American Medicine.* 1st ed. New York: W. W. Norton Co., 1934.

Sinai, Nathan, and Anderson, Odin W. *Emergency Maternity and Infant Care.* Ann Arbor: Bureau of Public Health Economics, University of Michigan, 1948.

Somers, Anne R. *Hospital Regulation: The Dilemma of Public Policy.* Princeton: Industrial Relations Section Princeton University, 1969.

Somers, Herman M. and Somers, Anne R. *Workmen's Compensation.* New York: John Wiley and Sons, Inc., 1954.

Somers, Herman M. and Somers, Anne R. *Doctors, Patients and Health Insurance: The Organization and Financing of Medical Care.* Washington, D.C.: Brookings Institution, 1961.

Somers, Herman M. and Somers, Anne R. *Medicare and the Hospitals.* Washington, D.C.: Brookings Institution, 1967.

Steiner, Walter Ralph. *Historical Address: The Evolution of Medicine in Connecticut, with the Foundation of the Yale Medical School As Its Notable Achievement.* New Haven: printed privately, 1915.

Stern, Bernhard J. *Social Factors in Medical Progress.* New York: Columbia University Press, 1927.

Stern, Bernhard J. *American Medical Practice in the Perspectives of a Century.* New York: Commonwealth Fund, 1945.

Stern, Bernhard J. *Medical Services by Government: Local, State and Federal.* New York: Commonwealth Fund, 1946.

Stern, Bernhard J. *Medicine in Industry.* New York: Commonwealth Fund, 1946.

Stevens, Rosemary. *Medical Practice in Modern England: The Impact of Specialization and State Medicine.* New Haven: Yale University Press, 1966.

Stewart, William H. *Report on Regional Medical Programs to the President and Congress.* U.S. Department of Health, Education, and Welfare, June 1967.

Sundquist, James L. *Politics and Policy: The Eisenhower, Kennedy, and Johnson Years.* Washington, D.C.: Brookings Institution, 1968.

Thatcher, Virginia S. *History of Anesthesia with Emphasis on the Nurse Specialist.* Philadelphia: Lippincott, 1953.

Thwing, Charles F. *A History of Higher Education in America.* New York: Appleton and Co., 1906.

Trussell, Ray E. *Hunterdon Medical Center.* Cambridge, Mass.: Published for the Commonwealth Fund by Harvard University Press, 1956.

U.S. Army Medical Service. *Personnel in World War II.* Washington, D.C.: Office of the Surgeon General, Department of the Army, 1963.

U.S. President's Commission on the Health Needs of the Nation. *Building America's Health: A Report to the President.* 5 vols. Washington, D.C.: U.S. Government Printing Office, 1952–53.

Van Ingen, P. *The New York Academy of Medicine: Its First Hundred Years.* New York: Columbia University Press, 1949.

Van Liere, Edward J., and Dodds, Gideon S. *History of Medical Education in West Virginia.* Morgantown, W. Va.: West Virginia University Library, 1965.

Viets, Henry R. *A Brief History of Medicine in Massachusetts.* Boston: Houghton Mifflin Co., 1930.

Washburn, Frederic A. *The Massachusetts General Hospital: Its Development, 1900–1935.* Boston: Houghton Mifflin Co., 1939.

Weiskotten, Herman G., and Johnson, Victor. *A History of the Council on Medical Education and Hospitals of the American Medical Association, 1904–1959.* Chicago: American Medical Association, 1959.

Weiskotten, Herman G., Schwitalla, Alphonse M., Cutter, William D., and Anderson, Hamilton H. *Medical Education in the United States, 1934–1939.* Commission on Medical Education. Chicago: American Medical Association, 1940.

Wheeler, Maynard C. *The American Ophthalmological Society: The First Hundred Years.* Toronto: University of Toronto Press, 1964.

Wilder, Lucy. *The Mayo Clinic.* Rev. ed. New York: Harcourt, Brace, and Co., 1939.

Williams, Ralph Chester. *The United States Public Health Service, 1798–1950.* Washington, D.C.: Commissioned Officers' Association of the U.S. Public Health Service, 1951.

Wolf, Stewart G., Jr., and Darley, Ward, eds. *Medical Education and Practice: Relationships and Responsibilities in a Changing Society.* Report of the Tenth Teaching Institute. Evanston, Ill.: Association of American Medical Colleges, 1965.

Yale Law Journal. "The American Medical Association: Power, Purpose, and Politics in Organized Medicine." Vol. 63 (1954).

Young, Hugh. *A Surgeon's Autobiography.* New York: Harcourt and Brace, 1940.

INDEX

Abdominal Surgery, 342; specialty board, 333–39

Abdominal Surgery (journal), 335

Advisory Board for Medical Specialties, 221, 228, 232, 233, 234, 242, 244, 245, 253, 257, 262, 302, 303, 308, 310, 324–27, 328–29, 330, 335, 339, 340, 341, 403, 404, 405, 407; established, 212–14, 217; general practice, 296; investigates graduate education, 260; strengthened, 345–46. *See also* American Board of Medical Specialties

Advisory Commission on Inter-governmental Relations, 487

Advisory Committee on Internships, 392

Advisory Council on Medical Education, Licensure, and Hospitals: established, 263–65

Aged, medical needs and care of, 433–43

Aiken, Senator, 483

Alabama medical legislation, 27

Alfano, Dr. Blaise, 333–34, 338*n*

Allergy, 179, 234; development as specialty, 339–40

AMA Committee on Medical Preparedness. *See* Committe on Medical Preparedness

American Academy of General Practice, 264*n*, 304, 304*n*, 311, 312, 313, 388, 391

American Academy of Ophthalmology and Otolaryngology, 101–02, 111

American Academy of Orthopaedic Surgeons, 235*n*

American Academy of Pediatrics, 207, 340*n*, 341; established, 219, 220–21

American Association of Clinical Immunology and Allergy: established, 340

American Association of Genito-Urinary Surgeons, 235*n*

American Association of Industrial Physicians, 331

American Association for Labor Legislation, health insurance investigation, 137

American Association of Obstetricians and Gynecologists, 160, 202

American Association for Thoracic Surgery, 242*n*

American Board of Abdominal Surgery: established, 333–35

American Board of Anesthesiology, 247, 321*n*, 322, 323*n*, 325

American Board of Clinical Immunology and Allergy, 340

American Board of Colon and Rectal Surgery, 328*n*, 336*n*

American Board of Dermatology, 207, 211, 325; curriculum standards, 259

American Board of Family Practice, 327, 345

American Board of Gastroenterology, 234

American Board of Internal Medicine, 245, 259, 297, 314, 321, 325, 325*n*, 326, 329, 344, 345, 391, 391*n*, 408; established, 232–35

American Board of Medical Specialties, 408–09, 533; established, 345–47

American Board of Neurological Surgery, 325, 344, 408

American Board of Obstetrics and Gynecology, 222, 281*n*, 322, 325, 336*n*, 344, 391; established, 202–04

American Board for Ophthalmic Examinations, 113

American Board of Ophthalmology, 113, 245, 252, 325, 332; curriculum standards, 259

American Board of Orthopaedic Surgery, 252, 325, 329, 344; established, 235, 235*n*

American Board of Orthopedics, 408

American Board of Otolaryngology, 321–22, 391

American Board of Pathology, 325, 342; established, 230–31, 230*n*